Preparing for the Occupational Therapy Assistant National Board Exam

45 DAYS AND COUNTING

Edited by

Rosanne DiZazzo-Miller, PhD, DrOT, OTR/L, CDP
Assistant Professor
Department of Health Care Sciences
Wayne State University
Detroit, Michigan

Guest Editor:
Tia Hughes, DrOT, MBA, OTR/L
Professor and Department Chair
Occupational Therapy and Occupational Therapy Assistant Program
Adventist University
Orlando, Florida
Vice Chairperson
Accreditation Council for Occupational Therapy (ACOTE)

Fredrick D. Pociask, PT, PhD, MSPT, OCS, OMT, FAAOMPT
Assistant Professor
Department of Health Care Sciences
Wayne State University
Detroit, Michigan

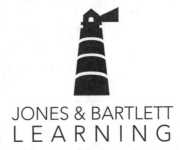

JONES & BARTLETT
LEARNING

World Headquarters
Jones & Bartlett Learning
5 Wall Street
Burlington, MA 01803
978-443-5000
info@jblearning.com
www.jblearning.com

Jones & Bartlett Learning books and products are available through most bookstores and online booksellers. To contact Jones & Bartlett Learning directly, call 800-832-0034, fax 978-443-8000, or visit our website, www.jblearning.com.

Substantial discounts on bulk quantities of Jones & Bartlett Learning publications are available to corporations, professional associations, and other qualified organizations. For details and specific discount information, contact the special sales department at Jones & Bartlett Learning via the above contact information or send an email to specialsales@jblearning.com.

13362-2

Production Credits

VP, Executive Publisher: David D. Cella
Publisher: Cathy L. Esperti
Acquisitions Editor: Sean Fabery
Associate Editor: Taylor Maurice
Editorial Assistant: Hannah Dziezanowski
Senior Vendor Manager: Sara Kelly
VP, Manufacturing and Inventory Control: Therese Connell
Composition and Project Management: S4Carlisle Publishing
  Services

Cover Design: Kristin E. Parker
Rights & Media Specialist: Merideth Tumasz
Media Development Editor: Shannon Sheehan
Cover Image (Title Page): © Mrs. Opossum/Shutterstock
Printing and Binding: Edwards Brothers Malloy
Cover Printing: Edwards Brothers Malloy

Library of Congress Cataloging-in-Publication Data
Names: DiZazzo-Miller, Rosanne, author. | Pociask, Fredrick D., author. |
  Hughes, Tia, author.
Title: Preparing for the occupational therapy assistant national board exam :
  45 days and counting / Rosanne DiZazzo-Miller, Fredrick D. Pociask, Tia
  Hughes.
Description: Burlington, MA: Jones & Bartlett Learning, [2018] | "Includes
  Navigate 2 preferred access." | Includes bibliographical references and
  index.
Identifiers: LCCN 2017022833 | ISBN 9781284072358
Subjects: | MESH: Occupational Therapy | Allied Health Personnel |
  Examination Questions
Classification: LCC RM735.32 | NLM WB 18.2 | DDC 615.8/515076--dc23 LC record available at https://lccn.loc.gov/2017022833

6048

Printed in the United States of America
21 20 19 18 17   10 9 8 7 6 5 4 3 2 1

"I can do all things through Christ who strengthens me." Philippians 4:23

To Carey, the love and joy of my life, and my children Joseph Alan, Victoria Rose, and Michael Anthony, my three pieces of Heaven on Earth.

To my parents Vittorio and Rosina who came to this country and taught me about hard work and perseverance, and my sisters Josie and JoAnne who taught me how to be tough!

To my dear friend Charity Anderson Stein, who has taught me all I'll ever need to know about true friendship and what's most veraciously important in life.

Carpe Diem!

To past, current, and future students—may this book help you pass this exam, but more importantly, guide you on your journey as a tireless patient advocate and client-centered occupational therapist.

Rosanne DiZazzo-Miller

To Juliana—my best friend and one true love.

To my parents Patricia and Fred; my grandmother Zina; my good friend John; my mentors and role models Gary, Rita, Jane, Kornelia, and Mrs. Brown; and everyone that has inspired me.

To healthcare professionals who have dedicated their life to helping others.

Fredrick D. Pociask

BRIEF CONTENTS

CONTENTS

Chapter 32 Health Promotion and Wellness 551

Michael A. Pizzi

Chapter 33 Occupational Rehabilitation and Ergonomics, and Low Back Pain 559

Regina Parnell and Jane Pomper DeHart

FOREWORD

"Never regard study as a duty, but as the enviable opportunity to learn to know the liberating influence of beauty in the realm of the spirit for your own personal joy and to the profit of the community to which your later work belongs."

Einstein

You survived your academic occupational therapy assistant program. You made it through fieldwork. You have dreamt about the day you would find out you were officially an occupational therapy assistant. You have longed to see yourself as a full member of this noble profession. Now, you are ready to embark on the final steps of your journey: The NBCOT COTA® certification exam.

Studying for the NBCOT® certification exam can feel like an overwhelming challenge. Like others in your shoes, you probably wonder: How do I begin? Where do I start? What do I do first? You are not alone. This book, *Preparing for the Occupational Therapy Assistant National Board Exam: 45 Days and Counting,* is more than a bank of multiple-choice questions or occupational therapy facts. It provides you with a plan and helps you organize your study by giving you an invaluable blueprint to guide you through the study process for the examination—your last hurdle to gain before entry into the occupational therapy profession.

You will find that the format, organized around a 45-day plan, is designed to lower your stress level and keep you on-task. It provides you with a review of critical information using the latest terminology. The authors provide you with opportunities to process questions and apply step-by-step clinical reasoning skills to solve case studies—a critical part of the exam content. Journaling questions provide you with insight into areas that need priority for further study. Electronic access to over 725 exam questions adds to your experience, helping you to practice in the format of the exam and easing you into the process.

So, begin following this plan and apply what you know to how you think about the world as an occupational therapist. Your future in the occupational therapy profession awaits you *45 Days and Counting . . .*

Barbara L. Kornblau, JD, OTR/L, FAOTA, DASPE, FNAP, CCM, CDMS, CPE
Past President of the American Occupational Therapy Association
Professor
Florida A&M University
Tallahassee, FL

*P*reparing for the Occupational Therapy Assistant National Board Exam: 45 Days and Counting is a comprehensive overview for occupational therapy assistant students preparing to take the National Board for Certification in Occupational Therapy Certified Occupational Therapy Assistant (NBCOT COTA®) exam. It utilizes a health and wellness focus and includes tips and self-assessment forms to develop effective study habits. Unlike other occupational therapy assistant (OTA) examination review guides, *Preparing for the Occupational Therapy Assistant National Board Exam: 45 Days and Counting* provides a more structured and holistic approach, including a detailed calendar and plan of study for the 45 days leading up to the exam.

This text was written to address identified gaps with currently available board exam review textbooks as expressed by students and graduates from multiple institutions via direct contact, focus groups, and through consultation with OTA programs. The need for a comprehensive and holistic board exam preparation textbook, as well as a structured study plan and resources, was clearly identified as essential to best ensure successful completion of the NBCOT COTA® examination. In response, *Preparing for the Occupational Therapy Assistant National Board Exam: 45 Days and Counting* was specifically designed to offer OTA students and institutions an all-inclusive approach to board exam preparation.

Each chapter is broken down into manageable and organized topics designed to be completed 45 days preceding the examination. This text offers a simplified, yet extensive, review with a calendar to guide students through each day of preparation. Each chapter was created using references and resources utilized in OTA curricula throughout the United States. At the end of each chapter, there are self-study learning activities with answers to check for knowledge and understanding. A journaling section includes questions using a reflective learning approach, where students learn individual areas to focus on and how to prioritize.

Furthermore, this text includes a special section for students who may find the NBCOT® exam challenging, in addition to advice from past students who had to retake the exam, including words of encouragement.

Resources for Students

In addition to the features found within the text, the accompanying digital component includes TestPrep software that features over 725 NBCOT® style multiple-choice practice questions that have been reviewed and edited by item-writing specialists in healthcare science education. The software allows you to create your own practice exams using questions linked to specific chapters in the text, as well as to the four exam domains.

The digital component also contains six-option multiple-choice answer questions, which are new to the NBCOT COTA® exam.

Resources for Educators

For educators and academic programs, this text can be used in a dual role as a course-ready capstone textbook with instructor-only materials, in addition to a means to ensure adequate board exam preparation for students during the academic portion of their study. The instructor materials include classroom worksheets and study questions, laboratory guides, and learning activities, as well as slides in PowerPoint® format for each chapter.

ACKNOWLEDGMENTS

I (Rosanne) am a person of great faith and so before I go on about the many incredible individuals whom I would like to thank for making this book possible, I would first like to thank God for the gifts and opportunities I have been given. I feel blessed to have the opportunity to work with students, both those who have passed and those who may need additional help to pass this incredibly stressful and challenging examination. I continue to learn every day from them and try to apply that learning into projects like this to help others.

To my husband Carey, for putting up with far more than any spouse should have to put up with since my PhD defense gave us 1 week of normalcy before deadlines for this book began to take effect. To my children, Joseph, Victoria, and Michael, for always being there, whether they were asleep by my side or cheering me on. My hope is that they learn what hard work and dedication can accomplish. I would also like to acknowledge my parents, Vittorio and Rosina DiZazzo, who came to this country to make a better life for their children. It was not easy and they were not treated very well, but rather than making excuses or taking the easy way out, they persisted and ultimately lived the great American Dream. I am a product of that as first-generation born in this country and thank them every day for the lessons they have taught me about work ethic, kindness, and charity, and for their without-fail advice to "Work hard and keep your head down"—words that have indubitably provided guidance throughout many aspects of my life. To my sisters, Josie and JoAnne, their husbands, and my nieces and nephews for reminding me of the importance of family and laughter. To my dearest friend Charity: your free spirit and relentless support will always inspire me. I was heart-broken for your wonderful spirit to leave this world, but smile when I think what Heaven must be like now that you're there!

This book would not be possible without the contributions and support of faculty and clinicians around the country who came together to provide a quality product that can support students in preparing for the ultimate challenge of their academics: passing the board examination. Thank you for your knowledge and expertise, for without them, this truly would not have been possible.

It means so much to have student input because they are ultimately the consumers of this endeavor. And so, to my incredible students—specifically the Wayne State University 2013 and 2014 Directed Study groups who helped formulate and trial test questions, and my 2016 professional year 1 students who reviewed the chapters prior to print and provided feedback—I can't thank you enough for taking part in this important project. A heartfelt thanks to Denise Rowe who read through the entire book and provided edits and suggestions from an exam candidate's point of view. Thank you for your invaluable perspective and hard work. I can't wait to support you with your first book!

I thank Joseph M. Pellerito, who coedited the companion text for occupational therapists with me. I will always remember and appreciate your mentoring and friendship throughout my years in academia.

Finally, to my coeditor Dr. Fredrick D. Pociask—my good friend and colleague—thank you for sharing your incredible knowledge and support with me and the many students who will benefit from our book. Your dry and sometimes questionable sense of humor has gotten me through many difficult times! A great many thanks to your wife Juliana, who endured many weeknight and weekend calls that would last hours on end in order to accomplish our goals—you are amazing and I so appreciate your support and kind heart.

Rosanne DiZazzo-Miller

I (Fredrick) wish to thank the following people for their contributions and help in creating this book:

To my wife Juliana, who made it possible for me to complete this project by helping me in countless ways too numerous to mention.

To the chapter authors, reviewers, item writers, and Wayne State University students for their countless contributions to making this book a reality.

Finally, to my good friend Dr. Rosanne DiZazzo-Miller, thank you for your seemingly endless enthusiasm and energy. Thank you Carey for your seemingly endless patience with this project, and thank you Victoria for taking care of your daddy and raising your brothers for the last 2 years—mommy will be back soon.

Last but not least, to the entire staff at Jones & Bartlett, for their guidance and expertise, and always for their understanding!

Fredrick D. Pociask

CONTRIBUTORS

Diane E. Adamo, PhD, MS, OTR
Assistant Professor
Wayne State University
Detroit, MI

Jessica Andrus, MOT, OTR/L
Occupational Therapist
Galaxy Brain and Therapy Center
Ann Arbor, MI

Beth Angst, OTR/L
Senior Occupational Therapist
Children's Hospital of Michigan
Detroit, MI
Part-Time Faculty
Baker College
Allen Park, MI

Shari Bernard, OTD, OTR/L, SCFES
Therapy Manager–Outpatient
Mayo Clinic
Rochester, MN

Thomas J. Birk, PT, PhD, MPT, FACSM
Associate Dean and Professor
University of Wisconsin–Milwaukee
Milwaukee, WI

Lori Bravi, MS, OTR/L, BCPR
Occupational Therapist, Level IV
Rehabilitation Institute of Chicago
Chicago, IL

Donna Case, PhD, OTL
Occupational Therapist
Cooke School/Northville Public Schools
Northville, MI

Jane Pomper DeHart, MA, OTR/L
Vice President of Operations
Work-Safe Occupational Health
Detroit, MI

Camille Dieterle, OTD, OTR/L, RYT
Assistant Professor
University of Southern California
Los Angeles, CA

Rosanne DiZazzo-Miller, PhD, DrOT, OTR/L, CDP
Assistant Professor
Wayne State University
Detroit, MI

Ken Eick, CP
Clinical Manager Prosthetics
Wright & Filippis
Rochester Hills, MI

Darren Gustitis, OTR/L, CHT
Clinical Manager and Occupational Therapist
Michigan Hand and Wrist, PC
Novi, MI

Piper Hansen, OTD, OTR/L
Occupational Therapist—Clinical Practice Leader
Rehabilitation Institute of Chicago
Chicago, IL

Doreen Head, PhD, OTR/L
Program Director and Assistant Professor
Wayne State University
Detroit, MI

Denise Hoffman, MSOT, OTR/L
Occupational Therapist
Occupational Therapy Plus
Portage, MI
Davenport University
Grand Rapids, MI
Handwriting without Tears
Cabin John, MD

Christine Johnson, MOT, OTR/L
Instructor
Lenoir-Rhyne University
Colombia, SC

Sophia Kimmons, OTR/L
Senior Occupational Therapist
Detroit Receiving Hospital
Detroit, MI

Kurt Krueger, OTR/L, CHT
Occupational Therapist
Michigan Hand and Sports Rehabilitation Center
Dearborn, MI

Deborah Loftus, MOT, OTR/L
Senior Occupational Therapist
Galaxy Brain and Therapy Center
Ann Arbor, MI

Bambi Lombardi, OTR/L
Clinical Therapy Specialist
Hanger Clinic Upper Limb Program
San Antonio, TX

Sheila M. Longpré, MOT, OTR/L
Director of Clinical and Community Relations
    and Assistant Professor
Nova Southeastern University
Tampa, FL

Moh H. Malek, PhD, FACSM, FNSCA, CSCS*D,
    NSCA-CPT*D
Associate Professor
Wayne State University
Detroit, MI

Sara Maher, PT, DScPT, OMPT
Program Director and Associate Professor
Wayne State University
Detroit, MI

Jennie McGillicuddy, MOT, OTR/L
Occupational Therapist III, Burn Rehabilitation Clinical
    Specialist
University of California at San Diego Regional Burn
    Center
San Diego, CA

Robin Mercer, MHS, OTR/L
Occupational Therapist
Wayne Westland Community School District
Westland, MI

Susan K. Meyers, EdD, MBA, OTR, FAOTA
Adjunct and Guest Faculty
Carmel, IN

Regina Parnell, PhD, OTR/L
Assistant Professor
Wayne State University
Detroit, MI

Marie Eve Pepin, PT, DPT, MSPT, OMPT
Assistant Professor
Wayne State University
Detroit, MI

Michael A. Pizzi, PhD, OTR/L, FAOTA
Associate Professor
Dominican College
Orangeburg, NY

Jeffrey Placzek, MD, PT
Board Certified Hand and Upper Extremity Surgeon
Michigan Hand and Wrist, PC
Novi, MI
Medical Director
Bone and Joint Surgery Center of Novi
Providence Park Medical Center
Novi, MI

Fredrick D. Pociask, PT, PhD, MSPT, OCS, OMT,
    FAAOMPT
Assistant Professor
Wayne State University
Detroit, MI

Kristina Reid, PT, MSPT, C/NDT
Lecturer
Wayne State University
Detroit, MI

Anne Riddering, OTR/L, CLVT, COMS
Rehabilitation Supervisor
Henry Ford Center for Vision Rehabilitation
    and Research
Livonia, MI

Susan Robosan-Burt, OTR/L
Consultant and Co-Advisor OTA Student Leadership
   Organization
Macomb Community College
Clinton Township, MI

Nicole Scheiman, MHS, OTR/L
Program Director and Associate Professor
Huntington University
Huntington, IN

Jennifer Siegert, OTR/L
Occupational Therapist
Michigan Hand and Wrist, PC
Novi, MI

Erin Skotzke, MOT, OTR/L
Occupational Therapist and Research Assistant
Wayne State University
Detroit, MI

Diane Thomson, MS, OTR/L, ATP
Senior Occupational Therapist
Rehabilitation Institute of Michigan
Detroit, MI

Jenna Tolmie, MOT, OTR/L
Pediatric Occupational Therapist
Beaumont Hospital
Grosse Pointe, MI

Rita E. Troxtel, OTD, OTR/L, CPAM
Assistant Professor
Tennessee State University
Nashville, TN

Patricia E. Tully, OTR
Occupational Therapist
TIRR Education Academy, TIRR Memorial Hermann
Houston, TX

Joyce Tyler, OTR/L, CHT
Clinical Therapy Specialist
Hanger Clinic Upper Limb Program
San Antonio, TX

Christine A. Watt, MS, OTR/L, CPAM
Assistant Professor
Tennessee State University
Nashville, TN

Item-Writing Contributors

Item-Writer Specialist and Editor

Sara Maher, PT, DScPT, OMPT
Item Writer Coordinator for the Federation of State
    Boards of Physical Therapy and Member of the Exam
    Development Committee
Program Director and Associate Professor
Wayne State University
Detroit, MI

Associate Item-Writer Specialist and Editor

Marie Eve Pepin, PT, DPT, MSPT, OMPT
Item Writer Coordinator for the Federation of State
    Boards of Physical Therapy and Member of the Exam
    Development Committee
Assistant Professor
Wayne State University
Detroit, MI

OTA Subject Matter Specialist

Nicole Scheiman, MHS, OTR/L
Program Director and Associate Professor
Huntington University
Huntington, IN

Multiple-Choice Item-Writer Contributors

Diane E. Adamo, PhD, MS, OTR
Assistant Professor
Wayne State University
Detroit, MI

Jessica Andrus, MOT, OTR/L
Occupational Therapist
Galaxy Brain and Therapy Center
Ann Arbor, MI

Beth Angst, OTR/L
Senior Occupational Therapist
Children's Hospital of Michigan
Detroit, MI
Part-time Faculty Baker College
Allen Park, MI

Shari Bernard, OTD, OTR/L, SCFES
Therapy Manager–Outpatient
Mayo Clinic
Rochester, MN

Thomas J. Birk, PT, PhD, MPT, FACSM
Associate Dean and Professor
University of Wisconsin–Milwaukee
Milwaukee, WI

Lori Bravi, MS, OTR/L, BCPR
Occupational Therapist, Level IV
Rehabilitation Institute of Chicago
Chicago, IL

Donna Case, PhD, OTL
Occupational Therapist
Cooke School/Northville Public Schools
Northville, MI

Jane Pomper DeHart, MA, OTR/L
Vice President of Operations
Work-Safe Occupational Health
Detroit, MI

Camille Dieterle, OTD, OTR/L, RYT
Assistant Professor
University of Southern California
Los Angeles, CA

Rosanne DiZazzo-Miller, PhD, DrOT, OTR/L, CDP
Assistant Professor
Wayne State University
Detroit, MI

Piper Hansen, OTD, OTR/L
Occupational Therapist—Clinical Practice Leader
Rehabilitation Institute of Chicago
Chicago, IL

Doreen Head, PhD, OTR/L
Program Director and Assistant Professor
Wayne State University
Detroit, MI

Denise Hoffman, MSOT, OTR/L
Occupational Therapist
Occupational Therapy Plus
Portage, MI
Davenport University
Grand Rapids, MI
Handwriting without Tears
Cabin John, MD

Christine Johnson, MOT, OTR/L
Instructor
Lenoir-Rhyne University
Columbia, SC

Sophia Kimmons, OTR/L
Senior Occupational Therapist
Detroit Receiving Hospital
Detroit, MI

Kurt Krueger, OTR/L, CHT
Occupational Therapist
Michigan Hand and Sports Rehabilitation Center
Dearborn, MI

Deborah Loftus, MOT, OTR/L
Senior Occupational Therapist
Galaxy Brain and Therapy Center
Ann Arbor, MI

Bambi Lombardi, OTR/L
Clinical Therapy Specialist
Hanger Clinic Upper Limb Program
San Antonio, TX

Sheila M. Longpré, MOT, OTR/L
Director of Clinical and Community Relations and
    Assistant Professor
Nova Southeastern University
Tampa, FL

Moh H. Malek, PhD, FACSM, FNSCA, CSCS*D,
    NSCA-CPT*D
Associate Professor
Wayne State University
Detroit, MI

Jennie McGillicuddy, MOT, OTR/L
Occupational Therapist III, Burn Rehabilitation
Clinical Specialist
University of California at San Diego Regional
    Burn Center
San Diego, CA

Robin Mercer, MHS, OTR/L
Occupational Therapist
Wayne Westland Community School District
Westland, MI

Susan K. Meyers, EdD, MBA, OTR, FAOTA
Adjunct and Guest Faculty
Carmel, IN

Kim Eberhardt Muir, MS, OTR/L
Adjunct Clinical Assistant Professor
University of Illinois at Chicago
Occupational Therapist
Rehabilitation Institute of Chicago
Chicago, IL

Regina Parnell, PhD, OTR/L
Assistant Professor
Wayne State University
Detroit, MI

Marie Eve Pepin, PT, DPT, MSPT, OMPT
Assistant Professor
Wayne State University
Detroit, MI

Michael A. Pizzi, PhD, OTR/L, FAOTA
Associate Professor
Dominican College
Orangeburg, NY

Fredrick D. Pociask, PT, PhD, MSPT, OCS, OMT,
    FAAOMPT
Assistant Professor
Wayne State University
Detroit, MI

Kristina Reid, PT, MSPT, C/NDT
Lecturer
Wayne State University
Detroit, MI

Anne Riddering, OTR/L, CLVT, COMS
Rehabilitation Supervisor
Henry Ford Health Care System's Center for Vision
    and Neuro Rehabilitation
Livonia, MI

Susan Robosan-Burt, OTR/L
Consultant and Co-Advisor OTA Student Leadership
    Organization
Macomb Community College
Clinton Township, MI

Preethy S. Samuel, PhD, OTR/L
Assistant Professor
Wayne State University
Detroit, MI

Nicole Scheiman, MHS, OTR/L
Program Director and Associate Professor
Huntington University
Huntington, IN

Erin Skotzke, OTR/L
Occupational Therapist and Research Assistant
Wayne State University
Detroit, MI

Diane Thomson, MS, OTR/L, ATP
Senior Occupational Therapist
Rehabilitation Institute of Michigan
Detroit, MI

Rita E. Troxtel, OTD, OTR/L, CPAM
Assistant Professor
Tennessee State University
Nashville, TN

Patricia E. Tully, OTR
Occupational Therapist
TIRR Education Academy, TIRR Memorial Hermann
Houston, TX

Joyce Tyler, OTR/L, CHT
Clinical Therapy Specialist
Hanger Clinic Upper Limb Program
San Antonio, TX

Chistine A. Watt, MS, OTR/L, CPAM
Assistant Professor
Tennessee State University
Nashville, TN

Pennie Wysocki-DuBray, COTA/L
Macomb Community College
Clinton Township, MI

Six-Option Multiple Answer Item-Writer Contributors

Aurelia K. Alexander, OTD, OTR/L
Assistant Professor
Florida A&M University
Tallahassee, FL

Kimberly R. Banfill, MOT, OTR/L
Part-Time Faculty, Pediatrics Instructor, Occupational
    Therapist
Wayne State University
Detroit, MI

Jane Pomper DeHart, MA, OTR/L
Vice President of Operations
Work-Safe Occupational Health
Detroit, MI

Heather Fritz, PhD, OTR/L, CHC
Assistant Professor of Occupational Therapy and
    Gerontology
Wayne State University
Detroit, MI

Beth Kuczma, OTR/L
Occupational Therapist
Henry Ford Hospital, Behavioral Medicine
Mount Clemens, MI

Deborah Loftus, MOT, OTR/L
Senior Occupational Therapist
Galaxy Brain and Therapy Center
Ann Arbor, MI

Claudia R. Morreale, OTR/L
Occupational Therapist

Sarah T. Mbiza, PhD, OTR/L
Assistant Professor
Florida A&M University
Tallahassee, FL

Denise Nitta, OT/L
Senior Clinician
Rehabilitation Institute of Michigan
Detroit, MI

Deb Olivieria, PhD, OTR/L, CRC
Program Director and Associate Professor
Florida A&M University
Tallahassee, FL

Alisha Reichenbach, MOT, OTR/L
Senior Specialist Occupational Therapy
Munson Hospital
Traverse City, MI

Preethy S. Samuel, PhD, OTR/L
Assistant Professor
Wayne State University
Detroit, MI

Meg Scaling, OTR/L
Chief Executive Officer
Galaxy Brain and Therapy Center
Ann Arbor, MI

Courtney Wang, MS, OTR/L, CBIS
Galaxy Brain and Therapy Center
Ann Arbor, MI

Jillian Woodworth, DrOT, OTR/L
Pediatric Occupational Therapist
Burger Baylor School for Students with Autism
Children's Hospital of Michigan
Detroit, MI

Preparing for the NBCOT® Examination Day 1

Getting Started

Rosanne DiZazzo-Miller and Fredrick D. Pociask

Learning Objectives

- Identify critical materials needed for exam review preparation.
- Differentiate between the three domains of the occupational therapy assistant board exam.
- Construct a reflective journal.
- Identify current stress score and strategies to address any potential challenges.

Introduction

Preparing for the Occupational Therapy Assistant National Board Exam: 45 Days and Counting is unlike any examination book currently available to occupational therapy assistant (OTA) students. Through research utilizing a focus group model, as well as individual interviews, we learned what students preparing for this examination need and want to optimize their success. Therefore, we have compiled a content review—based on a great majority of the most commonly used textbooks in OTA education, advice from an item-writing specialist, as well as an online bank of simulation test questions.

Guidebook at a Glance

The main theme of this book utilizes chapter content on subject matter that is learned throughout OTA curricula using a lexicon taken from the Occupational Therapy Practice Framework (OTPF) III (American Occupational Therapy Association, 2014). Each chapter is divided into topics taught throughout OTA curricula in the United States. From those topics—and using the National Board for Certification in Occupational Therapy (NBCOT®)

Practice Analysis (National Board for Certification in Occupational Therapy [NBCOT®], 2012) as a guide—this book was designed for you to begin the 45-day journey and, at the end, feel prepared and ready to take the NBCOT® examination. The *Practice Analysis* provides a summary of the research used to guide construction of the board exam. Therefore, it is highly suggested that you take time to review this document at this time. Focus on the areas of practice and diagnoses typically covered so you can better judge how much time to spend on specific areas. If followed according to the suggested study guide calendar (see **Table 1-1**), you could begin and end your preparation for the board exam within 45 days. Please note that the study guide calendar is a suggestion, and we encourage you to prepare for this exam based on your own specific contexts given work, family, and other obligations that may either expedite or impede you from completing within the given time frame. Nonetheless, this study guide calendar provides a plan on how to review much of the content covered within an OTA curriculum, while allowing for time to focus on test-taking practice and strategies. If you choose to use an alternate calendar, make sure to print one off so that it can provide you with a focus to stay on task during your exam preparation.

Although this book is structured to complete your studies within 45 days, it is important that you have a sense of confidence and security, which will result from your test preparation, before scheduling a date to take the examination. When you complete (or come close to completing) the 45 days of test preparation, you will have a better idea of when you should schedule your examination. It is important to check the NBCOT® website when planning your application process, since there is waiting period before you will receive your Authorization to Test letter. After you receive your letter, you can typically schedule your exam right away.

Table 1-1 Study Guide Calendar

Day 1	Day 2	Day 3	Day 4	Day 5
Chapters 1, 2, and 3	Chapters 4, 5, and 6	Chapter 7	Chapter 8	Chapter 9 Stress scale and reflection
Day 6	**Day 7**	**Day 8**	**Day 9**	**Day 10**
Chapter 10	Chapter 11	Chapter 12	Chapter 13	Chapters 14 and 15 Stress scale and reflection
Day 11	**Day 12**	**Day 13**	**Day 14**	**Day 15**
Chapters 16 and 17	Chapter 18	Chapter 19	Chapter 20	Chapters 21 and 22 Stress scale and reflection
Day 16	**Day 17**	**Day 18**	**Day 19**	**Day 20**
Chapters 23 and 24	Chapters 25 and 26	Chapter 27	Chapter 28	Chapter 29 Stress scale and reflection
Day 21	**Day 22**	**Day 23**	**Day 24**	**Day 25**
Chapter 30	Chapters 31 and 32	Chapter 33	Chapters 34 and 35	Chapters 36 and 37 Stress scale and reflection
Day 26	**Day 27**	**Day 28**	**Day 29**	**Day 30**
Chapters 38 and 39	Chapter 40	Chapters 41 and 42	Review any material that you feel necessary today	Complete your review today Stress scale and reflection
Day 31	**Day 32**	**Day 33**	**Day 34**	**Day 35**
Begin test-taking practice today! Take first practice test Locate the center you will be taking the test. Once you know the day and time, make sure to plan a visit at that day and time of the week!	Review correct and incorrect answers	Review correct and incorrect answers as well as the six-option multiple answer questions	Take second practice test Schedule test if you feel ready	Review correct and incorrect answers Stress scale and reflection
Day 36	**Day 37**	**Day 38**	**Day 39**	**Day 40**
Review correct and incorrect answers, as well as the six-option multiple answer questions	Take third practice test Review any content that was difficult during practice	Review correct and incorrect answers	Review correct and incorrect answers, as well as the six-option multiple answer questions	Take fourth practice test Stress scale and reflection
Day 41	**Day 42**	**Day 43**	**Day 44**	**Day 45**
Review correct and incorrect answers	Review correct and incorrect answers, as well as the six-option multiple answer questions	Final review areas of difficulty	Continue review until confident with the results and REST!	Downtime!

Additionally, each chapter includes self-study activities to help reinforce memorization and learning. The online component accompanying this text consists of interactive practice examinations. The questions cover content as specified in the chapter study guides and are appropriately distributed using the NBCOT® domain areas (NBCOT®, 2013). There are three COTA® domains that cover obtaining information on occupational performance throughout the Occupational therapy (OT) process, intervention implementation, and management. It is important to take time to review how these three domains are defined, as well as the percentage of the exam that each domain covers. Each exam question provides a rationale for correct answers along with references for your convenience. Furthermore, practice test results can be calculated to provide you with specific domain area percentage scores so you will know what areas you need to spend more time on. Evidence-based practice also guided the formation of each chapter. Furthermore, references used throughout this exam review book feature robust levels of evidence to provide the student with the most current and accurate information available.

Study Tools for Success

- Answer sheets to various self-study activities.
- Unique instructional materials that provide the learner with a creative means by which to learn and discover the content.
- Over 1,000 practice examination questions that can be taken to simulate the actual exam. Although it is not possible for us—or any other exam prep book that is not affiliated with NBCOT®—to receive item-writing assistance from past OTA item writers, we do have a physical therapist item-writing specialist who has edited all question content to ensure they meet the standards and guidelines that are comparable to NBCOT® standards.
- Multiple-step case studies are modeled after the clinical simulation test questions. Log onto the online portal and follow directions to the practice questions, tests, and multiple-step case studies.
- This text incorporates a holistic view of study skills and habits that contribute to a healthy examination preparation process. Wellness tips and the opportunity for self-assessment reinforce healthy lifestyle choices that are conducive to success. Every week you will be asked to perform a self-assessment

in the areas of sleep, nutrition, exercise, and stress. This will be completed using the Stress Vulnerability Scale (please see **Table 1-2**).

- If you begin to notice that your stress scale score is high or steadily increasing, please refer to **Table 1-3**, which provides suggestions on how to identify and manage your stress.
- You should consider getting at least one to two weeks of restorative or quality sleep (i.e., eight hours of uninterrupted sleep per day) leading up to the exam. These activities will serve as a reminder of the importance of taking care of yourself and are meant to reinforce key traits (e.g., flexibility, organization, and person-centeredness) that will enable you to become a productive and effective occupational therapist.
- A weekly reflective learning journaling section, courtesy of Live Wire Media, is provided using a three-question reflective learning approach with which students learn individual areas to focus on and prioritize. Research suggests that reflection "illuminates what has been experienced by [one's] self . . . providing a basis for future action" (Raelin 2001, p. 11). Each week you are asked to answer the following questions (see **Table 1-4**):
  1. **What?** What have I accomplished? What have I learned?
  2. **So what?** What difference did it make? Why should I do it? How is it important? How do I feel about it?
  3. **Now what?** What's next? Where do I go from here?
- Test-taking strategies and things to do prior to, and directly after, the exam are provided, with a focus on adult learning and test-taking strategies.
- Additionally, you will be directed to the NBCOT® website where you can download study tools to assist in the formulation of a personalized study plan to help keep you on track throughout this important process. This not only provides a focus, but will inevitably guide the identification of your strengths, weaknesses, and personal challenges. It is also very important to become familiar with the NBCOT® website (NBCOT®, 2015), where you will find the application and forms you need to complete in order to take the test, the certification handbook, practice analysis, guide for international students, special accommodations provisions, examination preparation tools, scoring calendar, and many other useful links and downloads.

Table 1-2 Stress Vulnerability Scale

In modern society, most of us cannot avoid stress. But we can learn to behave in ways that lessen its effects. Researchers have identified a number of factors that affect one's vulnerability to stress—among them are eating and sleeping habits, caffeine and alcohol intake, and how we express our emotions. The following questionnaire is designed to help you discover your vulnerability quotient and to pinpoint trouble spots. Rate each item from 1 (always) to 5 (never), according to how much of the time the statement is true of you. Be sure to mark each item, even if it does not apply to you—for example, if you do not smoke, circle 1 next to item six.

	Always	Sometimes			Never
1. I eat at least one hot, balanced meal a day.	1	2	3	4	5
2. I get 7–8 hours of sleep at least four nights a week.	1	2	3	4	5
3. I give and receive affection regularly.	1	2	3	4	5
4. I have at least one relative within 50 miles on whom I can rely.	1	2	3	4	5
5. I exercise to the point of perspiration at least twice a week.	1	2	3	4	5
6. I limit myself to less than half a pack of cigarettes a day.	1	2	3	4	5
7. I take fewer than five alcohol drinks a week.	1	2	3	4	5
8. I am the appropriate weight for my height.	1	2	3	4	5
9. I have an income adequate to meet basic expenses.	1	2	3	4	5
10. I get strength from my religious beliefs.	1	2	3	4	5
11. I regularly attend club or social activities.	1	2	3	4	5
12. I have a network of friends and acquaintances.	1	2	3	4	5
13. I have one or more friends to confide in about personal matters.	1	2	3	4	5
14. I am in good health (including eyesight, hearing, and teeth).	1	2	3	4	5
15. I am able to speak openly about my feelings when angry or worried.	1	2	3	4	5
16. I have regular conversations with the people I live with about domestic problems—for example, chores and money.	1	2	3	4	5
17. I do something for fun at least once a week.	1	2	3	4	5
18. I am able to organize my time effectively.	1	2	3	4	5
19. I drink fewer than three cups of coffee (or other caffeine-rich drinks) a day.	1	2	3	4	5
20. I take some quiet time for myself during the day.	1	2	3	4	5

Scoring Instructions: To calculate your score, add up the figures and subtract 20.

Score Interpretation: A score below 10 indicates excellent resistance to stress. A score over 30 indicates some vulnerability to tackling stress. A score over 50 indicates serious vulnerability to stress.

Self-Care Plan: Notice that nearly all the items describe the situations and behaviors over which you have a great deal of control. Review the items on which you scored three or higher. List those items in your self-care plan. Concentrate first on those that are easiest to change—for example, eating a hot, balanced meal daily and having fun at least once a week—before tackling those that seem difficult.

Table 1-3 Stress Busters

Tips and Techniques for Managing Stress and Introducing Relaxation into Your Life

What Is Stress?

Stress is the physiological and psychological response of the body to some sort of threat to our safety, self-esteem, or well-being. Stressors can be physical (e.g., illness), social (e.g., a relationship breakup or other loss), circumstantial (e.g., a poor exam grade or moving), or psychological (e.g., low self-esteem or worry). Often, transitions or changes, such as a new semester or new job, can bring on stress.

We are all under stress every day. A certain amount of stress helps us all to function better, keep ourselves safe from harm, and get things done during the day. Too much stress, however, can lead to physical illness, difficulty concentrating, or feelings of sadness or isolation.

Did You Know?

Most college campuses and communities have counseling and psychological services available for students and community residents at low cost. If the stress you experience interferes meaningfully with your ability to work, study, engage in positive social interactions, or feel okay, having an individual assessment and counseling for stress reduction and relaxation may be helpful. In a supportive environment, clients learn new stress reduction techniques and create an individualized plan to manage stress.

What Are the Symptoms of Stress?

Everyone responds to stress in different ways. What might be stressful for one person may be another person's hobby. In a similar way, everyone reacts differently to stress. Common stress reactions include

- Muscle tension or soreness in the back and shoulders
- Stomach troubles or digestive distress
- Difficulty falling asleep or waking early
- Increased heart rate or difficulty breathing
- Fatigue or exhaustion
- Lack of interest or boredom
- Engaging in destructive behaviors (e.g., drinking too much alcohol, overeating)
- Inability to concentrate
- Avoidance or fear of people, places, or tasks

In addition, stress can lead to more serious problems, such as depression, anxiety, hypertension, and other illnesses. These symptoms may also be caused by medical or psychological conditions other than stress.

Remember, chronic stress can have long-term effects on health and well-being, so if your symptoms are severe or prolonged, get outside support. If stress becomes too much to manage on your own, schedule a visit to see a qualified healthcare provider.

Questions to Ask Yourself About Your Stress

- What are the primary sources of stress in my life?
- What are the signs and symptoms in my body that let me know I am stressed?
- What have I done that worked in the past to manage my stress?
- What can I do to integrate more relaxation into my daily routine?
- What do I want to do today to resolve my stress and work toward relaxation?

Effective Ways to Manage Your Stress

- Think about possible causes of your stress and be active in reducing stress. Small shifts in your thinking, behaviors, or breathing can make a very big difference.
- Avoid stress-producing situations. Although it is not always possible, many stressful situations can be avoided. Watch for places where you can avoid inviting stress; seek out places to relax.
- Engage in some regular exercise, which has been shown to alleviate the impact of stress. Choose an assortment of tension-building and tension-releasing exercises; remember that even small doses help! Take a quick walk, stretch in your office, even simple stretches help!

(continues)

Table 1-3 Stress Busters (*continued*)

Tips and Techniques for Managing Stress and Introducing Relaxation into Your Life

- Examine if the way that you are thinking about your life (e.g., perfectionist thinking) is adding to or decreasing your stress. Are there other ways to think about the situation that is less stress inducing? Are there positive thoughts you could integrate into your daily thinking?
- Engage in activities that you enjoy and that give you an outlet for thinking about other things besides your stress.
- Increase your social connections. . . find other people who can relate to your experience. Do stress-busting activities together! Talk about the stressor and your plan to resolve your stress!
- Take good care of your body. . . eat well, get enough sleep, and avoid alcohol and drugs, which can increase stress.
- Use self-relaxation techniques like deep breathing, muscle relaxation, and visualizing successes or relaxing places (provided later).
- Download soothing music or music that makes you smile, and listen to it when you are feeling stressed.
- Search for meditation podcasts that are specific to your needs (e.g., pregnancy meditation, reducing test-taking anxiety). Many podcasts are available online and free!
- Consider writing a list of your stresses, including ways to address those stresses. Sometimes even the act of writing the list can ease worry. Start checking items off your list!
- Find your own optimal stress relievers. Is it changing your thoughts? A physical activity? A social occasion? Look for the healthy ways that help you to feel less stressed and do them!

From the Expert!

In his research, Stanford Professor and expert on stress Dr Robert Sapolsky has identified four important components of reducing stress, which include

1. Predictive information, such as a sign that the stress is going to be increasing (e.g., knowing a test date). That awareness gives us more control over our stress reactions.
2. Finding an outlet for dealing with stress (e.g., exercise, meditation, deep breathing).
3. Having a positive outlook or belief that life is going to get better, rather than get worse.
4. Having friends. Social support from others is an important component in keeping stress levels down.

Some Relaxation Techniques to Get You Started

- Try deep breathing exercises. Lie or sit in a comfortable position with your muscles relaxed, and take a few deep breaths. With your hand on your belly, feel your belly rise and fall as you inhale and exhale. Work toward breathing in to a slow count to five.
- 1 . . . 2 . . . 3 . . . 4 . . . 5 . . . Exhale slowly. Rely on this technique when you start to feel stressed.
- When your body feels tense, take 3 minutes to sit or lie down quietly and focus on calming all of the muscle groups in your body. Begin with the muscles in your feet and slowly work your way up your body. Relax your legs, back muscles, chest, arms, hands, cheeks, and forehead. You may wish to focus on areas that feel tense or where you are experiencing pain. Breathe air into those areas. Relaxing all of the major muscle groups will help your whole body feel at ease.
- If you are anticipating a stressful event, such as taking an exam or a difficult social interaction, take a few moments to visualize the event going well. See yourself experiencing success. Envision the details of what you might say or do that will result in positive outcomes. If negative thoughts or images occur, take a deep breath and refocus on the positive. Invite a successful outcome through visualization!
- After doing some breathing and muscle relaxation, or just taking time to rest, take a moment to calm your thoughts and visualize a peaceful place in your mind, either a place you have been or would like to go. Allow your body to relax more and your mind to calm. Take just 10 minutes! Recognize that you can go to that peaceful place in your mind and feel relief from life's stressors whenever you need a break!

Reproduced with permission of Shannon Casey-Cannon, PhD, Alliant International University.

Table 1-4 Reflection Journal
1. **What?** What have I accomplished? What have I learned?
2. **So what?** What difference did it make? Why should I do it? How is it important? How do I feel about it?
3. **Now what?** What's next? Where do I go from here?

Reproduced with permission of Live Wire Media.

Focus Group Transcript Results

Before planning of this examination guidebook began, we called on our alumni to attend a focus group or participate in surveys or individual interviews to provide us insight that we could implement into our book and pass along to future graduates. The results were as follows, beginning with themes and ending with specific questions.

Preparation

- Prepare for approximately six weeks at a minimum, and spend some time alone and some time together in small groups.
- Take tests repeatedly.
- Do not focus on studying what you already know.

Materials for Preparation

- NBCOT® materials are popular and similar to exam questions.
- Other materials were too vague and concrete, with only one-step questions.
- The national review course was helpful but overwhelming.
- Other materials were not helpful for critical thinking.
- The rationale for correct answers is very important.

Answering Multiple Choice Questions

- Practice combining diagnosis with treatment in multistep questions.
- Learn how to dissect questions.

Test Environment

- The environment was anxiety provoking.
- The room was cold.

Helpful Suggestions

- Most focus group students took off weekends from studying.
- Make sure you focus on spinal cord injury levels of function related to levels of injury and relevant equipment!
- Watch your caffeine intake.
- Go to the bathroom halfway through the test, even if you do not need to go.

- Take the clock off the computer screen if it is anxiety provoking.
- Visit the site the day before and walk in to get a feel for the environment.
- Dress in comfortable layers.
- Do not study the night before.
- Sleep eight hours the night before.
- Choose a time to take the exam that fits your personality.
- Volunteer at a site that you do not feel enough exposure to.

Questions and Answers

The following are some specific questions that were asked and answered by the students in the focus group:

Q: Are the questions presented one at a time?

A: Yes.

Q: Can you mark them and go back to them, and how does that work?

A: Yes, after you complete the questions, a list comes up of questions you marked to look at again.

Q: After you answer, can you change the answer later, even after you click on a selection?

A: Yes.

Q: What is the best piece of advice you can give a student who is preparing to answer the questions on this examination?

A: Eliminate two answers first from the options presented, and then reread the question to make sure your answer fits exactly what the question asks!

Q: Give your best description of your testing area or environment.

A: There were rows of computers with cubicle dividers, and you can wear headphones to block out sounds. Other people are writing different tests (e.g., Graduate Record Exam). The test room consisted of approximately 30 individuals.

Q: What are you allowed to bring into the testing center?

A: They give you a blank sheet of paper and a pen (some got a dry erase board). You cannot bring water, but you can take a break and leave for water or the bathroom. There were lockers where we had to leave our purses, etc., outside the testing room.

Q: Identify any mnemonics or charts that were helpful during your study preparation.

A: Charts and handouts with a short summary of infant and child reflexes/patterns were really helpful (e.g., Moro, Babinski, asymmetrical tonic neck reflex, symmetrical tonic neck reflex). Also, a synopsis of the most common splints was very helpful. It helped to have a page at a glance, with a picture of each splint and a short description, including the name and use for each. In addition, reviewing frames of reference for psychosocial and physical disabilities, manual muscle test, Ranchos, Glasgow Coma Scale, and range of motion norms/scales was very useful. Any kind of handout or page at a glance is helpful to reinforce the information into memory.

Q: Is there anything else you can remember about the exam and what was and was not allowed?

A: Be able to use clinical reasoning skills in terms of reading a treatment scenario and deciding on the best option. There were always one or two answers that were definitely wrong and two that seemed to be correct. I remember always having to narrow down out of the two, which was the *better* choice.

Q: Did you learn about how to take the test through a tutorial or as you went?

A: There were two tutorials (one for the multiple choice items and the other for the clinical simulation test items), and it did not take up any examination time.

Q: Please provide any additional comments regarding what you found helpful in preparing to take the exam.

A: The most helpful thing for me was to repeatedly take practice exams. I would go back and study the areas on the practice tests that I got wrong. I also spent a lot of time studying the basics and making sure those were embedded in my memory as a knowledge base for any type of question they might throw at me. Know the various scales, norms, reflexes, most common splints, contraindications for certain diagnoses, etc. Spend time studying with a few friends, quizzing one another, and discussing why an answer was wrong or right. It helped a lot to have feedback within a small group.

Final Thoughts

The following outline is based on our focus group findings and provides key considerations as you progress through your 45-day journey:

1. *Know your facts.*
   - Review, study, and become familiar with the facts presented, that is, what this entire book is about! If you do not know the facts, you cannot accurately critically reason through the question.

2. *Learn how to answer questions strategically.*
   - Keep in mind that the exam questions will contain a lot of information. You will need to focus on some of the information, but other information will not be relevant to the final question being asked. Remember to read each question statement one last time before selecting your answer. Do not get tripped up on answer options that make sense for only certain parts of the question. Make sure the answer you select addresses the central theme of the question being asked.

3. *Take at least two practice exams on a computer, and remember to keep time to simulate the actual testing environment.*
   - Get used to taking practice exams while being timed. Experience what answering one question per minute feels like in an environment where you hear people typing, fidgeting in their seats, and getting up to go to the restroom. Only bring items that are allowed in the testing environment. Complete at least two practice tests in this environment. You will find it very different than taking an exam at your leisure in your pajamas while munching on a snack!

4. *At the 2009 American Occupational Therapy Association Annual Conference in Texas, the NBCOT reported that test takers who took the full 10-minute tutorials during the exam performed better than students who did not. There are two tutorials, neither of which count against your exam time. Now. . . let's get started!*

Action Steps

1. Search, locate, and download the OTPF III and review the terminology, the operationalized OT process, and all the tables presented throughout the document. Focus specifically on the definitions and examples provided for the terminology used throughout the various areas of practice.

2. Search, locate, and download the most current version of the NBCOT® Practice Analysis. Pay special attention to the main areas of practice for primary employment, and the tables that list disorders and the percent of OT practitioners providing services in each area of practice. This will help guide your study with a better understanding of what you should focus on.

3. Search, locate, and download the most current version of the NBCOT® domain areas. Read through these and understand how the test is structured and the percentage of questions each domain covers.

4. Search, locate, and download the NBCOT® Certification Exam Handbook. Read through this to make sure you fully understand the processes and policies related to the NBCOT® examination.

References

American Occupational Therapy Association. (2014). Occupational therapy practice framework: Domain and process (3rd Edition). *American Journal of Occupational Therapy, 68,* S1–S48.

National Board for Certification in Occupational Therapy. (2012). *2012 Practice analysis of the certified occupational therapist assistant: Executive summary.* Retrieved from http://www.nbcot.org/assets/candidate-pdfs/2012-practice-analysis-executive-cota.

National Board for Certification in Occupational Therapy. (2013). *Validated domain, task, knowledge statements.* Retrieved from http://www.nbcot.org/assets/candidate-pdfs/cota_vdtks_2013

National Board for Certification in Occupational Therapy. (2015). *Connected. Current.* Certified. Retrieved from http://www.nbcot.org/.

Raelin, J. A. (2001). Public reflection as the basis of learning. *Management Learning, 32*(1), 11–30.

Learning as an Adult and Cognitive Factors in Learning

Fredrick D. Pociask

Learning Objectives

- Recognize principles and concepts of lifelong learning.
- Describe the key differences between entry-level and adult learners.
- Describe what we know about successful learners.
- List and describe key determinants of student success and failure.
- Recognize cognitive factors in learning and understanding.
- Describe the strengths and limitations of working and long-term memory.
- Describe the importance of monitoring comprehension.
- List and describe helpful metacognitive strategies.

Key Terms

- *Active learning*: Learners take an active role in their own learning and are in part responsible for learning outcomes.
- *Attention*: "Arousal and intention in the brain that influence an individual's learning processes. Without active, dynamic, and selective attending of environmental stimuli, it follows that meaning generation cannot occur" (Lee, Lim, & Grabowski, 2007, p. 112).
- *Human cognitive architecture*: The manner in which structures and functions required for human cognitive processes are organized (Sweller, 2007, p. 370).

- *Knowledge generation*: "Generation of understanding through developing relationships between and among ideas" (Lee et al., 2007, p. 112).
- *Long-term memory*: Component of the information-processing model of cognition that stores all knowledge and skills in hierarchical networks.
- *Meaning making*: "The process of connecting new information with prior knowledge, affected by one's intention, motivation, and strategies employed" (Lee et al., 2007, p. 112).
- *Memory*: The mental faculty of retaining and recalling past experiences (Seel, 2007, p. 40).
- *Motivation*: "The choice people make as to what experiences or goals they will approach or avoid and the degree of effort they will exert in that respect" (Crookes & Schmidt, 1991, p. 481).
- *Self-concept*: An individual's total picture of himself or herself (e.g., self-definition in societal roles, beliefs, feelings, and values) that is typically focused on societal and personal norms.
- *Self-efficacy*: An individual's belief that he or she can attain his or her goals or accomplish an identified task or tasks.
- *Sensory memory*: A component of the information-processing model of cognition that describes the initial input of information (e.g., vision and/or hearing) (Lohr & Gall, 2007, p. 80).
- *Working memory*: The structure that processes information coming from either the environment or long-term memory and transfers learned information for storage in long-term memory (Sweller, 2007, p. 370).

Introduction

If you are reading this page, you probably have completed or will soon complete an occupational therapy curriculum and will soon embark on a rewarding and challenging career as an occupational therapy assistant (OTA) and healthcare provider. The transition between an academic and a professional career is truly an exciting point in one's professional development and for the typical graduate, emotions may range from exuberance and extreme personal satisfaction to uncertainty and anxiousness over a pending national board examination. It is the intent of this chapter and this book to help the reader hold on to the extreme personal satisfaction that comes with completing a challenging academic program and to help manage any uncertainty and anxiousness that is so often typical for a new graduate who is facing a board examination.

This chapter has two sections. Section 1 introduces principles and concepts of lifelong learning, which includes a discussion of learning as an adult, the key differences between entry-level and adult learners, what we know about successful learners, and key determinants of student success and failure. Section 2 introduces cognitive factors in learning and understanding, which include memory and retention, strengths and limitations of working long-term memory, the importance of monitoring comprehension, and helpful cognitive learning strategies. The information in this chapter is intentionally presented in sufficient detail and with supporting evidence because comprehension and adoption of productive learning behaviors are only fostered by understanding and perceived usefulness.

Section 1: Lifelong Learning

It should be evident for individuals who are leaving the folds of an academic institution and embarking on lifelong careers as healthcare professionals that the transition from an academic to a professional career does not signify an end to formal learning. In contrast, graduation day simply signifies the official shift of ownership and responsibility for lifelong learning to the new graduate, a responsibility that will undoubtedly affect professional opportunities and define professional reputations. The following paragraphs will discuss lifelong learning as an adult and factors that can help account for student success.

Lifelong Learning as an Adult

Although there are numerous philosophies, theories, and models supporting adult learning, there is good consensus on the characteristics that make up the deliberative adult learner. Adult learning characteristics also comprise the emotional, psychological, and intellectual aspect of an individual and minimally include the following traits and behaviors (Knowles, Holton, & Swanson 1998; Merriam & Caffarella, 1999; Snowman & Biehler, 2006):

- *Experience*: The adult learner utilizes prior knowledge and experience as a vehicle for future learning, readily incorporates new knowledge into similar prior learning, and appreciates the application of knowledge in the context of real-life problems.
- *Self-concept*: The adult learner moves away from self-concept based on dependency toward a self-concept based on self-direction and personal independence.
- *Communication*: Adult learners become increasingly able to effectively express and exchange feelings, thoughts, opinions, and information through verbal and nonverbal modes of communication and varied forms of media.
- *Orientation to learning*: Adult learners increasingly move away from a subject-centered orientation toward knowledge that will be applied at some future point in time to a problem-specific application of knowledge in the context of real-world problems.
- *Motivation to learn*: Motivation toward learning shifts away from extrinsic incentives, such as course grades, and becomes increasingly directed toward intrinsic incentives, such as the completion of defined goals and tasks in the fulfillment of social and professional responsibilities.
- *Responsibility*: Adult learners are capable of reflective reasoning. They analyze knowledge, personal behaviors, and interactions on an ongoing basis; incorporate constructive feedback; and adapt knowledge, behaviors, and interactions to reflect ethical societal standards and values.
- *Intrapersonal and interpersonal skills*: Adult learners increasingly develop the ability to work independently and cooperatively with others and across varied circumstances and issues that affect the common well-being and one's own well-being in relationship to the world around them.

- *Critical inquiry and reasoning*: Adult learners increasingly develop the ability to examine and utilize reasoning and decision-making strategies to select, apply, and evaluate evidence in the context of real-world problems.

Although many characteristics of the model adult learner can be identified in adult learning philosophy and theory, we can certainly agree that seeking to achieve the previously described attributes would be a worthwhile endeavor. Now that we know important characteristics of an adult learner, let us make a simple comparison between college-level learning characteristics and adult learning characteristics, as depicted in **Table 2-1** (Knowles et al., 1998; Merriam & Caffarella, 1999; Snowman & Biehler, 2006).

Now that we have identified key characteristics of the adult learner and compared them to typical college-level learning, it should be apparent that the attributes identified in the right column of Table 2-1 are well aligned with lifelong professional development and achievement. Relative to the task at hand (i.e., successful completion of the National Board for Certification in Occupational Therapy [NBCOT®]) and in terms of common obstacles to learning and achievement, some of the greatest barriers to learning arise from discrepancies between learner behavior and expectations and authentic real-world expectations and anticipated outcomes. In practical terms, holding on to entry-level or college-level behaviors and expectations while preparing for the NBCOT® would be

expected to hinder preparedness and potentially limit achievement and confidence. The following paragraphs will describe why adult learning behaviors are well aligned with learner achievement, so regardless of where you fall on the spectrum of entry-level to adult learning behaviors, it is officially time to jump aboard the adult learning bandwagon.

What We Know About Successful Self-Directed Learners

Over the years, much effort has been directed toward understanding the complexity of the learning process and identifying the determinants or attributes that account for student success and failure (Alvarez & Risko 2009; Carroll, 1989; Morrison, Ross, Kalman, & Kemp, 2013; Rachal, Daigle, & Rachal, 2007; Spector, Merrill, Merrienboer, & Driscoll, 2007). Although it is obvious that there are many fixed factors that we cannot change in preparation for an examination, such as intelligence quotient (IQ), there are a number of adaptable factors or variables that will, in part, determine your successfulness on the NBCOT® exam, as specifically introduced and discussed as follows:

- *Understanding of task requirements*: Developing a thorough understanding of NBCOT® task requirements should be one of your first objectives. For example, very important task considerations include what is the structure and complexity of the

Table 2-1 Comparison of College-Level Learning and Learning as an Adult

Factor	College-Level Learning	Learning as an Adult
Instructor	The instructor is the source of knowledge, decides what is important and what will be learned	If present, the instructor is a facilitator or resource, and learners evaluate needs based on real-world goals and problems and decide what is important to be learned
Learning	Passive learners and individual work	Active learners, teamwork, and collaboration
	Accept learning experience and knowledge at face value	Validate learning experience and knowledge based on experiences and usefulness
Content	Homogeneous and stable content	Diverse and dynamic content
	Content learned in the abstract	Content learned in context
Organization	Learning is organized by subject and content area	Learning is organized around personal experiences, context, and problem solving
Orientation	Acquiring entry-level competencies	Acquiring real-world problem-solving competencies
Utility	Developing subject matter attitudes, knowledge, and fundamental skill sets	Developing lifelong learning attitudes, expertise, and advanced skill sets

Data from: Knowles et al. (1998), Merriam and Caffarella (1999), Snowman and Biehler (2006).

examination, how is the examination administered, when is the examination administered, how do you schedule the examination, what documentation needs to be completed by your university before you can schedule an examination date, when do you report on the day of the examination, can you find a testing center without getting lost, and what do you do if you need to reschedule. Additionally, a thorough understanding of task requirements will set your mind at ease and avoid any unnecessary panic attacks the day before the examination.

- *Ability to comprehend and follow instructions*: The ability to comprehend and follow instructions begins with the understanding of task requirements and continues throughout the examination preparation process. Because the brunt of the preparation for the NBCOT® exam will be through self-directed learning and preparatory lectures and/or courses, it is important to keep a running list of items that need clarification, principles and concepts you do not fully understand, and even simple task requirements that are not clear. Whether the need for further comprehension is related to the quality of information or gaps in knowledge, you will need to take deliberate action to seek help from resources such as your textbooks, journals, former professors, peers, clinical mentors, and/or the American Occupational Therapy Association.

- *Basic aptitudes and general abilities*: Regardless of fixed factors, such as IQ, basic aptitudes and general abilities can have a big effect on student success. These factors can encompass very manageable aptitudes and abilities, such as basic computer skills, library skills, and project management skills, to more challenging factors, such as verbal ability. Chapter 3 will offer much advice in terms of study tips, skills, and strategies, but it will be up to the self-directed learner to identify any weaknesses in general abilities and tackle them early on in the examination preparation process.

- *Time saved by prior learning*: Time saved by prior learning can be a substantial determinant in terms of student success or failure. Regrettably, courses that foster the use of rote recall strategies and fail to ask the learner to recall or apply knowledge beyond the examination or course conclusion have left many learners at a disadvantage. In simple terms, forgetting and relearning can be cognitively taxing

and will place additional constraints on available time and resources. This said, regardless of the degree of prior learning you are able to access when you begin preparing for the NBCOT®, you will need to use productive learning strategies to make sure the information gained on day 1 is still retained on day 45 (i.e., without forgetting and relearning).

- *Time allocated to learning*: The learner's decision to allocate suitable time to a given learning task is a very important consideration when preparing for the NBCOT®. In very simple terms, the time needed should clearly match the time allowed, and sufficient flexibility should be maintained in project management to address additional and unforeseen demands placed on your available time. In terms of examination preparation, if you find that you are frustrated or anxious because you cannot complete scheduled learning objectives in the time that you allowed for a given task, you are simply telling yourself that you have not allowed adequate time for the task.

- *Academically engaged time*: All learners probably realize that there can be small-to-colossal gaps between time allocated to a learning task and the amount of time actually devoted to learning with understanding. This said, academically engaged time is the time spent fully attending to a given learning task to meet prespecified learning objectives. For example, if a learner has scheduled a two-hour block of time to achieve a specific study objective and spends half of the time sorting and organizing materials to be learned, sending and receiving text messages, setting up a study playlist on the iPad, and allowing a friend to interrupt, academic engagement is, at best, 50%. From a more practical perception, remaining academically engaged during scheduled study periods would be expected to reduce undue frustration and anxiety levels, allow achievement of study objectives, and potentially open up free time to do activities that you enjoy.

- *Environmental characteristics*: Recommendations on how to control study environments will be discussed in Chapter 3; however, factors such as a distraction-free environment, location, time of day, and even temperature and lighting can affect study efficiency and effectiveness.

- *Quality and organization of instruction*: The clarity and adequacy of the instructional material to be learned can have a significant impact on student success. Because preparation for the NBCOT® will be predominantly self-directed learning, it will be important to identify and organize quality instructional materials in the initial stages of preparation and to note any gaps that will need to be filled through supplemental resources. The use of this board exam preparation text in combination with your course materials, course texts, acquired literature, and the Navigate 2 Preferred Access online resources should be more than sufficient for the task at hand.

Now that we have introduced some very important determinants of student success or failure, let us take a step back and identify the determinants that are fully or predominantly under the direct control of the learner, those that are partially controlled by the learner, and those for which the learner will have no control in preparation for the NBCOT®, by completing the determinant of student success or failure worksheet (**Table 2-2**).

Determinant of Student Success or Failure Worksheet Summary and Conclusions

In reflection, and in context of NBCOT® preparation, it should be apparent that attributes under direct learner control include (1) understanding of task requirements, (2) ability to comprehend and follow instructions, (3) basic aptitudes and general abilities, (4) time saved by prior learning, (5) time allocated to learning, and (6) academically engaged time. In fairness, (7) environmental characteristics

and (8) quality and organization of instruction are under partial to full learner control, and none of the attributes are outside of direct or partial learner control. In the grand scheme of things, this is great news because as a self-directed adult learner you will have considerable direct control over some of the most important determinants that will contribute to your success on the NBCOT® exam.

Common Obstacles to Learning

Now that we have discussed characteristics of the adult learner and determinants of learning that are readily modified to achieve successful outcomes, we can discuss common obstacles that can impede learning and performance. We hope that knowledge of these obstacles in combination with sound reflective reasoning will help the reader to avoid many learning obstacle pitfalls.

- *Attitude obstacles*: Attitude obstacles include making excuses, procrastination, decision avoidance, avoiding seeking help, task avoidance, approach-avoidance conflict behavior (i.e., the fear of something a person desires), lack of commitment or excessive commitment, requiring unattainable perfection, and lack of positive feedback and reinforcement. Although some learners may overlook or underestimate the impact of attitude obstacles, we should take a momentary pause to acknowledge that attitude obstacles can have a significant impact on both learning and performance under many circumstances (Anderson 2003; Elliot 1999; Elliot & Covington 2001; Ferrari, Johnson, &

Table 2-2 Determinant of Student Success or Failure Worksheet			
Determinant of Success or Failure	**Learner Control**	**Partial Learner Control**	**No Learner Control**
1. Understanding of task requirements	☐	☐	☐
2. Ability to comprehend and follow instructions	☐	☐	☐
3. Basic aptitudes and general abilities	☐	☐	☐
4. Time saved by prior learning	☐	☐	☐
5. Time allocated to learning	☐	☐	☐
6. Academically engaged time	☐	☐	☐
7. Environmental characteristics	☐	☐	☐
8. Quality and organization of instruction	☐	☐	☐

Data from: Alvarez and Risko (2009), Carroll (1989), Morrison et al. (2013), Rachal et al. (2007).

McCown, 1995; Levinger, 1957; Owens, 2001; Ryan, Pintrich, & Midgley, 2001; Steel, 2007).

- *Academic self-handicapping*: An excellent example of obstacle of attitude is cleverly coined as "academic self-handicapping" and is described as "creating impediments to successful performance on tasks that the individual considers important" (Urdan & Midgley, 2001, p. 116). Academic self-handicapping (1) is a conscious decision to pursue a behavior or establish an excuse before or alongside anticipated achievement activity, not after; (2) occurs prior to important situations where the probability of success is uncertain or in doubt; and (3) occurs as a consequence of both specific actions and lack of action (Schwinger, Wirthwein, Lemmer, & Steinmayr, 2014; Thomas & Gadbois, 2007; Urdan, 2004). Academic self-handicapping is noted in high- and lower-level performing college students, and common examples of academic self-handicapping include procrastination, excuses, over involvement in nonacademic activities, and choosing socializing in place of examination preparation (Schwinger et al., 2014; Urdan, 2004). The psychology behind academic self-handicapping is complex, but the cognitive affective and motivational factors driving academic self-handicapping are most likely a manifestation of avoidance motives driven by a fear of failure or fear of feeling less capable in the eyes of others (Urdan & Midgley, 2001). Additionally, high self-esteem learners may use self-handicapping to enhance success and failure (Tice, 1991). Regardless of your circumstances and motivation, academic self-handicapping and the NBCOT® exam do not make a good combination.

Let Us Take a Ridiculously Unscientific Quiz to See If You May Be an Academic Self-Handicapper

Before reading ahead, please complete **Table 2-3** by answering "yes" or "no" for each question.

Academic Self-Handicapper Quiz Worksheet Summary and Conclusions

Well, seeing as this is a ridiculously unscientific quiz, there are no passing or failing scores. However, if you found yourself answering yes to one or more questions without an authentic explanation, you may, in fact, be

Table 2-3 Academic Self-Handicapper Quiz

Questions (Answer "Yes" or "No" for Each Question)	Yes	No
I typically put off preparing for an examination until the last minute.	☐	☐
I typically put off completing homework until the last minute.	☐	☐
I allow my friends to distract me from paying attention in class.	☐	☐
I allow my friends to distract me from examination preparation.	☐	☐
When I do poorly on an exam it's typically because I didn't try.	☐	☐
When I do poorly on an exam it's typically because I'm involved in many activities and have numerous commitments.	☐	☐
I tend to procrastinate or I have been labeled as a procrastinator by those who know me best.	☐	☐
I've been known to socialize the night before an examination even though I am not fully prepared.	☐	☐
I know I could have gotten better grades in certain courses if I just spent the time studying.	☐	☐
I have difficulty performing well on exams because of lack of sleep.	☐	☐
I often tell my friends that I don't expect to do well on an examination for reasons such as illness and excessive commitment.	☐	☐
When I do poorly on an examination or homework assignment, I always have a good excuse for the poor performance.	☐	☐
I downplay examination and assignment performance because I feel like my friends and classmates will think of me as stupid if I do poorly.	☐	☐

Data from: Schwinger et al. (2014), Tice (1991), Urdan and Midgley (2001).

an academic self-handicapper. The good news is that because academic self-handicapping frequently occurs before an anticipated important event (e.g., NBCOT® exam), applicable individuals can seek to avoid these impediments to successful performance.

- *Lack of professional skill obstacles*: Unlike attitude obstacles, lack of professional skill obstacles does not reflect a conscious or counterproductive behavior; rather, it reflects general ability deficits, such as planning, goal setting, project management, technical skills (e.g., using a computer or conducting an online literature search), or writing skills. Lack of professional skill obstacles additionally includes soft skill sets, such as lack of professional networking and peer interactions and lack of professional contacts.

- *External obstacles*: External obstacles are usually unrelated to either attitudes or professional skill sets and may reflect highly personal, subjective, and multifactorial experiences. Examples of external obstacles can include the death of a loved one, chronic illness within a family, and financial hardships.

Section 2: Cognitive Factors in Learning with Understanding

Introduction

Have you ever completed a challenging two- or three-hour lecture composed of predominantly new material and felt like all of the important details and concepts quickly blurred into nothing more than the gist or general picture of the lecture? Additionally, have you ever left a learning experience with a solid framework for the lecture material only to find that by the time you go to study you have forgotten most details and are forced to relearn what was forgotten? If you answered yes to either or both questions, the good news is that you are 100% normal, and although there is no bad news, the implications are that we must recognize these limitations of our cognitive architecture and actively seek to overcome them. The following pages will discuss factors that have considerable impact on learning with both understanding and retention.

Memory and Retention

The previously mentioned three-hour lecture or forgetting-and-relearning scenario should sound familiar to most readers simply because human working memory is not capable of processing and effectively storing a three-hour lecture in long-term memory, especially if the information is both novel and cognitively demanding (Sweller, Ayres, & Kalyuga, 2011). Although human working memory is certainly amazing because it is able to temporarily store and manipulate information related to higher-level cognitive behaviors, such as understanding and reasoning, it presents with an unexpected limitation in that it can only process a few elements of information at any given time (Baddeley, 1992a; Becker & Morris, 1999). Miller (1956) established that working memory can only manage about seven elements of information at a time. This notion or acknowledgment of the number of elements a learner's working memory capacity can effectively manage has endearingly developed into the phrase "the magical number seven, plus or minus two" (Miller, 1956). In practical terms, human working memory is surprisingly prone to errors as the learning task becomes more complex, and under typical circumstances it can hold on to information only for a matter of seconds without rehearsal (Anderson, Reder, & Lebiere, 1996; Baddeley, 1992a; Miller, 1956; Shiffrin & Nosofsky, 1994). This is why we tend to appreciate the "gist" or essence of a learning experience, such as the previously described three-hour lecture, as opposed to remembering everything.

Let us take a little break to demonstrate capacity limitations of working Seven Plus or Minus Two: A Commentary on Capacity memory. Please solve the following questions solely in your head or working memory and without the use of any external aids, such as pen and paper; the answers are explained later, so please do not read ahead.

Question one: What is the four-digit number in which the first digit is one-third the second, the third is the sum of the first and second, and the last is three times the second?

Question two (from Cooper, 1998): Determine if either of the following statements could be true:

1. My father's brother's grandfather is my grandfather's brother's son.
2. My father's brother's grandfather is my grandfather's brother's father.

For the typical individual, trying to solve either or both questions without the use of external memory aids, such as paper and pen, would have likely exceeded the processing capacity of working memory. To explain, in situations involving serial processing of four or five independent items, little or no overlap exists between information, and the demands placed on working memory are low. Additionally, understanding or recall of one piece of information will have little or no bearing on the understanding or recall of another information element, and the learning task will not typically become difficult unless the number of independent elements is very high. For example, remembering the carpal bones is relatively simple because there are only eight bones, and forgetting the name of one bone will have no impact on the ability to recall the others (i.e., serial processing). Remembering all the bones in the human body is similar in that the items are unrelated; however, the high number of bones will make the task a bit more difficult. In contrast, the preceding questions require that all information be maintained in working memory and manipulated simultaneously to properly solve the problems (i.e., parallel processing). Incidentally, the answer to question one is 1,349; the answer to the first part of question two is false, and the answer to the second part of question two is true.

Understanding Sensory, Working, and Long-Term Memory

To manage complex cognitive tasks, individuals must be able to access large amounts of information. Long-term memory effectively stores all of our knowledge (e.g., content, skills, and strategies) on a permanent basis, with the ability to recall this information being somewhat more variable (Baddeley, 1992b; Ericsson & Kintsch, 1995). Furthermore, information may only be stored in long-term memory after first being processed by working memory; the activation of long-term memory can only occur by bringing the desired elements into working memory. It is additionally noted that knowledge elements that are activated with high regularity are activated automatically with little to no effort (Ericsson & Kintsch, 1995; Sweller, Ayres, & Kalyuga, 2011). The relationships between sensory, working, and long-term memory are depicted in **Figure 2-1**.

Within the constraints of the strengths and limitations of human memory, learning requires a change in the schematic structures of long-term memory (Cooper & Sweller, 1987). Schemata are cognitive constructs that allow an individual to treat multiple elements of information as a single element in terms of imposed working memory demands. Schemata are additionally hierarchical in nature and are usually made up of many interrelated elements, which include both the cognitive representation of the problem and the problem solution. Given that a schema can be managed in working memory as a single element, increased working memory can be left open to address the problem state at hand. A second and equally essential aspect of schemata is the principle of automation. Automation allows for the processing of a schema in an automated fashion in further reducing imposed demands on working memory (Cooper & Sweller, 1987; Sweller, 1999; Sweller, Ayres, & Kalyuga, 2011).

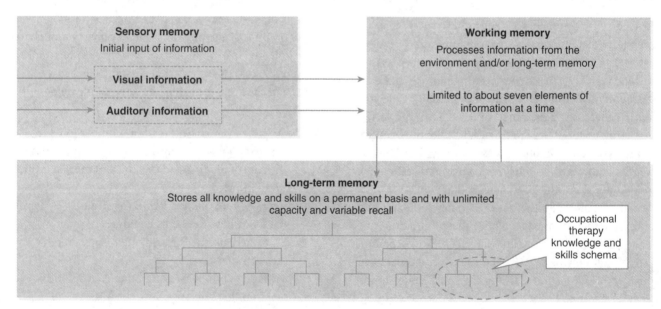

Figure 2-1 The relationships between sensory, working, and long-term memory.
Reproduced from: Fredrick D. Pociask.

For example, a skilled driver of an automobile will identify many elements associated with the task of driving a car as a single schema in working memory, which, in addition to being automated, imposes few to no cognitive demands on working memory. In contrast, a novice medical student examining a patient for the first time may be presented with considerable information. Assuming a lack of an adequate schema, important information will likely be dropped from working memory, and few (if any) cognitive resources will likely be available to diagnose the patient's condition.

What Is Learning?

Defining or describing learning may seem straightforward at first glance (e.g., the accumulation of knowledge), but it is somewhat difficult without first coming to agreement on the functions and outcomes of learning. The process of learning is often associated with relatively short-term classroom or university experiences, and the products of learning are often described in terms of credit hours and grades. In contrast to this perception is the idea that learning is fundamental and essential to individual and professional development, which encompasses the need for individuals to actively accept responsibility for their own learning and actively strive to develop themselves through the course of their lifetime. Robert Mayer (1982, p. 1040) offers a definition for learning that is well aligned with an adult learning perspective, which states "Learning is a relatively permanent change in a person's knowledge or behavior due to experience." This definition has three components, which describe that (1) the duration of change is long term as opposed to short term, (2) change entails the restructuring of the learner's cognitive architecture and/or the learner's behaviors, and (3) the catalyst for change is the learner's experience in the environment (Mayer, 1982). We will use Mayer's definition for learning because it matches quite well with our discussions on adult learning and memory.

What Is Metacognition?

In addition to being a very cool sounding word that you can use to impress your friends and family, metacognition is a very important concept for the adult learner and will certainly have great bearing on successful NBCOT® preparation. This said, metacognition simply means thinking about thinking and learning, or knowing how to learn (Winn, 2003). Metacognition

consists of two separate processes that occur simultaneously: (1) monitoring progress as you learn and (2) making necessary changes and adapting learning strategies when needed to achieve optimal learning outcomes (Holschuh & Aultman, 2009; Winn, 2003). **Figure 2-2** represents the minimal necessary skills needed to monitor comprehension of learning, which would additionally include factors such as motivation, attention, self-regulation, goal setting, and project management.

The development of metacognitive self-monitoring skills will play a critical role in the development of active and self-regulated learning behaviors, but it is highly unlikely that the skill set will develop if left to chance (Butler & Winne, 1995; Holschuh & Aultman, 2009; Stone, 2000). It has been shown that novice learners do not evaluate content comprehension or work quality, fail to examine problems in depth, and fail to analyze effectiveness and correct errors as they learn (Ertmer & Newby, 1996). In contrast, high metacognitive self-monitors are aware of when they need to check for errors, understand why they fail to comprehend, know how to redirect their efforts, and are more likely to use feedback from earlier testing experiences to further develop metacognitive skills and alter metacognitive self-judgments as compared to novice learners (Ertmer & Newby, 1996; Lin-Agler, Moore, & Zabrucky, 2004).

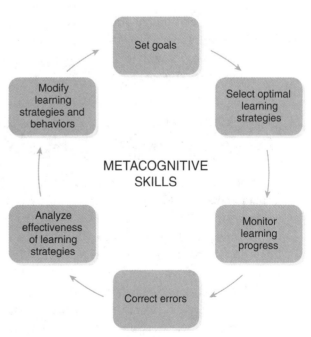

Figure 2-2 Metacognitive skills: the process of monitoring comprehension.

What Do We Know in a Nutshell in Case You Forgot?

1. Information about the world enters working memory through sensory information (e.g., vision, hearing, and touch).
2. There are monumental information processing and manipulation differences between the information entering working memory via the senses and information entering working memory via long-term memory.
3. Working memory is greatly limited in both capacity and duration, and these limitations can impede learning.
4. If the capacity of working memory is exceeded while processing information, some or all of the information will be lost.
5. The efficiency of memory is strongly linked to how we direct our attention. Lack of attention devoted to academic tasks will be expected to decrease learning efficiency and effectiveness to some degree.
6. The robust nature of long-term memory is a function of schemata that allow an individual to treat multiple chunks of information as a single element in terms of imposed demands placed on working memory.
7. Continued review and repetition will reinforce neural connections to information stored in long-term memory.
8. Knowledge that is activated with high regularity is activated automatically with little to no effort.
9. Learning will be more efficient and effective if learning tasks are matched to the strengths and limitations of working and long-term memory.

What Does All of This Mean in Terms of NBCOT® Exam Preparation?

1. *Learning requires comprehension*: Recalling information that you do not understand is highly unlikely. Monitor comprehension by building reflection points into your examination preparation. If information is not getting through or not making sense, adjust comprehension or modify applicable conditional factors accordingly. Conditional factors, such as sleep, nutrition, attention, motivation, anxiety, strategy selection, and study environments, can greatly affect learning recall and retention.
2. *Learning requires relationships, organization, and structure*: It is very difficult to recall random knowledge as compared to knowledge that is organized with some structure or in some pattern. Avoid line item or bullet point, book page, and flash card learning for complex principles and concepts because they are not an efficient or effective means for learning with understanding.
   a. Generate understanding by developing relationships between and among ideas.
   b. Actively associate or connect, and then add new information with, related prior knowledge to progressively construct robust schemata.
   c. Redefine new information in the context of practical real-world problems that can be solved using the knowledge being studied, or ask yourself how you will use the knowledge being studied in the clinic.
   d. Link new information to relevant personal experiences and/or historic events to enhance long-term memory storage and retention.
3. *Learning is layered*: Broad concepts can be remembered more easily than details, and if the broad concept is learned and anchored in memory first, details tend to readily fall into place. Conversely, it is much more difficult to learn and retain details if you do not understand how they fit into the big picture.
4. *Learning requires review and repetition*: Avoid learning–forgetting–relearning pitfalls by using multiple learning strategies, such as concept maps and imagery (i.e., as covered in Chapter 3), combined with continued review and repetition to reinforce neural connections to information stored in long-term memory.
5. *Learning is closely linked to metacognition*: Take control over the cognitive processes engaged in learning by actively thinking about thinking and learning. Monitor retention by thinking about how you think and learn: (1) set goals, (2) select learning strategies that best match the content to be learned and learn how to redirect cognitive efforts, (3) correct errors while you learn and understand why you fail to comprehend when it occurs, (4) analyze the effectiveness of your learning strategies after you complete a learning task, and (5) modify your learning strategies and behaviors when needed, and make certain to use feedback from earlier academic experiences.

Summary

This chapter introduced characteristics and behaviors to strive for in preparation for the NBCOT® and in preparation for what should be a long and rewarding career as a healthcare professional. Key determinants of student success and failure were then introduced and discussed in detail, and of most importance, we discovered that these determinants can readily be controlled by the learner in order to produce successful outcomes. Common obstacles to learning were then discussed of which many are recognizable and preventable or can be better managed using the information introduced in this chapter. The discussion of human memory and retention provided sound arguments for the use of learning strategies that do not readily succumb to the shortcomings of our cognitive architecture, and the importance of metacognitive skill development was made clear. Lastly, the chapter concluded with practical advice for matching learning with the strengths and limitations of human memory and for the development of important metacognitive skills. Chapter 3 will build on much of the information presented in Chapter 2 through the use of straightforward learning tips, skills, and strategies. Last, please always remember that learning how to learn is the ultimate capability that can be mastered by the adult learner and deliberative OTA; it is both self-fulfilling and self-perpetuating, and it is one of the few gifts that you can give to yourself that will truly last a lifetime.

References

Alvarez, M. C., & Risko, V. J. (2009). Motivation and study strategies. In R. F. Flippo, & D. C. Caverly (Eds.), *Handbook of college reading and study strategy research* (2nd ed., pp. 199–219). New York, NY: Routledge.

Anderson, C. J. (2003). The psychology of doing nothing: Forms of decision avoidance result. *Psychological Bulletin, 129*(1), 139–167.

Anderson, J. R., Reder, L. M., & Lebiere, C. (1996). Working memory: Activation limitations on retrieval. *Cognitive Psychology, 30*(3), 221–256.

Baddeley, A. (1992a). Working memory. *Science, 255*(5044), 556–559.

Baddeley, A. (1992b). Working memory: The interface between memory and cognition. *Journal of Cognitive Neuroscience, 4*(3), 281–288.

Becker, J. T., & Morris, R. G. (1999). Working memory(s). *Brain & Cognition, 41*(1), 1–8.

Butler, D. L., & Winne, P. H. (1995). Feedback and self-regulated learning: A theoretical synthesis. *Review of Educational Research, 65*(3), 245–281.

Carroll, J. B. (1989). The Carroll model: A 25-year retrospective and prospective view. *Educational Researcher, 18*(1), 26–31.

Cooper, G. (1998). *Research into cognitive load theory and instructional design at UNSW.* Retrieved from http://dwb4.unl.edu/Diss/Cooper/UNSW.htm

Cooper, G., & Sweller, J. (1987). Effects of schema acquisition and rule automation on mathematical problem-solving transfer. *Journal of Educational Psychology, 79*(4), 347–362.

Crookes, G., & Schmidt, R. W. (1991). Motivation: Reopening the research agenda. *Language Learning, 41*, 469–512.

Elliot, A. J. (1999). Approach and avoidance motivation and achievement goals. *Educational Psychologist, 34*(3), 169–189.

Elliot, A. J., & Covington, M. V. (2001). Approach and avoidance motivation. *Educational Psychology Review, 13*(2), 73–92.

Ericsson, K. A., & Kintsch, W. (1995). Long-term working memory. *Psychological Review, 102*(2), 211–245.

Ertmer, P. A., & Newby, T. J. (1996). The expert learner: Strategic, self-regulated, and reflective. *Instructional Science, 24*, 1–24.

Ferrari, J. R., Johnson, J., & McCown, W. G. (1995). *Procrastination and task avoidance: Theory, research, and treatment.* New York, NY: Plenum Press.

Holschuh, J. P., & Aultman, L. (2009). Comprehension development. In R. F. Flippo, & D. C. Caverly (Eds.), *Handbook of college reading and study strategy research* (2nd ed., pp. 121–144). New York, NY: Routledge.

Knowles, M. S., Holton, E., & Swanson, R. A. (1998). *The adult learner: The definitive classic in adult education and human resource development* (5th ed.). Houston, TX: Gulf Publishing Company.

Lee, H. W., Lim, K. Y., & Grabowski, B. L. (2007). Generative learning: Principles and implications for making meaning. In J. M. Spector, M. D. Merrill, J. V. Merriënboer, & M. P. Driscoll (Eds.), *Handbook of research on educational communications and technology* (3rd ed.). New York, NY: Taylor & Francis, Inc.

Levinger, G. (1957). Kurt Lewin's approach to conflict and its resolution: A review with some extensions. *The Journal of Conflict Resolution, 1*(4), 329–339.

Lin-Agler, L. M., Moore, D., & Zabrucky, K. M. (2004). Effects of personality on metacognitive self-assessments. *College Student Journal, 38*(3), 453.

Lohr, L. L., & Gall, J. E. (2007). Representation strategies. In J. M. Spector, M. D. Merrill, J. V. Merriënboer, & M. P. Driscoll (Eds.), *Handbook of research on educational communications and technology* (3rd ed.). New York, NY: Taylor & Francis, Inc.

Mayer, R. E. (1982). Learning. In H. E. Mitzel, J. H. Best, W. Rabinowitz, & A. E. R. Association (Eds.), *Encyclopedia of educational research* (5th ed., pp. 1040–1058). New York, NY: Free Press.

Merriam, S. B., & Caffarella, R. S. (1999). *Learning in adulthood: A comprehensive guide* (2nd ed.). San Francisco, CA: Jossey-Bass Publishers.

Miller, G. A. (1956). The magical number seven, plus or minus two: Some limits on our capacity for processing information. *Psychological Review, 63,* 81–97.

Morrison, G. R., Ross, S. M., Kalman, H. K., & Kemp, J. E. (2013). *Designing effective instruction* (7th ed.). Hoboken, NJ: Wiley.

Owens, R. G. (2001). So perfect it's positively harmful? Reflections on the adaptiveness and maladaptiveness of positive and negative perfectionism. *Educational Psychology Review, 13*(2), 157–175.

Rachal, K. C., Daigle, S., & Rachal, W. S. (2007). Learning problems reported by college students: Are they using learning strategies? *Journal of Instructional Psychology, 34*(4), 191–199.

Ryan, A. M., Pintrich, P. R., & Midgley, C. (2001). Avoiding seeking help in the classroom: Who and why? *Educational Psychology Review, 13*(2), 93–114.

Schwinger, M., Wirthwein, L., Lemmer, G., & Steinmayr, R. (2014). Academic self-handicapping and achievement: A meta-analysis. *Journal of Educational Psychology, 106*(3), 744–761. doi:10.1037/a0035832

Shiffrin, R. M., & Nosofsky, R. M. (1994). Seven Plus or Minus Two: A Commentary on Capacity Limitations. *Psychological Review, 101*(2), 357–361.

Seel, N. M. (2007). Empirical perspectives on memory and motivation. In J. M. Spector, M. D. Merrill, J. V. Merriënboer, & M. P. Driscoll (Eds.), *Handbook of research on educational communications and technology* (3rd ed.). New York, NY: Taylor & Francis, Inc.

Snowman, J., & Biehler, R. F. (2006). *Psychology applied to teaching* (11th ed.). Boston, MA: Houghton Mifflin Co.

Spector, J. M., Merrill, M. D., Merrienboer, J. V., & Driscoll, M. P. (Eds.). (2007). *Handbook of research for educational communications and technology* (3rd ed.). New York, NY: Routledge/Taylor & Francis, Inc.

Steel, P. (2007). The nature of procrastination: A meta-analytic and theoretical review of quintessential self-regulatory failure. *Psychological Bulletin, 133*(1), 65–94.

Stone, N. J. (2000). Exploring the relationship between calibration and self-regulated learning. *Educational Psychology Review, 12*(4), 437–475.

Sweller, J. (1999). *Instructional design in technical areas.* Camberwell, Australia: ACER Press.

Sweller, J. (2007). Human cognitive architecture. In J. M. Spector, M. D. Merrill, J. V. Merriënboer, & M. P. Driscoll (Eds.). *Handbook of research on educational communications and technology* (3rd ed.). New York, NY: Taylor & Francis, Inc.

Sweller, J., Ayres, P. L., & Kalyuga, S. (2011). *Cognitive load theory.* New York, NY: Springer.

Thomas, C. R., & Gadbois, S. A. (2007). Academic self-handicapping: The role of self-concept clarity and students' learning strategies. *British Journal of Educational Psychology, 77*(1), 101–119.

Tice, D. M. (1991). Esteem protection or enhancement? Self-handicapping motives and attributions differ by trait self-esteem. *Journal of Personality and Social Psychology, 60*(5), 711–725.

Urdan, T. (2004). Predictors of academic self-handicapping and achievement: Examining achievement goals, classroom goal structures, and culture. *Journal of Educational Psychology, 96*(2), 251–264.

Urdan, T., & Midgley, C. (2001). Academic self-handicapping: What we know, what more there is to learn. *Educational Psychology Review, 13*(2), 115–138.

Winn, W. (2003). Cognitive perspectives in psychology. In D. H. Jonassen (Ed.), *Handbook of research on educational communications and technology* (2nd ed., pp. 79–112). New York, NY: Lawrence Erlbaum Associates.

Study Tips, Methods, and Strategies

Fredrick D. Pociask and Sara Maher

Learning Objectives

- Describe strategies for maintaining focus, endurance, motivation, and self-confidence.
- Identify approaches for facilitating productive collaborative learning.
- Describe productive methods for project and time management, goal setting, and scheduling.
- Identify strategies and methods for identifying, collecting, and organizing study resources.
- Describe the key benefits of establishing a productive study environment.
- Describe eight comprehension strategies as presented in this chapter.
- List a minimum of four critical reading strategies as presented in this chapter.
- Describe the SQ3R (Survey–Question–Read–Recall–Review) and KWL (Know–Want to Know–Learned) methods of reading.
- List and describe six memorization methods or strategies as presented in this chapter.

Key Terms

- *Active learning*: Learners take an active role in their own learning and are in part responsible for learning outcomes.
- *Motivation*: "The choice people make as to what experiences or goals they will approach or avoid and the degree of effort they will exert in that respect."
- *Perseverance*: Following a course of action in spite of difficulties, obstacles, or discouragement.
- *Self-concept*: An individual's total picture of himself or herself (e.g., self-definition in societal roles, beliefs, feelings, and values) that is typically focused on societal and personal norms.

- *Self-efficacy*: An individual's belief that he or she can attain his or her goals or accomplish an identified task or tasks.
- *Self-regulation*: Active participation in one's own learning process in terms of behavior, motivation, and metacognition.

This chapter introduces important learning tips, skills, methods, and strategies, which include project and time management, collecting and organizing study resources, study environment management, study methods, and test-taking strategies.

Keep an open mind as you explore this chapter because as learners we often know what we like and what we want but not necessarily what we need in terms of optimal examination preparatory habits, strategies, and methods. For this reason, try to stick with objective measures of performance when evaluating a given learning tip, method, or strategy, such as completion of study goals in a timely fashion and performance of National Board for Certification in Occupational Therapy (NBCOT®)-style test items. Equally, it may be the case that the strategies and methods that are most helpful are the ones that require the most time, active engagement, motivation, and/or perseverance to adopt and stick with. Conversely, it will be wise to drop a particular strategy or method if it proves to be of little benefit when objectively scrutinized. The benefits of successful study habits include

- Improved self-concept, self-efficacy, and *self-regulation*
- Improved knowledge acquisition and retention
- Learning with understanding and academic engagement (i.e., as opposed to rote recall and forgetting or cyclic forgetting and relearning)
- Decreased frustration and procrastination

- More free time spent doing things you enjoy as you prepare for the NBCOT®
- Productive lifelong learning habits

Study Tips

Maintain Focus, Endurance, and Motivation

- Focus on the endgame, which is successful completion of the NBCOT® and beginning a career as a healthcare professional. Use imagery to clearly picture yourself achieving this goal.
- Focus on the task at hand instead of perseverating on the "colossal task" of preparing for the entire exam. This strategy is additionally true for individual tasks. For example, if you have 50 pages to study, go forward 1 page at a time and you will be done before you know it.
- Establish clear short-term and long-term study goals.
- Avoid procrastination and stay on task while studying.
- Change topics every couple of hours to add some variety to your study plan.
- Create study incentives, such as calling a friend, watching a television show, or exercise. Additionally, give yourself small rewards upon completion of primary study tasks.
- Take short 10 to 15-minute breaks during long study sessions, or even consider a 15-minute power nap to help maintain concentration and focus.
- Maintain healthy dietary habits and a consistent eating schedule.
- Maintain normal and healthy sleep patterns and a consistent sleep schedule.
- Have a few healthy snacks and water available for study periods.
- Maintain physical health and personal appearance.
- Manage stress and anxiety by scheduling time for relaxation and social interactions.

Maintain and Bolster Self-Confidence

- Establish and maintain a realistic exam preparation schedule. Successfully completing study tasks in a timely fashion is an excellent strategy for maintaining self-confidence.

- Use positive words or attributions to describe desired behaviors, such as "I can do this" as opposed to "I cannot do this."
- After you complete a given task, make sure to acknowledge the accomplishment before moving on to the next task.
- Avoid negative people, study groups, and study environments. . .period.

Actively Monitor Learning and Comprehension

- Schedule time to reflect on your learning progress and make certain to keep track of what works, what does not work, and what needs to be tweaked.
- Use self-questioning, self-testing, peer discussions, prior examinations and feedback, and NBCOT® preparatory questions to objectively evaluate learning.
- Use a notepad, electronic document, or similar tool to keep track of self-generated or peer feedback, important terminology, or any helpful information that needs to be recorded for later use.

Facilitate Productive Collaborative Learning

Strategies for group learning include collaborative goal setting and scheduling, selecting optimal learning strategies with emphasis on individual and group fairness, monitoring your progress, analyzing your effectiveness and efficiency, and modifying your learning strategies and behaviors as necessary. Attention given to the following will help facilitate optimal collaborative learning:

- Establish meeting schedules and ground rules while forming groups or at the beginning of the initial meeting. Everyone involved should agree that you are forming a study group and not a social club.
- Keep the group to a manageable size, and keep the number of groups that you participate into a manageable amount.
- Select group members that you can readily work with and that have a solid track record for preparedness and punctuality.
- Establish your unproductive study group exit strategy on day 1. Clearly state that you will not be able to participate in the study group if the group does not stay on task or fails to complete

established study objectives. Select a qualified group leader if individuals in the group have difficulty staying on task.

- Remember that primary reasons for forming the group are knowledge sharing, collaboration, and dissemination. Identify combined resources and a means for collection and dissemination of information and study resources early on.
- Preparing and disseminating assignments before meetings will likely be more productive in that meeting time can be used to seek clarification, discuss, debate, and further anchor knowledge in long-term memory.
- Remember that collaborative learning does not necessarily mean face-to-face learning. Take advantage of academic course management sites, email, blogs, Twitter, or even your Facebook page if it helps to achieve a collaborative learning goal.

Choose Study Companions and Study Groups Wisely

The study companions and groups that you collaborate with in preparation for the NBCOT® exam will most likely affect your preparedness and performance. If you associate with motivated, goal- and task-oriented, and overall well-rounded and positive colleagues, this will likely carry over into your self-confidence and preparedness. In contrast, if your collaborative learning experiences are plagued by more socializing and negative self-talk than examination preparation, it is time to break up and move on, but do not be sad because you can still be friends.

Study Skills

Project and Time Management

Project and time management will be very important factors in terms of NBCOT® preparation and preparedness. The following project and time management factors will be grouped together for the purposes of this chapter and will be further discussed in subsequent sections:

- Goal setting
- Collecting and organizing study resources
- Scheduling and planning time for studying, which includes the following:
  - Creating prioritized to-do lists
  - Establishing a study routine
  - Making use of free time
  - Scheduling regular reviews
  - Scheduling relaxation time
  - Identifying start and stop points or dates

Goal Setting and Scheduling

- Establish straightforward long-term goals and time frames before writing short-term goals. These goals should identify major start and stop points or dates, such as the final date for collecting and organizing study materials, the date you will begin studying, and the date of the examination.
- Short-term goals will typically span no more than one to four weeks based on your organization style, they should be kept simple and concise, and they should reflect specific study objectives and specific completion dates. For example, "Construct a study aid for all peripheral nerve compression neuropathies by Friday, May 5th."
- Break the exam preparation down into smaller and manageable tasks that can be readily accomplished in the time allotted.
- Reevaluate goals and time frames on a daily to weekly basis based on attainment of study objectives. Remember that the objective is learning with understanding and retention as opposed to poor learning outcomes and/or cyclic forgetting and relearning.
- Keep short-term goals and time frames challenging, but they should be realistic and consistent with the long-term goals and major start and stop points or dates.
- Take a few minutes to review and summarize your study objectives before beginning a study session or collaborative learning experience.
- Numerous short-term goals may be better managed by the use of daily and weekly prioritized to-do lists.
- Keep your short-term goals and to-do list in a highly visible location or multiple visible locations.
- Consider using a computer program or equivalent electronic resource specifically designed for project management, and make certain to back up frequently.
- Acknowledge the success of a given task because this will give you motivation to continue studying.

Identifying, Collecting, and Organizing Study Resources

Learners will predominantly have NBCOT® study resources available as a function of completing an accredited occupational therapy (OT) program. The wild cards will likely be the organization and ease of access to previous curricular materials and identifying and filling gaps in available resources. If you have an organization scheme that has served you well, you can jump to the next section; otherwise, following these guidelines will be helpful in collecting and organizing study resources.

- Identify and physically locate existing curricular resources, with specific emphasis placed on your primary OT textbooks as referenced throughout this textbook, as well as key course notes, previously constructed study tools that were particularly helpful, and key assigned journal readings.
- Hard-copy study resources may be ideally managed using three-ring binders organized by course name, content area, or study domain, and the side of each binder should be clearly labeled for quick access. Supplemental resources, such as photocopied journal articles and text chapters, can be organized in a similar fashion. If necessary, labeled tabs can be used to add additional levels of organization to existing course materials.
- Electronic resources (e.g., PDF) can be organized using folders and directories to match or as a substitution for hard-copy materials.
- Avoid the use of untrustworthy and non-peer-reviewed references. For example, Wikipedia is not the ultimate source of all knowledge and is, in fact, riddled with errors and unsubstantiated facts. For an examination such as the NBCOT®, you will want to stick with resources such as OT textbooks, peer-reviewed journals (e.g., *American Journal of Occupational Therapy*), and similar MEDLINE-accessible references.
- Store all materials in a safe location and in an organized fashion as previously suggested. If applicable, make certain your friends, family, and children know that there will be hell to pay if they even think about messing with your study materials. If at all possible, your safe storage location should be your preferred study environment as discussed later in this chapter.

- Identify supplemental resources that are presently of unidentified value and place them in a nearby location to be used only if necessary.
- If your curriculum requires the use of literature on the Web, create a single document or Web folder with all URLs clearly labeled and in one place.
- After you have completed the previous steps, additional management of study resources should be based on short-term objectives and study goals. For example, if you plan to spend next week studying anatomy, you should pull your anatomy text and course notes from compiled resources and return them when you are finished.
- As a general rule, this textbook will serve as your principal study resource, which you may need to supplement based on factors such as your individual learning attitude, general abilities, recall of previously learned OT curricula, and the quality of your OT program instruction and instructional materials.
- In terms of project management, only seek out supplemental resources based on identified gaps in your foundational or clinical knowledge (e.g., unable to recall anatomy, medical terminology, and basic patient care skills) and avoid the traps of constantly reorganizing, sorting, and resorting materials because this typically has little to do with studying and learning with understanding and retention.

Important Considerations for Electronic Resources

If your institution uses an electronic learning management system, such as Blackboard or Moodle, make certain to download and save applicable course materials because your access to campus learning management systems will typically expire upon or shortly after graduation. Lastly, because existing electronic resources, as well as those that you will generate in preparation for the examination, can be easily backed up, backups should be performed on a regular basis and ideally stored at two different locations.

Study Environment Management

Remember that what you like and want may not necessarily be what you need in terms of study times, study locations, and environmental factors. Pay close attention to your completion of study objectives and tasks, or lack of successful completion, and match your environmental factors to what works.

- *Select optimal study times*: Identify your best time of day to study, and try to arrange work and play around optimal study time. Optimal study times should reflect when you are most alert and when you make your greatest achievements toward your daily learning objectives, not simply when you like to study.
- *Select optimal study locations*: Identify the best location to study, and if applicable arrange work and play around access to your optimal study environment. Optimal study locations may range from a quiet library to a local coffee shop. Additionally, determine if you prefer to use the same study location whenever you sit down to study (i.e., typically recommended) or if you prefer some variety in your study locations.
- *Control environmental factors*: The following factors will help facilitate an optimal study environment:
  - Remove unnecessary distractions from the study environment, such as cell phones, audiovisual devices, friends, and family members. It is okay to tell mom and dad that you need peace and quiet so that you can pass the examination, get a job, and properly support them in their older years.
  - Determine the ideal lighting for your study environment. Low to moderate levels of indirect natural light are considered best for reading, followed by equivalent levels of indirect full-spectrum incandescent lighting, with equivalent levels of full-spectrum fluorescent lighting typically falling last on the list (Dunn, 1985; Hathaway, Hargreaves, Thompson, & Novitsky, 1992).
  - Determine the ideal temperature for your study environment. Room temperatures between 68°F and 72°F (20°C–22°C) are said to be best for learning and comprehension. Higher and lower temperatures have been shown to result in decreased performance and increased error rates (Canter, 1976; Harner, 1974; Herrington, 1952; Manning & Olsen, 1965).
  - Determine the ideal noise for your study environment, which may range from dead silence to quiet white noise or soft instrumental music.
  - Other environmental factors include humidity, air flow, drafts, room color, work space ergonomics, clutter, odors, or any other environmental factor that proves to be an annoyance or detrimental to concentration.

Study Methods and Strategies

This section will present commonly used reading, recall, and learning comprehension methods and strategies with brief descriptions for use when applicable. As always, remember to match the method or strategy to the content to be learned (e.g., recall of facts vs. application of complex concepts and principles). For example, prereading should be helpful for any new information or information that you did not grasp the first time it was read, an acronym or mnemonic should be a good memorization strategy for recalling the names and order of the carpal bones, and elaborative interrogation and self-explanation should be a good match for learning or relearning more complex concepts (Bellezza, 1981; Dunlosky, 2013; Dunlosky, Rawson, Marsh, Nathan, & Willingham, 2013; Flippo & Caverly, 2008; Roediger & Pyc, 2012).

Reading Comprehension Methods and Strategies

Reading and corresponding comprehension are best accomplished by use of systematic and reproducible methods and strategies. Conversely, simply skimming text in an arbitrary manner is less likely to result in comprehension, as well as the ability to quickly locate and utilize previously studied materials. The following section will introduce general reading comprehension strategies (i.e., good habits), as well as more systematic methods to maximize comprehension, retention, and productivity.

Prereading (Skim Before You Read)

1. Review the title and recall previous knowledge about the subject or content.
2. Review the subheadings and recognize the organizational structure of the content to be read.
3. Ask yourself what type of information is being presented.
4. Ask yourself what you expect to learn.

Understand Content Areas and Performance Expectations

Table 3-1, as adapted from Morrison, Ross, Kalman, and Kemp (2011), can be used to easily define content area(s) and level(s) of performance or to quickly give meaning

Table 3-1 Content Area and Level of Performance

Content	Performance	
	Recall (i.e., memorization for later recall or simple association)	**Application** (i.e., application of information to an abstract or actual case)
Fact (i.e., a statement that associates one item with another)	Simple associations between names, objects, symbols, locations, etc.	There is no such thing as application of a fact
Concept (i.e., concepts are categories we use for simplifying the world; a grouping of similar objects)	What are the characteristics of	Compare and contrast
Principle or rule (i.e., a principle or rule expresses a relationship between concepts, cause and effect, explanations and predictions)	What happens when	Explain why
Procedure (i.e., a procedure is a sequence of steps one follows to achieve a goal)	List the steps	Demonstrate the steps
Interpersonal (i.e., this category describes verbal and nonverbal interaction between two or more people)	List the steps	Demonstrate how to
Attitude (i.e., objectives that seek to change or modify a learner's attitude are classified in this category)	State the behaviors	Demonstrate the behaviors

Modified from Morrison, G. R., Ross, S. M., Kalman, H., & Kemp, J. E. (2011). Designing effective instruction (6th ed.). Hoboken, NJ: Wiley.

to an existing examination or study question. For example, if you are studying the application of a principle, you should be prepared to explain why the principle is or is not applicable to situations or circumstances in which the principle may apply (e.g., rationale, indication of contraindication for an intervention).

Read and Rereading Critically

Critical reading reflects the ability to analyze, evaluate, and synthesize what one reads, which minimally includes identifying relationships in linking new information with prior knowledge. Some suggestions for critical reading are as follows:

- Begin with prereading.
- Highlight, underline, and take notes as needed.
- Generate a terminology list as needed.
- Identify the purpose and central claims.
- Identify the source and credibility of the publication.
- Identify the author and his or her credentials and qualifications.

- Identify the context and intended audience.
- Distinguish the kinds of reasoning employed.
- Examine and evaluate the evidence.
- Identify strengths, weaknesses, and validity.
- Identify possible alternative conclusions.
- Write up notes immediately after reading.

Identify Emphasis Words

Pay close attention for words that signify primary ideas and important points such as those shown below:

"a central issue"	"especially relevant"	"the most distinctive symptom"
"a key feature"	"of most importance"	"the primary characteristic"
"above all"	"of particular value"	"the primary distinguishing factor"
"always document"	"the chief complaint"	"the principal item"

General Guidelines for Taking Notes from a Textbook

1. Begin with prereading as previously described.
2. Read the chapter or chapter section without taking notes and with the sole purpose of maintaining an understanding of the material.
3. Review the chapter or chapter section for a second time and locate the main ideas, emphasis words, and important points.
4. Paraphrase the information in your own words and without the use of the text. This step can be broken up into cognitively obtainable chunks, and the text can be used for review as long as you avoid copying directly from the text.
5. Now use the paraphrased ideas to generate the actual note pages, and again, do not copy any information directly from the textbook.

The SQ3R Method of Reading

The SQ3R method of reading (**Figure 3-1**) is intended for individual study but may also be applied to groups (Carlston, 2011; Robinson, 1970).

The KWL Method of Reading

The KWL method of reading as originally described by Ogle (1986) is intended as a learning exercise for study groups or classroom use and is composed of three stages:

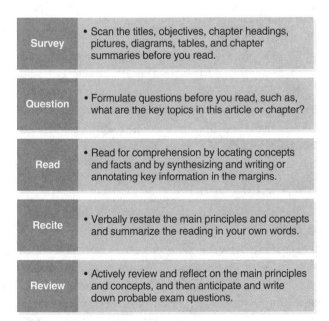

Figure 3-1 The SQ3R method of reading.
Data from Robinson, F. P. (1970). Effective Study (4 Ed.). New York: Harper & Row.

(1) what we **K**now, (2) what we **W**ant to know, and (3) what we **L**earned. For example, the three stages can be added as heading to a three-column table as pictured below (i.e., with rows added as needed, or used in an outline format).

What we know	What we want to know	What we learned

Learning and Comprehension Strategies

The following methods and strategies are typically helpful in improving comprehension and learning with understanding and retention. All methods and strategies should encompass active engagement on behalf of the learner in order to maximize potential benefits.

- *Question answering*: Answer preinstructional questions from textbooks, mock examination questions, and questions posed during study groups, to name a few.
- *Question generation*: Formulate questions during prereading or during any applicable stage of learning.
- *Self-explanation*: Constructing an explanation as to how new information is related to known information or explaining the steps that comprise or led to a problem solution.
- *Summarization*: Summarize text passages or applicable learning based on keywords, eliminate redundant and unnecessary information and information that does not satisfy study objectives, and always summarize in your own words.
- *Teaching (i.e., if you truly know it, you should be able to teach it)*: Teach something you believe you know to yourself using active imagery, or teach it to a mentor or a colleague in a study group. It is a very quick litmus test for knowing if you have mastered applicable content, and it will facilitate background processing to fill in the blanks and further anchor content in long-term memory. This strategy is helpful with broad concepts and principles that are cognitively demanding.
- *Elaborative interrogation*: Constructing an explanation or stating evidence as to why a given fact, principle, concept, or rule is true and under what conditions when applicable.
- *Graphic organizer, mind map, and concept map*: These tools are pictorial or graphic representations

of concepts, knowledge, or ideas. Graphic organizers are similar to an outline and show the organization and structure of concepts, as well as the relationships between concepts.

- *Mental imagery*: Create a mental visual image of a procedure or concept.
- *Text imagery*: Constructing a mental image of text materials while reading or listening in order to improve the likelihood or retention and recall.
- *Case studies*: Use case studies to integrate knowledge in the context of realistic or real-life scenarios.
- *Outline*: Outlines are a quick and effective means to organize main and subsidiary ideas for any subject, which is well matched to both simple and complex relationships and hierarchies.
- *Cooperative learning*: Use any of the preceding comprehension strategies and small groups.
- *Combine comprehension strategies*: Try to combine any or all of the preceding strategies individually or in small groups, with an emphasis on connecting principles and concepts, visualizing solutions to problem states, generating and answering questions, determining importance, and synthesis.

Memorization Methods and Strategies

Mnemonics

A mnemonic is a common memory aid used to facilitate retrieval in which each letter identifies or suggests what the learner wishes to remember. A mnemonic does not stand for a name, title, or phrase, and is typically recommended for up to 20 items. For example:

Cubital fossa contents from lateral to medial: "Really Need Brownies To Be At My Nicest."

1. Radial Nerve
2. Biceps Tendon
3. Brachial Artery
4. Median Nerve

Carpal bones list of proximal to distal and lateral to medial: "Some Lovers Try Positions That They Can't Handle."

1. Scaphoid
2. Lunate
3. Triquetrum
4. Pisiform
5. Trapezium
6. Trapezoid
7. Capitate
8. Hamate

Acronyms

Acronyms are similar to mnemonics with the exception that acronyms stand for an actual name, title, or phrase. For example:

- ADL
  - Activities of
  - Daily
  - Living
- FOGS (i.e., a method for mental status assessment)
  - Family story of memory loss
  - Orientation
  - General information
  - Spelling

Flash Cards

Flash cards are perhaps the most classic rote-recall memory aid known to the healthcare science student. Flash cards are ideal for a serial recall task where the number of items is relatively high and the text density on each flash card is relatively low. Flash cards are worth mentioning in this section because they are frequently and erroneously used with complex principles and concepts, for which they are not well suited.

Vocabulary Lists

Keep a hard copy or electronic medical dictionary close at hand. When you come across a term that you do not know or are uncertain about, look it up and make certain that you understand the use of the term in the context in which it is used. Lastly, add all referenced terms to a running terminology list to be used for quick access and ongoing study. A simple bulleted list maintained as an electronic document is recommended.

The Method of Loci

The method of loci (i.e., locations) is a classic memory aid, is typically recommended for lists up to 20 items, and is perhaps best suited for visual and kinesthetic learners. In this technique, the learner vividly imagines himself or herself in a fixed position or walking a fixed path within a very familiar environment (McCabe, 2015). For example, imagine walking into your study area and picturing the examination equipment that is required for cranial nerve examination evaluation laid out on your filing cabinet and desk.

Chaining

Chaining is a memory aid in which the learner creates a story in which each word that must be remembered acts as a cue for the next word or idea that needs to be recalled (Terry, 2009). For example, a learner trying to remember signs and symptoms that indicate the need for a neurological examination may create a story such as "My weakness led to asymmetries, which then caused my gait to become altered and unsteady, and this definitely raised some concerns for safety, which were probably appropriate because I neglected to see the wall as I ran into it, but it didn't hurt because I do not have any feeling in that arm," and so on.

Practice Testing and General Testing Tips

Completing NBCOT®-style practice questions such as those provided via online access with this textbook (i.e., self-testing) as you complete a given area of review and in final preparation for the NBCOT® exam will be of **Monumental Importance** in terms of preparation and success. Specific recommendations for taking a standardized examination will be covered in Chapter 42, and general tips for taking multiple-choice examinations are as follows:

- Read all testing directions carefully before beginning the examination.
- Remember that there is no such thing as a really obvious correct answer on a well-written multiple-choice examination.
- Read the question completely and concisely and then try to answer the question without reviewing the responses.
- Read the question completely and concisely and then read all responses in a similar manner. If you believe that you identified the correct response along the way, make a quick mental note and then read all responses completely and concisely one more time before recording your response.
- Eliminate responses that you know are incorrect before marking the correct answer.
- Pay very close attention to the wording of the question and identify conditional phrases, such as "which of the following interventions is most appropriate."

- Do not add or delete information from a question or bend a question or response to match knowledge that you know.
- Do not use answer-pattern strategies when taking a randomized examination.
- If the rare opportunity presents itself, use information found in other test questions to answer questions from which you do not know the answer.
- Keep track of time throughout the examination without obsessing about the remaining time.
- The best way to prepare for multiple-choice examinations is to practice taking multiple-choice examinations that best match the actual examination content, format, and testing environment.
- Do not guess unless absolutely necessary.

Changing an Answer on a Multiple-Choice Question

Please always remember that changing an answer to a multiple-choice question and guessing on the multiple-choice question are not the same. Additionally, advice that tells students never to change their first response on a multiple-choice examination under certain conditions is one of the most noted testing myths or urban legends in higher education. Specifically, the majority of time an answer is changed, it is changed from the incorrect to the correct answer, and most students who change their answers maintain or improve their test scores (Bauer, Kopp, & Fischer, 2007; Fischer, Herrmann, & Kopp, 2005; Ludy, Benjamin, Cavell, & Shallenberger, 1984). For example, you may wish to consider changing your initial response if

- You overtly made a mistake or misread the question.
- You find information in another test question that triggers a memory trace that shows your first choice was incorrect.
- You find information in another test question that shows your first choice was incorrect (i.e., uncommon on a well-written examination).
- You had no objective basis for your initial response.

References

Bauer, D., Kopp, V., & Fischer, M. R. (2007). Answer changing in multiple choice assessment change that answer when in doubt—And spread the word! *BMC Medical Education, 7*(28), 1–5.

Bellezza, F. S. (1981). Mnemonic devices: Classification, characteristics, and criteria. *Review of Educational Research, 51*(2), 247–275. doi:10.3102/003465430 51002247.

Canter, D. V. (1976). *Environmental interaction psychological approaches to our physical surroundings.* New York, NY: International University Press.

Carlston, D. L. (2011). Benefits of student-generated note packets: A preliminary investigation of SQ3R implementation. *Teaching of Psychology, 38*(3), 142–146. doi:10.1177/0098628311411786.

Dunlosky, J. (2013). Strengthening the student toolbox: Study strategies to boost learning. *American Educator, 37*(3), 12–21.

Dunlosky, J., Rawson, K. A., Marsh, E. J., Nathan, M. J., & Willingham, D. T. (2013). Improving students' learning with effective learning techniques: Promising directions from cognitive and educational psychology. *Psychological Science in the Public Interest, 14*(1), 4–58. doi:10.1177/1529100612453266.

Dunn, R. (1985). Light up their fives: A review of research on the effects of lighting on children's achievement and behavior. *Reading Teacher, 38*(9), 836–869.

Fischer, M. R., Herrmann, S., & Kopp, V. (2005). Answering multiple-choice questions in high-stakes. *Medical Education, 39*, 890–894.

Flippo, R. F., & Caverly, D. C. (2008). *Handbook of college reading and study strategy research* (2nd ed.). New York, NY: Routledge.

Harner, D. P. (1974). Effects of thermal environment on learning skills. *CEFP Journal, 29*(4), 25–30.

Hathaway, W. E., Hargreaves, J. A., Thompson, G. W., & Novitsky, D. (1992). A study into the effects of light on children of elementary school-age–A case of daylight robbery. Access ERIC: FullText (68). Edmonton, Alberta, Canada: Alberta Dept. of Education, Edmonton. Planning and Information Services.

Herrington, L. P. (1952). Effects of thermal environment on human action. *American School and University, 24*, 367–376.

Ludy, T., Benjamin, J., Cavell, T. A., & Shallenberger, W. (1984). Staying with initial answers on objective tests: It is a myth? *Teaching of Psychology, 11*(3), 133–141.

Manning, W. R., & Olsen, L. R. (1965). Air conditioning: Keystone of optimal thermal environment. *American School Board Journal, 149*(2), 22–23.

McCabe, J. A. (2015). Location, location, location! Demonstrating the mnemonic benefit of the method of loci. *Teaching of Psychology, 42*(2), 169–173. doi:10.1177/0098628315573143.

Morrison, G. R., Ross, S. M., Kalman, H., & Kemp, J. E. (2011). *Designing effective instruction* (6th ed.). Hoboken, NJ: Wiley.

Ogle, D. M. (1986). K-W-L: A teaching model that develops active reading of expository text. *The Reading Teacher, 39*(39), 564–557.

Robinson, F. P. (1970). *Effective study* (4th ed.). New York, NY: Harper & Row.

Roediger, H. L., III, & Pyc, M. A. (2012). Inexpensive techniques to improve education: Applying cognitive psychology to enhance educational practice. *Journal of Applied Research in Memory and Cognition, 1*(4), 242–248. doi:10.1016/j.jarmac.2012.09.002.

Terry, W. S. (2009). *Learning and memory: Basic principles, processes, and procedures* (4th ed.). Boston, MA: Pearson/AandB.

Factors in Occupational Functioning Days 2-5

Caregiving

Rosanne DiZazzo-Miller and Jessica Andrus

Learning Objectives

- Recall common terms and side effects associated with caregiving.
- Identify common positive and negative side effects of caregiving.
- Select appropriate assessments to perform with family caregivers.
- Select appropriate interventions to perform with family caregivers.
- Review ethical issues that may arise during caregiver education.

Key Terms

- *Advocacy*: Support to bring about awareness and education on available services and resources.
- *Co-occupation*: The physical and emotional aspects associated with an occupation shared between two or more people experiencing the same experience.
- *Informal caregiver*: Unpaid and not formally trained caregivers who tend to be family members or friends.
- *Quality of life*: Physical, psychosocial, psychological, and environmental feelings of health and comfort.

Introduction

Family caregivers play an important part throughout the **occupational therapy (OT)** process. The family context presents itself with many facilitators and barriers to patient outcomes. Throughout the current healthcare system, many patients are cared for in their home by family and friends. Caregiving has the potential to be one of the most rewarding occupations, yet at times it can cause stress, health concerns, and other complications. Caregiving is a broad term and can be used across many spectrums. There is a significant difference between family member caregivers and hired staff. Some of the differences include meaning, time and place of the care provided, compensation for the care provided, and the variance of emotional engagement in the occupation. Caregivers can be family members, friends, or hired staff; however, for the purpose of examination preparation, this chapter will focus on informal family caregivers including various relationships such as siblings, parents, adult children, and spouses.

Potential Effects of Caregiving

Caregiving has the potential to be one of the most rewarding occupations, yet at times can cause burden, depression, health concerns, and other complications that may lead to issues with quality of life (Canam & Acorn, 1999; Schulz & Beach, 1999). Caregiving is a broad term and can be used across many spectrums. Family caregivers have many additional roles to fill beyond caregiving, including some of the aforementioned as well as employee and parent. Unfortunately, when trauma or disease occurs, family members not only lose their loved ones as they once knew them, but they simultaneously take on a new, most likely unfamiliar, role as a caregiver while other roles intensify. For example, when a wife sustains a traumatic brain injury, the husband grieves the loss of his wife while becoming the primary caregiver for his wife and children. He must also take on increased responsibility at home in order to fill the roles that his wife participated in and performed prior to the injury. This may include items such as cooking, bill payment, and laundry all the while taking care of their two children.

A traumatic injury, for example, typically results in occupational dysfunction for a variable period of time, but is not limited to affecting the person who sustained the injury (Klinger, 2005). Injuries, disabilities, and illness in general tend to affect the entire family, but when it is traumatic, the changes that occur are sudden and magnified with emotion. Although traumatic injuries occur without warning, even diagnoses that intensify over time can catch families off guard and therefore, family caregivers tend to be unprepared for the significant effects of illness on their family and themselves. In addition, oftentimes, there is no training in specific skills needed to provide care. Variations and limitations after injury is not the main priority at the hospital in the acute phase. Caregivers and patients locate information through trial and error, support groups, the Internet, or questions to health professionals at follow-up appointment months, or even years, later. In fact, the World Health Organization (2012) identifies a lack of awareness and understanding of diagnoses as a barrier that impacts caregivers and families physically, psychologically, and economically.

Caregiving and OT

The OT literature points to the appropriateness of OT practitioners who are trained to influence the health and well-being of caregivers while taking into account the intricacies of family dynamics and client care (Moghimi, 2007). Within the **Occupational Therapy Practice Framework (OTPF)** III (American Occupational Therapy Association, 2014), it is clear to see the gravity of tasks that are required of family caregivers. In fact, caregiving is listed as an instrumental activity of daily living in the OTPF III and falls under social and environmental contexts (American Occupational Therapy Association, 2014). Specific to OT, practitioners must address issues related to family dynamics,

independent living services, and expectations of state and local agencies (American Occupational Therapy Association, 2014).

Caregiver Assessments

Although caregiver is a general term used to describe a wide variety of diagnoses, the specific diagnosis or type of trauma aids in determining the appropriate intervention. It is important to understand that different caregivers have different needs. For example, a study completed by Schulz and Sherwood (2008) showed that caring for a person with dementia—which is a chronic and progressive illness—tends to cause more negative health effects than for caregivers of other diagnoses. Caregiving has been linked to both positive and negative outcomes; therefore, assessments including social, personal, temporal, cultural, and environmental contexts are important as each caregiving situation is unique. These assessments may focus on the following:

- Stress
- Burden
- Confidence
- Knowledge/Competence
- Depression
- Quality of life
- Occupational performance and satisfaction

Caregiver Interventions

The intervention plan is set only after the treatment team, client and caregiver, and other appropriate stakeholders distinguish and prioritize the key factors needed for success in their caregiving role (American Occupational Therapy Association, 2014). Caregiver training is critical for families to become aware of both formal and informal services available to them in terms of education, support, coping skills, and increased knowledge of the disability and its impact on occupational functioning.

Common interventions may include the following:

- Psychosocial adjustment
- Behavior management techniques
- Environmental modifications
- Activities of daily living (ADL) training
- Advocacy
- Resources

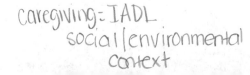

Co-occupation

Some argue that because caregiving involves two or more individuals at any given time it should always be considered a co-occupation, but in looking at the definition of occupation, we must reconsider. Schell, Gillen, and Scaffa (2014) describe occupations as "the things that people do that occupy their time and attention; meaningful, purposeful activity; the personal activities that individuals choose or need to engage in and the ways in which each individual actually expresses them" (p. 1237). Although numerous definitions of occupation exist, one common theme that emerges among each definition is meaningfulness. In order for an activity to change from a task or activity to an occupation, the individual must identify the activity as meaningful. The American Occupational Therapy Association (2014) describes caregiving as a co-occupation stating, "caregiving is a co-occupation that involves active participation on the part of both the caregiver and the recipient of care" (p. S6). With the crucial component of occupation being meaningfulness of the activity, one must also consider this in describing co-occupation.

Occupational Balance

Occupational balance is important in any person's life, but especially someone who is a primary caregiver. Many times, caregivers are lacking occupational balance. With decreased boundaries, no set hours, and the responsibility of care, family caregivers put in a significant amount of time and energy into their occupation. Social outlets and support circles or systems are extremely important for caregivers and can have a significant impact on health for both the recipient of care and the caregiver.

Effects of Caregiving on Family Dynamics

Expectations from other family members, health professionals, and friends can create tension and hardships as well. Health professionals, family members, and friends must recognize that caregiving is not only exhausting, but emotionally difficult to not only see the deficits, but also see the change in personality and mental health components. As healthcare providers, the most important piece of advice is to provide family-centered care. Influencing our patients is the first step, but in order to make that last and have a greater influence on recovery, we must influence and address those who spend every day with our patient in order to relay our therapeutic work throughout their daily lives. In many situations, we rely on caregivers to diffuse everyday situations and act appropriately when the patient feels stressed or overwhelmed. In order for the caregiver to have confidence in how to react in specific situations, especially in diffusing anger, we must educate, provide support, and be open to answering difficult questions at any point in time. If the caregiver is skilled at diffusing situations, this can cause less arguments and healthier experience for the patient. This will also create a better relationship between the caregiver and the patient.

Conclusion

Caregiving seems so general; however, it consists of many components. When the components are broken down into straightforward tasks, appropriately analyzed, one may see why the occupation can be so overwhelming and exhausting.

Caregiving influences family dynamics in a multitude of ways and the occupation of the family caregiver is specifically defined based on this diagnosis. Depending on prior involvement and knowledge, first-time family caregivers may experience a significant learning curve. In order to gain the skills to advocate for a family member, caregivers must be able to effectively communicate, build confidence through practice and questions to healthcare professionals, and participate in social support networks. It is just as important to the patient as it is to the caregiver to have a support system and plan as it keeps both individuals in a healthier mental state of mind.

Over time and through multiple trials, caregivers tend to navigate the system well and become advocates for their family members. Oftentimes, healthcare providers give advice by prefacing it with "If this were my family member, this is what I would do." This quote oftentimes brings great comfort and reassurance to caregivers when facing difficult decisions. Unfortunately, many times caregivers do not feel that they have relationships with healthcare providers in order to get that reassurance they are seeking.

Chapter 4 Self-Study Activities (Answers Are Provided at the End of the Chapter)

1. Match the following terms with the appropriate definition:

Occupational balance (D)	A. The physical and emotional aspects associated with an occupation shared between two or more people experiencing the same experience
Co-occupation (A)	B. Support to bring about awareness and education on available services and resources
Quality of life (C)	C. Physical, psychosocial, psychological, and environmental feelings of health and comfort
Advocacy (B)	D. Daily occupations and their relationship to overall well-being

Choose the best answer for the following case scenario.

2. Bill is the primary caregiver for his wife, Doris, who is in mid-stage Alzheimer's disease. You are an OT assistant working with Doris secondary to a hip fracture she received as a result of a fall. You notice that she is having difficulty completing ADL; however, Bill states that she is independent and does not need his help. Prior to discharging Doris home to live alone with Bill, the OT team should first
   A. Meet with both Bill and Doris to discuss her functional status and needs.
   B. Meet with Doris alone and make sure she achieved her goals prior to discharge.
   C. Meet with Bill alone to ask about family dynamics.

Chapter 4 Self-Study Answers

Question 1

Occupational balance	D
Co-occupation	A
Quality of life	C
Advocacy	B

Question 2

The answer is A. It is important to meet with both the caregiver and care recipient to establish their needs from both perspectives and provide the training and resources necessary to transition home safely.

References

American Occupational Therapy Association. (2014). Occupational therapy practice framework: Domain and process (3rd Edition). *American Journal of Occupational Therapy*, 68(1 Suppl), S1–S48. doi:10.5014/ajot.2014.682006

Canam, C., & Acorn, S. (1999). Quality of life for family caregivers of people with chronic health problems. *Rehabilitation Nursing*, 24(5), 192–196, 200. Retrieved from http://www.ncbi.nlm.nih.gov/pubmed/10754909

Klinger, L. (2005). Occupational adaptation: Perspectives of people with traumatic brain injury. *Journal of Occupational Science*, 12(1), 9–16. doi:10.1080/14427591.2005.9686543

Moghimi, C. (2007). Issues in caregiving: The role of occupational therapy in caregiver training. *Topics in Geriatric Rehabilitation*, 23(3), 269–279.

Schell, B. A. B., Gillen, G., & Scaffa, M. E. (2014). *Willard & Spackman's occupational therapy* (12th ed.). Philadelphia: Wolters Kluwer Health/Lippincott Williams & Wilkins.

Schulz, R., & Beach, S. R. (1999). Caregiving as a risk factor for mortality: The Caregiver Health Effects Study. *JAMA*, 282(23), 2215–2219. Retrieved from http://www.ncbi.nlm.nih.gov/pubmed/10605972

Schulz, R., & Sherwood, P. R. (2008). Physical and mental health effects of family caregiving. *American Journal of Nursing*, 108(9 Suppl), 23–27; quiz 27. doi:10.1097/01.NAJ.0000336406.45248.4c

World Health Organization. (2012). *Dementia: A public health priority*. Retrieved from http://whqlibdoc.who.int/publications/2012/9789241564458_eng.pdf

Roles and Context: Personal, Social, Physical, and Cultural

Jessica Andrus and Rosanne DiZazzo-Miller

Learning Objectives

- Describe the importance of context in occupational performance assessment.
- Compare and contrast the components of personal, social, physical, and cultural context that influence occupational therapy assessment and guide treatment planning.
- Identify major theories and models that guide occupational therapists' use of assessments of context.
- Identify appropriate assessments of context in all three areas (i.e., personal, social, and cultural).
- State the importance of how assessment knowledge is applied to clinical situations.

Key Terms

- *Cultural context*: The manner in which culture affects values, behaviors, and attitudes.
- *Disability*: A physical or mental condition that impacts occupational performance.
- *Personal context*: Internal factors such as age, gender, and cultural identity.
- *Social context*: Factors related to personal roles and social networks.
- *Therapeutic use of self*: The ability to establish trust and rapport in a therapeutic relationship and use it as an effective tool throughout the assessment and intervention process.

Introduction

Occupational therapy (OT) treatment interventions are more productive when therapists understand the background of their clients and their real-life situations and environments. This chapter will review key concepts and assessment tools that therapists use to assess and incorporate the personal context and the broader social, physical, and cultural environment.

The Importance of Assessing Context

Assessing context is an important tool for occupational therapists, as it is a client-centered, holistic profession. A dynamic array of contextual factors influences occupational performance. Assessing these factors allows the therapist to plan, conduct, and interpret the results of the OT assessment. Context is a vital part within the OT process as it provides the therapist with a more complete picture of the client, guides selection of assessments, shapes the focus of intervention, and allows the therapist to fit into the client's world instead of vice versa.

OT assessment must go beyond the physical body and impairments to include personal attributes of individuals and the life roles they assume at various points across the life span. Assessing a person's occupational performance context is multidimensional. Assessment of context must include

- Unique personal attributes (e.g., gender and age)
- Personal life roles (e.g., worker, mother, and spouse)
- The various physical, social, and cultural contexts in which people live and interact with one another (e.g., one's home and neighborhood, and one's society)

There are models and frameworks to help therapists organize how they understand and assess context, as well as well-accepted criteria, including reliability and validity, which help therapists identify useful assessments of context. OT practitioners live and work in a personal, social, physical, and cultural context too. It is essential to be familiar with the various forces that shape occupational therapists' perceptions of their clients. These will be discussed in detail within this chapter. Contextual factors may change the meaning behind occupations, the level of function, approaches to treatment, and more (Radomski & Roberts, 2014).

Personal, Social, Physical, and Cultural Context

Personal context refers to a person's internal unseen environment that is derived from, among other things, age, gender, personal beliefs and values, cultural background and identity, and psychological state of mind. Some of the factors in the personal context are fixed, like age, while others are dynamic and changeable, such as pain, adaptation to illness, or one's emotional state, which is often altered in response to positive and negative conditions (Burnett, 2013; Radomski & Roberts, 2014).

Social context refers to factors in the human environment that influence people but are external to the person. Social context refers to a person's social roles, social networks, and also to the socioeconomic resources a person has along with the social position one holds in the social groups to which the person belongs (Burnett, 2013; Radomski & Roberts, 2014).

Physical context refers to the natural and human-made or -built environment we live in. People's homes and the objects within them, as well as neighborhoods and buildings, are examples of the physical context. Physical contexts can facilitate occupational engagement and participation, but the environment can also pose barriers (Burnett, 2013; Radomski & Roberts, 2014).

Cultural context is broader than personal and social contexts and refers to the influence of norms, beliefs and values, and standards of behavior that are expected and accepted in a particular person's community or society. The effect of cultural context is often very subtle and not easy to measure because we are so much a part of our society's rules and practices and beliefs that it is difficult to have the ability to stand back and realize how it could be different (Burnett, 2013; Radomski & Roberts, 2014).

Models and Theories

Models and theories help us organize how we view, interpret, and measure concepts. The following models and theories used in OT include context; however, this list is not all-inclusive. Many of the theories and models in OT aim to encompass context in some form. These theories and models stress that the whole situation or context is relevant to understanding occupational performance (Radomski & Roberts, 2014):

- *Ecology of Human Performance Model* (Dunn, Brown, & McGuigan, 1994): In this model, the interaction between the person and the environment affects his or her behavior and performance. Within the Ecology of Human Performance Model, human performance can only be understood through context, which operates externally from the person. In this model, the interrelationship between person and context determines which tasks fall within the individual's expected performance range.
- *Person–Environment Occupational Model of Occupational Performance* (Law et al., 1996): In this model, occupational performance is defined as a transactive relationship among people, their occupations and roles, and the environments in which they live, work, and play. This model emphasizes the interdependence of persons and their environments and the changing nature of occupational roles over time (Law et al., 1996).
- The World Health Organization's (WHO) *International Classification of Functioning, Disability and Health (ICF) Model* (World Health Organization, 2002): The ICF model views a person's functioning and disability as a dynamic interaction between health conditions and contextual factors. In this model, contextual factors are divided into personal and environmental factors. Personal factors are internal influences on functioning like age and gender. Environmental factors are external influences on functioning that include features of the physical and social environment (World Health Organization, 2002).

Occupational Therapy Practice Framework

The Occupational Therapy Practice Framework III states that the goal of OT is to facilitate clients' engagement in occupation to support participation in the unique context of their life situations (American Occupational Therapy Association, 2014). In the framework, one of the major sections consists of five aspects including occupations, client factors, performance skills, performance patterns, contexts, and environments. They are all of equal value and affect the client's occupational identity, health, and well-being (American Occupational Therapy Association, 2014). Client factors include values, beliefs, and spirituality. The area of performance patterns includes habits, routines, rituals, and roles. The category context and environments include cultural, personal, physical, social, temporal, and virtual (American Occupational Therapy Association, 2014). "Temporal context includes stage of life, time of day or year, duration or rhythm of activity, and history" (American Occupational Therapy Association, 2014, p. S9). Virtual context is becoming more important as technology use increases. It refers to interactions that occur in simulated or real-time situations that are absent of physical contact. Clients must be able to function and engage within their world, which consists of both contexts and environments, in order to achieve full participation (American Occupational Therapy Association, 2014).

Personal Context and Factors

Fixed personal attributes include age, gender, and sexual orientation. A person's age may influence the length of stay, outcome of rehabilitation, and interventions used. The temporal aspect of a person's life is important as people experience occupational shifts throughout life that lead to changes in roles, activities, and goals. Generational cohorts may impact attitudes and beliefs and therefore must be taken into account while assessing the client (Radomski & Roberts, 2014). Gender is personally adopted, but socially constructed from social/cultural norms, roles, behaviors, and activities; sex is biologically determined. Sexual orientation refers to an individual's sexuality, usually related to romantic, emotional, and/or sexual attraction to persons of a particular gender (Boyt-Schell, Gillen, Scaffa, & Cohn, 2014). Personality traits influence not only the assessment and implementation of OT, but also how the individual copes with and responds to the injury or illness (Solet, 2014). Dynamic personal attributes to assess include educational background, marital status, employment status, life roles, perceived health and function, stress and the ability to cope, fatigue, and pain.

Occupational performance and competence in valued life roles are assessed with various tools, some of which are described below. Competence in performance areas such as activities of daily living (ADLs), instrumental activities of daily living (IADLs), and work is evaluated over time and across varying environments such as a hospital, workplace, rehabilitation center, or school (Fasoli, 2014).

- *Role checklist* (Oakley, Kielhofner, Barris, & Reichler, 1986): Assesses productive roles in adulthood, including motivation to assume roles and perceptions of role shifting
- *Interest checklist* (Klyczek, Bauer-Yox, & Fiedler, 1997): Assesses interest patterns and characteristics (i.e., adolescence to adulthood), including ADL, sports, social, educational, and recreational activities
- *Occupational Performance History Interview-II (OPHI)* (Kielhofner et al., 2004): Assesses occupational adaptation over time (i.e., adolescence to adulthood), with a focus on critical life events, daily routines, and occupational behavior roles and settings
- *Canadian Occupational Performance Measure* (Carswell et al., 2004): A client-centered tool for persons aged 7 years and older that evaluates clients' perceptions of their occupational performance over time
- *Worker Role Interview* (Braveman et al., 2005): Gathers data on adults regarding the psychosocial and environmental factors that affect work and the workplace.

Perceived health and functioning (e.g., independence) influence a person's roles and the abilities to participate within their environment. The occupational therapist assesses function and the impact that a disability has on an individual's function for ADLs. Two common assessments used include the Functional Independence Measure (FIM) and the Barthel Index.

- FIM (Keith, Granger, Hamilton, & Sherwin, 1987): A very well-known 18-item measure of disability consisting of 13 motor items and 5 cognitive/communication items.
- Barthel Index (Mahoney & Barthel, 1965): A combination of self-reported information and observation for 10 ADLs with a total score ranging from 0 (total dependence) to 100 (independence).

Personal and social contexts of disability include stress, coping, and adjustment to the disability.

An individual's reactions are influenced not only by the time and type of onset, severity, functions impaired, and visibility of disability, but also by the person's age, gender, interests, values and goals, inner resources, personality and temperament, self-image, and environmental factors (Burnett, 2013). According to Burnett (2013), there is a four-stage process of adjustment or adaptation to a disability. The four stages include vigilance, disruption, enduring the self, and striving to regain self.

Individuals going through adjustment or adaptation to a disability should also be assessed and screened for the following symptoms. Depression can be measured using the Beck Depression Inventory, which assesses the intensity of depression in persons aged 13–80 years (Beck, Steer, Ball, & Ranieri, 1996). Possible signs of clinical depression include significant declines in functioning for the last two weeks or more, feelings of worthlessness or self-doubt, and diminished interest in virtually all activities, even those that were once enjoyable. Anxiety can be measured with an array of tools. An example includes the Hospital Anxiety and Depression Scale, consisting of a self-administered questionnaire composed of 16 questions. There are many assessments to test for specific stressors. One example is the CAGE screening for alcoholism, consisting of four questions (i.e., Have you felt the need to **C**ut down on drinking? Have you been **A**nnoyed by complaints about your drinking? Have you felt **G**uilty about drinking? Have you experienced an **E**ye-opener in terms of needing a drink first thing in the morning?) and only takes approximately 5–10 minutes to administer.

Fatigue and pain are common problems and each have several tests to measure factors such as the effect they have on function or the intensity of each symptom. The Fatigue Severity Scale is a brief scale that relates fatigue to daily function and the McGill Pain Questionnaire is a five-minute test that allows a client to describe the intensity and quality of pain that he/she is experiencing. Many times, a numeric pain rating scale or visual pain rating scale can be used to quickly assess pain from 0 (i.e., no pain) to 10 (i.e., pain as bad as it could be) (Radomski & Roberts, 2014).

Coping strategies are important to maintain psychosocial adaptation during times of stress. Anyone can learn active coping strategies; however, typically during the initial phases of rehabilitation the coping strategies can be maladaptive, and rehabilitation professionals promote and support appropriate coping strategies to maximize treatment (Radomski & Roberts, 2014).

According to Egan and Swedersky (2003), *spirituality* refers to beliefs and practices about one's place in the world that give a person transcendent meaning in life and may be expressed as a religious faith or directed toward nature, family, or community. Physical context can facilitate spiritual experiences. For example, many individuals find spirituality through experiences in nature. For some, home may also be a place that facilitates spirituality, but for others, it may be the opposite if they have a negative experience associated with the house. According to Hasselkus as cited in Billock (2014), the social context can also influence spiritual experiences because meaning is both personally and socially constructed.

The following include some aspects to consider when assessing and treating an individual in regard to social context considerations:

- *Socioeconomic status (SES) and social class*: Socioeconomic resources are not always distributed evenly in society. When certain groups systematically have less, their health appears to be much worse. Visible minorities, women, and children are vulnerable groups who, in some situations, have less. Over many years, the disadvantages associated with having fewer economic resources can accumulate and lead to higher rates of disability (Lysack & Adamo, 2014).
- *SES and poverty*: Poverty can increase the exposure to factors that make people sick, and decrease the chances of having quality medical insurance. There are working poor and new poor. Working poor are those working full time, but their wages do not exceed above the poverty line, while new poor are those that have fallen into poverty because of a sudden circumstance.
- *Health inequalities and disparities:* Each can put people at greater health risks with decreased health and life expectancy. Therapists should become educated about economic and structural barriers to treatment to increase their ability to provide individualized treatment plans (Lysack & Adamo, 2014).
- *Social network and social support*: Research shows all people need access to tangible hands-on help and emotional support if they wish to have good health throughout their lives. Caring for the caregivers is also critical because caregiving itself can put a stress on one's health. All of the contextual factors discussed in this chapter can also be applied to the occupational functioning as

a caregiver. A family-centered approach to care is important and allows the therapist to address the family's priorities and contributions to client care and recovery (Radomski & Roberts, 2014).

Independent living philosophy: Many times, treatment is focused on modifying the individual to the existing environment through means of medical interventions (e.g., surgery and rehabilitation) and is therefore considered a biomedical approach. The healthcare provider and physicians are often the primary decision makers. With the independent living model, the person receiving services is considered the consumer and is the primary decision maker. The services are related to the consumer's current abilities and focus is on modifying the environment, on the attitudes held by others regarding disability, and assistive devices that are chosen by the consumer. The independent living philosophy is similar to the social model of disability, which includes the therapist working as a consultant, advocate, and helper rather than a diagnostician or prescriber. The OT practitioner works to remove community barriers (Burnett, 2013).

- *Client-centered practice*: This is facilitated by the use of interviews and semistructured questionnaires. OT practitioners shape the interaction with their clients through communication and behaviors. Effective occupational therapists manage their own stresses so that personal needs do not influence social interactions with clients (Radomski & Roberts, 2014). The interaction and relationship between the therapist and the client should be based on mutual cooperation and should not consist of an active therapist and passive client (Burnett, 2013).
- *Person-first language*: This is the use of language that recognizes that the person comes first and is not defined solely as a disability or disease. It recognizes that the person is a human being before being someone with a disability. Instead of terms such as "the disabled," "quad," "para," or "amputee," descriptions should begin with "a person with" a disability, such as a person with a spinal cord injury or a person with a below-the-knee amputation.

Physical context is assessed in many different environments including home, work, and the community. As people live longer, the incidence of disability increases and therefore, disability should not be viewed as an abnormality. As individuals age, they have increasing concerns about using assistive devices because of social acceptability and aesthetics. Universally designed devices, aids, and environments may be one way to reduce the stigmatization attached (Burnett, 2013). Universal housing would allow for aging in place (Seamon, 2014). The Americans with Disabilities Act Accessibility Guidelines regulate the design of public buildings, enforcing barrier-free and universal design such as ramps. With universal design, the needs of more people are met including those with rolling luggage, parents pushing children in strollers, and staff rolling carts (Burnett, 2013). The following sections include a list of commonly used assessments for home, work, and the community.

Home Accessibility

- *Safety Assessment of Function and the Environment for Rehabilitation (SAFER) and SAFER Home* (Chiu et al., 2006): Evaluates home safety for older adults
- *Westmead Home Safety Assessment* (Clemson, 1997): Evaluates potential fall hazards in the home

Access to the Workplace

- *Workplace Environment Impact Scale (Moore-Corner, Kielhofner, & Olson, 1998): Semistructured interview to evaluate a person's perceptions of his or her work environment*

Access to the Community

Physical and Environmental Barriers

- *Craig Handicap Inventory of Environmental Factors (CHIEF)* (Han et al., 2005): A brief assessment of perceived environmental barriers
- *Measure of the Quality of the Environment* (Fougeyrollas, Noreau, St-Michael, & Boschen, 2008): Developed in the context of spinal cord injury but used to measure facilitators and obstacles to social participation for all persons with disabilities
- *Accessibility checklist*: An assessment that identifies problems in community access, including compliance to Americans with Disabilities Act policies and regulations (American with Disabilities Act, 1995)

Community Integration and Participation

- *Community Integration Measure (CIM)* (McColl, Davies, Carlson, Johnston, & Minnes, 2001): A 10-item assessment focused on feelings of belonging and independence in one's community
- *Community Integration Questionnaire* (Dijkers, Whiteneck, & El-Jaroudi, 2000): A 15-item survey relevant to home integration, social integration, and productive activities
- *Reintegration to Normal Living Index (RNL)* (Wood-Dauphinee, Opzoomer, Williams, Marchand, & Spitzer, 1988): Assesses how well a person reintegrates into normal living after severe disability

Cultural Context

The cultural context is defined by Radomski and Roberts (2014, p. 71) as "stable and dynamic norms, values, and behaviors associated with the community or societal environments in which occupational functioning occurs." A culturally aware OT practitioner resists characterizing or stereotyping clients based on ethnicity or geographical background. Instead, occupational therapists must attempt to recognize and step away from their own cultural backgrounds in order to appreciate and accept the client's individual culturally based values, customs, and beliefs (Radomski & Roberts, 2014).

Societal Context

Western (i.e., dominant) culture: Ideas of full adult personhood, self-sufficiency (i.e., independence), and individualism that may be difficult to fulfill if a person is living with a chronic illness or disability

Culture of Disability

Social status and disability, and disability as a collective experience: There is an idea of disability as a deficit and a deficiency. Many, even healthcare providers, form common assumptions of those with disabilities. There are many stereotypes from a person who is helpless secondary to his or her disability, to an inspiring overachiever. Some feel that those with a disability have less credibility and are not as capable. At times, people with a disability have to put excess effort into establishing themselves as autonomous and worthy individuals (Burnett, 2013). In addition, there are some who feel that the aim of rehabilitation emphasizes the burden and devastation of disability, and some individuals, quite simply, do not have a desire to change the status of their disability. It is important to seek these alternative views to better understand our clients and families. Viewing client experiences through these various lenses can improve awareness and quality of care for both clients and their caregivers (DiZazzo-Miller & Pociask, 2015). Therefore, it is crucial for OT practitioners to consider the many contexts that surround each individual client.

Referrals and Discharge Considerations

Understanding and integrating each unique personal, social, physical, and cultural context into the therapeutic experience can ultimately enhance therapeutic rapport and outcomes. In addition, it is critical for occupational therapists to consider appropriate referral sources in addition to the appropriate discharge environment to ensure inclusivity of personal, social, physical, cultural, and environmental influences (i.e., facilitators and barriers) that may affect each individual client's success.

Management and Standards of Practice

Context is everything. Occupational therapists and occupational therapist assistants must understand and apply the various contexts and situations that can both enhance and inhibit occupational performance. This begins with a thorough assessment of each client and their unique circumstance and situation, followed by interventions that target their strengths while addressing their challenges. Therapeutic use of self is a key factor that occupational therapists can use in order to reduce doubt, fear, and anxiety while building client trust and respect that can contribute to a more meaningful therapeutic journey (Mosey, 1986). Through better understanding of each client's unique perspective and situation, occupational therapists can affect change.

Chapter 5 Self-Study Activities (Answers Are Provided at the End of the Chapter)

Please match each assessment with its *most* appropriate category. Assessments will be used more than once.

		Assessment options
1. OPHI		**A.** Occupational performance
2. SAFER		**B.** Roles and community integration
3. CIM		**C.** ADL
4. Interest checklist		**D.** IADL
5. KTA		**E.** Work
6. CHART		**F.** Leisure
7. Barthel		
8. AMPS		
9. Katz		
10. Worker role interview		
11. Klein-Bell		
12. KELS		
13. Role checklist		
14. RNL		
15. Rabideau		
16. VALPAR		
17. FIM		
18. COPM		

Data from: Radomski, M. V., & Roberts, P. (2014). Assessing context: Personal, social, cultural, and payer-reimbursement factors. In M. V. Radomski & C. A. T. Latham (Eds.), Occupational therapy for physical dysfunction (7th ed., pp. 50–75). Philadelphia: Wolters Kluwer Health/Lippincott Williams & Wilkins.

An occupational therapist is evaluating a 65-year-old who immigrated from Greece with a moderate traumatic brain injury to determine safety, problem-solving, and impulsivity. The occupational therapist brings the client into the kitchen area and asks him to complete a simple hot meal prep activity. The client reports that he does not cook at home.

19. How should the occupational therapist proceed?
   A. Ask the client to simply try his best.
   B. Provide client education on the status of his injury.
   C. Provide client education on the importance of this evaluation.
   D. Ask the client about his interests.
20. Later on that week the occupational therapy assistant (OTA) begins an upper and lower body dressing session with a client. The client states that his wife will help him with that and he does not want the OTA to help him. The OTA should
   A. Tell the client that he needs to complete the dressing task because that is an area of difficulty for him.
   B. Ask the client why he feels this way and follow up with his wife with permission.
   C. Provide client education on why dressing is an important ADL.

Chapter 5 Self-Study Answers

1. A
2. D
3. B
4. F
5. D
6. B
7. C
8. D
9. C
10. E
11. C
12. D
13. B
14. B
15. D
16. E
17. C
18. A
19. The correct response is D. The occupational therapist should ask the client about his interests so that a more appropriate and contextually relevant task can be used to assess safety, problem-solving, and impulsivity. Although it is important to provide client education, at this point the occupational therapist needs to determine what task is most appropriate to use for evaluation purposes. If the client has never cooked before and the task of cooking is not meaningful to the client, then the assessment results may be invalid.
20. The correct response is B. The OTA should find out why the client does not want to get dressed,

and if his wife is willing and able to complete the task for him based on both of their wishes, then the OTA should shift the focus to joint client and caregiver education. Although this is an ADL, the therapist cannot force what they think is important or necessary on the client as that may conflict with their values and culture. The OTA would never tell a client they need to complete tasks, and although client education is always good, it is more important to find out why the client feels like this so that the client education can be targeted at their specific reason(s).

References

American Occupational Therapy Association. (2014). Occupational therapy practice framework: Domain and process (3rd ed.). *American Journal of Occupational Therapy*, 68(Suppl._1), S1–S48. doi:10.5014/ajot.2014.682006

American with Disabilities Act. (1995). *Checklist for existing facilities version 2.1*. Retrieved from http://www.ada.gov/racheck.pdf

Beck, A. T., Steer, R. A., Ball, R., & Ranieri, W. (1996). Comparison of Beck depression inventories-IA and -II in psychiatric outpatients. *Journal of Personality Assessment*, 67(3), 588–597. doi:10.1207/s15327752jpa6703_13

Billock, C. (2014). Personal values, beliefs, and spirituality. In M. E. Scaffa, B. A. B. Schell, G. Gillen, & E. S. Cohn (Eds.), *Willard & Spackman's occupational therapy* (12th ed., pp. 225–232). Philadelphia, PA: Wolters Kluwer Health/Lippincott Williams & Wilkins.

Boyt-Schell, B., Gillen, G., Scaffa, M. E., & Cohn, E. S. (2014). Individual variance: Body structures and functions. In M. E. Scaffa, B. A. B. Schell, G. Gillen, & E. S. Cohn (Eds.), *Willard & Spackman's occupational therapy* (12th ed., pp. 225–232). Philadelphia, PA: Wolters Kluwer Health/Lippincott Williams & Wilkins.

Braveman, B., Robson, M., Velozo, C., Kielhofner, G., Fisher, G., Forsyth, K., & Kerschbaum, J. (2005). *Worker role interview*. Chicago, IL: University of Illinois at Chicago.

Burnett, S. E. (2013). Personal and social contexts of disability: Implications for occupational therapists. In L. W. Pedretti, H. M. Pendleton, & W. Schultz-Krohn (Eds.), *Pedretti's occupational therapy: Practice skills for physical dysfunction* (7th ed., pp. 83–103). St. Louis, MO: Elsevier.

Carswell, A., McColl, M. A., Baptiste, S., Law, M., Polatajko, H., & Pollock, N. (2004). The Canadian Occupational Performance Measure: A research and clinical literature review. *Canadian Journal of Occupational Therapy*, 71(4), 210–222.

Chiu, T., Oliver, R., Ascott, P., Choo, L. C., Davis, T., Gaya, A., . . . Letts, L. (2006). *Safety assessment of functional and the environment for rehabilitation-health outcome measurement and evaluation (SAFER-HOME), version 3 manual*. Toronto, ON: COTA Health.

Clemson, L. (1997). *Home fall hazards*. West Brunswick, Victoria: Co-ordinates Therapy Services.

Dijkers, M. P., Whiteneck, G., & El-Jaroudi, R. (2000). Measures of social outcomes in disability research. *Archives of Physical Medicine and Rehabilitation*, 81(12 Suppl. 2), S63–S80. Retrieved from http://www.ncbi.nlm.nih.gov/pubmed/11128906

DiZazzo-Miller, R., & Pociask, F. D. (2015). Dementia in the context of disability. *Physical & Occupational Therapy in Geriatrics*, 33(2), 139–151. doi:10.3109/02703181.2015.1014126

Dunn, W., Brown, C., & McGuigan, A. (1994). The ecology of human performance: A framework for considering the effect of context. *American Journal of Occupational Therapy*, 48(7), 595–607. doi:10.5014/ajot.48.7.595

Egan, M., & Swedersky, J. (2003). Spirituality as experienced by occupational therapists in practice. *American Journal of Occupational Therapy*, 57(5), 525–533. Retrieved from http://www.ncbi.nlm.nih.gov/pubmed/14527114

Fasoli, S. E. (2014). Assessing roles and competence. In M. V. Radomski & C. A. T. Latham (Eds.), *Occupational therapy for physical dysfunction* (7th ed., pp. 76–102). Philadelphia, PA: Wolters Kluwer Health/Lippincott Williams & Wilkins.

Fougeyrollas, P., Noreau, L., St-Michael, G., & Boschen, K. (2008). *Measure of the quality of the environment*. Quebec, Canada: RIPPH/INDCP.

Han, C. W., Yajima, Y., Lee, E. J., Nakajima, K., Meguro, M., & Kohzuki, M. (2005). Validity and utility of the Craig Hospital Inventory of Environmental Factors for Korean community-dwelling elderly with or without stroke. *Tohoku Journal of Experimental Medicine*, 206(1), 41–49. Retrieved from http://www.ncbi.nlm.nih.gov/pubmed/15802874

Keith, R. A., Granger, C. V., Hamilton, B. B., & Sherwin, F. S. (1987). The functional independence measure: A new tool for rehabilitation. *Advanced Clinical Rehabilitation*, 1, 6–18.

Kielhofner, G., Malinson, T., Crawford, C., Nowak, M., Rigby, P., Henry, A., & Walens, D. (2004). *Occupational performance history interview-II (version 2.1).* Chicago, IL: MOHO Clearinghouse.

Klyczek, J. P., Bauer-Yox, N., & Fiedler, R. C. (1997). The interest checklist: A factor analysis. *American Journal of Occupational Therapy, 51*(10), 815–823.

Law, M., Cooper, B., Strong, S., Stewart, D., Rigby, P., & Letts, L. (1996). The person–environment–occupation model: A transactive approach to occupational performance. *Canadian Journal of Occupational Therapy, 63*(1), 9–23.

Lysack, C. L., & Adamo, D. E. (2014). Social, economic, and political factors that influence occupational performance. In M. E. Scaffa, B. A. B. Schell, G. Gillen, & E. S. Cohn (Eds.), *Willard & Spackman's occupational therapy* (12th ed., pp. 188–201). Philadelphia, PA: Wolters Kluwer Health/Lippincott Williams & Wilkins.

Mahoney, F. I., & Barthel, D. (1965). Functional evaluation: The Barthel Index. *Maryland State Medical Journal, 14,* 56–61.

McColl, M. A., Davies, D., Carlson, P., Johnston, J., & Minnes, P. (2001). The community integration measure: Development and preliminary validation. *Archives of Physical Medicine and Rehabilitation, 82*(4), 429–434. doi:10.1053/apmr.2001.22195

Moore-Corner, R., Kielhofner, G., & Olson, L. (1998). *Work environment impact scale (WEIS) version 2.0.* Chicago, IL: Model of Human Occupation Clearinghouse, Department of Occupational Therapy.

Mosey, A. (1986). *Psychosocial components of occupational therapy.* New York, NY: Raven Press.

Oakley, F., Kielhofner, G., Barris, R., & Reichler, R. K. (1986). The role checklist: Development and empirical assessment of reliability. *Occupational Therapy Journal of Research, 6*(3), 157–170.

Radomski, M. V., & Roberts, P. (2014). Assessing context: Personal, social, cultural, and payer-reimbursement factors. In M. V. Radomski & C. A. T. Latham (Eds.), *Occupational therapy for physical dysfunction* (7th ed., pp. 50–75). Philadelphia, PA: Wolters Kluwer Health/Lippincott Williams & Wilkins.

Seamon, D. (2014). Physical and virtual environments: Meaning of place and space. In M. E. Scaffa, B. A. B. Schell, G. Gillen, & E. S. Cohn (Eds.), *Willard & Spackman's occupational therapy* (12th ed., pp. 202–215). Philadelphia, PA: Wolters Kluwer Health/Lippincott Williams & Wilkins.

Solet, J. M. (2014). Optimizing personal and social adaptation. In M. V. Radomski & C. A. T. Latham (Eds.), *Occupational therapy for physical dysfunction* (7th ed., pp. 925–973). Philadelphia, PA: Lippincott Williams & Wilkins.

Wood-Dauphinee, S. L., Opzoomer, M. A., Williams, J. I., Marchand, B., & Spitzer, W. O. (1988). Assessment of global function: The reintegration to normal living index. *Archives of Physical Medicine and Rehabilitation, 69*(8), 583–590.

World Health Organization. (2002). *Towards a common language for functioning, disability, and health ICF.* Geneva: World Health Organization. Retrieved from http://www.who.int/classifications/icf/training/icfbe ginnersguide.pdf

Sensation, Range of Motion, Strength, and Coordination

Christine Johnson, Sara Maher, and Rosanne DiZazzo-Miller

Learning Objectives

- Describe common standardized and nonstandardized assessment methods for sensation, range of motion (ROM), strength, and coordination.
- Describe normal and abnormal sensation, ROM, strength, and coordination assessment findings.
- State precautions and contraindications for the assessment and intervention of sensation, ROM, strength, and coordination.
- Discuss how abnormal sensation, ROM, strength, and coordination findings impact areas of occupation, activity demands, performance patterns, and performance skills.
- Given a case study, select appropriate sensation, ROM, strength, and coordination assessment measures and interventions.

Key Terms

- *Aesthesiometer*: Measures two-point discrimination.
- *Desensitization*: These exercises are used to help decrease hypersensitivities.
- *Hyperesthesia*: An abnormal underreaction to sensory stimulation.
- *Hypersensitivity*: An abnormal overreaction to sensory stimulation.
- *Monofilament*: Nylon wire that is measured in grams of force for more accurate touch sensitivity measurements.
- *Neuropathy*: Weakness, numbness, or pain associated with damage to peripheral nerves.

Introduction

This chapter will provide a comprehensive review on assessment and intervention for sensation, range of motion (ROM), strength, and coordination. The following sections will cover pertinent information in the definitions and process of how to complete each assessment. The corresponding worksheets at the end of the chapter will help to reinforce understanding of principles, concepts, and application of knowledge.

Etiology and Pathology

Conditions or injuries to the central nervous system (CNS) and/or peripheral nervous system (PNS) can affect normal functioning related to sensation, ROM, strength, and coordination. There are various procedures recommended for screening, assessing, and treating areas of motor control. When performed correctly, occupational therapy (OT) practitioners (and occupational therapy assistant [OTAs]) can provide appropriate assessment and intervention for individuals to regain or compensate for injuries that limit their occupational functioning.

CNS Injuries

The sensory cortex receives information from the periphery for interpretation, which is received and organized by the somatosensory cortex somatotopically. Different areas of the body have more and less sensitivity. Examples of the body that have higher sensitivity are the tips of the fingers and lips. A homunculus is often used to represent the proportions of the sensory cortex utilized by various body areas (Cooper & Canyock, 2013; Theis, 2014). The homunculus indicates the location and amount of the cortex devoted to each part of the body.

Peripheral Nervous System Disorders

Spinal nerves combine to form peripheral nerves, which are outside of the brain and the spinal cord. The brachial and lumbar plexuses regroup these sensory neurons into peripheral nerves. Sensory information from the peripheral nerves is sent to the brain through tracts. An injury to a peripheral nerve may result in motor or sensory impairments or a combination of both. Pain, temperature, and crude touch travel along the anterolateral spinothalamic tracts, whereas conscious proprioception, discriminatory touch, and vibration travel along the column–medial lemniscus pathway. A person with a PNS injury is more likely to have deficits in touch pressure awareness and two-point discrimination. Individual spinal nerves contribute to several peripheral nerves, and each peripheral nerve contains fibers from several spinal nerves. Each spinal nerve has a dermatomal distribution, referring to the area of skin supplied by sensory fibers of a single dorsal root through the dorsal and ventral rami of its spinal nerve (Cooper & Canyock, 2013; Theis, 2014).

Cerebellar disorders: Cerebellar disorders can cause incoordination that may affect any body region and cause a variety of clinical symptoms including the client's inability to maintain body position resulting in leaning and spinal curvature. The resting position of the eye, as well as reflexive and voluntary eye movements, may be affected as well. Ataxia, a common cerebellar disorder, is characterized by delayed initiation of movement responses resulting in jerky, and poorly controlled movements. Clients with ataxia typically have a wide-based gait with decreased arm swing, and step length that may be uneven. The client's extremity will often stray from the normal trajectory while reaching for an object. Additional challenges may include the following:

- *Adiadochokinesia*: The inability to perform rapid alternating movements such as pronation and supination simultaneously.
- *Dysmetria*: The inability to estimate the ROM required to reach a target.
- *Hypermetria*: Overshooting a target.
- *Hypometria*: Undershooting a target.
- *Dyssynergia*: The decomposition of movements in which voluntary movements are broken down into their component parts and appear jerky.
- *The Rebound Phenomenon of Holmes*: The inability to stop motion quickly to avoid hitting something.
- *Nystagmus*: The involuntary movement of the eyeballs in a vertical, horizontal, or rotating direction. This can interfere with the small adjustments required for balance.
- *Dysarthria*: Explosive or slurred speech (Gillen, 2013; Woodson, 2014).

Extrapyramidal disorders: Extrapyramidal disorders are characterized by hypokinesia and hyperkinesia (i.e., an increase in muscle movement). These disorders are typically difficult to measure and therefore rating scales are commonly used, which include the Simpson–Angus Scale (SAS), the Barnes Akathisia Rating Scale (BARS), the Abnormal Involuntary Movement Scale (AIMS), and the Extrapyramidal Symptom Rating Scale. Additional challenges may include the following:

- *Chorea*: Involuntary, coarse, quick, jerky, and dysthymic movements that usually subside during sleep.
- *Huntington's disease and tardive dyskinesia*: Two diagnoses in which chorea may be present.
- *Athetoid movements*: Continuous, slow, wormlike, and arrhythmic movements that affect the distal portion of the extremities. Athetoid movement that occurs with chorea is called choreoathetosis.
- *Dystonia*: Results in persistent posturing of the extremities with concurrent torsion of the spine and twisting of the trunk. These movements are often seen in conjunction with spasticity.
- *Ballism*: A rare movement disorder that is produced by continuous abrupt contractions of the axial and proximal musculature of the extremity. This disorder causes undesired flailing and ballistic movements of the limbs.
- The three most common types of tremors include the following:
  1. Intention tremor occurs during voluntary movement.
  2. Resting tremor occurs at rest and subsides when voluntary movement is attempted.

3. Essential familial tremor is inherited as an auto-somal dominant trait and is most visible when the client is carrying out a fine precision task (Gillen, 2013; Woodson, 2014).

Typical interventions for incoordination include weight-bearing exercises, sensorimotor approaches, casting, physical agent modalities, distal-to-proximal approaches, pharmacologic agents, nerve blocks, and surgical methods. A specific description for each of these interventions and information regarding supporting research can be found in the main OT textbooks on adult physical disabilities (i.e., Early, 2012; Pendleton & Schultz-Krohn, 2013; Radomski & Latham, 2014).

Somatosensory

A client with sensory dysfunction should be evaluated to determine the impact on the ability of the client to perform occupation-based activities. There are a variety of different sensory impairments that can be identified by specific sensory tests. Anesthesia is a complete loss of sensation. Paresthesia is a sensation that is typically described as pins and needles, tingling, or an electric shock. Hypersensitivity is used to describe increased sensitivity. Hyperalgesia is used to describe increased pain sensation. Allodynia is a painful response to a nontissue-damaging stimulus that would not be expected to evoke pain. Diminished or inaccurate sensation is used to describe sensation that may be present, but is not consistent or may be misinterpreted (Cooper & Canyock, 2013; Theis, 2014).

Sensation is a body function, which is a client factor that plays an important role in motor and processing aspects of performance skills. Sensation and sensory dysfunction has a large impact on a person's ability to participate in each area of occupation. The somatosensory system allows the client to receive information regarding objects in the external environment through touch and proprioception with the stimulation of muscles and joints, which is vital in the completion of activities of daily living (ADLs) such as locating clothes and getting dressed. It also monitors the temperature of the body and provides information about painful, itchy, and tickling stimuli, particularly important in the occupation of cooking (Cooper & Canyock, 2013). Tests and measures selected to assess sensory impairment depend on whether the person has experienced an injury in either their CNS or PNS (Cooper & Canyock, 2013).

It is important to select assessment and interventions based on the individual's level of sensory awareness.

Detection is an individual's most basic skill and allows the person to be aware of sensation. Discrimination is the ability of a person to distinguish between two or more different stimuli without using vision. Quantification is the ability to perceive different intensities of sensory stimuli. Recognition is the ability to meaningfully interpret a combination of sensory stimuli. These levels of sensory awareness are described with increasing difficulty and each level should be mastered before progressing to the next.

The OT practitioner should ensure the client understands the procedure before beginning screening and assessment. It is recommended that the OT practitioner explain and demonstrate the procedure for the client with his or her eyes open and on the area of skin that has intact sensation. Next, have the client respond to the test procedure to confirm understanding. Responses may differ depending on the client's communication skills and/or limitations. Make sure that there are no extraneous cues that the client may use to respond to the testing. The OT's or OTA's hand should be limited to the lateral borders of the body segment to limit pressure cues. Make sure that clothes, bedding, or other similar objects do not touch the body segment being tested. Use alternate patterns when testing and avoid predictable patterns. Minimize distractions in the environment. Apply the stimulus in a consistent manner. All of the testing should be done with the client's vision occluded after directions are understood (Cooper & Canyock, 2013; Theis, 2014).

Somatosensory Precautions and Contraindications

Prior to somatosensory testing, it is crucial for the OT practitioner to assess the following areas:

- Hearing
- Language skills (i.e., receptive and expressive)
- Mental function
- Verbal skills
- Vision

Impairment in any of these areas can inadvertently alter the results of somatosensory testing, thereby producing false and inaccurate data. In addition, it is important for the OT practitioner to reduce extraneous environmental and physical cues such as unnecessary visual, auditory, and tactile input. This will allow the client to focus on the stimulus and provide a more accurate representation of the specific somatosensory area under examination.

Somatosensory Screening and Assessments

1. *Pain*: Pain is a protective sensation that a person uses for safety. The OT practitioner will need a sterilized safety pin to perform this assessment. The OT or OTA will alternate between sharp and dull sides of the safety pin and document the accuracy of responses. Document if pain perception is intact, impaired, or absent, or if hyperalgesia is present (Cooper & Canyock, 2013; Theis, 2014).

2. *Temperature*: Temperature is also a protective sensation. The ability to detect temperature is vital in the completion of ADLs such as bathing or cooking tasks without compensatory techniques. The OT practitioner will preferably need two equal-sized test tubes; one will be filled with warm water and one with cold water. If test tubes are unavailable, objects such as wash cloths run under warm or cold water temperatures may be used. The OT practitioner will touch the client with each test tube in a random order and ask the client to identify which tube is warm and which one is cold. Document the accuracy of responses and if temperature sensation is intact, impaired, or absent (Cooper & Canyock, 2013; Theis, 2014).

3. *Touch*: Touch supports abilities and skills, such as grasping and releasing of objects, and is required for competence in handling and manipulating objects. It is also a means of communication and a source of pleasure. Touch can be measured in a variety of ways and at a variety of levels of discrimination (Cooper & Canyock, 2013; Theis, 2014).

4. *Touch sensation*: Touch sensation is measured by a two-point discrimination test. This is the minimum distance between two points in which the individual can accurately perceive the distinct two points. The OT practitioner will need a Boley gauge or Disk-Criminator. The OT or OTA will alternate between touching the client with one point or two points. The test should continue until there is a distance presented in which the client is unable to identify the two distinct points. If the client indicates that the two points are one, this is an incorrect response. Document the minimum distance for accurate perception of the two points at specific areas of the skin (Cooper & Canyock, 2013; Theis, 2014).

5. *Touch pressure*: Light touch is perceived by receptors in the superficial skin, whereas pressure is perceived by receptors in the subcutaneous and deeper tissues. Touch pressure is tested with a set of 20 monofilaments that vary in thickness. The OT determines through the testing procedure, the thinnest filament at which the client can reliably determine that he or she is being touched. The client replies "touch" when he or she perceives that they feel a monofilament. Document the smallest size monofilament that the client can perceive at various sites (Cooper & Canyock, 2013; Theis, 2014).

6. *Touch localization*: Localization of touch is a test of functional sensation because it is highly correlated between this test and the test of two-point discrimination. This helps determine the client's baseline and projected functional prognosis. The OT practitioner will use a cotton ball, thinnest monofilament, or very fine tipped gel pen. The OT practitioner will lightly touch an area and ask the client to point to the area that was touched. Document the accuracy of the responses. Make sure to record the distance between where the client was touched and where he or she indicated the touch was felt (Cooper & Canyock, 2013; Theis, 2014).

7. *Proprioception*: Conscious proprioception stems from receptors found in muscles, tendons, and joints and is defined as the awareness of a joint in its position in space. When proprioception is impaired, an individual can have a difficult time gauging how much pressure is required to hold an object. The OT practitioner will hold the lateral aspects of the elbow, wrist, or digit. The OT practitioner then moves the body into flexion or extension and the client reports if the body part is being moved up or down. The term kinesthesia is sometimes used interchangeably with proprioception. However, if the OT practitioner is testing kinesthesia, it is recommended that the OT practitioner move the unaffected limb into a certain posture and have the client copy the movement with the affected side. Document the accuracy of responses and if proprioception is intact, impaired, or absent at each joint (Cooper & Canyock, 2013; Theis, 2014).

8. *Stereognosis*: Stereognosis requires the use of both proprioceptive information and touch information in order to identify a familiar object. It would be very difficult to identify an item in a pocket or pick up a fork from a soapy sink if stereognosis was impaired. The OT or OTA should use common

objects such as a key, nut, bolt, closed safety pin, coin, paper clip, and dice. The OT practitioner places the items into the client's hand one object at a time and asks the client to identify the object by stating the name or pointing to a picture. Document the accuracy of the responses and whether stereognosis is intact, impaired, or absent (Cooper & Canyock, 2013; Theis, 2014).

9. *Graphesthesia*: Graphesthesia is demonstrated through the ability to identify a number or letter drawn on the skin. The OT practitioner uses a dull-pointed pencil to trace letters, numbers, or geometric figures on the fingertips or palms of the client's hand. The OT practitioner will orient the bottom of the letter proximally. The client identifies the letter or the number by saying it or pointing to a picture. Document the percentage of correct responses (Cooper & Canyock, 2013; Theis, 2014).

10. *Desensitization*: Hypersensitivity can limit the use of a body part and prevent a person from engaging in sensory reeducation. The goal is to reduce hypersensitivity through habituation. A graded stimulation is utilized. The stimuli are upgraded to be slightly more noxious as the client's tolerance increases. There are specific protocols that can be used depending on the severity of the hypersensitivity; however, OT can be creative in incorporating desensitization into routines, for example, rubbing textured materials or clothing against the client's skin during dressing (Cooper & Canyock, 2013; Theis, 2014).

11. *Sensory reeducation*: The cortical map is affected by stimulation and the use of different body parts. Training can help improve functional sensibility over time. It is important to identify if the client requires protective or discriminative reeducation. Protective sensation impairments can put clients at risk for burns, blisters, and cuts. Several compensatory techniques should be utilized for clients without protective sensation. Intact protective sensation allows a client to be a candidate for discriminative sensory training. Localization of moving touch tends to return before localization of constant touch. The OT practitioner can use the eraser end of a pencil or finger in the client's midline of one zone of the hand to make the task easier. Having the client touch the area that the OT practitioner touches can also increase awareness. Presenting the client with two different objects is one way

to perform graded discrimination. As the client's sensation improves, the OT team can use objects that are similar (e.g., progressing from a utensil and coin to a penny and dime) (Cooper & Canyock, 2013; Theis, 2014).

Somatosensory Interventions

Somatosensory interventions are aimed at either remediating or compensating for diminished or absent sensation caused by paresthesia, hyperalgesia, dysesthesia, or allodynia (Cooper & Canyock, 2013). They vary depending on the type and degree of injury. For example, a loss of sensation secondary to a complete spinal cord injury (SCI) would focus on remediating weaker muscles above the level of the lesion and compensating for the loss of sensation below the level of the lesion. Alternately, interventions from a peripheral nerve injury due to brief nerve compression may focus more so on remedial techniques. Specific remedial interventions commonly include the following:

- Sensory reeducation through desensitization for hypersensitivity typically includes a tuning fork, paraffin, massage, electrical vibrators, texture and object identification, and work and daily activities (Latham & Bentzel, 2014). There are two types of sensory reeducation:

  1. Protective sensory reeducation—typically indicated for clients who have diminished or absent pinprick or hot/cold sense. Cooper and Canyock (2013) discuss the following interventions:
     - Address any edema and skin integrity.
     - Use built-up handles to decrease grip force.
     - Protect the skin from hot/cold and sharp items.

  2. Discriminative sensory reeducation for clients with limited touch sensation enough to feel but not localize input and intact protective sensation. Cooper and Canyock (2013) discuss the following interventions:
     - Retraining through moving touch localization.
     - Graded discrimination through identification of the object in addition to whether the object is the same or different, as well as the degree to which they are similar or different.

Additional interventions include mirror visual feedback; weight bearing; fluidotherapy or immersion of a hand or foot into rice, beans, or popcorn; massage (e.g., scar massage); transcutaneous electrical nerve stimulation (TENS); and incorporation of affected body parts into everyday living and graded functional tasks (Latham & Bentzel, 2014).

Common compensatory interventions focus on ADLs and environmental modifications. For example, it is important to prevent injury with items that are hot and cold such as setting the water temperature to a maximum of 120°. Insulation of exposed water pipes and other hot or sharp household objects will protect lower extremities from harm, in addition to special attention to wrinkles and seams in clothing to prevent pressure ulcers (James, 2014). Additional modifications can be made as follows:

- Visual compensation
- Stabilization during tasks
- Tactile, proprioceptive, and kinesthetic cues
- Adaptive equipment that provides visual, verbal, auditory, or tactile cues
- Environmental adaptation to minimize and organize spaces

Joint Range of Motion

Functional ROM refers to the amount of joint range necessary to perform essential ADLs and instrumental activities of daily living (IADLs) without special equipment.

Joint ROM is the amount of movement that is possible at a specific joint. ROM can be measured through active range of motion (AROM) in which the joint is moved by the muscles that act on the joint. Passive range of motion (PROM) occurs when an external force, such as when an OT practitioner, moves the joint. It is important to maintain consistent methods of measurement to ensure high intratester reliability and validity. Reliability refers to the consistency of accurate test outcomes under the same conditions in a repeated scenario with the same tester (i.e., intratester) or a different tester (i.e., intertester). The validity refers to how well the measurement represents the true value of the variable of interest. It is appropriate to complete goniometric measurements on joints in which an OT detects limitations in the ability to perform daily occupations. Before beginning a ROM assessment, it is important to be familiar with the above ways of measurements, precautions and contraindications, joint end-feel, testing procedures, and correct limb positioning (Killingsworth, Pedretti, & Pendleton, 2013b; Whelan, 2014).

Joint end-feel: End-feel is the sensation the examiner feels in the joint as it reaches the end of its ROM. Passive movement carried out from the point where resistance is first met to the final stop in the range of movement is called end-feel. The end of PROM is normally limited by joint structures and soft tissue surrounding the joint. There are normal end-feels associated with specific joints. These end-feels are expected to occur at the end of normal ROM (i.e., each joint has a characteristic end-feel). Joint end-feel is categorized as hard (e.g., bone contacting bone), soft (e.g., soft tissue contacting muscle), or firm (e.g., springy with some give such as a dorsiflexed ankle with the knee in extension) (Killingsworth et al., 2013b; Whelan, 2014). An end-feel is considered abnormal when it is different than the end-feel expected for a joint and/or when it occurs at a point in the range that is different than what is normal for a joint.

Precautions and Contraindications

ROM assessment should not be conducted (i.e., contraindicated) on a joint with a dislocation or unhealed fracture, on a joint where soft tissue surgery was recently performed, or if myositis ossification or ectopic ossification is present near the joint (Killingsworth et al., 2013b). ROM assessment may occur cautiously (i.e., precaution) in the presence of inflammation or infection in the joint; if medications are being taken to fight pain or relax muscles; if a joint has been diagnosed with osteoporosis, hypermobility, or subluxation; if the client has hemophilia; if a hematoma or sustained soft tissue injury occurred near the joint; in the presence of a newly united fracture or following, prolonged immobilization of a joint; or if bony ankyloses or carcinoma is suspected in the area.

Screening and Assessments

The primary purpose of goniometry is to measure joint ROM of the musculoskeletal system. The goniometer consists of a body, stationary arm, and moveable arm. The general procedure for goniometric measurements using the 360° method is the most common and will be described; however, there are various types and sizes of goniometers available for different joints. The fulcrum of the goniometer is placed over the approximate axis of the joint being measured using anatomic landmarks. The stationary arm is typically aligned parallel to the longitudinal axis of the proximal segment of the joint, and the distal arm is typically aligned parallel to the distal segment of the joint. The OT practitioner reports the number of degrees at the starting position (i.e., do not assume it is 0) and the number of degrees at the final position (Killingsworth et al., 2013b; Whelan, 2014). It is important for the OT to use proper body mechanics, proper client positioning, a goniometer suited for the joint to be measured, and standardized goniometric techniques (Killingsworth et al., 2013b; Whelan, 2014). For example, the OT must reproduce the same measurements under the same conditions in order to measure change. In addition, any change of ±5° is generally the accepted margin of error. Commonly tested joints for upper and lower extremity ROM include the following:

1. Shoulder
   a. Flexion and extension.
   b. Abduction and adduction.
   c. External and internal rotation.
   d. Horizontal abduction and adduction.
2. Elbow
   a. Flexion and extension.
3. Forearm
   a. Pronation and supination.
4. Wrist
   a. Flexion and extension.
   b. Radial and ulnar deviation.
5. Hand
   a. Metacarpophalangeal (MCP), proximal interphalangeal (PIP), distal interphalangeal (DIP) flexion and extension. MCP refers to the joint between the metacarpal bone and phalanges of the finger. PCP refers to the joint between the first and second phalanges, and DIP is the joint between the second and third phalanges.
   b. MCP abduction and adduction.
   c. Total active motion (TAM) for the finger joints are taken by adding extension deficits and subtracting from flexion measurements. For example, digit #3 MCP = 20 − 50; PIP = 10 − 70; DIP = 0 − 5; TAM = 95.
6. Thumb
   a. Flexion and extension.
   b. Opposition.
   c. Abduction and adduction.
7. Hip
   a. Flexion and extension.
   b. Abduction and adduction.
   c. External and internal rotation.
8. Knee
   a. Flexion and extension.
   b. Foot and ankle.
   c. Dorsiflexion and plantar flexion.
   d. Inversion and eversion.

Interventions

Functional ROM is necessary to participate in daily activities. ROM may be limited due to a variety of neurological, muscular, systemic, or other conditions that impact muscle function or cause damage to a joint. In addition, inactivity, scarring, or immobilization can lead to a loss of motion. Some significant limitations in ROM can be improved or corrected with exercise and occupational therapy. Other challenges cannot be changed by these techniques and include ankylosis or arthrodesis, long-standing contractures with fibrotic changes, and severe joint destruction (Whelan, 2014). Deficits found in functional ROM require treatment to focus on either maintaining existing motion or regaining motion that has been lost.

1. *Decreasing edema*: A variety of techniques can prevent ROM limitations due to edema and include elevation, cryotherapy, compression, massage, electrical stimulation, and gentle motion of the joint involved.
2. *Minimizing contractures*: Contractures are shortening of muscle and connective tissue, often permanent, resulting in reduced joint mobility and an increase in resistance to passive joint movement (Whelan, 2014). To help prevent contractures and the accompanying loss of ROM, techniques of therapeutic positioning and splinting may be used.
3. *Moving through full ROM*: Moving a joint through its full available ROM. This can be done actively by the client (i.e., AROM), passively by another person (i.e., PROM), or with just enough assistance by another person to allow the client to achieve the desired motion (i.e., AAROM). A continuous passive motion (CPM) device may also be used to continually move a joint through a controlled ROM.
4. *Stretching*: Stretching is a process where a muscle is lengthened either actively or passively to help increase ROM. Active stretching involves contracting the muscle(s) opposite to the direction of limitation (i.e., antagonist(s)). This can be done by the use of slow, repetitive isotonic contractions of the antagonist(s) or by prolonged contractions of the same muscle(s). Proprioceptive neuromuscular

facilitation (PNF) techniques such as contract relax and/or agonist contraction may be used by resisting a manual force for 5–10 seconds and then allowing the muscle to relax. During relaxation, the joint is moved in the opposite direction to the contraction and held for a stretch. Passive stretching utilizes the application of an external force. Typical forces include manual therapy, splinting, casting, or external equipment. Additionally, longer durations of tissue stretching may be associated with greater gains in ROM.

Manual Muscle Testing

Manual muscle testing (MMT) is the maximal contraction of a muscle or muscle group. Gravity is a form of resistance in testing strength. The specific measurement within certain muscles can assist in diagnosing certain neuromuscular conditions such as peripheral nerve injuries and SCIs and indicating whether the involvement is partial or complete. Establishing a baseline measurement for the client will help determine to what extent weakness is limiting the client's performance in meaningful occupations, prevent deformities resulting from muscle imbalances, identify assistive devices needed to compensate for weak muscles, and evaluate the overall effectiveness of intervention strategies over time (Killingsworth, Pedretti, & Pendleton, et al., 2013a).

Precautions and Contraindications

MMT is contraindicated when the client has inflammation or pain in the region to be tested, a dislocation or unhealed fracture, recent surgery of the musculoskeletal structures, or myositis ossificans. Special consideration should be taken if the client has osteoporosis, subluxation or hypermobility of a joint, hemophilia or any type of cardiovascular risk disease, abdominal surgery, or fatigue that exacerbates a condition. Unlike some of the ROM procedures, MMT requires the client's complete involvement and requires the OT to be mindful of the client's willingness to expend true efforts (Killingsworth et al., 2013b; Whelan, 2014).

Screening and Assessments

The OT practitioner should demonstrate and describe the test motion to the client and ask him or her to perform the test motion and return to the starting position. This allows the OT or OTA to note general observation of the quality of movement and difficulties the client may have

before resistance is applied. The following procedure should be followed when testing each muscle group: (1) position, (2) stabilize, (3) palpate, (4) observe, and (5) grade. The OT practitioner should first position themselves and the client in the correct way (Killingsworth et al., 2013b; Whelan, 2014). The OT practitioner should stabilize proximal to the joint being tested and isolate the muscle group, to ensure for the correct test motion and to eliminate substitution from other muscle groups. To palpate, the OT or OTA places his or her fingers on the muscle group being tested and asks the client to repeat the motion. The OT practitioner asks the client to stop just before the end range and hold the position. The break test is used to apply resistance in the opposite direction (Killingsworth et al., 2013a). Helpful terms such as "do not let me move you" can help the client to understand his or her role during the break test. A client with scores 2+ or below should be positioned in a gravity-eliminated position. See **Table 6-1** for score interpretation.

Table 6-1 MMT Score Interpretation	
Grades of Muscle Strength	
Grade	**Description**
5 or N	Full ROM against gravity and full resistance for the client's size, age, and sex
N–	Slight weakness
G+	Moderate weakness
4 or G	Movement against gravity and moderate resistance at least 10 times without fatigue
F+	Movement against gravity several times or mild resistance one time
3 or F	Full range against gravity
F–	Movement against gravity and complete ROM one time
P+	Full ROM with gravity eliminated but some resistance applied
2 or P	Full ROM with gravity eliminated
P–	Incomplete ROM with gravity eliminated
1 or T	Evidence of contraction (i.e., visible or palpable) but no joint movement
0	No palpable or visible contraction and no joint movement

N = normal; G = good; F = fair; P = poor; T = trace.
Data from: Moroz (2015).

It is crucial for the OT practitioner to follow correct techniques for each motion, as well as proper positioning of the OT practitioner and client (Killingsworth et al., 2013a, pp. 540–573; Whelan, 2014, pp. 191–225). Commonly tested joints for upper and lower extremity MMT include the following:

1. Neck
   a. Flexion and extension
   b. Right and left lateral flexion
2. Scapula
   a. Abduction and adduction
   b. Elevation and depression
3. Shoulder
   a. Flexion and extension
   b. Abduction and adduction
   c. External and internal rotation
   d. Horizontal abduction and adduction
4. Elbow
   a. Flexion and extension
5. Forearm
   a. Pronation and supination
6. Wrist
   a. Flexion and extension
   b. Radial and ulnar deviation
7. Hand
   a. MCP, PIP, DIP flexion and extension
   b. MCP abduction and adduction
8. Thumb
   a. Flexion and extension
   b. Opposition
   c. Abduction and adduction
9. Hip
   a. Flexion and extension
   b. Abduction adduction
   c. Internal and external rotation
10. Knee
    a. Flexion and extension
11. Foot and ankle
    a. Dorsiflexion and plantar flexion
    b. Inversion and eversion

Interventions

Strengthening involves working a muscle or muscle group against resistance to increase the amount of force that can be attained. Strengthening is most warranted if a client has weakness that is preventing participation in an occupation or ADLs or weakness that may lead to a deformity. Strengthening involves repetitive muscle contractions and can include biofeedback, electrical stimulation, muscle reeducation, and progressive resistance exercises (Whelan, 2014). Isometric exercises involve contraction of a muscle with no changes in joint angle or muscle length. Concentric exercises occur with muscle contraction, resulting in shortening of the muscle. Eccentric exercises occur when a muscle is lengthening while it is under load. Strengthening interventions are developed based on the tasks the client needs to accomplish and the physical abilities of the client, such as those below:

1. *Isometric*: A weak muscle (1) is contracted maximally and held.
2. *Dynamic assistive (i.e., active assistive ROM)*: A weak muscle is concentrically or eccentrically contracted through as much ROM as a client can achieve, and/or an external force provides assistance to allow the client to complete the desired motion. The muscle is placed in a gravity-eliminated position (i.e., 2–) or against gravity (i.e., 3–).
3. *Dynamic active (i.e., active ROM)*: Client contracts muscle to move through full ROM. This is done in a gravity-eliminated plane (2) or against gravity (3).
4. *Dynamic active resistive (i.e., active resistive ROM)*: Client contracts muscle to move through full available ROM against resistance. This can be done in a gravity-eliminated plane (i.e., 2+ and 3) or against gravity (i.e., 3+ and above) (Whelan, 2014).

Exercise programs can be progressed or made less difficult by changing any of the following: the amount of time a contraction is held, the number of repetitions performed, the number of sets required, the amount of rest between exercises, the type and velocity of contractions, the amount of resistance provided, and the frequency of exercise. In addition, muscle endurance (i.e., the ability of a muscle to maintain performance over time) may be a treatment goal by using parameters focusing on low-intensity muscle contractions, a large number of repetitions, and a prolonged time period (Whelan, 2014).

Coordination

Coordination is required to complete accurate and controlled movements. The cerebellum controls the coordination of muscle action. Coordinated movements require all elements of the neuromuscular system to be intact. Clients demonstrating difficulty with timing, sequencing, direction, accuracy, speed, force, and smoothness may require further assessment of coordination deficits (Anderson-Preston, 2013).

Precautions and Contraindications

Precautions for clients with dysfunction in coordination revolve around safety. The OT is responsible for identifying the level of dysfunction within the coordination difficulty in order to provide a recommendation and/or a safe environment for the client to succeed. Safety features to keep in mind include sharp objects, electric appliances, and wet/slippery surfaces. Facilitators such as adaptive equipment should be incorporated into the client's environment and barriers should be removed.

Screening and Assessments

People experiencing difficulty in one or more element(s) of coordination should be assessed for coordination dysfunction. An OT or OTA can complete a screening of coordination through administration of a finger–nose test, which includes instructing the client to touch his or her finger to his or her nose. The knee pat test includes instructing the client to rotate forearms between pronation and supination. Finger wiggling and drawing of spirals can also assess coordination. These screenings can reveal dysmetria, dyssynergia, adiadochokinesis, tremors, and ataxia (Anderson-Preston, 2013). Further assessment should be completed through occupation-based activities. The OT practitioner can observe coordination difficulties through ADL assessment (Anderson-Preston, 2013; James, 2014). The OT practitioner should observe for irregularity in time, accuracy (e.g., overshooting or undershooting targets), or jerky movements while completing ADL tasks (Anderson-Preston, 2013). There are several standardized assessments that can be performed to assess coordination, including the Purdue Pegboard, the Minnesota Rate of Manipulation Test, the Pennsylvania Bimanual Work Sample, the Crawford Small Parts Dexterity Test, the Jebsen-Taylor Hand Function Test, the Motor Assessment Scale, the Nine-Hole Peg Test, the Tinetti Performance Oriented Mobility Assessment, and the Wolf Motor Function Test (Amini, 2014).

Interventions

When implementing treatment for coordination disorders, it is important to understand motor learning and control principles. Activities should aim at focusing on proximal stability first and grading activities to challenge the client in working toward reaching the highest level of mobility within the client's capacity. There is an additional emphasis on modulating reflexes and abnormal synergy patterns through exercises in which the client can practice postural control, as well as righting and equilibrium reactions (James, 2014). As the client masters these skills, the focus should switch to incorporating the ability of the client to practice the skills in the natural environment through occupation-based activities. If restoration is not an option for the client, interventions allowing for compensation and adaption may be necessary.

Referrals and Discharge Considerations

The OT is responsible for determining if additional tests and/or measures are indicated given the client's current status. Safety is always a consideration for discharge, and most important to note, given any limitations in sensation, ROM, strength, and/or coordination. Ultimately, the OT must ensure that the discharge setting is conducive to the client's unique abilities and limitations. Tests and measures discussed in this chapter are intended to assist with the diagnosis provided by the physician or as a screen to provide further information to the diagnosis in addition to potential referrals.

Management and Standards of Practice

Although the OT is responsible for the treatment plan, the OTA can assist with evaluations and carry out treatment plans. During examination procedures, the OT practitioner must ensure complete and precise testing as they relate to sensation, ROM, strength, and coordination. An inability to follow proper protocol can result in inaccurate data and therefore a potentially negative effect on the client's function. In addition, OTs and OTAs must work within their standards of practice. For example, when physical agent modalities are utilized, the OT practitioner must have the appropriate training and utilize the modality as a preparatory tool prior to clients engagement into a functional activity related to their impairments. Furthermore, the OT practitioner must communicate with other team members to ensure treatment is complimentary and not duplicative with other disciplines.

Chapter 6 Self-Study Activities (Answers Are Provided at the End of the Chapter)

1. The client is a 5-year-old child who sustained a C6 SCI secondary to a motor vehicle accident. The injury occurred to the right side of his spinal cord. The OT begins the evaluation knowing that the sensation *MOST LIKELY* to be impaired on the left side of the body, below the level of the lesion, is:
   a. Two-point discrimination
   b. Touch localization
   c. Temperature
   d. Joint motion or kinesthesia

2. The OT receives orders to evaluate and treat a client with a T2 SCI. What will be the focus of the sensory testing?
   a. Peripheral nerve distribution
   b. Dermatomal distribution
   c. CNS distribution

3. The OT receives orders to evaluate and treat a 72-year-old client with left hemiplegia secondary to a cerebrovascular accident (CVA). Should the OT include a peripheral nerve, dermatomal, and/or CNS distribution? Please explain the rationale for your response.

4. A 40-year-old client with a newly acquired mild traumatic brain injury and history of diabetes mellitus is referred to the OT for evaluation and treatment. She complains of numbness throughout the thumb region of her right hand. Should the OT include a peripheral nerve distribution, dermatomal distribution, and/or CNS distribution? Please explain the rationale for your response.

5. Use different colors to fill in the different dermatomal distributions (see **Figure 6-1**) and quiz yourself on their locations.

6. Use different colors to fill in the different peripheral nerve distributions (see **Figure 6-2**) and quiz yourself on their locations.

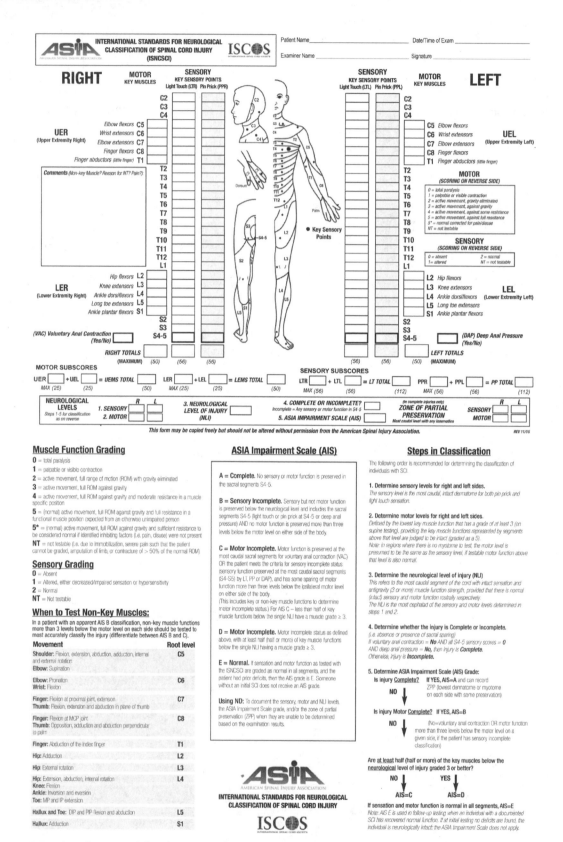

Figure 6-1 UE and LE dermatomal distribution learning activity.

Peripheral Nerve Learning Activity

Color in the following peripheral nerve distributions and then practice completing all peripheral nerve testing for each nerve distribution.

Upper Extremities

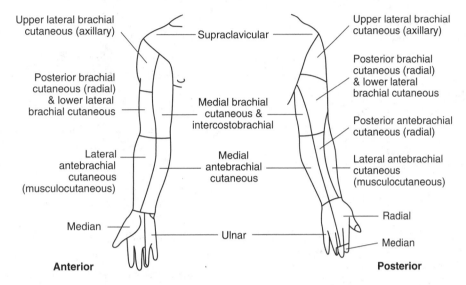

Figure courtesy of The Merck Manual of Diagnosis and Therapy, Edition 18, p. 1754, edited by Mark H. Beers. Copyright 2006 by Merck & Co., Inc., Whitehouse Station, NJ. Available at http://www.merck.com/mmpe. Accessed (February 26, 2009). Please visit all of the Merck Manuals free online at www.MerckManuals.com

Lower Extremities

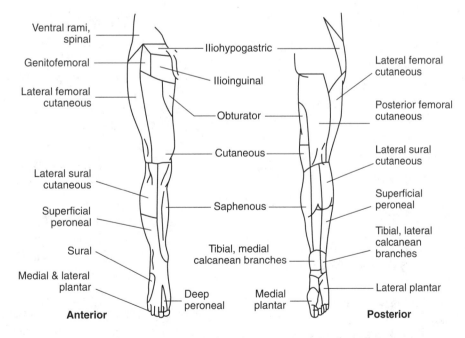

Figure reprinted with permission from The Merck Manual of Diagnosis and Therapy, Edition 18, p. 1754, edited by Mark H. Beers. Copyright 2006 by Merck & Co., Inc., Whitehouse Station, NJ. Available at http://www.merck.com/mmpe. Accessed (February 26, 2009). Please visit all of the Merck Manuals free online at www.MerckManuals.com

Figure 6-2 Peripheral nerve learning activity.

Modified with permission of the authors from: Basic Human Anatomy. O'Rahilly, Müller, Carpenter, & Swenson.

Chapter 6 Self-Study Answers

1. *Correct answer*: C. Pain and temperature will be absent on the left side of the body below the level of the lesion to the right half of the spinal cord. Joint motion, touch localization, and two-point discrimination will likely remain intact.

2. *Correct answer*: B. Peripheral nerve distributions are used for clients who experience trauma to the peripheral nerves either by injury or by disease, and CNS distributions occur when clients sustain head injuries or some other trauma to the brain.

3. Somatosensory examination to evaluate CNS is indicated for this example. The client had a CVA, which commonly affects sensory and motor functions.

4. The OT should assess for somatosensory losses in peripheral nerve distributions secondary to peripheral neuropathies associated with diabetes, in addition to CNS distribution secondary to the traumatic brain injury.

5–6. Please refer to the learning Figures 6-1 and 6-2 for answers.

References

American Spinal Injury Association. (2013). *International Standards for Neurological Classification of Spinal Cord Injury (ISNCSCI)*. Retrieved from http://asia-spinalinjury.org/wp-content/uploads/2016/02/International_Stds_Diagram_Worksheet.pdf

Amini, D. (2014). Motor and praxis assessments. In I. E. Asher (Ed.), *Asher's occupational therapy assessment tools* (4th ed., pp. 441–500). Bethesda, MD: AOTA Press.

Anderson-Preston, L. (2013). Evaluation of motor control. In L. W. Pedretti, H. M. Pendleton, & W. Schultz-Krohn (Eds.), *Pedretti's occupational therapy: Practice skills for physical dysfunction* (7th ed., pp. 461–488). St. Louis, MO: Elsevier.

Beers, M. H., Porter, R. S., & Jones, T. V. (2006). *The Merck manual of diagnosis and therapy* (18th ed.). Whitehouse Station, NJ: Merck Research Laboratories.

Cooper, C., & Canyock, J. D. (2013). Evaluation of sensation and intervention for sensory dysfunction. In L. W. Pedretti, H. M. Pendleton, & W. Schultz-Krohn (Eds.), *Pedretti's occupational therapy: Practice skills for physical dysfunction* (7th ed., pp. 575–589). St. Louis, MO: Elsevier.

Early, M. B. (2012). Physical dysfunction practice skills for the occupational therapy assistant (3rd ed.). St. Louis, MO: Mosby.

Gillen, G. (2013). Cerebrovascular accident/stroke. In L. W. Pedretti, H. M. Pendleton, & W. Schultz-Krohn (Eds.), *Pedretti's occupational therapy: Practice skills for physical dysfunction* (7th ed., pp. 844–880). St. Louis, MO: Elsevier.

James, A. B. (2014). Restoring the role of the independent person. In M. V. Radomski & C. A. T. Latham (Eds.), *Occupational therapy for physical dysfunction* (7th ed., pp. 753–803). Philadelphia, PA: Wolters Kluwer Health/Lippincott Williams & Wilkins.

Killingsworth, A. P., Pedretti, L. W., & Pendleton, H. M. (2013a). Evaluation of muscle strength. In L. W. Pedretti, H. M. Pendleton, & W. Schultz-Krohn (Eds.), *Pedretti's occupational therapy: Practice skills for physical dysfunction* (7th ed., pp. 529–574). St. Louis, MO: Elsevier.

Killingsworth, A. P., Pedretti, L. W., & Pendleton, H. M. (2013b). Joint range of motion. In L. W. Pedretti, H. M. Pendleton, & W. Schultz-Krohn (Eds.), *Pedretti's occupational therapy: Practice skills for physical dysfunction* (7th ed., pp. 497–528). St. Louis, MO: Elsevier.

Latham, C. A. T., & Bentzel, K. (2014). Optimizing sensory abilities and capacities. In M. V. Radomski & C. A. T. Latham (Eds.), *Occupational therapy for physical dysfunction* (7th ed., pp. 681–698). Philadelphia, PA: Wolters Kluwer Health/Lippincott Williams & Wilkins.

Moroz, A. (2015). Physical Therapy (PT): Grades of muscle strength. *Merck manual professional version*. Retrieved from http://www.merckmanuals.com/professional/special-subjects/rehabilitation/physical-therapy-pt

Pendleton, H. M., & Schultz-Krohn, W. (2013). Pedretti's occupational therapy practice skills for physical dysfunction (7th ed.). St. Louis, MO: Elsevier.

Pierre, J. M. (2005). Extrapyramidal symptoms with atypical antipsychotics: Incidence, prevention and management. *Drug Safety*, *28*(3), 191–208. Retrieved from http://www.ncbi.nlm.nih.gov/pubmed/15733025

Radomski, M. V., & Latham, C. A. T. (2014). Occupational therapy for physical dysfunction (7th ed.). Philadelphia, PA: Wolters Kluwer Health/Lippincott Williams & Wilkins.

Theis, J. L. (2014). Assessing abilities and capacities: Sensation. In M. V. Radomski & C. A. T. Latham (Eds.), *Occupational therapy for physical dysfunction* (7th ed., pp. 276–305). Philadelphia, PA: Wolters Kluwer Health/Lippincott Williams & Wilkins.

Whelan, L. R. (2014). Assessing abilities and capacities: Range of motion, strength, and endurance. In M. V. Radomski & C. A. T. Latham (Eds.), *Occupational therapy for physical dysfunction* (7th ed., pp. 145–241). Philadelphia, PA: Wolters Kluwer Health/Lippincott Williams & Wilkins.

Woodson, A. M. (2014). Stroke. In M. V. Radomski & C. A. T. Latham (Eds.), *Occupational therapy for physical dysfunction* (7th ed.). Philadelphia, PA: Wolters Kluwer Health/Lippincott Williams & Wilkins.

The Visual System

Anne Riddering

Learning Objectives

- Describe the key function of each structure of the eye.
- Describe the key function of the visual pathway.
- Describe the impact on vision when a structure of the eye or the visual pathway is injured.
- Describe the eye diseases and injuries covered in this chapter and their impact on vision.
- Compare and contrast the eye diseases and injuries covered in this chapter.
- Summarize occupational therapy low-vision assessment and intervention (i.e., including clinical observations, standardized tests, impact on activities of daily living, and interventions) for the following deficit areas: visual acuity, visual field, contrast sensitivity, oculomotor function, and visual perceptual deficits.

Key Terms

- *Accommodation*: The ability to quickly change focus from near to far (Kaldenberg, 2014; Scheiman, Scheiman, & Whittaker, 2007; Warren, 2013; Weisser-Pike, 2014; Zoltan, 2007).
- *Age-related macular degeneration*: An eye disease caused by deterioration of the eye's macula; resulting in the gradual loss of vision; frequently described as blurriness in the center of vision, and/or darker, lighter, or missing areas of vision (Meibeyer, 2014; Whittaker, Scheiman, & Sokol-McKay, 2015). Visual acuity and contrast sensitivity are affected, causing functional challenges with near-vision tasks, such as reading, writing, and dialing the phone.
- *Contrast sensitivity*: The ability to detect grayness from a background and detect an object that is on a similar color background (Meyers & Wilcox, 2011; Mogk, 2011).
- *Diabetic retinopathy*: Systemic disease of diabetes that affects the blood vessels of the eyes that supply the retina and is typically caused by elevated and fluctuating blood glucose levels (Mogk, 2011; Whittaker et al., 2015).
- *Fixation*: The process of locating and focusing on an object on the fovea; foundation of oculomotor control (Kaldenberg, 2014; Warren, 2013; Weisser-Pike, 2014; Zoltan, 2007).
- *Glaucoma*: An eye disease causing increased intraocular pressure. Increased intraocular pressure causes tissue damage in the retina near the optic nerve (Kaldenberg, 2014; Meibeyer, 2014; Mogk, 2011; Whittaker et al., 2015).
- *Legally blind*: Visual acuity at a level of 20/200 or less (i.e., best-corrected vision in the best eye) or a visual field of 20° or less in the best eye is classified as legal blindness (Meibeyer, 2014).
- *Low vision*: Loss of vision is severe enough to interfere with performance, but allowing some usable vision to be used in daily tasks. There are approximately 1.5 million Americans, aged 45 and older, who have been diagnosed with low vision (Weisser-Pike, 2014). In such instances, loss of visual function is severe enough to interfere with performance, but allows some usable vision to be used in daily tasks. The vision is no longer correctable by conventional measures, such as a change in the prescription of glasses, surgery, or medication. Among adults 85 years and older, 27% report vision issues which impact their ability to complete activities of daily living (Weisser-Pike, 2014).
- *Normal vision*: Visual acuity is defined as 20/30 or better vision and/or the ability to read standard print. The visual field measures

horizontally at approximately 150° and vertically at approximately 120° (Whittaker et al., 2015).

- *Saccades*: Quick, small movements of the eye (i.e., oscillations), used when scanning, allowing us to move from word to word (e.g., reading) or object to object (e.g., searching for object on shelf or driving) (Kaldenberg, 2014; Scheiman et al., 2007; Warren, 2013; Weisser-Pike, 2014; Zoltan, 2007).
- *Snellen chart*: U.S. standard measurement chart, big "e" chart, with the standardized measure based on a ratio of the size of a letter or symbol that a client can read over the distance the client's eyes are from the chart (Meyers & Wilcox, 2011; Mogk, 2011).
- *Visual field*: The visual field is the entire area that the eyes are able to see; normal horizontal field (i.e., left to right) 150°; normal vertical field (i.e., superior to inferior) 120° (Mogk, 2011; Whittaker et al., 2015).

Description

The visual system and how it is applicable to the practice of occupational therapy (OT) is discussed here. The visual system allows us to see an image and interpret or process the image in order to adapt in our environment. The visual system and our ability to "see" can be impacted in several ways:

1. The eye can be injured or a disease can affect a structure or structures in the eye causing a visual impairment;
2. The cranial nerves can be damaged, usually causing oculomotor deficits;
3. The visual pathway can be damaged causing different types of visual field loss based on the location of injury; or
4. A neurologic injury to a specific area in one of the lobes of the brain can cause limitations of visual field, oculomotor deficits, or a visual perception impairment, which will be addressed in Chapter 8.

In this chapter, key regions of the eyeball, cranial nerves, and visual pathway, as well as their corresponding impact on vision, will be discussed. Chapter content will additionally include low-vision assessment, key functions of vision, common vision deficits, and interventions for the entry-level occupational therapy assistants (OTAs).

Vision has several key roles in our daily life. Vision allows us to interact with others (e.g., see facial expressions, observe nonverbal gestures, and see body movements) and our environment by allowing for adaptation of visual motor activities and speed during activities of daily living (ADLs) such as walking. Vision aids in memory and learning and allows us to enjoy our surroundings (e.g., observation of color and details during ADLs, including leisure activities). Vision also helps us to remain safe in our environment by providing information on orientation and spatial relations, as well as allowing us to adapt to maintain balance and respond to early warning signs of danger (e.g., walking on uneven surfaces, medication management, and kitchen safety) (Warren, 2013).

Low-Vision Healthcare Professionals

- *Low-vision professionals*: There are various low-vision professionals involved in the diagnosis and treatment of low vision.
- *Eye care physicians*: Evaluate and diagnose vision deficits and diseases; recommend treatment, including medication, surgery, optical changes, and assistive devices (Warren, 2011; Weisser-Pike, 2014; Whittaker et al., 2015).
- *Ophthalmologist*: A medical doctor who evaluates, treats, and manages structures, functions, and diseases of the eye (Weisser-Pike, 2014; Whittaker et al., 2015).
- *Optometrist*: Professionals with a postgraduate education and training to evaluate the eye's function and ability to diagnose and correct refractive errors with glasses or contact lenses (Warren, 2011; Weisser-Pike, 2014; Whittaker et al., 2015).

Other practitioners involved in low-vision care include the following:

- *Occupational therapist, generalist*: May train clients in some general adaptations for low vision, such as increased lighting and contrast; refers to specialists for more extensive training (Warren, 2011; Whittaker et al., 2015).
- *OTA, generalist: May train clients in some general adaptations for low vision, such as increased lighting and contrast; collaborates with the occupational therapist on therapy strategies.*

- *Occupational therapist, specialist—Specialty Certification in Low Vision (SCLV)*: Professionals who have become involved in the process of ongoing, focused, and targeted professional development in the area of low-vision rehabilitation. An OT specialist may train clients in the use of residual vision to complete ADL; training includes environmental adaptation, compensatory techniques, community training, client and family training, and training with optical and nonoptical devices (Warren, 2011; Weisser-Pike, 2014; Whittaker et al., 2015).
- *Certified low-vision therapist (CLVT)*: Trains clients to use vision more effectively to complete daily activities, with and without devices (Warren, 2011; Weisser-Pike, 2014; Whittaker et al., 2015).
- *Certified vision rehabilitation therapist (CVRT) (i.e., formerly rehabilitation teacher)*: Emphasis of training is on blind techniques (e.g., teaching Braille), assistive technology, and device use for persons who are blind or have low vision (Warren, 2011; Weisser-Pike, 2014; Whittaker et al., 2015).
- *Certified orientation and mobility specialist (O&M; COMS)*: Teach clients in systematic, efficient techniques to remain oriented and safe when traveling using long canes, a sighted guide, or dog guide (Warren, 2011; Weisser-Pike, 2014; Whittaker et al., 2015).

Warren's Visual Perceptual Hierarchy

Picture a pyramid or a house. On the bottom, there is a base or the foundation. Similarly, there are basic skills that need to be mastered before moving to higher levels. We want to build upon previously mastered skills, similar to putting the second story on the house and then the roof (Warren, 2013; Zoltan, 2007). This hierarchy is a very important piece to study because you may need to identify functional activities and skills that are appropriate given a client's hierarchical status. Basic level or foundational skills include the following:

- Oculomotor control is defined as efficient movement of the eyes in a coordinated manner allowing for perceptual stability; includes eye alignment, accommodation, convergence and divergence, saccadic eye movements, and smooth pursuit eye movements (i.e., tracking) (Warren, 2013; Weisser-Pike, 2014; Zoltan, 2007). In both eyes together, there are 12 muscles (i.e., motor) and 6 cranial nerves (i.e., sensory) that contribute to these skills.
- The visual field is the entire area that the eyes are able to see; the normal horizontal field (i.e., left to right) 150°; and the normal vertical field (i.e., superior to inferior) 120° (Whittaker et al., 2015) (described in more detail in the low-vision section of this chapter).
- Visual acuity is the ability of the eye to distinguish the fine details of what is seen (Warren, 2013).
- Intermediate-level skills include components of visual attention, which is the identification of the body, the environment around one's body, and the relationship between the two; the ability to search, scan, and identify an object and filter out unnecessary details (Warren, 2013; Weisser-Pike, 2014). Alertness is the most basic type of attention (Zoltan, 2007). Attention allows us to determine the gross features of a task or of the environment (i.e., the "what" and "where" of the task or environment). Attention has several categories, including the following:
  - Ambient or peripheral attention is the detection in the peripheral environment and relationship to the person.
  - Selective or focal attention involves the visual details (Gillen, 2009; Warren, 2013).
- *Scanning or visual search*: The ability to search the environment, focus on the most important details to interpret and correctly identify; accomplished using saccadic eye movements; scanning is a result of visual attention (Warren, 2013).
- *Pattern recognition*: Recognition of relevant details of an object; uses specific details to discriminate an object from its background (Warren, 2013; Zoltan, 2007).
  - Identification of general characteristics includes shape and outline.
  - Identification of specific characteristics includes color, shape, and texture.
  - Disorders include lack of visual discrimination.

Advanced-level skills facilitate complex visual analysis and form the basis for academic learning (e.g., reading, writing, and mathematics). Disorders include agnosia, alexia, visual closure, figure ground, and spatial relations (Zoltan, 2007). Advanced-level skills include the following:

- Visual memory, which involves proficiency in taking, retaining, and processing a mental picture of an object; includes storing and retrieving images from short- and long-term memory (Warren, 2013; Zoltan, 2007).
- Visual cognition is defined as "The ability to manipulate and integrate visual input with other sensory information to gain knowledge, solve problems, formulate plans, and make decisions" (Warren, 2013, p. 597).

Highest on the pyramid are mastery-level skills, which include adaptive responses as listed below:

- Adaptation through vision occurs when one is able to filter, organize, and process information acquired through the visual system to adapt to the environment. This adaptive response requires one to use visual perceptual skills, other pertinent sensory information, and cognitive concepts throughout the integrated central nervous system (CNS) process (Warren, 2013; Zoltan, 2007).

Anatomical and Physiologic Structures Related to Vision

Prior to discussing assessments and interventions for low vision, it is important to become familiar with the key anatomical structures related to vision. The key structures of the eyeball are as follows:

- *Cornea*: Outermost transparent layer protecting the eye; assists in light refraction
- *Iris*: Colored part of the eye; muscular ring that controls the amount of light that enters the eye by dilating and constricting the pupil
- *Lens*: Biconvex structure that bends light to focus rays on the retina
- *Ciliary body*: Muscle and fluid that aid the focusing of the lens
- *Vitreous*: Clear gel-like substance that maintains the shape of the eye
- *Sclera*: Tough coating of the eye that protects the inner structures

- *Choroid*: Layer between the sclera and the retina that contains the blood vessels of the eye
- *Retina*: Multilayer, sensory structure for the eye that contains rods and cones; initiates impulses to the visual cortex via the optic nerve
- *Macula*: Area of the retina that is the area of best vision
- *Fovea*: Center of the macula where the focus area of vision is located
- *Optic nerve*: Carries the picture to the brain for interpretation (Mogk, 2011; Warren, 2013; Whittaker et al., 2015)

There are four rectus muscles and two oblique muscles around the eye. The rectus muscles adduct and abduct, and depress and elevate the eye, while the oblique muscles move the eye inward and down, as well as outward and up. The extraocular muscles are as follows:

- *Rectus muscles* (4):
  1. *Medial*: Function is adduction.
  2. *Lateral*: Function is abduction.
  3. *Inferior*: Function is depression.
  4. *Superior*: Function is elevation (Gillen, 2009; Whittaker et al., 2015).
- *Oblique muscles* (2):
  1. *Superior*: Function is turning inward and down; longest, thinnest muscle.
  2. *Inferior*: Function is turning outward and up (Gillen, 2009; Whittaker et al., 2015).

Cranial Nerves

There are six cranial nerves that impact vision and the cranial nerves and their contributions to vision are as follows:

1. *Optic nerve (II)*: Tract of brain; cells originate in the retina and axon fibers group together to form the optic nerve; optic nerves travel posteriorly then cross at the optic chiasm with neurons leading to the visual cortex in the occipital lobe.
2. *Oculomotor nerve (III)*: Controls four eye muscles: medial rectus (adduction), inferior rectus (i.e., depression), superior rectus (i.e., elevation), and inferior oblique (i.e., outward and upward).
   - Controls dilation and constriction of the pupil.
   - Controls positioning of eyelid.
   - Controls the accommodation process or focusing of the eye.

3. *Trochlear nerve (IV)*: Controls the superior oblique muscle (i.e., inward and downward).
4. *Trigeminal nerve (V)*: Ophthalmic branch supplies sensory fibers to the upper eyelid, eyeball, and skin surrounding the eyes.
5. *Abducens nerve (VI)*: Controls the lateral rectus muscle (i.e., abduction of the eye).
6. *Facial nerve (VII)*: Controls closing your eyelid (Gillen, 2009; Whittaker et al., 2015).

Visual Pathway

In order to understand visual pathways, you must first gain a basic understanding of the structures and roles they play in vision. The visual pathways are as follows:

- *Optic nerve*: Cranial nerve II carries the visual message beginning in the retina and contains fibers from one eye.
- *Optic chiasm*: The point at which the optic nerve fibers cross; the medial half of each eye crosses to the opposite side and travels along with the information from the other eye.
- *Optic tract*: Carries the visual message from the optic chiasm to the thalamus of the brain and contains fibers from both eyes.
- *Lateral geniculate nucleus of the thalamus*: Structure at which fibers of the optic tract synapse, assists the CNS to filter out input that is not needed and refines the image.
- *Visual cortex*: Area of the occipital lobe in which enhancement of an image occurs before it is cortically processed (Gillen, 2009; Mogk, 2011; Warren, 2013; Whittaker et al., 2015; Zoltan, 2007).

When some of these structures are damaged, patterns of vision loss may include deficits by either a partial or complete lesion in the optic tract (see **Figure 7-1**). The following list outlines the impact of lesions with structures involved in the visual pathway as previously described:

- Lesions to the optic nerve, located between the eyeball and the optic chiasm, will cause a partial or total loss of vision on the side of the lesion (i.e., the right optic nerve causes loss of vision of the right eye).
- Lesions to the optic chiasm will cause a loss of vision to the temporal half of the visual field in both eyes (i.e., the outer half of vision in both eyes).

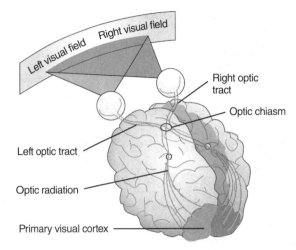

Figure 7-1 The visual system.

- Lesions on the optic tract, between the optic chiasm and the lateral geniculate body, causes opposite half of the visual field to be lost in both eyes (i.e., the right optic tract causes loss of the left visual field in both eyes).
- Lesions to the optic radiations can cause a quadrant loss, called a quadrantanopia (Gillen, 2009; Zoltan, 2007).

The Lobes of the Brain

In addition to the previous background on the visual system, the lobes of the brain have specific roles and functions as well. For example, the occipital lobe contains the visual cortex, which is responsible for scanning, identification of objects, awareness, and discrimination. Visual field deficits (i.e., partial to complete visual field loss), scanning deficits, and agnosia may be present (Gillen, 2009; Whittaker et al., 2015). The frontal lobe is responsible for attention and initiation of movement. Fixation and saccade deficits, slowed responses in periphery, and reduced speed in visual motor tasks may be observed (Gillen, 2009; Whittaker et al., 2015). The parietal and temporal lobes may present with visual field loss as a result of damage in these lobes (Gillen, 2009; Whittaker et al., 2015). The thalamus, cerebellum, and brainstem have additional specific functions as outlined below:

- *Thalamus*: Eye movement; integration of visual and cognitive information (Gillen, 2009; Zoltan, 2007).
- *Cerebellum*: Eye control and coordination (Gillen, 2009; Whittaker et al., 2015).
- *Brainstem*: Protective eye responses; the cranial nerves run through it.

Eye movement deficits (i.e., eye control and coordination), visual and cognitive processing deficits, and praxis (i.e., motor perception) are deficits that could be observed based on damage to these areas of the brain (Gillen, 2009; Zoltan, 2007).

Basic OT Intervention Approaches

OT intervention approaches fall into two categories including restorative or remedial and adaptive or compensatory.

1. *Restorative or remedial approach*: Using a restorative or remedial approach, the goal of the therapy is to develop increased organization in the brain by enhancing brain recovery in order to improve the client's abilities during completion of ADLs (Warren, 2013; Zoltan, 2007). Activities are chosen that meet the client's current level of function, and more difficult tasks are slowly introduced to improve independence. Repetition of exercises working on a particular component skill can help increase organization.

2. *Adaptive or compensatory approach*: The goal when using an adaptive or compensatory approach is to encourage adaptation to the environment for ADL completion by using compensatory techniques, based on activity analysis, or by modifying the environment or activity to change client performance (Warren, 2013; Zoltan, 2007). Adaptations are practiced in a variety of settings so they become automatic.

Visual Impairments

This next section of the chapter will focus on specific visual impairments in terms of a brief description, clinical presentation, and common prognosis and treatment.

Refractive Errors

Refractive errors are not diseases. They are caused by the shape of the eyeball and affect approximately 42 million Americans older than age 40. These are usually correctable with glasses or by surgery such as Lasik (laser-assisted in situ keratomileusis) (Nowakowski, 2011; Scheiman et al., 2007; Warren, 2013; Whittaker et al., 2015).

- *Myopia (nearsightedness)* is the result of an elongated eyeball, front to back, causing light rays entering to converge focus before they get to the retina. Near objects are clear while distant objects are blurred. This is corrected with a concave lens (Nowakowski, 2011; Scheiman et al., 2007; Warren, 2013; Whittaker et al., 2015).
- *Hyperopia (farsightedness)* is the result of a short eyeball, front to back, which causes light rays entering the eye to reach the retina before they have converged to a point of focus (i.e., they pass the retina before converging) (Nowakowski, 2011; Scheiman et al., 2007; Warren, 2013; Whittaker et al., 2015). This is corrected with a convex lens.
- *Astigmatism* is the result of a cornea that is oval instead of round, causing light rays to converge at more than one point of focus (Nowakowski, 2011; Scheiman et al., 2007; Warren, 2013; Whittaker et al., 2015).
- *Presbyopia*: In childhood, near and distance vision is clear because the lens can change its shape to converge light rays. In adulthood (i.e., older than 40 years) people may experience blurred images in near, more than distant, vision, because the lenses become stiff and the ability to focus is diminished or lost (Nowakowski, 2011; Scheiman et al., 2007; Warren, 2013; Whittaker et al., 2015).

People with nearsightedness older than 40 years can see near as long as they are not wearing their distance glasses; with glasses they need a bifocal to see near, which may be clear glass. People with farsightedness older than 40 years need more power to see near than they do for distance. Others who may not need a bifocal are those who have one eye nearsighted and the other eye normal for distance (i.e., natural monovision) or people who are nearsighted and take their glasses off to read. If a client has not had a recent comprehensive (i.e., dilated) eye exam, the OT should refer the client to an optometrist or ophthalmologist. Refractive errors are correctable with glasses.

Diseases Causing Peripheral Vision Loss

Peripheral vision impacts one's peripheral visual field, often causing difficulty with mobility tasks. Contrast sensitivity may also be decreased, glare sensitivity may be increased, and the ability to see at night may be decreased (i.e., night blindness) while light/dark adaptation may be slowed (Kaldenberg, 2014; Meibeyer, 2014; Mogk, 2011).

Retinitis Pigmentosa (RP)

- *Description*: A hereditary condition causing slow, progressive field loss that may lead to blindness (Kaldenberg, 2014; Meibeyer, 2014; Mogk, 2011).
- *Clinical presentation*: Decreased visual acuity; sensitivity to light (i.e., photophobia); constriction of the peripheral visual field; night blindness (Kaldenberg, 2014; Meibeyer, 2014; Mogk, 2011). Functional problems may include near, intermediate, or distance vision tasks, depending on the stage of the disease.
- *Common prognosis and treatment of disease*: No known cure; optical aids, long cane techniques, substitution techniques, and visual rehabilitation training depending on the extent of the deficit (Kaldenberg, 2014; Meibeyer, 2014; Mogk, 2011).

Glaucoma

- *Description*: Acute attack due to the inability of aqueous humor to drain, causing increased intraocular pressure. Increased intraocular pressure causes tissue damage in the retina near the optic nerve (Kaldenberg, 2014; Meibeyer, 2014; Mogk, 2011; Whittaker et al., 2015).
- *Clinical presentation*: Severe redness, pain in the eye, headache, or nausea (Kaldenberg, 2014; Meibeyer, 2014; Mogk, 2011). Functional problems may include near, intermediate, or distance vision tasks, depending on the stage of the disease.
- *Common prognosis and treatment of disease*: Emergency surgery, either large laser hole or an incision to allow the aqueous humor to drain quickly and intraocular pressure to drop. If left untreated for too long, permanent damage can result, causing loss of visual acuity and field (Kaldenberg, 2014; Meibeyer, 2014; Mogk, 2011).

Chronic Open Angle Glaucoma (COAG)

- *Description*: Blockage in the drainage system of the eye (i.e., trabecular meshwork) that increases the pressure in the eye and puts pressure on the optic nerve (i.e., chronic episode is the most common type) (Kaldenberg, 2014; Meibeyer, 2014; Mogk, 2011; Whittaker et al., 2015).
- *Clinical presentation*: Decreased visual acuity and peripheral fields; light sensitivity in some cases; no pain (Kaldenberg, 2014; Meibeyer, 2014; Mogk, 2011). Functional problems may include near, intermediate, or distance vision tasks, depending on the stage of the disease. With progression, glaucoma may cause difficulty with night vision, mobility deficits, and eventually central field loss, affecting near-vision tasks.
- *Common prognosis and treatment*: Eye drops or several different types of drops to decrease production of the aqueous humor. Eye tissue damage is preventable with regular monitoring and treatment of intraocular pressure; decreased visual acuity or peripheral fields result if the disease is left untreated. Progression of vision loss is from mid-peripheral vision to outer vision and lastly the central visual field (Kaldenberg, 2014; Meibeyer, 2014; Mogk, 2011).

All types of glaucoma affect approximately 2 million Americans but in many people, the disease is controlled and does not cause low vision (Kaldenberg, 2014; Meibeyer, 2014; Mogk, 2011; Whittaker et al., 2015).

Diseases affecting central vision most often affect one's visual acuity. Visual acuity is the ability to detect the details of an object. Visual acuity can be affected at different distances: near, intermediate, and far. Contrast sensitivity may also be decreased; glare sensitivity may be increased; ability to see at night may be decreased (e.g., night blindness); and light/dark adaptation may be slowed (Kaldenberg, 2014; Meibeyer, 2014; Mogk, 2011).

Diseases Causing Central Vision Loss

Age-Related Macular Degeneration (ARMD or AMD)

- *Description*: Leading cause of visual impairment in adults 60 years and older, with an estimated 1.8 million Americans affected (Meibeyer, 2014). The incidence of ARMD is likely to rise because the number of seniors is increasing. Risk factors for macular degeneration may include smoking, air pollution, sunlight, and deficient nutrition (e.g., diets low in green leafy vegetables, fish, and fruit) (Whittaker et al., 2015).

- *Clinical presentation*: Gradual loss causes a blurry area in the center of vision that some people describe as a black area, missing area, or lighter area (Meibeyer, 2014; Whittaker et al., 2015). Visual acuity and contrast sensitivity are affected. Functional problems usually include near-vision tasks such as reading, writing, and dialing the phone. Decreased contrast sensitivity causes difficulty with tasks such as curbs, steps, seeing faces, and pouring milk into a light-colored cup.
- *Common prognosis and treatment of two types*:
  1. *Dry AMD*: Drusen deposits form in the retina, increasing in number to form scotomas (i.e., scarred areas) in the macula (Meibeyer, 2014; Mogk, 2011).
  2. *Wet AMD*: Abnormal vessel growth under the retina; the vessels leak fluid, causing damage to the cells of the macula (Meibeyer, 2014; Mogk, 2011).

Both types cause deterioration of the retinal cells in the macula and fovea. Only the central vision of the macula is affected, causing scotomas (i.e., scarred areas); reduced contrast sensitivity and visual acuity (Meibeyer, 2014; Mogk, 2011). Nutritional supplements are recommended for people who are diagnosed with wet or dry types to slow the progression of the disease. Current treatment for wet-type AMD uses antivascular endothelial growth factor (anti-VEGF) drugs to retard the progression of the disease (Meibeyer, 2014; Mogk, 2011). Since AMD is considered a progressive disease, clients with AMD will benefit from vision rehabilitation, starting at the early stages, in order to learn to use residual vision, compensatory strategies, and nonoptical and optical devices for completion of ADLs.

Retinal Degenerations Affecting Central Vision

- *Description*: There are several different degenerative diseases that affect the retinal tissue. Best disease is an autosomal dominant disease, usually diagnosed in childhood and affects central vision. Stargardt disease is an autosomal recessive disease, usually diagnosed in childhood that affects central vision

(Meibeyer, 2014). Other less common diagnoses might include myopic degeneration or macular hole.

- *Clinical presentation*: Affects central vision with functional problems relating to near-vision tasks and contrast sensitivity (Meibeyer, 2014).
- *Common prognosis and treatment of disease*: This varies depending on the disease but most clients with these diseases will have remaining vision that may or may not progressively worsen (Meibeyer, 2014). Rehabilitation emphasizes using the remaining vision efficiently during ADLs.

Diseases Causing Nonspecific Vision Loss

Nonspecific vision loss does not have one pattern of vision loss, which can affect central vision, peripheral vision, or both (Mogk, 2011).

Cataracts

- *Description*: Typically caused by age-related clouding and hardening of the lens of the eye, but may also result from disease, trauma, and/or congenital (e.g., hereditary) factors (Mogk, 2011; Whittaker et al., 2015).
- *Clinical presentation*: Decreased acuity, progressively blurred, hazy, or unclear vision in both the central and peripheral visual fields (Mogk, 2011; Whittaker et al., 2015). The client may complain of dulled colors, increased sensitivity to glare indoors and/or outdoors. Near vision may be better than distance vision.
- *Common prognosis and treatment of disease*: Treatment options include lens replacement with an artificial lens and the use of prescription glasses and/or contact lenses (Mogk, 2011; Whittaker et al., 2015). In the United States, prognosis is good and cataracts rarely cause permanent blindness. In less-developed countries, where surgery may not be readily available, cataracts cause a higher rate of visual impairment and blindness. After surgery, a person will not have the ability to accommodate for near-vision tasks, but this is usually correctable with glasses or a prescription in the intraocular lens (Mogk, 2011; Whittaker et al., 2015).

Retinopathy of Prematurity (ROP)

- *Description*: ROP, also called retrolental fibroplasia, occurs when premature birth interrupts the process of developing blood vessels to the retina (Mogk, 2011). Normal vessels may stop growing. The edges of the retina may not get enough oxygen and nutrients. Blood vessels may constrict and new abnormal and fragile blood vessels can leak into the vitreous or cause a retinal detachment (Mogk, 2011).
- *Clinical presentation*: Decreased visual acuity, scarring, and retinal detachment can cause possible field loss or blindness (Mogk, 2011).
- *Common prognosis and treatment of disease*: Permanent vision loss of varying degrees may occur but usually does not progressively get worse (Mogk, 2011). Secondary complications include glaucoma, increased occurrence of retinal detachment, inflammation of the uvea, increased risk for strabismus (i.e., crossed eyes), and amblyopia (i.e., lazy eye). Vision rehabilitation starting at a young age includes the use of optical aids, glare control, long cane techniques, substitution techniques, and visual rehabilitation training (Mogk, 2011).

Albinism

- *Description*: Albinism (i.e., a total or partial loss of pigment) is a hereditary disease causing an underdeveloped macula of the retina (Mogk, 2011).
- *Clinical presentation*: The disease causes decreased acuity, usually between 20/70 and 20/200, nystagmus (i.e., involuntary oscillation of the eyeballs), and extreme light sensitivity (Mogk, 2011). The person with ocular albinism may have a high refractive error and astigmatism, and the impact on the visual field may vary.
- *Common prognosis and treatment of disease*: A nonprogressive disease; however, individuals will benefit from corrective glasses and/or contacts, glare control, and optical aids, and training for ADLs should start at an early age (i.e., school age) (Mogk, 2011).

Diabetic Retinopathy

- *Description*: Systemic disease of diabetes, affects the blood vessels of the eyes that supply the retina, and

is typically caused by elevated and fluctuating blood glucose levels (Mogk, 2011; Whittaker et al., 2015). Background diabetic retinopathy (BDR): Changes in the small retinal vessels also cause macular edema (Mogk, 2011; Whittaker et al., 2015). Proliferative diabetic retinopathy (PDR): New, abnormal vessels grow as a replacement for the damaged vessels (i.e., neovascularization). The new vessels tend to be weak and bleed, causing further damage (Mogk, 2011; Whittaker et al., 2015).
- *Clinical presentation*: Common symptoms include spotted areas of vision (i.e., Swiss cheese effect); fluctuations in vision based on glucose levels; decreased visual acuity, contrast sensitivity, color vision, and night vision; temporary diplopia (i.e., neuropathy affecting CN III or VI) (Mogk, 2011; Whittaker et al., 2015).
- *Common prognosis and treatment of disease*: Individuals with diabetic retinopathy are at increased risk for cataracts, glaucoma, and retinal detachments (Mogk, 2011). Treatments vary but may include surgery or procedures to retard the progression of the disease. The disease is progressive and can affect both the central and/or peripheral vision. If left untreated, it can cause blindness. It is important to rigorously monitor glucose daily, exercise regularly, and follow a diet to help maintain glucose levels. Individuals with diabetic retinopathy will benefit from individualized rehabilitation to address ADL limitations at near, intermediate, and far distances (Mogk, 2011; Whittaker et al., 2015).

Screening and Assessment

Measuring distance and near visual acuity: Visual acuity is the ability to recognize the small details of the object; good acuity allows for speed and accuracy in processing what is seen and aids in decision making (Freeman, 2015; Mogk, 2011).

Snellen charts: A standardized measure based on a ratio of the size of a letter or symbol a client can read over the distance the client's eyes are from the chart (e.g., U.S. standard measurement chart or the big "e" chart) (Meyers & Wilcox, 2011; Mogk, 2011). A person with 20/70 vision can see the same size object at 20 feet that a person with normal vision can see at 70 feet. Test the client with the best correction (e.g., wearing glasses). Test one eye at a time, then both eyes together. Test near acuity (i.e., reading distance) at 16 inches and distance acuity at approximately 20 feet.

Other charts: Single-letter charts may include single letters, numbers, symbols, or tumbling "e" charts (e.g., for clients with aphasia, non-English speaking, and children) (Meyers & Wilcox, 2011; Mogk, 2011). Examples include the Colenbrander, EDTRS, and SK Read charts (i.e., standardized). Continuous print (i.e., words and sentences) charts measure a person's ability to see multiple letters at one time to read continuous print (Meyers & Wilcox, 2011; Mogk, 2011). Examples include the Colenbrander continuous print chart and MNREAD chart (i.e., standardized).

Informal Measures and Clinical Observations

Near acuity deficits include activities involving reading, writing, and fine motor coordination (e.g., reading labels on medication or food, setting appliance dials, threading a needle, reading bills, writing checks, identifying money, and pouring). Difficulty may be apparent through socialization and communication with others (e.g., dialing the phone, writing a letter, and reading newsletters). Clients may be embarrassed by difficulty eating, such as cutting and seasoning food. Safety during ADLs may include the following: cooking (e.g., cutting, chopping, and slicing); and accessing emergency assistance (e.g., via phone) (Gillen, 2009; Kaldenberg, 2014; Meibeyer, 2014; Meyers & Wilcox, 2011; Warren, 2013; Weisser-Pike, 2014; Zoltan, 2007).

Near acuity deficits: The following are examples of clinical observations that are typically seen with near acuity deficits:

- The client moves the reading material to one side of midline (i.e., horizontal or vertical) and/or toward the eyes, then away as if trying to bring the print into focus (Mogk, 2011).
- The client changes head position often to try to locate a clear area.
- The client is unable to stay on a line when writing or loses track of the tip of the pen. Complaints include needing more light, print being too faint, too small, blurred, or fuzzy, and difficulty reading small print.

Distance and intermediate acuity deficits typically include activities involving reading, writing, and fine motor coordination (e.g., reading room numbers, street signs, and store signs, seeing the television, bowling pins, or a ball on golf course, difficulty driving, seeing cards on the middle of a table, playing board games, reading computer screens, or seeing letters on a keyboard). Socialization and communication with others may be difficult (e.g., difficulty emailing, seeing food at a buffet, reading directions, or restroom signs). Safety during ADLs may include difficulty with driving, reading signs for emergency exit procedures, and stove and oven safety (Gillen, 2009; Kaldenberg, 2014; Meibeyer, 2014; Meyers & Wilcox, 2011; Warren, 2013; Weisser-Pike, 2014; Zoltan, 2007).

Distance and intermediate acuity deficits: The following are examples of clinical observations typically seen with distance and intermediate acuity deficits:

- The client has difficulty navigating or driving, seeing bowling pins, or following a ball on a golf course.
- Visual acuity and occupational performance deficits include complaints of difficulty reading signs, seeing stop lights, seeing the television, reading the computer monitor or sheet music, or playing cards or bingo.

Interventions

Lighting: When possible, increase available room lighting. Increase task lighting; explore use of different types of lighting (e.g., incandescent and fluorescent, light-emitting diode (LED), halogen, full spectrum, and natural lighting from a window). For near tasks, position lighting closest to the better eye; for fine motor tasks, place the light opposite the writing hand to minimize shadows. Control glare, such as adjusting blinds and window shades; yellow sunglasses may help indoor, and yellow and amber sunglasses, hats, and visors may help control glare outdoors.

Magnification: Relative size magnification: Use large-print books, clocks, checks and check registers, playing cards and board games, pillboxes, and glucose monitors. Relative distance magnification involves moving objects closer to the eyes (e.g., print closer to the face, or eyes and body closer to the object) (Freeman, 2015; Kaldenberg, 2014; Nowakowski, 2011). Low-vision physicians usually recommend optical devices. Handheld devices are small enough to hold or fit inside pockets.

Illuminated and nonilluminated versions must be held at a specific distance to maintain focus, which is difficult for individuals with tremors.

Stand magnifiers:

- Set focus distance.
- Illuminated and nonilluminated versions.
- Not portable.
- Easier to use for individuals with hand problems (e.g., arthritis and tremors).
- Head-worn devices, including microscopic glasses, high-powered spectacles, and clip-on lenses.
- Offer a wide field of view, and hands are free for tasks.
- Many models are portable.
- Binocular viewing and increased reading speed for some models.
- Must hold reading materials close to the eyes to maintain focus, but light may be obstructed when held close (Kaldenberg, 2014; Nowakowski, 2011).

Electronic magnification devices or closed-circuit televisions (CCTVs):

- Greatest range of magnification and largest field of view.
- Digital technology allows for optimal adjustments, clear and crisp magnification.
- Desktop and portable color models.
- Can change background color, contrast, and magnification.
- More expensive than standard handheld and stand magnifiers.
- Improving features, such as automatic scroll of reading material, optical character recognition (OCR) readers built into CCTV, and interfaces with a computer (Kaldenberg, 2014; Nowakowski, 2011).

Telescopic devices are used mainly for spotting in the distance; some can be used at intermediate or near distance and include the following types:

- *Monocular*: Portable, although difficult to use with tremors or with large scotomas. May require manual focusing for changes in distance.
- *Binocular*: Portable, lightweight, and allows for a wider field of view (i.e., as compared to monocular).
- *Bioptics*: Individually fitted telescope (e.g., monocular or binocular style) that are mounted on the upper portion of glasses. The individual dips their head and spots objects. In some states, bioptics can be used for driving (e.g., with one eye only) (Kaldenberg, 2014; Nowakowski, 2011).

To use magnifiers correctly and efficiently may require extensive practice; especially before a task such as driving.

Visual Field

The visual field is the entire area that the eyes are able to see (Mogk, 2011). Normal visual field is classified by the following: superior 60°; inferior 75°; nasal side 60°; temporal side 100° (Warren, 2011). Damage can occur to the retina or along the optic pathway [e.g., cerebrovascular accident (CVA) or traumatic brain injury (TBI)] with the location determining the pattern of vision loss.

Central visual field: The center 10° is called the fovea and is responsible for identifying details. When the fovea is damaged, an individual will have visual acuity deficits (Mogk, 2011) (see previous section). Scotomas, or scarred areas, form in the central vision. The pattern of vision loss can impact performance during ADLs and individuals may not be aware of a scotoma due to the brain's ability to perceptually complete or fill in the blind area (Mogk, 2011). Physicians who specialize in low vision can assess scotomas, as well as OT practitioners who specialize in low vision (Whittaker et al., 2015).

Peripheral visual field: Peripheral field (i.e., all of the field except the fovea) is responsible for identification of shapes, forms, and movement in the environment. Peripheral fields aid mobility.

Assessments for Central Field

- The automated macular perimetry is an automated central field (i.e., macular perimetry) test, usually administered at a large low-vision center (e.g., scanning laser ophthalmoscope with macular perimetry, Macular Integrity Assessment (MAIA) or Nidek MP-1) (i.e., standardized) (Barstow & Crossland, 2011; Weisser-Pike, 2014; Whittaker et al., 2015).
- The California Central Field Test uses a laminated field template placed on a reading stand and laser pointer to plot out the seeing and nonseeing areas with scotomas (i.e., nonstandardized) (Barstow & Crossland, 2011).
- The Damato 30-Point Campimeter is a portable test card that measures the central 30° of the visual field and is included as part of the Brain Injury Visual Assessment Battery for Adults (biVABA) (i.e., standardized) (Warren, 2013).
- The Pepper Visual Skills for Reading Test (VSRT) is a functional standardized test that indicates scotomas and their impact on function (Barstow & Crossland, 2011).

Assessments for Peripheral Visual Field

- The Goldmann Visual Field Test is a manual bowl perimetry administered at the office of an optometrist or ophthalmologist (i.e., standardized) (Warren, 2013).
- The Humphrey Visual Field Test is an automated bowl perimetry administered at the office of an optometrist or ophthalmologist (i.e., standardized) (Warren, 2013).
- Confrontation testing involves gross examination of visual fields in which a therapist sits in front of the client and instructs the client to focus on the therapist's eyes while the therapist brings in two targets from different areas in the field (Weisser-Pike, 2014; Whittaker et al., 2015). The client indicates if targets are seen and where they are seen. Confrontation testing can also be administered with two therapists; the person standing behind the client presents the targets. This is not a reliable visual field test but rather a gross assessment (i.e., nonstandardized) (Weisser-Pike, 2014; Whittaker et al., 2015).
- A tangent screen includes the use of a black felt screen with a grid visible only to the examiner. The client is 1 meter away and asked to fixate on a target affixed to the center of the screen. A white target (i.e., affixed to a black wand) is moved around the screen. The client indicates when the target is seen. The client's indication of when the target is seen, and unseen, allows the therapist to plot visual field deficits (i.e., nonstandardized) (Warren, 2013; Whittaker et al., 2015).
- The Pepper VSRT is a functional standardized test that can indicate peripheral vision loss, especially with central field involvement (Whittaker et al., 2015).
- The Dynavision 2000 is an automated machine that allows for objective assessment of a person's ability to execute scanning strategies, speed and accuracy of scanning, visual motor performance, and one's ability to shift and divide attention. The Dynavision is frequently used for training, but can be used to establish quantitative baseline function (Warren, 2013).

Clinical Observations for Visual Field Deficits

Central field deficits usually impact near acuity or vision tasks (i.e., as discussed in the previous section of this chapter, which explains visual acuity deficits).

Peripheral visual field clinical observations may be present during reading, as clients may omit letters or words, consistently lose their place on one side of the page or when finding the next line, or require the use of their finger to maintain their place on the page (Warren, 2013). Mobility can provide cues for the therapist. Many clients watch their feet when walking, may have poor navigational skills and get lost easily, avoid obstacles in familiar areas but collide or come close to obstacles in unfamiliar areas, stay close to one side of the hallway, use their fingers to trail the wall as a tactile guide, experience difficulty navigating in crowded areas, stop walking when approaching or passing another person, and/or refuse to take the lead when ambulating as they prefer to follow others. Additional ADLs that may be affected include having poor or absent eye contact, complaints of seeing one-half of an image or darker objects on one side, difficulty judging distances, reluctant to change head position or holds head to one side, displace writing to one side when completing a form or drift off line, and/or become upset with others who leave items out or return them to a different location.

Peripheral Visual Field Deficits and Occupational Performance

Due to reduced perceptual span, reading speed, and accuracy, clients frequently miss letters, have difficulty reading long words or difficulty locating the next line when reading or writing, and may lose his or her place when writing. Superior field cuts tend to cause more difficulty with reading (i.e., near and distance), writing, and tabletop activities (e.g., cutting, chopping, stove top, cards, and medication management) (Warren, 2013). Deficits involving mobility may include difficulty walking, shuffling feet, frequent bumps, trips, stumbles, and falls that may cause difficulty walking in unfamiliar areas. Inferior field loss can also cause decreased balance, difficulty seeing steps or curbs, and identifying visual landmarks. Socialization and communication with others may be evident with difficulty entering a room, locating a friend in a restaurant, locating an empty chair in a room, navigating in crowded rooms and stores, and eventual reluctance to use a long cane for mobility due to social stigma. Safety during ADLs may also place the individual at greater risk for falls secondary to visual field deficits (Whittaker et al., 2015).

Interventions

Lighting

When possible, increase available room lighting. Increase task lighting by exploring the use of different types of lighting (e.g., incandescent, fluorescent, LED, halogen, full spectrum, and natural lighting from window). For near tasks, position lighting closest to the better eye. For fine motor tasks, place light opposite of the writing hand to minimize shadows (Kaldenberg, 2014; Whittaker et al., 2015).

Control Glare

Adjust blinds and window shades; yellow sunglasses may help indoors, and yellow and amber sunglasses, hats, and visors may help control glare outdoors (Kaldenberg, 2014; Whittaker et al., 2015).

Scanning Training

Educate the client about field boundaries and perceptual completion or a CNS process in which a visual scene is completed although only part of the information is seen visually (Warren, 2013). Train the use of organized search patterns (e.g., left to right, up and down); increase speed, scope, organization, and accuracy; generalize patterns into everyday ADLs (Riddering, 2011). Functional activities include card searches, word searches, locating items in a cupboard or on a grocery shelf, wiping off counters, sorting laundry, and scanning courses.

Safety Adaptations

Educate the client and caregiver about safety hazards in the home and how to maximize safe completion of ADLs. Provide both physical and verbal cues.

Contrast Sensitivity

Definition: The ability to detect grayness from a background and detect an object that is on a similar color background. This skill tends to decrease with age (Meyers & Wilcox, 2011; Mogk, 2011).

Screening and Assessments
Formal Standardized Assessments

The following are charts used in a clinic environment to evaluate a contrast sensitivity deficit: Vistech, Pelli-Robson, ETDRS LEA Numbers, Evans Letter Contrast Test (ELCT) (i.e., not portable and more expensive) (Meyers & Wilcox, 2011; Whittaker et al., 2015). The following are portable charts used to evaluate a contrast sensitivity deficit: LEA portable chart, Hiding Heidi, Low Contrast Face Test, LEA Symbols, and Colenbrander Mixed Contrast Card (i.e., smaller and inexpensive).

Informal Assessment and Clinical Observations

There is a clinical observation list available in the biVABA. An example of a task used for assessment purposes is to have the client pour water into a clear glass and have the client pour cold coffee into a white mug. Compare the client's ability to complete both tasks. Is the glass underfilled or overfilled? Does the client use his or her fingers with the glass? Other observations or complaints may include difficulty recognizing faces, trimming fingernails, distinguishing similar colors (e.g., black, navy, brown, and dark green); hesitation with a subtle change in support surface; difficulty with stairs and curbs; difficulty cutting food or eating when the food, plate, or cutting surface is of a similar color; and reports of an increased number of falls, trips, and stumbles. Gilbert and Baker (2011), Weisser-Pike (2014), and Whittaker et al. (2015) report other functional outcome assessments used for visual impairments, which include the following:

- Self-Reported Assessment of Functional Vision Performance (SRAFVP)
- National Eye Institute Visual Function Questionnaire (NEI-VFQ) 2014
- Melbourne Low Vision ADL Index

Contrast Sensitivity and Occupational Performance

Functional activities with the best or highest contrast are those activities that are white on black or black on white

(Meyers & Wilcox, 2011; Warren, 2013; Weisser-Pike, 2014; Zoltan, 2007), for example, black coffee in a white mug, mashed potatoes on a dark plate, and black felt-tipped pen on white paper. Examples of low-contrast functional activities include facial features used to recognize and identify someone and are usually similar in color (e.g., high cheekbones blend in with nose shape), reading a newspaper that has grayish paper with slightly darker ink, and negotiating curbs and steps.

Limitations related to contrast sensitivity can cause challenges with activities involving reading, writing, and fine motor tasks, including the following: difficulty reading low-contrast or colored print; difficulty reading or writing with pencil, blue, or red pens; difficulty with disorganized space, clutter, or patterned backgrounds; difficulty with sewing, pouring, trimming fingernails, putting on makeup evenly; and difficulty cleaning up spills. Decreased contrast sensitivity can also cause challenges with activities involving mobility and typically include difficulty with curbs, stairs, steps, and detecting subtle changes in surfaces. Challenges related to socialization and communication with others may include difficulty recognizing others and distinguishing faces. Difficulty cutting food or seeing food on a similar color plate can also occur with contrast sensitivity deficits. Safety during ADLs may present challenges when reaching into the oven and negotiating steps, stairs, curbs, and obstacles on the floor or ground that are the same color as the floor/ground, as well as a greater risk of cuts when trimming cuticles or nails.

Interventions
Change Color to Increase Contrast

Strategies for increasing color contrast include changing background colors and having a light and dark-colored plate, cutting board, and cups available for use (Kaldenberg, 2014; Meibeyer, 2014; Warren, 2013). Men can use a blue tablet in the water of a white commode. Other strategies include hanging a contrasting colored towel in the bathroom to see hair in a mirror. When sewing, place a solid-colored towel on the table; it should contrast with the material being sewn. Add high-contrast marks on appliances, letters on a keyboard, and numbers on a telephone; for example, use a black felt-tipped pen and bold-lined paper for writing.

Decrease Patterns

Use solid color on backgrounds and support surfaces (Gilbert & Baker, 2011; Warren, 2013). Examples of contrast-reducing patterns include pencil on a flowered tablecloth, fork or spoon on a plaid placemat, or coins on a patterned carpet.

Reduce Clutter

Clutter creates a pattern and makes items more difficult to locate (Warren, 2013). Organize spaces (Gilbert & Baker, 2011; Kaldenberg, 2014; Warren, 2013). Clean off counters. In the kitchen, organize the spice rack and cupboards, organize medications and grooming tools, throw out unused items, and recycle or throw out junk mail and old newspapers. Clean out clothes closet with this rule in mind: "If you have not worn it in 1 year, you probably will not wear it again." This rule can be adapted throughout the house. Finally, return items to their storage place after using them.

Environmental Adaptations for Safety

Add a contrasting stripe to the edges of steps, use black electrical tape to stripe a white pull cord, use liquid-level indicators for pouring hot liquids, or pull the oven rack out when placing items in or removing them from the oven (Gilbert & Baker, 2011; Meibeyer, 2014).

Other options to consider for low-vision deficits which impact occupational performance include paying special attention to glare sensitivity, which impacts safety during ADLs both indoors and outdoors (Meibeyer, 2014). Observe if the client squints or shades his or her eyes; a hat, visor, or sun filters can decrease glare (Kaldenberg, 2014). A light/dark adaptation can impact safety during ADL completion. Does the client pause, hesitate, or move slower when moving from a bright sunny area to a darkened area? For instance, glare when walking from outdoors into a church or store can create difficulty with mobility tasks.

General Low-Vision Intervention Strategies

General guidelines for strategies to address low vision include visual skills training and compensatory training. Visual skills training includes scanning and eccentric viewing involving training where the scarred, nonseeing, or impaired areas of vision should be addressed in addition to training the client to locate the areas of good vision (Barstow & Crossland, 2011; Kaldenberg, 2014;

Warren, 2013; Whittaker et al., 2015). Compensatory strategies using other senses that are often helpful for individuals with visual impairments include auditory, tactile, and olfactory cues that can be used in the completion of ADLs (Gilbert & Baker, 2011; Kaldenberg, 2014; Meibeyer, 2014). Training should include maximizing lighting while decreasing glare; strategies to increase contrast sensitivity include decreasing patterns and clutter or changing the background color, and magnification using optical (i.e., magnifiers) and nonoptical strategies (i.e., moving closer to something) and devices (i.e., large-print checks, books, or telephone) (Gilbert & Baker, 2011; Kaldenberg, 2014; Weisser-Pike, 2014; Whittaker et al., 2015).

Oculomotor Deficits

Recommendations for Assessments and Interventions

It is important to involve an optometrist or ophthalmologist in the assessment process. The optometrist or ophthalmologist will direct treatment to be provided by the OT team. The main goal of treatment is for the client to be able to complete ADLs. The main categories for intervention include adaptive interventions that might involve compensatory strategies for safety, occlusion, or the use of prisms; and restorative interventions that might involve eye exercises or surgery for some oculomotor deficits that may also be present in clients with low vision (e.g., fixation and saccades) (Kaldenberg, 2014; Scheiman et al., 2007; Warren, 2013; Weisser-Pike, 2014; Zoltan, 2007).

Foveation

Foveation creates and sustains a clear, precise image (Kaldenberg, 2014; Warren, 2013; Weisser-Pike, 2014; Zoltan, 2007). The skills needed to achieve foveation are fixation, saccades, and smooth pursuits or tracking and are described below including an outline of their description, clinical presentation, and approaches to assessment and intervention.

Fixation

- *Description*: The process of locating and focusing on an object on the fovea is the foundation of oculomotor control (Kaldenberg, 2014; Scheiman et al., 2007;

Warren, 2013; Weisser-Pike, 2014; Zoltan, 2007). Deficits may be a result of acuity loss or binocular vision problems. Nystagmus (i.e., rapid, involuntary, and oscillating eye movements) may be present.

- *Clinical presentation/observations*: Clients will have difficulty attaining, changing, or sustaining gaze, especially at varying locations in the visual field, causing decreased vision, and the client will have binocular vision problems (Kaldenberg, 2014; Scheiman et al., 2007; Warren, 2013; Weisser-Pike, 2014; Zoltan, 2007). Fixation deficits may give the therapist a false impression that the client has an attention or motivation issue. The client usually has low endurance for visual tasks.

- *Assessment*: The biVABA. In addition, the OT or OTA can assess for fixation by holding two different targets 16 inches from the face and approximately 8 inches apart. Ask the client to look from one to the other when verbally cued (Kaldenberg, 2014; Warren, 2013; Weisser-Pike, 2014; Zoltan, 2007). Repeat for a total of 10 fixations (i.e., five complete cycles). Observe the ability to complete all cycles, accuracy of eye movements (i.e., overshoot/ undershoot), and movements of the head or body.

- *Intervention*: Interventions for deficits with fixation include using activities that will force the client to fixate, refixate, and hold fixation at different distances (Kaldenberg, 2014; Warren, 2013; Weisser-Pike, 2014; Zoltan, 2007). Activities may include two columns of letters or numbers on a piece of paper, a chalkboard, or doorframe, or card-type games. To grade the activities, the OT practitioner might control the density of information and adjust lighting, contrast, and size. Interventions for fixation deficits can be incorporated into interventions for deficits in saccades and smooth pursuits or tracking.

Saccades

- *Description*: Saccades are quick, small movements of the eye (i.e., oscillations); used when scanning; moves us from word to word (i.e., reading) or object to object (e.g., searching for an object on a shelf or driving) (Kaldenberg, 2014; Scheiman et al., 2007; Warren, 2013; Weisser-Pike, 2014; Zoltan, 2007). Saccadic eye movements can be disrupted as the result of cranial nerve damage, visual field cut, visual inattention, cerebellar damage, fixation deficit, or a complicated optic pathway.

- *Clinical presentation/observation*: The client may experience difficulty reading, especially longer words or sentences (e.g., may lose his or her place on a page or have difficulty with page navigation) (Kaldenberg, 2014; Scheiman et al., 2007; Warren, 2013; Weisser-Pike, 2014; Zoltan, 2007). Other challenges may include difficulty watching sports, writing, searching and locating objects, and driving. Clients may have decreased concentration or visual memory.

- *Assessment*: The OT practitioner holds two target sticks or objects approximately 6 inches apart, about 12–16 inches away from the bridge of the nose of the client. Ask the client to look quickly from one object to the other and back again. The client should be able to smoothly shift gaze from one object to the other and back. In a person who is functioning within normal limits, you should observe no head turning, a slight undershooting, overshooting, or refixating (Kaldenberg, 2014; Scheiman et al., 2007; Warren, 2013; Weisser-Pike, 2014; Zoltan, 2007).

- *Intervention*: Interventions for deficits with foveation include using activities that will force the client to fixate, refixate, and hold fixation for stationary and moving tasks (Kaldenberg, 2014; Warren, 2013; Weisser-Pike, 2014; Zoltan, 2007). Activities may include two columns of letters or numbers on a piece of paper, chalkboard, or doorframe, scanning activities, flashlight tag, or a Marsden ball (i.e., small suspended ball with letters or numbers on it). To grade the activities, the OT practitioner might control the density of information, adjust lighting, contrast, and size, and allow the client to use an "anchor" or line guide when reading. Tasks should be completed in a number of distances (e.g., near, intermediate, and far), and treatment should progress from stationary to moving both the objects and the client's head and body. Interventions for deficits in saccades can be done in conjunction with interventions for fixation deficits and deficits in smooth pursuits or tracking.

Smooth Pursuits/Tracking

- *Description*: Smooth pursuits or tracking is the ability to follow a moving object with the fovea (Kaldenberg, 2014; Scheiman et al., 2007; Warren, 2013; Weisser-Pike, 2014; Zoltan, 2007). Deficits

may be the result of cranial nerve damage, visual field cut, visual inattention, cerebellar damage, fixation deficit, or a complicated optic pathway.

- *Clinical presentation/observation*: Unable or impaired ability to track across the visual field or coordinate both eyes to move in the same direction symmetrically (Kaldenberg, 2014; Scheiman et al., 2007; Warren, 2013; Weisser-Pike, 2014; Zoltan, 2007). Additional challenges include playing and watching sports; problems staying on line when reading and writing; difficulty driving; difficulty with page navigation; inability to follow a moving object, such as a person, ball, or car; and decreased concentration or visual memory.

- *Assessment*: The biVABA can be used, in addition to holding a target 16 inches from the client's face. Tell the client to focus on the target and follow it without taking his or her eyes off it. Move the target in a clockwise direction; repeat twice. Move the target in a counterclockwise direction; repeat twice. Record the number of rotations completed and how many times the client loses and reestablishes fixation (Kaldenberg, 2014; Warren, 2013; Weisser-Pike, 2014; Zoltan, 2007). Record any head or body movement.

- *Intervention*: Interventions for deficits with foveation include using activities that will force the client to fixate, refixate, and hold fixation for stationary and moving tasks (Kaldenberg, 2014; Warren, 2013; Weisser-Pike, 2014; Zoltan, 2007). Activities may include two columns of letters or numbers on a piece of paper, chalkboard, or doorframe, scanning activities, flashlight tag, or a Marsden ball. To grade the activities, the OT practitioner might control the density of information, adjust lighting, contrast, and size, and allow the client to use an "anchor" or line guide when reading. Tasks should be completed in a number of distances (e.g., near, intermediate, and far), and treatment should progress from stationary to moving for both objects and the client's head and body.

Sensory Fusion

- Sensory fusion is the ability to merge two images into one for binocular vision, which requires intact CNS functioning (Kaldenberg, 2014; Warren, 2013;

Weisser-Pike, 2014; Zoltan, 2007). Skills include vergence (i.e., convergence and divergence), accommodation, and extraocular range of motion. These skills are presented below in terms of their description, clinical presentation, and appropriate assessment and intervention.

Vergence

- *Description*: Convergence is described as focusing on an object and maintaining the image as it moves toward the face (Kaldenberg, 2014; Warren, 2013; Weisser-Pike, 2014; Zoltan, 2007). The eyes move medially toward the nose. Divergence involves focusing on an object and maintaining the image as it moves away from the face (Kaldenberg, 2014; Warren, 2013; Weisser-Pike, 2014; Zoltan, 2007). The eyes move laterally away from the nose.
- *Clinical presentation*: The client may complain of diplopia (i.e., double vision) at distances greater than 4 inches from the eye (Kaldenberg, 2014; Warren, 2013; Weisser-Pike, 2014; Zoltan, 2007). There may be intermittent diplopia, blurred vision, headache, eyestrain, or fatigue when reading. Clients may complain of eyes stinging or burning, or they may squint or close one eye. They may lose their place when reading, or have difficulty sustaining their focus at specific distances (e.g., sewing, cutting, computer use, and driving). Balance, depth perception or judgment, and mobility may be impacted along with eye–hand coordination tasks.
- *Assessment*: Slowly move the target toward the client's bridge of the nose. The client indicates when two targets are seen (i.e., when diplopia occurs) and the distance is measured. Next, move the target inward approximately 1 inch farther, and then slowly move the target away from the client's nose. The client reports the distance at which one image is seen, and that distance is measured (Kaldenberg, 2014; Warren, 2013; Weisser-Pike, 2014; Whittaker et al., 2015; Zoltan, 2007).
- *Intervention*: The client needs to be able to recognize and monitor symptoms. The OT practitioner will need to consider compensatory techniques, such as environmental modification or frequent breaks, to reduce visual stress during ADL completion (Kaldenberg, 2014; Warren, 2013; Weisser-Pike, 2014; Zoltan, 2007). OTs

and OTAs should control or grade the density of information, the space it is presented in, and the cognitive demands.

Accommodation

- *Description*: Ability to quickly change focus from near to far (Kaldenberg, 2014; Warren, 2013; Weisser-Pike, 2014; Zoltan, 2007). Uses both saccades and vergence skills and requires convergence, lens thickening, and pupil constriction.
- *Clinical presentation/observation*: Clients may blink excessively or experience light sensitivity, blurring when changing the focal distance, swirling or moving print, blurred vision, headaches, eyestrain, or fatigue (Kaldenberg, 2014; Warren, 2013; Weisser-Pike, 2014; Zoltan, 2007). They may have difficulty with near tasks (e.g., sewing, cutting, and reading), dialing the phone from a written number (e.g., phone directory), buttoning, shaving, and copying from a chalkboard.
- *Assessment*: Same test as for convergence. Hold a pen at near point of convergence (i.e., the point at which fixation is broken and usually one eye moves outward). Ask the client to look at your face, then look at the pen, and focus on it. Record the amount of time before the client loses fixation or looks away (Kaldenberg, 2014; Warren, 2013; Weisser-Pike, 2014; Zoltan, 2007).
- *Intervention*: The client needs to be able to recognize and monitor symptoms. The OT practitioners will need to consider compensatory techniques, such as environmental modifications or frequent breaks to reduce visual stress during ADL completion (Kaldenberg, 2014; Warren, 2013; Weisser-Pike, 2014; Zoltan, 2007). The OT practitioner should control or grade the density of information, the space it is presented in, and the cognitive demands.

Extraocular Range of Motion

- *Description*: Motor process of moving the eyes in a symmetrical manner throughout all nine cardinal directions; strabismus (i.e., tropia) is the misalignment of the eyes (Kaldenberg, 2014; Scheiman et al., 2007; Warren, 2013; Weisser-Pike, 2014; Zoltan, 2007).

- *Clinical presentation/observation*: The OT or OTA may observe slow or unequal eye movements, overshooting or undershooting during eye–hand or eye–foot coordination tasks, clumsiness, difficulty focusing, frequently closing one eye, diplopia, and difficulty with depth perception (Kaldenberg, 2014; Scheiman et al., 2007; Warren, 2013; Weisser-Pike, 2014; Zoltan, 2007). The client may complain of nausea, motion sickness, and vertigo.
- *Assessment*: The biVABA.
- *Intervention*: The client needs to be able to recognize and monitor symptoms. The OT practitioner will need to consider compensatory techniques, such as environmental modifications or frequent breaks to reduce visual stress during ADL completion. The OT practitioner should control or grade the density of information, the space it is presented in, and the cognitive demands. The goal is to increase the visual endurance, density of information, visual field, and cognitive demands of tasks (Kaldenberg, 2014; Warren, 2013; Weisser-Pike, 2014; Zoltan, 2007).

Diplopia

- *Description*: Double vision occurs when the fovea of both eyes are not aligned on the same target, so the brain is not able to fuse the image (Kaldenberg, 2014; Scheiman et al., 2007; Warren, 2013; Weisser-Pike, 2014; Zoltan, 2007). Diplopia can present either horizontally or vertically, as a double image, blurred vision, or with shadows, and may be present at near, intermediate, or far distances.
- *Clinical presentation/observation*: Clients with tropias will complain of constant diplopia when viewing objects and often must close one eye to complete tasks (Kaldenberg, 2014; Scheiman et al., 2007; Warren, 2013; Weisser-Pike, 2014; Zoltan, 2007). Clients with phorias will complain of diplopia that comes and goes and is most noticeable with fatigue. Additional areas of difficulty include spatial judgment, disorientation, eye–hand coordination, mobility (e.g., difficulty with stairs), reading, pouring, measuring, weeding, golfing, getting in and out of the bathtub, hammering, threading a needle, cutting, and writing.
- *Assessment*: Question the client on the following in terms of the presence of diplopia:

  - When? Near, far, constant, or intermittent?
  - Where? Straight ahead, right, left, up, or down?
  - How? Vertical, horizontal, shadows, or ghosting?

Tropia

- *Description*:
  - *Esotropia*: Inward deviation of the eye when the other is focusing on an object.
  - *Exotropia*: Outward turning of the eye when the other is focusing on an object.
  - *Hypertropia*: Upward turning of the eye when the other is focusing on an object.
  - *Hypotropia*: Downward turning of the eye when the other is focusing on an object (Kaldenberg, 2014; Scheiman et al., 2007; Warren, 2013; Weisser-Pike, 2014; Zoltan, 2007).
- *Assessment*: The Cover–Uncover Test is appropriate when a tropia is suspected. Ask the client to fixate on a target held at eye level. Cover one eye while observing the movement of the other eye. Record if there is movement. The uncovered eye will maintain fixed (i.e., very little to no movement).
- *Intervention*: See general interventions for oculomotor deficits below.

Phoria

- *Description*:
  - *Esophoria*: Tendency for eyes to turn inward when both eyes are fixating on an object; controlled by fusion.
  - *Exophoria*: Tendency for eyes to turn outward when both eyes are fixating on an object; controlled by fusion.
  - *Hyperphoria*: Tendency for eyes to turn upward when both eyes are fixating on an object; controlled by fusion.
  - *Hypophoria*: Tendency for eyes to turn downward when both eyes are fixating on an object; controlled by fusion (Kaldenberg, 2014; Scheiman et al., 2007; Warren, 2013; Weisser-Pike, 2014; Zoltan, 2007).
- *Assessment*: Alternate the Cover–Uncover Test when a phoria is suspected: ask the client to fixate on a target held at eye level. Occlude one eye then the other every 2 seconds. Record the direction of movement. The covered eye will move to obtain

fixation when it is uncovered. The client needs to be able to recognize and monitor symptoms. Refer to an eye care physician for possible intervention, including prisms, occlusion, or surgery (Kaldenberg, 2014; Scheiman et al., 2007; Warren, 2013; Weisser-Pike, 2014; Zoltan, 2007). Communicate with the physician how diplopia affects daily tasks and client complaints. Targets can be placed in areas where fusion occurs and the OT practitioner can gradually move the target away. Teach clients the range or distance where fusion occurs so ADL items can be placed within range.

- *Intervention*: See general interventions for oculomotor deficits next.

General Interventions for Oculomotor Deficits

Refer clients to ophthalmologists or optometrists. Provide your clinical observations and impact on ADL performance, if possible. Monitor visual fatigue, stress, and endurance during activities. Eye movement activities and visual–motor coordination tasks, such as tracing exercises on paper or a chalkboard, bird watching, or tracking children running and playing, playing video games, crossword puzzles, laser pointer tag, reading a map, sweeping, balloon activities, finding a car in a parking lot, coloring, or painting, are appropriate tasks for oculomotor deficits. It is also important to increase visual endurance during tasks, density of information, and space tasks. Most treatment activities will incorporate tasks, visually guided hand or foot tasks, or depth perception activities.

Referrals and Discharge Considerations

It is important for the OT to refer clients to an eye care practitioner when an older adult has not had his or her eyes checked and/or disease managed for 1 year. Provide referrals to a low-vision physician (i.e., ophthalmologist or optometrist) when the client's acuity is moderately or severely impaired (i.e., moderately impaired starts at 20/70; severely impaired starts at 20/200).

Screen for depression using a measure such as the Geriatric Depression Scale. Individuals with visual impairments are at risk for depression due to social isolation, adjustment issues, and loss of independence (Meibeyer, 2014).

Refer to a community agency serving the blind and persons with visual impairments (e.g., private nonprofit agency, state agency, or, if appropriate, school system department of special education). The Library of Congress provides large-print materials and talking resources, including books, magazines, and sheet music. Large-print books and audio books are also available from local libraries or bookstores as well as book clubs that individuals can join. Radio reading services are often used in conjunction with university radio stations, where information such as local and national newspapers, advertisements, and magazines is read over the air.

Operator assistance is available for dialing and looking up a number; however, it is only available from some phone companies. Voice-operated cell phones may be an option but consider how much difficulty a person will have viewing and/or using the keys or touch screen. Refer to local support groups and community transportation services. Refer to an orientation and mobility specialist for training in mobility specifically for clients with significant field loss and clients who need to travel in special or complicated environments, crossing streets with traffic lights, multiple lanes, or traffic moving at speeds greater than 25 miles per hour, and travel in areas without sidewalks (Riddering, 2011). Referral to a mobility specialist may also be appropriate for specific challenges or needs, such as detecting curbs, steps, drop-offs, frequently getting lost or unable to establish a relationship between themselves and objects, use of a long cane, difficulty walking at night or on moving walkways and escalators, and difficulty with buses, subways, or crowded areas (Riddering, 2011).

Management and Standards of Practice

The OTA needs to have an understanding of the patterns of vision loss, occupational performance deficits related to each pattern, and other limitations due to low vision, such as contrast sensitivity loss. After evaluating the client, the OT will identify the client's limitations, needs, and goals in order to direct the intervention priorities. In collaboration with the OTA, the OT should develop the intervention plan, delegating the aspects that will be carried out by the OT. For instance, the OT may be responsible for training related to scotoma awareness and using the remaining vision, while the OTA may be responsible for implementing interventions related to occupational performance activities, such as increasing lighting and contrast, decreasing glare, and increasing magnification. The OT and OTA should collaborate with the client on final recommendations for equipment (e.g., lighting, magnifiers, glare control, talking clocks, and large-print materials), community resources (e.g., talking books and community transportation), and referrals to other professionals (e.g., orientation and mobility specialist and certified driver rehabilitation specialist).

Chapter 7 Self-Study Activities (Answers Are Provided at the End of the Chapter)

Case Scenario: Multiple Short Answer Response

Mrs. Paul, a 78-year-old housewife, has come to the outpatient clinic after hospitalization for a recent fall after missing an unpainted curb in front of a friend's apartment. During the evaluation, she reports to the OT that she has arthritis, high blood pressure, is hard of hearing, and was diagnosed with diabetes "several years ago." The OT asks Mrs. Paul if she has had her eyes examined recently. Mrs. Paul states that she has not seen an eye doctor in a number of years because Medicare will not pay for new glasses. She had her cataracts removed 12 years ago and Medicare paid for one pair of glasses after the surgery, which she is still currently using, although she reports, "they do not really help." She reports that occasionally she uses a magnifier when the book print is "very, very small." She reports if she still cannot see it, she asks her husband or tries to read it on another day. Mrs. Paul reports she is still driving, "but only during the day."

1. What are four to six clinical observations the OT might watch for when working with Mrs. Paul?
2. What type of assessments, if any, related to the visual system should the OT generalist complete with Mrs. Paul?
3. What, if any, intervention should the OT provide regarding decreased vision?
4. Should Mrs. Paul be referred for services elsewhere? If yes, where?

Functional Limitations: Fill in the Blanks

1. Central vision impairments typically impact _____ vision tasks, including reading, writing, setting dials, and using the phone.
2. Peripheral vision impairments typically impact _____ tasks, including locating objects and obstacles, identifying drop-offs, crossing the street, and driving.

Chapter 7 Self-Study Answers

1. Since diabetes can affect the entire visual field, Mrs. Paul may complain of problems related to both central field issues (i.e., near-vision tasks) and peripheral field issues (i.e., mainly mobility). Some challenges may include any of the following:
   - Needing more light
   - Print appearing fuzzy
   - Difficulty reading small print
   - Sitting close to the television
   - Getting lost
   - Experiencing difficulty in crowded areas
   - Difficulty seeing the edge of step(s)
   Some observations may include
   - Moving a page around or her head around when trying to read
   - Leaning toward a window or light source
   - Staying close to one side of a hallway
   - Watches her feet when walking
   - Using her finger to maintain her place on a line
   - Difficulty recognizing her friend's faces
2. Visual acuity: Snellen chart for distance, possibly a letter or continuous print chart for near reading; visual field: confrontation testing; contrast sensitivity: either chart or functional tasks.
3. Training during functional activities to increase lighting and contrast, decrease glare and increase safety in the home.
4. Mrs. Paul should be referred to an eye care physician, preferably an ophthalmologist (i.e., medical doctor), since she has already been diagnosed with diabetes, for an eye exam to determine if and how the diabetes has affected her vision. The OT may refer her to the Library of Congress talking book program or offer alternatives for driving (e.g., community transportation options).

Functional Limitations: Fill in the Blank Answers

1. Near
2. Mobility

References

Barstow, E. A., & Crossland, M. D. (2011). Intervention and rehabilitation for reading and writing. In M. Warren, E. A. Barstow, & American Occupational Therapy Association (Eds.), *Occupational therapy interventions for adults with low vision* (pp. 105–151). Bethesda, MD: AOTA Press.

Freeman, P. B. (2015). Overview and review of optometric low vision evaluation. In S. Whittaker, M. Scheiman, & D. A. Sokol-McKay (Eds.), *Low vision rehabilitation: A practical guide for occupational therapists* (2nd ed., pp. 97–105). Thorofare, NJ: SLACK Incorporated.

Gilbert, M. P., & Baker, S. S. (2011). Evaluation and intervention for basic and instrumental activities of daily living. In M. Warren, E. A. Barstow, & American Occupational Therapy Association (Eds.), *Occupational therapy interventions for adults with low vision* (pp. 227–267). Bethesda, MD: AOTA Press.

Gillen, G. (2009). *Cognitive and perceptual rehabilitation: Optimizing function.* St. Louis, MO: Mosby/Elsevier.

Kaldenberg, J. (2014). Optimizing vision and visual processing. In M. V. Radomski & C. A. T. Latham (Eds.), *Occupational therapy for physical dysfunction* (7th ed., pp. 699–724). Philadelphia, PA: Wolters Kluwer Health/Lippincott Williams & Wilkins.

Meibeyer, E. (2014). Appendix I common conditions, resources and evidence: Visual impairment. In B. A. B. Schell, G. Gillen, & M. E. Scaffa (Eds.), *Willard & Spackman's occupational therapy* (12th ed., pp. 1187–1189). Philadelphia, PA: Wolters Kluwer Health/Lippincott Williams & Wilkins.

Meyers, J. R., & Wilcox, D. T. (2011). Low vision evaluation. In M. Warren, E. A. Barstow, & American Occupational Therapy Association (Eds.), *Occupational therapy interventions for adults with low vision* (pp. 47–74). Bethesda, MD: AOTA Press.

Mogk, L. G. (2011). Eye conditions that cause low vision in adults. In M. Warren, E. A. Barstow, & American Occupational Therapy Association (Eds.), *Occupational therapy interventions for adults with low vision* (pp. 27–46). Bethesda, MD: AOTA Press.

Nowakowski, R. W. (2011). Basic optics and optical devices. In M. Warren, E. A. Barstow, & American Occupational Therapy Association (Eds.), *Occupational therapy interventions for adults with low vision* (pp. 75–104). Bethesda, MD: AOTA Press.

Riddering, A. T. (2011). Evaluation and intervention for deficits in home and community mobility. In M. Warren, E. A. Barstow, & American Occupational Therapy Association (Eds.), *Occupational therapy interventions for adults with low vision* (pp. 269–300). Bethesda, MD: AOTA Press.

Scheiman, M., Scheiman, M., & Whittaker, S. (2007). *Low vision rehabilitation: A practical guide for occupational therapists.* Thorofare, NJ: SLACK Incorporated.

Warren, M. (2011). An overview of low vision rehabilitation and the role of occupational therapists. In M. Warren, E. A. Barstow, & American Occupational Therapy Association (Eds.), *Occupational therapy interventions for adults with low vision* (pp. 1–26). Bethesda, MD: AOTA Press.

Warren, M. (2013). Evaluation and treatment of visual deficits following brain injury. In H. M. Pendleton & W. Schultz-Krohn (Eds.), *Pedretti's occupational therapy: Practice skills for physical dysfunction* (7th ed., pp. 590–626). St. Louis, MO: Elsevier.

Weisser-Pike, O. (2014). Assessing abilities and capabilities: Vision and visual processing. In M. V. Radomski & C. A. T. Latham (Eds.), *Occupational therapy for physical dysfunction* (7th ed., pp. 103–119). Philadelphia, PA: Wolters Kluwer Health/Lippincott Williams & Wilkins.

Whittaker, S., Scheiman, M., & Sokol-McKay, D. A. (2015). *Low vision rehabilitation: A practical guide for occupational therapists* (2nd ed.). Thorofare, NJ: SLACK Incorporated.

Zoltan, B. (2007). *Vision, perception, and cognition: A manual for the evaluation and treatment of the adult with acquired brain injury* (4th ed.). Thorofare, NJ: SLACK Incorporated.

Perception and Cognition

Anne Riddering

Learning Objectives

- Describe key areas of the brain and the effects on perception when injured.
- Compare and contrast the following cognitive functions: attention, memory, executive function (i.e., inhibition and initiation, planning and organization, problem solving, self-awareness, and mental flexibility), generalization and transfer.
- Summarize occupational therapy (OT) assessment and intervention (i.e., including clinical observations, standardized tests, effect on activities of daily living [ADLs], and intervention) for the following perception deficits: inattention, apraxia, agnosia, visual spatial perception deficits, deficits of tactile perception, and body scheme disorders.
- Summarize OT low-vision assessment and intervention (i.e., including clinical observations, standardized tests, effect on ADLs, and intervention) for the following cognitive functions: attention, memory, executive function (i.e., inhibition and initiation, planning and organization, problem solving, self-awareness, and mental flexibility), generalization and transfer.

Key Terms

- *Agnosia*: A failure to recognize familiar objects perceived by the senses. "Gnosis" means knowing; therefore agnosias are not a sensory issue, but rather a perception/processing issue (Gillen, 2009).
- *Apraxia*: The inability to perform a movement even though the sensory system, muscles, and coordination are intact (Zoltan, 2007).

- *Attention*: The process of alerting and orienting to relevant incoming information (Zoltan, 2007). Visual attention is the ability to observe and discriminate visual information related to objects and their environment (Warren, 2013).
- *Executive function*: Higher-level mental functions involving decision making, planning, sequencing, and executing (Gillen, 2009; Zoltan, 2007). Skills include initiation, planning and organization, safety and judgment, mental flexibility and calculations, self-awareness, and problem solving.
- *Figure ground*: The ability to recognize the foreground from the background based on differences in color, luminance, depth, texture, or motion (Gillen, 2009; Whittaker, Scheiman, & Sokol-McKay, 2015; Zoltan, 2007).
- *Memory*: The process by which an individual attends, encodes, stores, and retrieves information (Gillen, 2009; Radomski & Morrison, 2014; Toglia, Golisz, & Goverover, 2014; Zoltan, 2007).
- *Orientation*: The recognition and/or attentiveness to self, others, environments, and time (Zoltan, 2007).
- *Perception*: The way the brain interprets information received by the body's sensory systems. There are motor and sensory perception systems. Sensory perception includes vision, auditory, and tactile perception. Both the right and left areas of the brain are responsible for perception (Scheiman, 2011; Zoltan, 2007).
- *Problem solving*: The active process of making a decision by integrating information using several cognitive skills, including memory, attention, planning, organization and categorization, initiation, inhibition and impulse control, and mental flexibility and reasoning (Zoltan, 2007).

- *Self-awareness*: The ability to perceive the self objectively, as well as the knowledge and recognition of one's own abilities and limitations (Radomski & Morrison, 2014; Toglia et al., 2014; Zoltan, 2007).
- *Spatial relations*: The ability to perceive the position of one's self in relation to objects in the environment (Gillen, 2009; Scheiman, 2011; Zoltan, 2007).
- *Visual spatial perception (i.e., visual discrimination)*: The ability to distinguish the space around one's body, objects in relation to the body and environment, and the relationship between objects in the environment (Gillen, 2009; Scheiman, 2011; Zoltan, 2007).

Perception Deficits

In this chapter, you will learn about sensory and motor perception systems, cognition, and how both are applicable to the practice of occupational therapy (OT). Key areas of the brain will be discussed, as well as perceptual and cognitive assessment and intervention strategies for the entry-level OT.

Perception is the way the brain interprets information received by the body's sensory systems. There are motor and sensory perception systems. Sensory perception includes vision, auditory, and tactile perception. Both the right and left areas of the brain are responsible for perception. The right hemisphere's focus is on the whole (e.g., holistic thinking) and the left hemisphere's focus is on the details.

Damage to the right hemisphere includes visual inattention (i.e., visual neglect or visual attention deficit) which includes both visual field loss and hemi-inattention, visual spatial deficits, left-sided motor apraxia, and visual spatial perception disorders (Gillen, 2009). Conversely, damage to the left hemisphere typically results in difficulty identifying objects (i.e., agnosias), difficulty attending to details of an object, and right-sided motor apraxia, which may also be present with right hemisphere damage (Gillen, 2009).

Deficits are also noted throughout the various lobes of the brain; these are delineated as follows:

- *Occipital lobe*: Contains the visual cortex and is responsible for scanning, the identification of objects, awareness, and discrimination. Visual field deficits (i.e., partial to complete visual field loss), scanning deficits, and agnosia may also be present (Gillen, 2009; Whittaker et al., 2015).
- *Frontal lobe*: Responsible for attention and may present with reduced speed in visual motor tasks (Gillen, 2009; Whittaker et al., 2015).
- *Parietal and temporal lobes*: The right parietal lobe is responsible for visual spatial relations and the right temporal lobe is responsible for visual recognition and memory. Common deficits include visual spatial perception, body scheme, visual memory, visual discrimination, visual attention, visual field, and agnosia (Gillen, 2009; Whittaker et al., 2015).
- *Thalamus*: Responsible for eye movement and integration of visual and cognitive information. Damage may result in visual and cognitive processing deficits and praxis. Specifically, right-side damage may present with visual neglect, anosognosia, and visual spatial deficits, while left-side damage may result in anomia (Gillen, 2009).

Attention Deficits

Attention is the process of alerting and orienting to relevant incoming information (Zoltan, 2007). Attention is a skill that is required for the CNS to use information during an adaptive response or compensatory strategy. Visual attention is the ability to observe and discriminate visual information related to objects and their environment (Warren, 2013). There are two types of visual attention deficits: sensory and motor neglect. Both result in impaired scanning (Warren, 2013; Zoltan, 2007).

Sensory Neglect

Description: Sensory neglect may also be called attention deficit, unilateral neglect, visual neglect, visual inattention, or hemi-inattention (Gillen, 2009; Kaldenberg, 2014; Warren, 2013; Weisser-Pike, 2014; Zoltan, 2007). It is characterized by a lack of or impaired awareness of information to one side of the body or in the space to one side of the body. The goals of the visual attention system include careful observation of objects, obtaining information about specific features, relationships of self to environment, and shifting focus from one object to another (Warren, 2013).

Clinical presentation/observation: Sensory neglect typically includes the following:

- Difficulty scanning into personal and extrapersonal space
- Disorganized, asymmetrical, and quick scanning during a task
- Sidetracked by motion on the right
- Impulsive behavior; does not rescan or recheck work
- Breakdown of scanning to the left
- Loses items
- Difficulty with grooming and dressing
- Difficulty finding way in familiar environments (Warren, 2013; Weisser-Pike, 2014; Zoltan, 2007)

Screening and Assessments

Standardized assessments include the following:

- Brain Injury Visual Assessment Battery for Adults (biVABA) (Warren, 2013; Zoltan, 2007)
- Catherine Bergego Scale (Gillen, 2009)
- Arnadottir Occupational Therapy-ADL Neurobehavioral Evaluation (A-ONE) (Gillen, 2009)
- Assessment of Motor and Process Skills (AMPS (Gillen, 2009)
- Behavioral Inattention Test (BIT) (Gillen, 2009; Zoltan, 2007)

Nonstandardized assessments include the following:

- Cancellation tests (e.g., star and letter)
- Design copying tests
- Figure drawing tests (e.g., house, clock, and flower)
- Line bisection test (Zoltan, 2007)

Interventions

During the intervention phase, it is important to emphasize scanning to the left using organized search patterns and to correct errors through careful inspection (Toglia et al., 2014; Warren, 2013). Slowly increase cognitive demands during activities of daily living (ADLs). Scanning needs to be automatic, spontaneous, and integrated into all aspects of ADLs. Use anchoring techniques or cuing to redirect the client's attention back to the impaired side (Kaldenberg, 2014). Total or partial occlusion should be carried out under the direction of the eye care physician, and as scanning to the neglected side automatically increases, the occluded area is decreased. Prisms prescribed by an eye care physician use a lens to bend light and move an image to a specific area of the fovea (Kaldenberg, 2014; Warren, 2013; Zoltan, 2007). A Fresnel prism is a temporary, inexpensive plastic sheet adhered to a client's glasses (Kaldenberg, 2014; Whittaker et al., 2015).

Motor Neglect

Description: Motor neglect (i.e., output or intentional) refers to the breakdown of the ability to begin or perform a purposeful movement (Toglia et al., 2014; Weisser-Pike, 2014). Praxis is a performance skill and therefore, deficits interfere with the completion of ADLs (Gillen, 2009; Toglia et al., 2014; Zoltan, 2007). There are several different types of motor neglect that are classified under praxis and apraxia. Praxis refers to the ability to perform a movement while apraxia is the inability to carry out a movement, even though the sensory system, muscles, and coordination are intact (Zoltan, 2007). The various types of apraxia are as follows:

- *Limb apraxia*: Difficulty with purposeful movement (Gillen, 2009; Toglia et al., 2014; Zoltan, 2007)
- *Ideational apraxia*: Difficulty with sequencing steps within a task (Gillen, 2009; Toglia et al., 2014; Zoltan, 2007)
- *Ideomotor apraxia*: Production error; can use tools but appears awkward or clumsy (Zoltan, 2007)
- *Conceptual apraxia*: Difficulty with use of tools (Zoltan, 2007)
- *Constructional apraxia*: Difficulty copying, drawing, and constructing designs (Gillen, 2009; Toglia et al., 2014; Zoltan, 2007)
- *Dressing apraxia*: The inability to complete dressing tasks (Toglia et al., 2014; Zoltan, 2007)
- *Limb akinesia*: Absence of the ability to move a limb (Gillen, 2009; Toglia et al., 2014; Zoltan, 2007)
  - *Hypokinesia*: Delayed movement of limb(s)
  - *Hypometria*: Decreased amplitude of movement
  - *Impersistence*: Difficulty sustaining movement or posture
  - *Motor perseveration*: Difficulty ending or terminating movement
  - *Extinction*: Lack of awareness of one object when objects are presented to both sides of the body at a time, even though they are recognized when presented individually

Clinical presentation/observation: This type of apraxia may depend on the exact location of the lesion or damage.

Apraxia may be present alone or in addition to aphasia. Difficulties due to apraxia may be negligible or very obvious with many clients becoming extremely frustrated. The client may also present as clumsy (Gillen, 2009; Zoltan, 2007).

Screening and Assessments

Standardized tests may include the following:

- Florida Apraxia Test–Revised (Gillen, 2009)
- Cambridge Apraxia Battery (Gillen, 2009)
- Lowenstein Occupational Therapy Cognitive Assessment (LOTCA) (Cooke & Kline, 2007; Radomski & Morrison, 2014; Toglia et al., 2014; Zoltan, 2007)
- A-ONE (Gillen, 2009, 2013; Radomski & Morrison, 2014; Toglia et al., 2014)
- Brief Neuropsychological Cognitive Examination (Cooke & Kline, 2007)
- Structured Observational Test of Function (SOTOF) (Gillen, 2009)

Nonstandardized tests include observation during ADLs such as feeding, grooming, hygiene, dressing, and mobility (Gillen, 2009).

Interventions

Verbal and physical cues are commonly used with interventions pertaining to motor neglect. The following approaches and strategies may be used during intervention:

- Provide and combine tactile, kinesthetic, and proprioceptive feedback during tasks (Gillen, 2009; Zoltan, 2007).
- Use hand-over-hand guidance during tasks (Gillen, 2009; Toglia et al., 2014; Zoltan, 2007).
- Use specific and simple verbal directions (Gillen, 2009; Zoltan, 2007).
- Use chaining techniques during tasks. Chaining is a method of breaking the task into smaller steps. The client then relearns the task by completing steps and sequencing the steps together. Backward chaining, or allowing the client to first complete the last step and then the second-to-the-last step, can also be used (Gillen, 2009).
- Establish a routine for activities and perform training during an appropriate time (Gillen, 2009; Toglia et al., 2014; Zoltan, 2007).
- Use cue cards for daily tasks with step-by-step instructions (Zoltan, 2007).

- Maximize safety and ease of completion by modifying the environment (Toglia et al., 2014; Zoltan, 2007).

Agnosia

Agnosia results in difficulty recognizing and identifying objects using only visual means, which is caused by lesions to the right occipital lobe (Gillen, 2009; Zoltan, 2007).

Description: In general, agnosia results in a failure to recognize familiar objects perceived by the senses. "Gnosis" means knowing; therefore, agnosias are not a sensory issue, but rather a perception/processing issue (Gillen, 2009).

Clinical presentation/observation: Individuals with agnosias will not have word-finding deficits in conversation or language impairments (Gillen, 2009; Zoltan, 2007). They can supply words when hearing a definition. They can often follow one-, two-, or three-step directions and generate lists of specific categories (Zoltan, 2007). They can demonstrate the use of objects not in their presence (Zoltan, 2007). For example, an appropriate request from the OT may include, "show me what you do with a hair brush." Primary senses and reception remain intact. Hearing is typically adequate in order to hold a conversation, and visual acuity and visual fields are usually normal or near normal.

Screening and Assessments

Standardized assessments typically include the following:

- LOTCA (Cooke & Kline, 2007; Radomski & Morrison, 2014; Toglia et al., 2014; Zoltan, 2007)
- A-ONE (Gillen, 2009, 2013; Radomski & Morrison, 2014; Toglia et al., 2014)
- Ayres Manual Form Perception (i.e., subset of Southern California SI test) (Zoltan, 2007)

Nonstandardized assessments typically include various tasks that are observed by the OT, which may include the following:

- Have the client identify familiar objects used in ADLs (e.g., fork, cup, pencil, and comb).
- Identify well-known celebrities, family, and friends from pictures.
- Read or identify words or letters.
- Identify colors in a magazine or from a color palette (Zoltan, 2007).

Types of Agnosias

There are many types of agnosias that differ slightly among description, assessments, and interventions. Several more common types are outlined as follows.

Color Agnosia

Description: Color agnosia involves the inability to recognize or remember specific colors for common objects, although clients should be able to state if two colors are the same or different (Gillen, 2009; Zoltan, 2007). For example, clients may confuse two fruits that are of similar size such as a lemon and a lime, or an apple and an orange (Gillen, 2009).

Screening and Assessments

A nonstandardized approach to assessment includes presenting the client with two common items that are correctly colored and two that are incorrectly colored. Ask the client to pick out the two inaccurately colored items. An incorrect answer indicates color agnosia (Zoltan, 2007).

Interventions

Ask the client to recognize, identify, and name various colors of objects within the environment during functional tasks or ADL training (Zoltan, 2007).

   Additional information: Color anomia is the inability to name the specific color of the objects. Color agnosia and color anomias should be distinguished. To determine a color anomia, ask the client to name the color of various objects in the environment. An inability to correctly identify the color of the object indicates a color anomia. OTs can provide clients with aphasia color choices and ask them to answer "yes" or "no."

Object Agnosia and Metamorphopsia

Description: Object agnosia is the inability to recognize objects using only vision, while metamorphopsia is the visual distortion of objects, although they might be recognizable to the client (Gillen, 2009; Zoltan, 2007). The client cannot locate needed items in the cabinet, drawer, store shelf, or refrigerator by vision alone (Gillen, 2009).

Screening and Assessments

A standardized test for object agnosia includes the A-ONE (Gillen, 2009). A nonstandardized assessment includes placing various common objects (e.g., comb, key, glass, and ball) of different weights, sizes, or colors on the table in front of the client and asking them to identify each object and demonstrate its use.

Interventions

Provide items in their natural environments, allowing clients to use other senses to identify them. Provide an auditory description of the object and allow the client to feel it (Zoltan, 2007). Progress from simple to complex objects. Provide real objects before line drawings or objects in their functional environments rather than at a clinic table. Identify the object itself before the larger group to which it belongs (e.g., fork vs. utensil) (Zoltan, 2007).

Prosopagnosia

Description: Prosopagnosia (i.e., facial agnosia) is the inability to recognize or identify a known face or individual (Gillen, 2009; Zoltan, 2007).

Screening and Assessments

Using family photographs (i.e., facial agnosia) are a nonstandardized approach to assessment. Have the client identify the people pictured. Using photographs from magazines, ask the client to identify the famous people pictured (Zoltan, 2007). Examples of famous people may include a political or religious person who has recently been in the news, a famous talk show host, or a movie actor. The family may confirm if the client should recognize the famous person. A deficit is indicated if the client cannot make a visual identification (Gillen, 2009).

Interventions

Provide pictures of family members, friends, and famous people and assist the client in identifying unique physical characteristics or mannerisms. Provide face-matching exercises. Teach the client how to make a mental list of features when they are introduced to others (Zoltan, 2007).

Simultanagnosia

Description: Simultanagnosia is the inability to recognize and interpret an entire visual array (e.g., more than one thing) at a time, usually due to damage to the right hemisphere of the brain (Gillen, 2009; Zoltan, 2007). The client may be unable to read and to count the number of objects on a table or people in a room and may have difficulty getting needed items for a recipe from the refrigerator or cupboards (Gillen, 2009).

Screening and Assessments

Present the client with a photograph that includes a detailed visual array (e.g., a picture with several people, animals, and details). Ask the client to describe what is seen. A deficit is indicated if the client can identify one particular object, person, or detail at a time but cannot describe the meaning of the entire scene (nonstandardized) (Gillen, 2009).

Interventions

Assist the client in learning to see the whole picture by offering verbal feedback and by questioning the client about the details and how they relate to the entire picture (Toglia et al., 2014). Start simple, then move to more complex situations (e.g., home or work then community outings) (Gillen, 2009; Zoltan, 2007). Other agnosias include auditory agnosias, body scheme agnosias, and tactile agnosias. Body scheme agnosias, such as somatognosia and anosognosia, will be discussed under the body scheme disorders. Tactile agnosias are discussed under their own section.

Visual Spatial Perception Deficits

Description: Visual spatial perception deficits (i.e., visual discrimination deficits) are defined as the ability to distinguish the space around one's body, objects in relation to the body and environment, and the relationship between objects in the environment (Gillen, 2009; Scheiman, 2011; Zoltan, 2007). Visual spatial perception deficits include limitations of figure ground, form constancy or discrimination, spatial relations, depth perception or stereopsis, and topographical orientation.

Clinical presentation/observation: Processes are controlled by the right hemisphere, and quick responses are a result of intact functioning. Deficits may include an absent response or a slowed response, although the response may be correct (Gillen, 2009; Zoltan, 2007). Slowed responses can still affect ADL functioning such as driving. Visual spatial perception uses proprioception, tactile, and pressure input (Zoltan, 2007). Sometimes visual discrimination issues such as right/left discrimination and finger agnosia are categorized as visual spatial deficits.

There are different types of visual spatial perception deficits that differ slightly among description, assessments, and interventions. They are outlined as follows.

Figure Ground

Description: Figure ground refers to the ability to recognize the foreground from the background based on differences in color, luminance, depth, texture, or motion (Gillen, 2009; Whittaker et al., 2015; Zoltan, 2007).

Clinical presentation/observation: Difficulty with ADLs such as dressing and self-care activities primarily presents with difficulty locating objects in cluttered environments (Gillen, 2009; Whittaker et al., 2015).

Screening and Assessments

Various standardized assessments for figure ground include the following:

- Ayres' Figure-Ground Visual Perception Test (i.e., subset of Southern California Sensory Integration Test) (Zoltan, 2007)
- Overlapping Figures Subtest of the LOTCA (Cooke & Kline, 2007; Radomski & Morrison, 2014; Toglia et al., 2014; Zoltan, 2007)
- Developmental Test of Visual Perception (DTVP)—adolescent and adult (Scheiman, 2011; Zoltan, 2007)
- Motor-Free Visual Perception Test (MVPT), third edition (Gillen, 2009; Zoltan, 2007)
- DTVP—adult and pediatric (Frostig DTVP-2) (Cooke & Kline, 2007)
- A-ONE (Gillen, 2009, 2013; Radomski & Morrison, 2014; Toglia et al., 2014)
- SOTOF (Gillen, 2009)

Nonstandardized assessments include observing the client during functional tasks. Some examples may include locating a white washcloth on a white sink or locating a cooking or eating utensil in a cluttered drawer.

Interventions

Approaches to intervention include remedial, adaptive, and multicultural. They are as follows:

- *Remedial approach*: An example of a remedial approach includes placing a number of objects in front of the client and asking them to pick out particular objects of similar color to the background, and increasing the number of objects on the table as the client improves (Zoltan, 2007).

- *Adaptive approach*: Environmental modification may include organization of items and removal of objects that are not necessary for the task. Labeling or marking commonly used items so they are easily identified is another adaptive approach (Zoltan, 2007).
- *Multicultural approach (Toglia)*: Assist the client in increasing recognition of compensatory strategies such as scanning and organization, as well as learning to integrate general skills to other ADL situations (Zoltan, 2007).

Form Constancy or Discrimination Deficits

Description: Form constancy is the ability to distinguish a form, shape, or object despite its location, position, color, or size (Scheiman, 2011; Zoltan, 2007).

Clinical presentation/observation: Form constancy impacts the ability to recognize common objects needed to complete ADLs. Safety is also affected with form constancy (Zoltan, 2007).

Screening and Assessments

Various standardized assessments for form constancy include the following:

- DTVP—adolescent and adult (Scheiman, 2011; Zoltan, 2007)
- MVPT, third edition (Gillen, 2009; Zoltan, 2007)
- Form Board Test (Zoltan, 2007)
- DTVP—pediatric (Frostig DTVP-2) (Cooke & Kline, 2007)

Nonstandardized assessments include asking the client to locate and identify different objects of similar forms, such as eating utensils in a kitchen or a cup on its side. A deficit is indicated if the client cannot identify an object in a different position, color, or location (Zoltan, 2007).

Interventions

There are both remedial and adaptive approaches to interventions. Remedial approaches seek to improve the client's condition and adaptive approaches seek to compensate for the condition through adaptive techniques or equipment. Zoltan (2007) provides the following remedial and adaptive approaches for form constancy:

- *Remedial approach*: Have the client practice sorting commonly used items in different forms, and encourage identification of differences and similarities using tactile cues.

- *Adaptive approach*: Necessary objects should be placed in upright positions and should be labeled so they are easily identified. Organization strategies should be implemented.

Spatial Relations

Description: Spatial relations (i.e., position in space) refer to the ability to perceive the position of one's self in relation to objects in the environment (Gillen, 2009; Scheiman, 2011; Zoltan, 2007).

Clinical presentation/observation: You may observe a client unable to align a zipper or buttons, difficulty determining the front or back of clothing, unsafe transfers, and/or difficulty ambulating through crowds (Gillen, 2009; Zoltan, 2007).

Screening and Assessments

Various standardized assessments for spatial relations include the following:

- Ayres' Space Visualization Test (i.e., subtest of the Southern California Sensory Integration Test) (Zoltan, 2007)
- MVPT (Gillen, 2009; Toglia et al., 2014; Zoltan, 2007)
- LOTCA (Cooke & Kline, 2007; Radomski & Morrison, 2014; Toglia et al., 2014)
- Preschool Visual Motor Integration Assessment (PVMIA) (Cooke & Kline, 2007)
- A-ONE (Gillen, 2013; Radomski & Morrison, 2014; Toglia et al., 2014)
- SOTOF (Gillen, 2009)

The cross test is a nonstandardized approach to assessing spatial relations (Zoltan, 2007). The OT can ask the client to place an object in a certain position using terms such as up/down, above/below, on/off, top/bottom, and over/under. Deficits are indicated if the client is unable to complete the task. The OT can also have the client copy two-dimensional designs such as a flower or a house drawing (Zoltan, 2007).

Interventions

Remedial and adaptive approaches to intervention are noted below:

- *Remedial approach*: Present the client with opportunities to follow directions during ADLs (Zoltan, 2007). Use directional terms (e.g., up/down, and on/off). Ask the client to point to objects in the room and describe their location in relation to themselves or other objects. Incorporate the use of tactile and kinesthetic senses to demonstrate position or distances (Zoltan, 2007).

- *Adaptive approach*: Arrange the client's environment so that items needed for ADLs have a designated, consistent location (Zoltan, 2007).

Depth Perception and Stereopsis

Description: Depth perception is the ability to judge distances and stereopsis is the ability to see things in three dimensions (Gillen, 2009; Zoltan, 2007). A lack of stereopsis can affect depth perception and make the environment appear flat. Depth perception can be impaired without any signs of diplopia and may be the result of eyes that are misaligned (i.e., strabismus present). Other visual functions may also affect depth perception, such as visual acuity and contrast sensitivity (Zoltan, 2007). If the client has one eye patched for diplopia or does not have use of one eye, depth perception will be affected (Gillen, 2009).

Clinical presentation/observation: Difficulty ambulating up or down stairs, difficulty transferring, driving, threading a needle, sewing, knitting, stabbing food with a fork, pouring, hammering, or placing a denture adhesive on teeth are common signs of depth perception (Gillen, 2009).

Screening and Assessments

Various semistandardized assessments for depth perception include the following:

- Clinic Depth Perception Test (Zoltan, 2007)
- SOTOF (Gillen, 2009)

Nonstandardized approaches to assessment include the following:

- Ask the client to estimate distances of several objects on a table. Which is closer? Farther away? A deficit is indicated if the client cannot complete the task and demonstrates similar difficulties in ADLs (Zoltan, 2007).
- Place an object on a table and ask the client to pick it up. Hold the object in front of the client and ask him or her to take it from you. A deficit is indicated if the client cannot complete the tasks and demonstrates similar difficulties with ADLs (Zoltan, 2007).

Interventions

They include the following:

- *Remedial approach*: During ADLs, allow the client to use tactile and kinesthetic senses to increase awareness (Zoltan, 2007).
- *Adaptive approach*: Modify the environment and label objects to maximize safety. Use other senses and provide verbal cues to compensate for deficits. Train the client and family in order to maximize safety (Zoltan, 2007).

Topographical Orientation

Description: Topographical orientation involves the ability to navigate from one place to the next. Requirements include the ability to determine current location, goal location, and problem solving to implement an action (Zoltan, 2007).

Clinical presentation/observation: Clients present with difficulty completing a return trip, difficulty locating rooms, buildings, and so forth in familiar or unfamiliar environments, and easily gets lost when driving or walking (Gillen, 2009; Zoltan, 2007).

Screening and Assessments

After being shown a route several times, ask the client to find his or her way to a specific place (e.g., clinic to room, clinic to outside door, and room to clinic) (Gillen, 2009; Zoltan, 2007). This task is dependent on intact cognition, such as memory (i.e., nonstandardized) (Zoltan, 2007).

Interventions

Assist the client in learning landmarks on a route. Landmarks should be consistently available, and not change from day to day, and should be easily identified (e.g., high in contrast). Verbally describe the route plan to the client prior to beginning a task (Gillen, 2009; Zoltan, 2007).

Tactile Perception Deficits

Description: Stereognosis (i.e., astereognosis, tactile agnosia) involves the ability to identify everyday objects using their tactile properties without the use of visual input (Gillen, 2009; Zoltan, 2007). The inability to complete the task is called astereognosis (i.e., tactile agnosia), which requires the integration of tactile information (e.g., temperature, texture, weight, and contour) for task completion (Zoltan, 2007).

Ahylognosia is the inability to discriminate materials, while amorphagnosia is the inability to discriminate forms or shapes (Zoltan, 2007). Agraphesthesia is the inability to identify forms, numbers, or letters written on the palm of the hand.

Clinical presentation/observation: Tasks that require sensation in the hands as a guide are difficult to complete. These tasks typically include locating something in a drawer, a pocket, or a bag without using vision; knitting while watching television; stabbing food with a fork while talking; locating a light switch in the dark or at night; and meal preparation tasks. Objects cannot be located without the use of vision (Gillen, 2009; Zoltan, 2007). Persons with deficits in tactile perception may have difficulty with clothing fasteners even with intact motor function (Gillen, 2009).

Screening and Assessments

The main standardized assessment used for stereognosis includes the Ayres' Manual Form Perception Test (Zoltan, 2007).

Nonstandardized assessment typically includes the OT occluding the client's vision or objects from vision and asking the client to identify common objects without looking (Zoltan, 2007). The OT should record the number of trials, as well as the number of errors. A correct response would include identification of the object within five seconds. Also important is to record a description of the response to the object (e.g., quickly/slowly identified, object described but name not identified and only one property of an object). Objects that could be used include pen, key, screw, safety pin, fork, dime, penny, button, playing card, small ball, banana, or a pair of glasses.

Interventions

Graded intervention programs can be used in which the client looks, feels, and listens to the object (Zoltan, 2007). The vision is occluded and the client identifies the object. The client then locates and identifies objects in sand or rice. Lastly, the client is required to pick out a small item from a group of items. It is important to provide interaction with different textures, awareness and safety training, and visual/auditory compensations as necessary (Gillen, 2009; Zoltan, 2007). The focus should be on the properties of the object.

Body Scheme Disorders

There are four main types of body scheme disorders. These vary in terms of description, assessments, and interventions. They are as follows.

Autotopagnosia or Somatognosia

Description: Autotopagnosia involves the inability to identify body parts on themselves or someone else, as the relationship between parts (Zoltan, 2007). Proposagnosia is the inability to recognize faces or people even though cognition and the ability to recognize other stimuli are intact (Gillen, 2009).

Screening and Assessments

A semistandardized assessment for autotopagnosia includes the Draw-A-Man Test (Goodenough–Harris Drawing Tests) (Cooke & Kline, 2007; Zoltan, 2007). The OT gives the client a blank sheet of paper and pencil, and asks him or her to draw a man. Scoring in its simplest form includes 10 body parts: head, trunk, right arm, left arm, right leg, left leg, right hand, left hand, right foot, and left foot. A score of intact is given if all 10 are noted; minimally impaired results in the drawing of 6–9 body parts; severely impaired is noted when 5 or less body parts are drawn correctly (Zoltan, 2007).

Typical nonstandardized measures to assess for autotopagnosia include asking the client to follow your directions by pointing or identifying the body part named on his or her body, your body, or on a doll (e.g., show me your right foot, touch your left eye with your right hand, and show me your knee). The client imitates the OT's movements or mirror images. The OT can make up his or her own movements and commands. An intact result is noted if the client can answer all questions in a reasonable length of time (Zoltan, 2007).

Interventions

It is important to provide opportunities to reinforce identification of body parts on themselves and someone else, especially during self-care activities such as dressing or grooming. Combine tactile input/stimulation with naming body parts. Bilateral integration tasks will help reinforce learning. Safety awareness and precautions should be a part of the intervention (Zoltan, 2007).

Finger Agnosia

Description: Finger agnosia results in the inability to recognize which finger is touched or is being used (Zoltan, 2007).

Clinical presentation/observation: Clients may have difficulty identifying fingers when asked and may display clumsiness with fingers (Zoltan, 2007).

Screening and Assessments

Occlude the client's eyes and ask him or her to tell you which finger was touched (nonstandardized) (Zoltan, 2007).

Interventions

Provide opportunities to reinforce the identification of fingers in ADLs (Zoltan, 2007). Examples might include asking the client to point to an object with a specific finger, or ask the client to identify which fingers he is using to hold the pencil, utensil, or other object. Other professionals may also have an opportunity to reinforce learning, such as a nurse or certified diabetic educator during training to use a glucometer.

Anosognosia

Description: Anosognosia results in a lack of recognition or awareness of one's deficits and includes both cognitive and sensory (i.e., proprioception) impairments (Zoltan, 2007). The term anosognosia may be used interchangeably with the term self-awareness deficit (Gillen, 2013), which is discussed at length later in this chapter.

Clinical presentation/observation: It is important to monitor hands during ADLs; specifically safety in regard to burns and cuts (Zoltan, 2007).

Interventions

The focus should be on providing reinforcements of body parts using tactile and proprioceptive awareness. The client should integrate the use of affected body parts during functional ADL tasks (Zoltan, 2007).

Right/Left Discrimination

Description: Right and/or left discrimination affecting the ability to identify, discriminate, and understand the concept of right and left. Short-term memory and aphasia can affect the client's accuracy (Gillen, 2009; Zoltan, 2007).

Clinical presentation/observation: Typically presents with difficulty following directions during ADLs, especially dressing, grooming, and functional mobility tasks (Gillen, 2009; Zoltan, 2007).

Screening and Assessments

The main standardized assessment used for right/left discrimination includes the Ayres' Right/Left Discrimination Test (i.e., subtest of Southern California Sensory Integration Test) (Zoltan, 2007).

Nonstandardized assessment involves asking the client to identify body parts or to do something with a particular body part (e.g., show me your left foot, touch your right ear, and take the paper with your left hand). The client should be able to follow directions in a reasonable amount of time (Zoltan, 2007).

Interventions

The focus should be on providing reinforcements of body parts using tactile and proprioceptive awareness. The client should integrate the use of the affected body parts during functional ADL tasks, with special attention to the potential for safety concerns in regard to burns and cuts (Zoltan, 2007). A watch or bracelet on one wrist may help clients discriminate between their right and left sides. As the client progresses, the OT can discontinue use of the bracelet and use cueing instead.

Management and Standards of Practice

After evaluating the client, the OT will identify the client's limitations, needs, and goals in order to direct the intervention priorities. In collaboration with the occupational therapy assistant (OTA), the OT should develop the intervention plan, delegating the aspects that will be carried out by the OTA. For instance, the OT may be responsible for training related to oculomotor deficits, while the OTA may be responsible for implementing intervention strategies for visual inattention related to occupational performance activities, such as emphasized scanning using organized search patterns during therapeutic activities and ADL, or increasing or decreasing cognitive demands during tasks. The OTA needs to have an understanding of the vision deficits and visual perception deficits caused by neurological injuries. The OT and OTA should collaborate with the client on final recommendations for safety and/or caregiver assistance, community resources, and referrals to other professionals.

Cognition

Cognition is defined as mental skills and processes, including the ability to organize, interpret, and apply the information (Radomski & Morrison, 2014; Toglia et al., 2014). Metacognition is the ability to choose and use specific mental skills to complete a task. Each area of the brain is responsible for different cognitive functions, which are classified into right and left hemispheres and then further classified into the various lobes of the brain (Gillen, 2009). Damage to the right hemisphere of the brain will result in attention deficits and reduced insight and judgment, whereas damage to the left hemisphere may result in deficits with organization, sequencing, and planning (Gillen, 2009). The regions of the brain and primary cognitive functions are as follows:

- *Frontal lobe*: Planning, initiation, organizing, attention, appropriate behavior, problem solving, short-term memory, and emotions (Gillen, 2009; Gutman, 2008).
- *Parietal lobe*: Alertness, judgment, perseveration, right side—visual spatial relations, left side—spoken and written language (Gillen, 2009; Gutman, 2008).
- *Temporal lobes*: Memory (i.e., visual and verbal) and emotion (Gillen, 2009).
- *Occipital lobe*: Interpretation of visual stimuli (Gutman, 2008).
- *Brainstem*: Composed of the midbrain, pons, and medulla oblongata and is responsible for automatic reflexive behaviors with vision and audition, and functions such as breathing, heart rate, cough/gag reflexes, pupillary responses, and the swallowing reflex (Gutman, 2008).
- *Thalamus*: Visual, auditory, and tactile/sensory processing (Gutman, 2008).
- *Hypothalamus*: Regulates the autonomic nervous system, temperature, hunger, sleep–wake cycles, and expression of emotion (Gutman, 2008).
- *Basal ganglia*: Composed of the caudate nucleus, putamen, and globus pallidus and is responsible for unconscious motor patterns as well as motor planning and appropriate movement (Gutman, 2008). This portion of the brain works closely with the frontal lobe and therefore contributes to orientation, initiation, and memory (Gillen, 2009).

General Screening and Assessments

Assessments and interventions with cognitive deficits should focus on relevant occupations (Gillen, 2009, 2013; Radomski & Giles, 2014). It is important to consider the level of the cognitive skills required to complete specific ADLs or instrumental activities of daily living (IADLs) within the chosen assessments or interventions. Information from the caregiver's family and the results of self-reports may provide insight into deficits and goals. OT practitioners should practice the same strategy across multiple tasks in natural environments. Grading of strategies should occur slowly to ensure a transfer of skills (e.g., change one to two characteristics of a task, then three to four characteristics, and eventually change the task, but keep the approach similar) (Gillen, 2009; Radomski & Giles, 2014; Toglia et al., 2014; Zoltan, 2007).

Cognition Hierarchy

The cognitive hierarchy begins with a foundational level of the most basic to most complex skills beginning with attention and orientation and resulting in the ability to generalize and transfer knowledge.

1. Attention and orientation
2. Memory
3. Lower-level executive functions including initiation and inhibition, planning, and organization
4. Higher-level executive functions including problem solving, self-awareness, and mental flexibility
5. Generalization and transfer of knowledge (Gillen, 2009)

Cognitive Interventions

The goal of OT intervention is to improve ADL performance and the quality of life for the individual with cognitive deficits (Gillen, 2009, 2013; Radomski & Morrison, 2014; Toglia et al., 2014). The following factors should be considered during assessments and intervention:

- Affective, emotional, and motivational factors (e.g., anxieties, pain, depression, fatigue, and adjustment issues) (Radomski & Giles, 2014; Radomski & Morrison, 2014; Zoltan, 2007)

- Sensory loss (e.g., vision and hearing) (Radomski & Giles, 2014; Radomski & Morrison, 2014; Zoltan, 2007)
- Sleep disorders (Radomski & Morrison, 2014; Zoltan, 2007)
- Chronic and acute illness (Radomski & Giles, 2014; Radomski & Morrison, 2014)
- Family or social problems (Gillen, 2009; Zoltan, 2007)
- Environment (Gillen, 2009; Zoltan, 2007)

Remedial approaches to cognitive deficits center on the restoration of cognitive abilities by using exercises to increase abilities. Increasing the complexity and demands of the intervention are methods used to grade each task. It is important to note that one deficit can be treated independently from another (Gillen, 2009; Radomski & Giles, 2014; Toglia et al., 2014).

Adaptive approaches use changes in context, habits, routines, and strategies so that the client can perform everyday occupations (Zoltan, 2007). Context changes involve lower cognitive demands and are effective with dementia. Physical context involves the modification of physical properties, such as a decrease in the tools used, items in the environment, distractions, or an increase in physical cues. Social context may involve training a caregiver or family members in methods to assist the client. Habits and routines are another adaptive approach and involve changing automatic behaviors (Gillen, 2009; Toglia et al., 2014; Zoltan, 2007).

Interventions require practice and repetition in order to develop new habits and routines. This is often an effective approach for ADL independence. Formal models incorporate remedial approaches, adaptive approaches, or a combination of both. They are as follows:

- *Dynamic interactional/multicontext approach*: Investigates the underlying conditions influencing performance such as self-awareness, acquisition of new information, processing strategies, and addresses the person, activity, and environment to facilitate modification of performance (Gillen, 2009, 2013; Radomski & Giles, 2014; Toglia et al., 2014; Zoltan, 2007).
- *Quadraphonic approach (i.e., functional/occupation-based approach)*: Uses analysis of performance skills with a synthesis of meaningful human occupations from medical and social perspectives, and focuses on remediation of subskills and functional ADL skills (Gillen, 2009, 2013; Toglia et al., 2014; Zoltan, 2007).

- *Cognitive compensatory strategy (i.e., retraining)*: Improves self-awareness through anticipation, acquisition, application, and adaptation by teaching strategies based on a client's abilities through remedial, procedural, and learning techniques (Gillen, 2009; Radomski & Giles, 2014).
- *Neurofunctional approach*: Trains clients to use specific strategies by focusing on retraining skills, not the functional limitation. Generalization to other situations is not expected when the neurofunctional approach is used. The neurofunctional approach is often used in the most severe cases (Gillen, 2009, 2013; Toglia et al., 2014).

Cognitive Deficits

Alertness, orientation, and attention are three main areas of cognitive deficits related to attention. Each of these varies in terms of their description, clinical presentation, assessment, and intervention processes as outlined below.

Alertness

Description: Alertness is the state of responsiveness when stimulated through a variety of senses such as visual, auditory, and tactile (Gillen, 2009; Zoltan, 2007).

Clinical presentation/observation: Typically, the client responds by maintaining open eyes, using sounds or by movement, and eventually begins to follow simple directions.

Screening and Assessments

There are two main standardized assessments for alertness.

1. Glasgow Coma Scale is a scale used to record a person's conscious state using three tests (i.e., eye, verbal, and motor response) resulting in a score between 3 and 15.
2. Rancho Levels of Cognitive Functioning—Revised is an assessment used to grade a person's cognitive status, starting with "no response, total assistance" and progressing through 10 levels to "purposeful, appropriate, modified independence."

It is important to record the response given by the client along with the amount of time the client maintained a response (Gillen, 2009).

Orientation

Description: Orientation refers to the recognition and/or attentiveness to self, others, environments, and time (Zoltan, 2007).

Clinical presentation/observation: Multiple areas of the brain control the function of orientation (Toglia et al., 2014; Zoltan, 2007). There are three subsets of orientation, which include person, place, and time (i.e., date and time of day). Deficits may be temporary or last longer with disorientation reflected verbally or behaviorally. The dimension of time seems to be recovered last and breaks down the easiest, possibly because it is multidimensional (Radomski & Morrison, 2014; Toglia et al., 2014; Zoltan, 2007). Orientation may also be associated with memory limitations such as the recall and retention of information (Radomski & Morrison, 2014; Toglia et al., 2014; Zoltan, 2007).

Screening and Assessments

There are various standardized assessments appropriate for orientation. They are as follows:

- LOTCA (Cooke & Kline, 2007; Radomski & Morrison, 2014; Toglia et al., 2014)
- Test of Orientation for Rehabilitation Patients (TORP) (Toglia et al., 2014)
- Montreal Cognitive Assessment (MoCA) (Cooke & Kline, 2007; Radomski & Morrison, 2014; Toglia et al., 2014)
- Brief Neuropsychological Cognitive Examination (Cooke & Kline, 2007)
- Mini-Mental State Examination (MMSE) (Radomski & Morrison, 2014; Toglia et al., 2014)

Interventions

Deficits in orientation can cause confusion, agitation, and other behavioral issues. Disorientation often causes difficulty with orienting oneself in the environment causing a person to get lost and experience an altered sense of time. Appropriate interventions include daily orientation in group and individual settings with consistent reminders and external orientation aids, such as personal items from home (Toglia et al., 2014; Zoltan, 2007). Keeping the client organized with a predictable and consistent schedule and minimizing unfamiliar or unexpected change are also important intervention strategies (Zoltan, 2007). The OT practitioner should introduce himself or herself and incorporate information on orientation into conversation. Use redirection techniques to decrease agitation and confusion (Zoltan, 2007). It is also critical to train family and caregivers with strategies to maintain orientation using all senses, including auditory, tactile, and visual (Toglia et al., 2014; Zoltan, 2007).

Attention

Description: Attention involves the active process that assists in determining what a person focuses on. It allows a person to receive incoming information from another person or their environment. Components of attention involve the ability to narrow focus, sustain focus, and shift focus in a voluntary manner requiring effort (Gillen, 2013; Zoltan, 2007).

Clinical presentation/observation: Components of attention include consciousness, awareness, arousal, memory, motivation, and information processing (Toglia et al., 2014; Zoltan, 2007). The lesion site is mainly centered on the frontal lobe and/or parietal lobe in the right hemisphere, although multiple areas of the brain control different aspects of attention (Gillen, 2009; Radomski & Morrison, 2014; Zoltan, 2007). The various types of attention are as follows:

- *Focused attention*: The ability to attend to different stimuli and involves alertness (Radomski & Morrison, 2014; Zoltan, 2007).
- *Sustained attention*: A conscious effort to maintain one's attention over a period of time (Gillen, 2009; Radomski & Morrison, 2014; Toglia et al., 2014; Zoltan, 2007).
- *Selective attention*: Ability to maintain attention on an item while ignoring competing stimuli, such as ignoring fighting children when driving, which is needed for goal-directed behavior. It is needed for adequate perception and adequate visual attention (Gillen, 2009; Radomski & Morrison, 2014; Toglia et al., 2014; Zoltan, 2007).
- *Alternating attention or attentional flexibility*: The ability to switch back and forth between multiple tasks, for instance, reading signs while driving (Gillen, 2009; Radomski & Morrison, 2014; Toglia et al., 2014; Zoltan, 2007).
- *Divided attention*: The ability to maintain attention on multiple tasks at the same time, requiring decision making for time-sharing (Gillen, 2009; Radomski & Morrison, 2014; Toglia et al., 2014; Zoltan, 2007).

- *Concentration*: The ability to do mental work while attending, which requires one to actively encode information in one's working memory (Zoltan, 2007).

Screening and Assessments

Standardized assessments: Various standardized assessments are appropriate for attention. They are as follows:

- Test of Everyday Attention (TEA)—adult and children version (Cooke & Kline, 2007; Gillen, 2013; Radomski & Morrison, 2014; Toglia et al., 2014)
- A-ONE (Gillen, 2013; Radomski & Morrison, 2014; Toglia et al., 2014)
- AMPS (Gillen, 2013; Toglia et al., 2014)
- Cognitive Assessment of Minnesota (CAM) (Cooke & Kline, 2007; Radomski & Morrison, 2014; Toglia et al., 2014)
- Cognistat (Neurobehavioral Cognitive Status Examination) (Cooke & Kline, 2007; Radomski & Morrison, 2014; Toglia et al., 2014)
- MoCA (Cooke & Kline, 2007; Radomski & Morrison, 2014; Toglia et al., 2014)
- MMSE (Cooke & Kline, 2007; Radomski & Morrison, 2014; Toglia et al., 2014)
- Brief Neuropsychological Cognitive Examination (Cooke & Kline, 2007)
- Kettle Test (Gillen, 2013; Toglia et al., 2014)
- Moss Attention Rating Scale (Gillen, 2013)
- Rating Scale of Attentional Behavior (Gillen, 2013)
- Allen Cognitive Level Test (Toglia et al., 2014)
- Comprehensive Trail-Making Test (Toglia et al., 2014)
- Dementia Rating Scale (Cooke & Kline, 2007)

Nonstandardized assessments include clinical observations involving distractibility, difficulty focusing, poor concentration, fatigue, irritability, headache, sensitivity to noise, difficulty completing a task, more time to complete a task, symptoms of overload, and difficulty remembering what he or she is doing (Zoltan, 2007). Informal assessments include observing the client in different settings and performing different ADLs (Gillen, 2009; Zoltan, 2007). Letter cancellation tests and a Dynavision scanning task may allow for observation of attention deficit. OT practitioners should also consider other limitations that may impact attention, such as vision, memory, and processing. Questions to ask include the following: When can a person attend and for how long? With what types of tasks does attention break down (Zoltan, 2007)?

Interventions

Restorative approach: The restorative approach uses occupational and client-centered activities. The specific type of attention is targeted in the chosen task. Sensory and motor involvement is also incorporated into the intervention. Some restorative interventions incorporate the following:

- Use warm-up activities before ADLs such as mazes and cancellation tasks.
- Assist the client in organizing new information.
- Motivate the client using a reward system if needed.
- Alter task or environment to change the level of attention required for success by grading the intervention.
- Develop the client's active listening skills (Gillen, 2009, 2013; Toglia et al., 2014; Zoltan, 2007).

Adaptive approach: In terms of interventions using an adaptive approach, it is important to structure the environment for success by reducing clutter, noise, hunger, fatigue, and pain. Some additional adaptive strategies include the following:

- The client should prepare to listen and engage by using techniques such as self-talk.
- The client can vocalize task step by step and practice discriminating important components of task.
- The OT practitioner should slow the client down to aid with processing and repetition (Gillen, 2009, 2013; Toglia et al., 2014; Zoltan, 2007).

Regardless of the intervention approach used, it is important to provide training to caregivers and family members in the following areas:

- Reduce stimulation, distraction, and clutter, and control the rate of incoming information.
- Organization strategies for the environment and client's time, using techniques such as self-pacing, labels, schedules, and lists.
- Encourage and prompt the client to ask for help (Gillen, 2009, 2013; Toglia et al., 2014; Zoltan, 2007).

Memory

Description: Memory is the process by which an individual attends, encodes, stores, and retrieves information (Gillen, 2009; Radomski & Morrison, 2014; Toglia et al., 2014; Zoltan, 2007).

Clinical presentation/observation: Memory is controlled in the frontal lobe, parietal lobe, and the thalamus (Gillen, 2009, 2013). Memory deficits can also be seen as a result of insult such as anoxia, encephalopathy/meningitis, dementia/Alzheimer's disease, traumatic brain injury, cerebral vascular accidents, or concussions (Gillen, 2013). Chronic stress or depression and some medications may also cause memory loss (Zoltan, 2007). Memory can be affected by personality, awareness, motivation, anxiety, depression, lifestyle, mood, and level of motivation (Zoltan, 2007). Memory deficits can affect short-term memory, working memory, long-term memory, implicit (i.e., procedural or nondeclarative) memory, explicit (i.e., declarative) memory, episodic memory, semantic memory, and prospective memory (Gillen, 2009; Radomski & Morrison, 2014; Zoltan, 2007). The following provides a list of the different types of memory:

- *Short-term memory*: The memory that is considered temporary storage (Gillen, 2009; Radomski & Morrison, 2014; Zoltan, 2007).
- *Primary memory*: Simple storage of information in *short-term memory*; little processing occurs here (Gillen, 2009).
- *Working memory*: Interim storage and manipulation of information with conscious or controlled recovery of information (Gillen, 2009, 2013; Zoltan, 2007).
- *Long-term memory*: The memory that is permanent storage (Gillen, 2009, 2013; Radomski & Morrison, 2014; Zoltan, 2007).
- *Implicit memory*: Related to the steps of doing something (i.e., nondeclarative memory or procedural memory). Becomes automatic and effortless (i.e., automatic process and habitual). It is the most extensive and permanent memory and aids motor or mental functions (Gillen, 2009, 2013; Zoltan, 2007).
- *Explicit*: Learned or experienced (i.e., declarative memory) (Gillen, 2009, 2013; Zoltan, 2007).
- *Episodic*: Personal knowledge of an event; linked to a person, place, and time (Gillen, 2009, 2013; Zoltan, 2007).
- *Semantic*: General wisdom of factual information that is not dependent on episodic memory and uses visual perception and visual spatial information (Gillen, 2009, 2013; Zoltan, 2007).
- *Procedural memory*: Most complex form of memory used to complete a task and includes a combination of skills from many of the body's systems (Gillen, 2009, 2013; Zoltan, 2007).
- *Prospective memory*: Related to carrying out future activities (Gillen, 2009, 2013; Toglia et al., 2014).

Screening and Assessments

Various standardized assessments are appropriate for memory. They are as follows:

- Rivermead Behavioral Memory Test (Cooke & Kline, 2007; Gillen, 2009, 2013; Radomski & Morrison, 2014; Toglia et al., 2014)
- Cognistat (Neurobehavioral Cognitive Status Examination) (Cooke & Kline, 2007; Gillen, 2013; Radomski & Morrison, 2014; Toglia et al., 2014)
- Contextual Memory Test (Cooke & Kline, 2007; Gillen, 2009; Radomski & Morrison, 2014; Toglia et al., 2014; Zoltan, 2007)
- Everyday Memory Questionnaire (Gillen, 2009, 2013; Toglia et al., 2014)
- Cambridge Prospective Memory Test (Cooke & Kline, 2007; Gillen, 2009, 2013; Toglia et al., 2014)
- A-ONE (Gillen, 2009, 2013; Radomski & Morrison, 2014; Toglia et al., 2014)
- AMPS (Gillen, 2009, 2013)
- Galveston Orientation and Amnesia Test (GOAT) (Cooke & Kline, 2007; Radomski & Morrison, 2014)
- CAM (Cooke & Kline, 2007; Radomski & Morrison, 2014; Toglia et al., 2014)
- MoCA (Cooke & Kline, 2007; Radomski & Morrison, 2014; Toglia et al., 2014)
- Dementia Rating Scale (Cooke & Kline, 2007)

Nonstandardized assessments include observation of clients in a variety of environments and with a variety of ADLs in order to observe which sensory systems are impaired and may be affecting memory (i.e., vision impacts visual memory) (Gillen, 2009; Zoltan, 2007).

Interventions

ADL completion depends on information retrieval. A lack of awareness may impact a client's ability to be left home alone. In addition, memory deficits can lead to paranoia or anger toward others. General suggestions for interventions include the following:

- Identify learning styles or preferences.
- Utilize pictures to assist the client in remembering.

- Place external cues strategically to ensure success.
- Assist clients in developing appropriate strategies.
- Treat the client in his or her natural environment when possible, such as dressing tasks in bathroom or bedroom.
- Monitor the client for information overload.
- Base goals on client's needs, keeping them realistic and relevant. Make use of old routines.
- To ensure generalization of concepts, provide opportunities for repetition and practice.
- The more severe the impairment, the more you may need to structure the environment (Gillen, 2009; Zoltan, 2007).

Restorative approach: In terms of a restorative approach for memory interventions, there is little evidence available suggesting that memory can be restored and whether restoration strategies should be task specific or generalized to other tasks (Gillen, 2009; Zoltan, 2007). The OT practitioner should monitor the effectiveness of strategies. Deficits should be addressed in the following order: attention, short-term memory, and long-term memory. Repetition with vanishing cues often improves success, although rehearsals should be spaced out for retention. Strategies should be ADL specific and built around preserved memory (Zoltan, 2007).

Adaptive approach: Evidence-based success using adaptive strategies indicates compensatory strategies may be the preferred approach (Zoltan, 2007). Internal aids are person centered and utilize the person with the deficit(s). External aids utilize resources outside of a person's brain (Radomski & Giles, 2014; Zoltan, 2007).

Types of strategies that may be effective for OTs and OTAs to use during intervention include the following internal and external strategies. Internal strategies include the following:

- Internal strategies include a mental moment (i.e., think for a minute to jog memory) and association (i.e., pairing with something else so that you are able to remember at a later time, new or old associations or sensory, emotional, and location associations).
- Repetition: repeating to one's self.
- Mnemonics: a word, sentence, or song that assists in remembering something. This can also be used with pictures. Pegging is a type of mnemonic strategy and is used when things need to be recalled in a particular order.

- Visual imagery: picturing in your head what to remember later (Gillen, 2009, 2013; Radomski & Giles, 2014; Toglia et al., 2014; Zoltan, 2007).

External strategies include the following:

- Electronic aids and reminders, including clock/watch/phone alarms, recorders (e.g., audio or video), answering machines/voice mail, electronic pill-boxes, microwave with preset buttons, automatic shut-off appliances, programmable phones, and voice-activated aids; should be portable, able to store many cues, and be simple for clients to use.
- Cuing from other people allows for immediate feedback, assists in using retrieval cues in original process, and allows for active questioning.
- Write reminders and take notes, including paper or email.
- Calendars: paper and electronic (Gillen, 2009, 2013; Radomski & Giles, 2014; Toglia et al., 2014; Zoltan, 2007).

As with any intervention, it is critical to educate and train family and caregivers in compensatory strategies and safety concerns. Listen to concerns of the client, family, and caregivers. Give direction in order to help with future preparations. Emphasize the need for consistency in routines and implementation of strategies and teach caretakers to take advantage of incidental learning (Gillen, 2009, 2013; Radomski & Giles, 2014; Toglia et al., 2014; Zoltan, 2007).

Executive Function

Description: Executive functions are defined as higher-level mental functions involving decision making, planning, sequencing, and executing (Gillen, 2013; Zoltan, 2007). They can be divided into two groups: lower-level tasks and higher-level tasks. The lower-level tasks include initiation, planning, and organization tasks (Zoltan, 2007). The higher-level functions include safety and judgment, mental flexibility and calculations, self-awareness, and problem solving (Gillen, 2009, 2013; Zoltan, 2007). Since OT often addresses self-awareness and problem solving, they are described individually below. Generalization, the ability to apply learned compensatory strategies to new situations or environments, occurs with intact executive function and short-term memory. There is also a self-correction component required for generalization (Gillen, 2009; Zoltan, 2007). Initiation is the ability to start a task or activity while termination is the ability to stop or end the task (Gillen, 2013; Zoltan, 2007). Inhibition is the ability to slow or delay an impulse or the slowing down of an activity or occurrence (Gillen, 2009; Zoltan, 2007). Planning and organization includes sequencing and categorization and the ability to use multiple steps in a process to achieve a goal (Gillen, 2009; Zoltan, 2007). Planning and organization includes the ability to organize the steps into action (i.e., sequencing), as well as assemble the needed materials, identify skills required to complete a task, and recognize the limits and/or restrictions, which is a precursor to problem solving. The following skills are prerequisites to master skills of planning and organization: adequate memory, sustained attention, volition (i.e., power to make one's own choices), impulse control, and the ability to perform complex actions (Gillen, 2009; Zoltan, 2007). Executive function deficits are associated with frontal lobe damage (Gillen, 2009; Toglia et al., 2014; Zoltan, 2007).

Clinical presentation/observation: A person with deficits of initiation or termination may be observed as slow to respond, lacking spontaneity, showing little or no initiative, and/or requiring verbal cuing for when and where to do something (Gillen, 2009; Zoltan, 2007). This deficit can be misinterpreted as an intentional lack of motivation. These clients may have trouble getting started on homework or chores. They can usually plan, organize, and carry out complex tasks but only with cuing. They may repeatedly voice a plan but never carry it out (Zoltan, 2007). A person with inhibition deficits may be observed interrupting others, getting out of a seat at the wrong time, and saying whatever is on their mind (i.e., no filter). They may exhibit behavior that is more "out of control" than peers (Gillen, 2009; Zoltan, 2007). Observations of a person with planning and organization deficits may include a lack of foresight; demonstration of poor, unrealistic, or illogical plans; setting unrealistic goals; and having difficulty prioritizing or estimating time requirements (Zoltan, 2007). Perseveration may be observed or clients may follow the "routine" even when it is not productive. Fragmented sequences may also be observed. Deficits in executive function may be more apparent in unfamiliar settings or nonclinical settings, such as at home, at work, at school, or in the community (Radomski & Morrison, 2014; Toglia et al., 2014).

Screening and Assessments

Various standardized assessments are appropriate for executive functioning skills. They are as follows:

- Executive Function Performance Test (EFPT) (Gillen, 2009, 2013; Radomski & Morrison, 2014; Toglia et al., 2014; Zoltan, 2007)
- Behavior Rating Inventory of Executive Function (BRIEF), versions for pediatric, adolescent, and adult (Gillen, 2009; Radomski & Morrison, 2014; Toglia et al., 2014)
- A-ONE (Gillen, 2009, 2013; Radomski & Morrison, 2014; Toglia et al., 2014)
- Dementia Rating Scale (Cooke & Kline, 2007)
- Behavioral Assessment of Dysexecutive Syndrome (BADS) (Cooke & Kline, 2007; Gillen, 2009, 2013; Toglia et al., 2014)
- Multiple Errands Test (Gillen, 2009, 2013; Radomski & Morrison, 2014)
- Routine Task Inventory (Cooke & Kline, 2007; Toglia et al., 2014)
- CAM (Cooke & Kline, 2007; Radomski & Morrison, 2014; Toglia et al., 2014)
- Cognistat (Neurobehavioral Cognitive Status Examination) (Cooke & Kline, 2007; Radomski & Morrison, 2014; Toglia et al., 2014)
- LOTCA (Cooke & Kline, 2007; Radomski & Morrison, 2014; Toglia et al., 2014)
- Executive Function Route-Finding Task (EFRT) (Gillen, 2013; Toglia et al., 2014)
- Observed Tasks of Daily Living—Revised (OTDL-R) (Radomski & Morrison, 2014; Toglia et al., 2014)

Interventions

Restorative approach: Restorative interventions for initiation may include the use of habits and routine daily tasks, where the end of one step triggers the next step (Gillen, 2013; Zoltan, 2007). Initial steps may need to be mastered before a routine for ADLs is successful. Sensory input may also elicit initiation. The OT practitioner may also use nonverbal tactile or kinesthetic guiding to cue the client. Incentive training may be a valuable motivator (Zoltan, 2007). Restorative interventions for planning and organization include relating information into a meaningful structure for the client, such as dividing tasks into categories. Recognition and rehearsal of strategies is important including training in the elements of organization such as how to do things that relate to each other (Radomski & Giles, 2014). Clients should take an active role or have responsibility in planning activities. Clients should also be trained to verbalize, plan, and utilize self-questioning (Gillen, 2009; Zoltan, 2007).

Adaptive approach: Adaptive or compensatory training begins with external cues and prompts and moves to internal strategies and self-monitoring. External strategies may include attentional kicks (e.g., "Just do it", "Get going"), alarms, calendar reminders, audiocassettes, to-do lists, and checklists (Gillen, 2009; Toglia et al., 2014; Zoltan, 2007). Clients can write steps down and practice mental rehearsals before the actions. OTs typically initiate organization strategies, accessibility, consistency, grouping, and separation and proximity (Zoltan, 2007). The OT practitioner may begin with verbal cuing and progress to written cues and then self-reminders. Arranging items in order of sequence before beginning the task may be helpful for clients.

Other therapeutic activities include categorization games where the client needs to identify the items, words, or pictures that belong together or the one that does not. Helpful games include *Apples-to-Apples Junior*, *Sequencing* or *Sequence for Kids*, *Simon*, and *Mastermind*, in addition to identifying and recognizing patterns, and dot-to-dots or alphabet mazes. To practice more complex activities, write out scenario-based activities such as the schedule for the day or a list of errands for today—which you would do first (e.g., if you are moving into a new apartment, which task needs to be done first) or make a list of the items that are needed to accomplish the task.

Considerations for referral and discharge include the identification of safety concerns. Although the client may be able to perform in a clinic environment, the client may not be able to transfer skills to the home environment without supervision (Gillen, 2009; Radomski & Morrison, 2014; Toglia et al., 2014).

Problem Solving and Reasoning

Description: Higher-level (i.e., executive function) problem solving is the active process of making a decision by integrating information using several cognitive skills, including memory, attention, planning, organization and categorization, initiation, inhibition and impulse control, and mental flexibility and reasoning (Zoltan, 2007). In basic problem-solving tasks, a problem is easily identified and solved, and if something is done incorrectly in the process, it is immediately apparent (Zoltan,

2007). Complex or advanced problem-solving tasks require the ability to plan, test, and reject what does not work and formulate alternatives. Incorrect solutions are not obvious and solutions require an active process (Zoltan, 2007). There are various steps required in the problem-solving process.

Reasoning is one step of problem solving. It is the ability to use information to reach a conclusion and involves the formulation and manipulation of the mental image of the relationship of objects (Zoltan, 2007). Reasoning involves making hypotheses, inferences, and justifying conclusions. Decision making is another part of problem solving which requires a client to actively choose from several known options to make a decision (Toglia et al., 2014; Zoltan, 2007). There are two types of decision making. In traditional decision making, the correct response is intrinsic or inherent to the external situation, and there is a right and wrong answer. Many executive functioning assessments evaluate this type of decision making (Zoltan, 2007). Adaptive decision making is client centered or priority based. This type of decision making is used in real-life situations. Safety and judgment involves an evaluation of the solution that was developed for the problem. Was the problem solved? Were there consequences to the solution, including safety issues (Toglia et al., 2014)? This often involves applying compensatory strategies, such as for safety to ADLs. Flexibility is the ability to switch actions appropriately depending on feedback from the environment related to these actions. Other key skills impacting problem solving include the following:

- *Abstract thinking*: Ability to differentiate between pertinent and nonpertinent information, as well as recognize the relationships within the situation (i.e., events, people, objects, and thoughts), or thinking symbolically
- *Concrete thinking*: Tangible, specific ideas or thoughts and literal definitions (i.e., opposite of abstract thinking)
- *Convergent thinking*: Central idea
- *Divergent thinking*: Conflicting or alternative ideas (Zoltan, 2007)

Clinical presentation/observation: People with reasoning and decision-making deficits may exhibit impulsive behavior, be confused on where to start, and have difficulty identifying best options and difficulty learning from mistakes (Zoltan, 2007). The person may repeat the decisions or behaviors with negative outcomes. People with deficits may have sequencing issues or have difficulty applying learned skills to new situations. Flexibility deficits will often present with rigid, inflexible behavior; they may perseverate, may continue to respond or react to irrelevant cues, and may be unable to shift a response although they know it is incorrect (Gillen, 2009; Toglia et al., 2014; Zoltan, 2007). Individuals with deficits in flexibility may continue to give the same response to various situations, even though the situation may be dangerous (Zoltan, 2007).

Screening and Assessments

Various standardized assessments are appropriate for problem solving and reasoning. They are as follows:

- A-ONE (Gillen, 2009, 2013; Radomski & Morrison, 2014; Toglia et al., 2014)
- CAM (Cooke & Kline, 2007; Radomski & Morrison, 2014; Toglia et al., 2014)
- Cognistat (Neurobehavioral Cognitive Status Examination) (Cooke & Kline, 2007; Radomski & Morrison, 2014; Toglia et al., 2014)
- BADS (Cooke & Kline, 2007; Gillen, 2009, 2013; Toglia et al., 2014)
- MoCA (Cooke & Kline, 2007; Radomski & Morrison, 2014; Toglia et al., 2014)
- Multiple Errands Test (Gillen, 2009, 2013; Radomski & Morrison, 2014)
- EFPT (Gillen, 2009, 2013; Radomski & Giles, 2014; Toglia et al., 2014; Zoltan, 2007)
- The main nonstandardized assessment being the Odd–Even Cross Out (i.e., flexibility) approach to problem solving and reasoning

Interventions

Deficits with problem solving include reasoning, decision making, judgment, and flexibility, and will impact independence and safety during ADLs. Clients may only be able to perform tasks in one structured environment. Clients may require cues (e.g., verbal or written) when there is a slight change to a task. The OT team and caregivers should constantly monitor the client for safety issues.

Restorative approach: Restorative interventions for problem-solving deficits should incorporate the following:

- Train the client to read and reread directions.
- The client should be able to describe task steps or main points in his or her own words; he or she should be able to ask questions to clarify.

- Train the client to identify goals of the task and recognize parts of the task that may cause problems. Clients should be able to list alternative solutions and discuss advantages and disadvantages.
- During the task, the client should be trained to recognize mistakes, identify the correct step, and return to the task.
- Problem-solving worksheets or scenarios and games such as *Mastermind* may be helpful to use in training.
- Chaining parts of activities together may be an effective strategy.
- Verbalization of steps and strategies slows the client down (Gillen, 2009, 2013; Toglia et al., 2014; Zoltan, 2007).

Adaptive approach: Adaptive interventions for problem-solving deficits should include the following:

- Modify the environment based on the client's level of functioning:
  - Reduce the amount of irrelevant information (i.e., stimulus reduction and distractions).
  - Organize and simplify tasks.
  - Set an adequate pace for the client's level of functioning.
- Provide external and internal cues including self-guidance, self-coaching, and self-questioning:
  - Instruct the client to check and recheck for errors.
  - Identify key areas of impairment and provide step-by-step instructions.
  - Train the client to ask for assistance and provide scenarios to practice this skill (Gillen, 2009, 2013; Toglia et al., 2014; Zoltan, 2007).

A combined approach of restorative and adaptive interventions should address the following:

- Examine processes affecting problem solving (e.g., reasoning and decision making).
- Identify other deficits that may contribute to problem-solving deficits (e.g., memory, and sequencing).
- Address areas in OT that have the most overlap and are most likely to respond well to interventions.
- Identify variables related to the task, such as steps, strategies, environment, and alternative solutions, and how to advance as the client improves.
- Utilize techniques in many different situations (Gillen, 2009, 2013; Toglia et al., 2014; Zoltan, 2007).

Generalization and Transfer of Problem-Solving Skills

Description: Generalization is the ability to use a newly learned strategy in a novel situation (Gillen, 2009; Zoltan, 2007). Transfer of learning is the ability to use the same knowledge in a similar way in successive tasks (Gillen, 2009, 2013; Zoltan, 2007).

Continuum of skill progression, as first described by Toglia, includes the following:

- Near transfer is when one to two task characteristics have changed.
- Intermediate transfer is when three to six elements differ. Although the new task will share some physical characteristics, other characteristics may be less identifiable.
- Far transfer is a conceptually similar task, but it is completely different or shares only one surface characteristic.
- Very far transfer or generalization occurs when the application of a strategy is spontaneous and can be carried over from treatment to ADLs (Gillen, 2009; Radomski & Giles, 2014; Toglia et al., 2014; Zoltan, 2007).

Interventions

The OT practitioner should grade tasks by changing task elements while keeping the adaptive strategy the same (i.e., organization). The client should be able to apply adaptive strategies across a variety of environments for a variety of tasks (Gillen, 2009; Radomski & Giles, 2014; Zoltan, 2007). The OT practitioner should provide a variety of different practice situations and environments while assisting the client to recognize how a new situation is similar to an old one (Gillen, 2009; Zoltan, 2007). Create simulated environments and scenarios for overlearning and verification of skills while using occupations relevant to the client (Zoltan, 2007).

The goal of executive dysfunction is for the client to be able to generalize strategies and apply them to any situation (Toglia et al., 2014). With higher-level cognitive deficits such as executive function deficits, it is crucial to constantly monitor for safety. Consider a living situation at home and whether or not the client can generalize and transfer skills to new environments and tasks (Zoltan, 2007).

Self-Awareness

Description: Self-awareness is the ability to perceive the self objectively, as well as the knowledge and recognition of one's own abilities and limitations (Radomski & Morrison, 2014; Toglia et al., 2014; Zoltan, 2007). There are two levels of awareness: awareness of deficits and awareness of consequences related to these deficits. There are three components of awareness, as defined below, which build upon each other for mastery:

- Intellectual awareness is the foundational or basic component or skill and is the ability to understand at some level that function is impaired (Gillen, 2009, 2013; Radomski & Morrison, 2014; Zoltan, 2007).
- Emergent awareness is the middle component or skill and involves the ability to recognize a problem as it is happening (Gillen, 2009, 2013; Radomski & Morrison, 2014; Zoltan, 2007).
- Anticipatory awareness, the most advanced component or skill, is defined as the ability to anticipate that problems will occur as the result of a particular impairment in advance of action (Gillen, 2009, 2013; Radomski & Morrison, 2014; Zoltan, 2007).

Clinical presentation/observation: The client with deficits in self-awareness may exhibit impulsive behavior, have difficulty adjusting to unexpected change, and be unable to control temper or handle arguments (Gillen, 2009; Zoltan, 2007). They may present as confused, perplexed, or surprised when they are given feedback. They may fabricate or outright deny when someone points out deficits (Toglia et al., 2014). They may continually focus (or overfocus) on irrelevant information, fail to recognize all aspects of the task, lose track of the goal, or lack the motivation to monitor progress or mistakes (Gillen, 2009; Toglia et al., 2014; Zoltan, 2007). The person with deficits of self-awareness will not initiate self-checking, does not tend to recognize errors, and will not adjust speed when errors are made (Gillen, 2009; Toglia et al., 2014). The client may have limited or poor awareness of appropriate interpersonal boundaries, exhibit poor self-care and grooming, or display poor/inappropriate manners (Zoltan, 2007). Clients may verbalize false judgments or beliefs about one's own abilities, have difficulty identifying and accepting their own deficits, and fail to recognize the need to use compensatory strategies (Gillen, 2009).

Screening and Assessments

Various standardized assessments are appropriate for self-awareness. They are as follows:

- A-ONE (Gillen, 2009, 2013; Radomski & Morrison, 2014; Toglia et al., 2014)
- Patient Competency Rating Scale (PCRS) (Gillen, 2009, 2013; Toglia et al., 2014)
- Self-Awareness of Deficits Interview (SADI) (Cooke & Kline, 2007; Gillen, 2009, 2013; Radomski & Morrison, 2014; Toglia et al., 2014)
- Toglia Category Assessment and Contextual Memory Test (Cooke & Kline, 2007)

Semistandardized assessments for self-awareness include the following:

- Self-Regulation Skills Interview (Gillen, 2009, 2013)
- Assessment of Awareness of Disability used in conjunction with AMPS (Gillen, 2009, 2013; Toglia et al., 2014)
- Awareness Questionnaire (Gillen, 2009, 2013; Toglia et al., 2014)

Nonstandardized assessment may include the evaluation of the three levels of awareness (Zoltan, 2007).

Interventions

Self-awareness deficits impact every ADL, as well as one's ability to participate in rehabilitation and learn compensatory strategies (Toglia et al., 2014; Zoltan, 2007). Clients may be unable to correct mistakes and display poor safety awareness, which may cause injury or increased frustration during ADLs (Zoltan, 2007).

Restorative approach: Restorative interventions are appropriate for deficits in emergent awareness and anticipatory awareness; it is not appropriate for intellectual awareness deficits (i.e., foundational or basic level of awareness) (Zoltan, 2007). Some strategies include allowing the client to predict performance, and perform and reevaluate the predictions (Gillen, 2009; Radomski & Giles, 2014; Toglia et al., 2014; Zoltan, 2007). Additional strategies include performing role reversal where the OT practitioner performs and the client identifies mistakes, uses self-talk strategies to improve performance, and rewards the client for completion of a task or for making accurate predictions (Gillen, 2009; Zoltan, 2007). Process each activity by identifying the purpose, defining the boundaries, skills, and limitations; relate to other relevant situations; and collaborate on new goals (Zoltan, 2007).

The OT practitioner should remain nonjudgmental when identifying behaviors and mistakes, and plan practice so that compensatory strategies become automatic. For an emergent awareness deficit, provide specific and direct feedback during and after a task (Gillen, 2009; Radomski & Giles, 2014; Zoltan, 2007). Use consistent terminology and cuing throughout the task. A self-rating scale that allows for comparisons between the client's scores and family or OTs scores may be helpful (Gillen, 2009; Toglia et al., 2014; Zoltan, 2007). For anticipatory awareness, guide the client to plan for deficits and anticipate needed compensatory strategies (Gillen, 2009). Slowly reduce cuing or use the "vanishing cue" technique (Zoltan, 2007).

Adaptive approach: Adaptive techniques for intervention of self-awareness deficits include the following:

- Provide alternative strategies, such as the use of a microwave instead of the oven or stove.
- Use a checklist for each task that may start as a written checklist but progress to a mental checklist.
- Teach verification strategies.
- Use role reversal to practice techniques.
- Have the client use a self-reflection journal to document what went wrong, how it can be changed, and what was learned or could be done differently in the future.
- For intellectual awareness deficits (e.g., foundational or basic level), use repetitive education of the deficit and how it affects performance. External cues and environmental modification strategies should be used during interventions while always attending to safety.
- For an emergent awareness deficit, practice and repetition for "situational awareness" will be helpful along with checklists.
- For anticipatory awareness (i.e., the highest level) deficits, the client will need to practice anticipation of errors or limitations in order to compensate effectively. Practice recognition of cues, strategy identification, and planning. The client should also be allowed to practice evaluating the strategy and planning how it could be modified in the future (Gillen, 2009, 2013; Radomski & Giles, 2014; Toglia et al., 2014; Zoltan, 2007).

Referrals and Discharge Considerations

When planning discharge and possible referrals, it is critical to train caregivers to consistently point out limitations and provide cues for the appropriate use of compensatory strategies. Caregivers must learn to protect client's safety first and foremost. Without adequate, consistent, or effective awareness, supervision is required.

Management and Standards of Practice

After evaluating the client, the OT will identify the client's limitations, needs, and goals in order to direct the intervention priorities. In collaboration with the OTA, the OT should develop the intervention plan, delegating the aspects that will be carried out by the OT. For instance, the OT may be responsible for the initial training to implement a compensatory strategy, while the OTA may be responsible for implementing the compensatory strategies during functional occupational performance interventions. The OTA needs to have an understanding of different cognitive deficits. The OT and OTA may collaborate on grading the cognitive demands of the tasks, as well as collaboration with the client and his or her caregivers on recommendations for carryover of techniques. Effective communication between the OT and OTA is critical in order to protect the client's safety once discharge occurs.

Chapter 8 Self-Study Activities (Answers Are Provided at the End of the Chapter)

Please read the following case study and answer the questions provided.

Mr. Greene, an 82-year old, who was widowed 9 months ago, recently had a stroke. He is alert and oriented to person, place, and time. He was able to attend to the OT's conversation and questions in his room, even though a nurse and OT were talking and laughing with his roommate in the next bed. Mr. Greene stated that he was living at home independently in a house he had lived in for 50 years. His chart stated that he has been in an assisted living facility near his daughter for 2 months. He could not recall what he had for breakfast. In a quick ADL assessment, the OT decided to have Mr. Greene get dressed for the day. Mr. Greene had difficulty verbalizing the steps required to get ready in the morning and he could not prioritize what needed to be done first, second, and so forth. Once Mr. Greene's clothes were sitting on the bed, he needed multiple verbal cues to get started.

1. What deficits do you suspect based on the client complaints and clinical observations mentioned in the case study?
2. Where in the brain (lobe and hemisphere) do you suspect the infarct to be?
3. Name two to three appropriate assessments that could be completed with the client based on suspected deficits. Could any assessments be used to identify multiple deficits that this client may have?
4. Name two to three intervention strategies for each suspected deficit. Identify the general approach to each intervention.

Chapter 8 Self-Study Answers

1. Organization, sequencing and planning, and short-term memory. It would be correct to also identify problem solving as an issue, which can also be a result of a frontal lobe injury.
2. The left hemisphere and frontal lobe.
3. Parts a and b are as follows:
   a) *Short-term memory*: Several examples follow: Rivermead Behavioral Memory Test, Cognistat, Contextual Memory Test, Everyday Memory Questionnaire, Cambridge Prospective Memory Test, CAM, MoCA, A-ONE, Dementia Rating Scale.
   b) *Sequencing, planning, and organization*: EFPT, A-ONE, Dementia Rating Scale, Multiple Errands Test, BADS, Routine Task Inventory, CAM, Cognistat, LOTCA, EFRT, OTDL-R.
      a. For both a and b: Cognistat, CAM, A-ONE, Dementia Rating Scale.
4. For short-term memory, there are any number of interventions that are listed within this chapter. General suggestions for interventions include the following:
   - Utilizing pictures and strategically hanging them
   - Working in natural environments
   - Monitoring for overload
   - Making use of old routines and allowing time for practice and repetition

Restorative approaches to intervention include addressing short-term memory issues after attention and before long-term memory issue, role playing, and repetition using ADL-specific strategies. Adaptive approaches to intervention include internal aids (e.g., mental moment, association, repetition or repeating to one's self, mnemonics, and visual imagery) and external strategies such as electronic aids and reminders, cuing from others, writing reminders or taking notes, or using calendars. For initiation, planning, and organization, there are any number of interventions that are listed within this chapter:

Initiation:

- *Restorative approach*: Use habits and routines to trigger the next step; sensory input to elicit initiation; incentive training may motivate.
- *Adaptive approach*: External cues and prompts first progressing to internal cues and self-monitoring; attentional kicks, alarms, calendar reminders, and audio cassettes.

Planning and organization:

- *Restorative approach*: Relate information into a meaningful structure for the client; recognition and rehearsal of strategies on how things relate to each other; the client should take an active role in planning; verbalization of the plan, and self-questioning.
- *Adaptive approach*: External aids (e.g., calendars and to-do lists); write steps down before doing, mental rehearsals, organizational strategies, arrange materials before starting, and progressive cuing. Other interventions/therapeutic activities: categorization and sequencing games, such as *Apples to Apples*, *Sequencing*, *Simon*, and *Mastermind*, and practice complex scenario-based activities.

References

Cooke, D. M., & Kline, N. F. (2007). Assessments of process skills and mental functions, part 1: Cognitive assessments. In I. E. Asher (Ed.), *Occupational therapy assessment tools: An annotated index*. Bethesda, MD: AOTA Press.

Gillen, G. (2009). *Cognitive and perceptual rehabilitation: Optimizing function*. St. Louis, MO: Mosby/Elsevier.

Gillen, G. (2013). Evaluation and treatment of limited occupational performance secondary to cognitive dysfunction. In H. M. Pendleton & W. Schultz-Krohn (Eds.), *Pedretti's occupational therapy: Practice skills for physical dysfunction* (7th ed., pp. 648–673). St. Louis, MO: Elsevier.

Gutman, S. A. (2008). *Quick reference neuroscience for rehabilitation professionals: The essential neurologic principles underlying rehabilitation practice* (2nd ed.). Thorofare, NJ: SLACK Incorporated.

Kaldenberg, J. (2014). Optimizing vision and visual processing. In M. V. Radomski & C. A. T. Latham (Eds.), *Occupational therapy for physical dysfunction* (7th ed., pp. 699–724). Philadelphia, PA: Wolters Kluwer Health/Lippincott Williams & Wilkins.

Radomski, M. V., & Giles, G. M. (2014). Optimizing cognitive performance. In M. V. Radomski & C. A. T. Latham (Eds.), *Occupational therapy for physical dysfunction* (7th ed., pp. 725–752). Philadelphia, PA: Wolters Kluwer Health/Lippincott Williams & Wilkins.

Radomski, M. V., & Morrison, M. T. (2014). Assessing abilities and capacities: Cognition. In M. V. Radomski & C. A. T. Latham (Eds.), *Occupational therapy for physical dysfunction* (7th ed., pp. 121–143). Philadelphia, PA: Wolters Kluwer Health/Lippincott Williams & Wilkins.

Scheiman, M. (2011). *Understanding and managing vision deficits: A guide for occupational therapists* (3rd ed.). Thorofare, NJ: SLACK Incorporated.

Toglia, J. P., Golisz, K. M., & Goverover, Y. (2014). Cognition, perception, and occupational performance. In B. A. B. Schell, G. Gillen, & M. E. Scaffa (Eds.), *Willard & Spackman's occupational therapy* (12th ed., pp. 779–815). Baltimore, MD: Lippincott Williams & Wilkins.

Warren, M. (2013). Evaluation and treatment of visual deficits following brain injury. In H. M. Pendleton & W. Schultz-Krohn (Eds.), *Pedretti's occupational therapy: Practice skills for physical dysfunction* (7th ed., pp. 590–626). St. Louis, MO: Elsevier.

Weisser-Pike, O. (2014). Assessing abilities and capabilities: Vision and visual processing. In M. V. Radomski & C. A. T. Latham (Eds.), *Occupational therapy for physical dysfunction* (7th ed., pp. 103–119). Philadelphia, PA: Wolters Kluwer Health/Lippincott Williams & Wilkins.

Whittaker, S., Scheiman, M., & Sokol-McKay, D. A. (2015). *Low vision rehabilitation: A practical guide for occupational therapists* (2nd ed.). Thorofare, NJ: SLACK Incorporated.

Zoltan, B. (2007). *Vision, perception, and cognition: A manual for the evaluation and treatment of the adult with acquired brain injury* (4th ed.). Thorofare, NJ: SLACK Incorporated.

Motor Control

Diane Adamo and Erin Skotzke

Learning Objectives

- Define motor control theory and motor learning.
- Describe the proprioceptive neuromuscular facilitation (PNF), neurodevelopmental treatment (NDT), task-oriented approach (TOA), and Rood approach principles utilized in occupational therapy (OT) intervention.
- Compare and contrast PNF, NDT, TOA, and Rood approach to OT intervention.
- Describe the evaluations and assessments used to assess motor function.
- Appraise the evidence for the various theories, assessments, and interventions used in OT practice for motor control dysfunction.

Key Terms

- *Adaptation*: The ability to alter or change course when necessary
- *Functional assessment*: Typically includes observation of task completion within a natural or simulated setting
- *Learned nonuse*: The result of injury to an extremity that is oftentimes not used, and therefore the person adapts his or her behavior by learning how to carry out daily activities without the use of the affected extremity
- *Motor skills*: The manner in which individuals move and interact within their environment
- *Occupational engagement*: Occupational functioning and mental awareness within specific environments

Description

This chapter describes the nature and control of movement as it relates to the rehabilitative process in humans. The goal of this chapter is to educate its reader about motor control dysfunction as well as to provide information about various evaluations used to assess deficits related to motor dysfunction. This section discusses principles used in the neurodevelopmental treatment (NDT), proprioceptive neuromuscular facilitation (PNF), Rood approach, and task-oriented approach (TOA) to motor recovery used in neurorehabilitation.

Etiology and Pathology

Motor control describes how the human nervous system uses sensory and motor information to process, organize, and execute conscious and unconscious movements. When a condition or disease affects the nervous system, the body's normal pattern of movement may be altered and lead to motor dysfunction. The various signs of motor dysfunction are dependent on the part of the nervous system that has been affected by the injury or disease. The disruption of a person's normal movement pattern may cause the person to exhibit difficulties carrying out activities of daily living (ADL). This chapter focuses on the various theories, assessments, and interventions that encompass evidence-based occupational therapy (OT) intervention for motor control dysfunction.

Sensorimotor Frames of Reference and Sensorimotor Approaches

OT process and practice corresponding to the application of motor control principles are based on the sensorimotor frame of reference. PNF, NDT, and the Rood approach are used to treat individuals who have suffered a central nervous system (CNS) insult that results in upper motor neuron (UMN) disorders such as cerebral palsy (CP), stroke, and head injury. Damage to the UMNs disrupts the regulation and control of the lower motor neurons and corresponding movements. The sensorimotor approach (PNF, NDT) uses activities to facilitate or inhibit specific movement patterns.

Motor Control Theory

Motor control theory is based on the principle that the brain organizes and plans one's ability to perform purposeful activity. Motor control is the ability to make dynamic postural adjustments and direct body and limb movements in purposeful activity (Umphred, 1995). Components necessary for motor control include normal muscle tone, normal postural tone and postural mechanisms, and selective movement and coordination.

Alterations and disruptions to sensory and motor information that occur between the brain and the corresponding limb and body segments may be due to the progression of a disease (e.g., Parkinson's [PD] and multiple sclerosis [MS]) or the onset of brain injury (cerebrovascular accident [CVA]). Ultimately, these disruptions lead to deficits in sensory and motor processing and subsequent movement disorders. Functional recovery depends on the initial amount of neurological damage, early treatment interventions, and whether the disease process is static or dynamic.

Plasticity is an important concept in neurologic rehabilitation because it helps to explain why recovery is possible after brain injury or lesion. Neuroplasticity is defined as "anatomic[al] and electrophysiologic[al] changes in the central nervous system" (Umphred, 1995). Cortical reorganization is based on the concept that the adult brain has a neoplastic ability to alter or modify synaptic connections in the context of performance.

OT interventions aim to increase occupational engagement and reduce movement deficits by teaching individuals to practice new movement patterns that, in turn, reinforce the activation of specific cortical regions. A control parameter is a term that pertains to anything that shifts a motor behavior from one manner of performance to another type of performance. A shift in performance can be driven by internal (i.e., strength and vision) and/or external (i.e., object location and lighting) changes.

Motor Learning/Relearning

Motor learning is defined as a "set of processes associated with practice or experience leading to relatively permanent changes in the capability for skilled movement" (Schmidt & Lee, 2011, p. 327). Motor learning may include tapping into existing neural pathways (unmasking) and/or developing new neural connections (sprouting) (Nudo, Wise, SiFuentes, & Milliken, 1996). Evaluating body functions and performances and utilizing specific treatment approaches facilitate this process. Motor relearning programs are specific to the rehabilitation of patients following a stroke. The program is based on four factors: (1) elimination of unnecessary muscle activity, (2) feedback, (3) practice, and (4) the interrelationship of postural adjustment and movement (Carr & Shepherd, 1987).

Carr and Shepherd (1987) present a four-step sequence followed for skill acquisition:

1. Analysis of the task, including observation
2. Practice of missing components, including goal identification, instruction, practice, and feedback with some manual guidance
3. Practice of the task with the addition of reevaluation and encouraging of task flexibility
4. Targets transfer of training

Task-Oriented Training/ Task-Oriented Approach

Following an injury or insult to the brain, task-oriented training/TOAs lead to an interaction between intended movements and changes in the brain. The TOA is also described as a task-specific training, repetitive task practice, goal-directed training, and functional task practice

(Timmermans, Spooren, Kingma, & Seelen, 2010). In this top-down approach, movement emerges as an interaction between many systems in the brain and is organized around a goal that is constrained by the environment (Shumway-Cook & Woollacott, 2012). Support for using a TOA is based on assumptions of the Occupational Therapy Task-Oriented Approach and Systems Model of Motor Behavior (Mathiowitz, 2010). A major focus of task-oriented training is arm training using functional tasks, such as grasping objects and constraint-induced movement therapy (CIMT) (Wolf et al., 2006).

Wolf et al. (2006) discuss the following assumptions:

1. Functional tasks help to organize behavior.
2. Personal and environmental systems, including the CNS, are hierarchically organized.
3. Behavioral changes reflect attempts to compensate and to achieve task performance.

Repetition and practice are important components of the TOA and neuromuscular facilitation. However, occupational therapists (OTs) and occupational therapy assistants (OTAs) need to be aware that utilizing compensatory movement patterns during the relearning process may introduce complications. For example, a patient who presents with an inability to reach and grasp an object following a stroke may compensate by hiking his or her shoulder to assist with hand placement. Repeated practice of such movements may lead to maladaptive movement patterns and subsequent overuse syndromes. Skilled application of the TOA/task-specific training reduces the potential for developing maladaptive movement patterns and enhances the potential for developing effective movement patterns. Timmermans et al. (2010) discuss training components of the TOA that include the following:

- *Functional movements*: A movement that is directed toward a specific ADL.
- *Clear functional goals*: Everyday life activities (e.g., dressing or feeding oneself).
- *Client-centered patient goal*: Patient's input and considerations determine therapy goals.
- *Overload*: Determined by the total time spent on a therapeutic activity, number of repetitions, difficulty of the activity, and intensity level.
- *Real-life manipulation*: Integrates the use of everyday objects during manipulation.
- *Context-specific environment*: A training environment that mimics the natural environment for a specific task.

- *Exercise progression*: Increases in exercise intensity are presented in a graded manner specific to the patient's abilities.
- *Exercise variety*: Different exercises are offered to enhance motor skills.
- *Feedback*: Information to the patient to increase motor learning.
- *Multiple movement planes*: Movements that occur in more than one place.
- *Patient-customized training load*: Designed to meet the needs of the patient.
- *Total skill practice*: Includes practice in total.
- *Random practice*: Performance of tasks randomly assigned.
- *Distributed practice*: Task performance with built-in rest periods.
- *Bimanual practice*: Tasks that require the use of both arms and hands.

Timmermans et al. (2010) also discuss the five main areas to assess using the TOA:

1. Role performance (social participation)
2. Occupational performance of tasks
3. Task selection and analyses
4. Person (e.g., client factors, performance skills, and patterns)
5. Environment (e.g., context and activity demands)

Neurodevelopmental Treatment Approach

Berta and Karel Bobath first introduced the "Bobath" concept in the 1940s, which later came to be known as the NDT approach. This approach is most applicable to restoration of movement and participation for individuals with UMN lesions, specifically CP and hemiplegia. Deficits result from combined neurological dysfunction due to damage of the CNS, musculoskeletal changes, and learned movement strategies. The primary objectives when using the NDT approach include normalizing tone, inhibiting primitive reflexes, and facilitating normal postural reactions (Sabari, Capasso, & Feld-Glazman, 2014; Schultz-Krohn, Pope-Davis, Jourdan, & McLaughlin-Gray, 2013).

In order to achieve the objectives, specific techniques are used:

- Handling techniques.
- Weight bearing over the affected limb.

- Use of positions that encourage bilateral use of the body.
- Avoid any sensory input that may adversely affect muscle tone (Sabari et al., 2014; Schultz-Krohn et al., 2013).
- *General principle*: NDT is based on restoring normal movement and postural control using a bottom-up approach. This approach refers to the evaluation and treatment of the underlying cause of dysfunction, which then leads to improved occupational function. Specific attention to postural alignment, movement strategy, and underlying deficits are recorded (Sabari et al., 2014; Schultz-Krohn et al., 2013).

Evaluation using the NDT approach follows four steps as outlined below (Sabari et al., 2014; Schultz-Krohn et al., 2013):

1. Assess the client's ability to maintain alignment and postures required for occupation.
2. Analyze movements in terms of the whole body and the stability–mobility relationship between body segments during task performance.
3. Analyze movements while performing basic motor skills for reaching, sit–stand, and transferring.
4. Assess potential underlying impairments such as changes in muscle strength, muscle tone, muscle activation and sensory processing and their potential contribution to movement dysfunction, and compensatory movements.

Assess the client's ability to maintain alignment and postures required for occupation. The therapist evaluates the client's ability to maintain postural alignment while standing and reaching for objects, to transition between seated and standing postures based on the stability-mobility tradeoff, and to identify potential underlying impairments in strength, muscle tone, muscle activation, and changes in sensory processing. Identifying potential impairments in strength and muscle tone, for example, may help to reduce secondary impairments such as changes in orthopedic alignment and mobility, edema, and pain (Sabari et al., 2014; Schultz-Krohn et al., 2013).

Intervention: Intervention is structured according to the preparation–movement–function sequence of events (Sabari et al., 2014; Schultz-Krohn et al., 2013):

- *Preparation*: (1) Analyze movement components and the flow of movement that occurs between body segments required for the task or occupational goal, (2) set up the environment to promote active participation and encourage use of symmetric distribution of body segments, and (3) provide mobilization techniques.
  1) *Analyze movements*: Therapy practitioner uses manual cues and handling techniques to position the patient symmetrically to improve posture.
  2) *Set up environment*: Therapy practitioner provides cues to help position the patient to perform a task; foster symmetric postures.
  3) *Provide mobilization*: Therapy practitioner instructs the patient to use a mobilization technique to reduce the flexor tone prior to starting a task.
- *Movement*: (1) Implement graded handling and guiding techniques to promote more efficient movements and reduce unwanted motor responses or alignments and (2) limb movements should progress from closed to open chain patterns of movement.

  1) *Implement graded handling techniques*: The therapy practitioner uses his or her hands to apply support, also referred to as "key points of control," to position the client more symmetrically while seated.
  2) *Limb movements progress from closed to open chain movements*: Instruct the client to use a closed chain movement by placing in weight-bearing position, standing, or pressing hand/arm toward the ground. A more symmetric posture facilitated by improved standing balance will allow for graded movements where the hand reaches into a cupboard (e.g., open chain).
- *Function*: (1) Eventual withdrawal of forms of handling techniques and support and (2) incorporating learned movement patterns into the occupational or functional task.

  1) *Withdrawal of handling techniques and using learned movement patterns*: By following the guidelines for preparation and movement as indicated above, the client will show improved ability to perform self-care tasks.
  2) *Incorporating learned movement patterns into the occupational or functional task*: Closely monitor progress to reduce the likelihood of using maladaptive compensatory movement patterns.

Neurodevelopmental Treatment Approach for Stroke

Is using the NDT approach the best approach for treating stroke? According to a systematic review (Kollen et al., 2009), using the NDT approach did not prove to be superior to other approaches, although this study had noted limitations.

Neurodevelopmental Treatment Approach for Traumatic Brain Injury (TBI)

Individuals with TBI may present with numerous types of impairments that include spasticity, rigidity, soft tissue contractures, presence of primitive reflexes, diminished or lost postural reactions, muscle weakness, impaired sensation, and an inability to perform ADLs.

Common principles of an intervention for neuromuscular impairments are to

- Facilitate control of muscle groups, progressing from proximal–distal.
- Encourage symmetric posture.
- Facilitate integration of both sides of the body into activities.
- Encourage bilateral weight bearing.
- Introduce normal sensory experiences.

Major principles of NDT include the following (Sabari et al., 2014; Schultz-Krohn et al., 2013):

- Facilitate trunk alignment.
- Stimulate reciprocal trunk muscle activity.
- Encourage the individuals to weight-shift out of a stable posture into multiple directions (e.g., bending, turning, and lateral reaching).
- Once the trunk is stable, interventions may progress to the upper extremities (UEs).

PNF Approach

The PNF approach is grounded in the reflex and hierarchic models of motor control (Sabari et al., 2014; Schultz-Krohn et al., 2013). Emphasis is placed on the developmental sequencing of movement and the interplay between agonist and antagonist in producing volitional movement. This approach uses diagonal motor movement patterns and sensory stimulation (i.e., tactile, auditory, and visual) to promote a motor response.

The PNF approach originated with Dr. Herman Kabat in the 1940s and Voss presented 11 principles of PNF interventions in 1966. This approach draws from principles based on normal motor development, which proceeds in a cervicocaudal and proximodistal direction, integrates primitive reflexes, balances motor responses (e.g., flexion and extension), and incorporates various developmental motor patterns (Sabari et al., 2014; Schultz-Krohn et al., 2013).

Approximation is a special technique done by creating compression between the joint surfaces and activating the joint receptors. This, in turn, promotes stability and postural control of limb movements. Approximation is usually superimposed on a weight-bearing posture. For example, while in a prone on elbow posture, pushing down on the shoulders facilitates approximation because the joint receptors are compressed. This will promote stability in the shoulders.

The PNF approach builds on the premise that movement patterns, unilateral, bilateral, and reciprocal diagonal are taken from the patterns of movements used to perform most functional tasks. Two diagonal motions are present for each major part of the body (Sabari et al., 2014; Schultz-Krohn et al., 2013):

- Head and neck
- Upper and lower parts of the trunk
- Extremities

Each pattern has a flexion and extension component, together with rotation and movement toward or away from the midline. Here is a detailed explanation of each type of pattern of movement and associate functional activities.

Unilateral Patterns

- UE D_1 flexion (shoulder flexion–adduction–external rotation) = scapular elevation, abduction, and rotation; shoulder flexion, adduction, and external rotation; elbow in flexion or extension; forearm supination; wrist flexion to radial side; finger flexion and adduction; thumb adduction (Sabari et al., 2014; Schultz-Krohn et al., 2013). *Examples of functional activity:* hand-to-mouth motion in feeding, tennis forehand, and combing hair on the left side of the head with the right hand.

- UE D_1 extension (shoulder extension–abduction–internal rotation) = scapular depression, adduction, and rotation; shoulder extension, abduction, and internal rotation; elbow in flexion or extension; forearm pronation; wrist extension to the ulnar side; finger extension and abduction; and thumb in palmar abduction (Sabari et al., 2014; Schultz-Krohn et al., 2013). *Examples of functional activity:* pushing a car door open from the inside, tennis backhand stroke, and rolling from prone to supine.

- UE D_2 flexion (shoulder flexion–abduction–external rotation) = scapular elevation, adduction, and rotation; shoulder flexion, abduction, and external rotation; elbow in flexion or extension; forearm supination; wrist extension to the radial side; finger extension and abduction; and thumb extension (Sabari et al., 2014; Schultz-Krohn et al., 2013). *Examples of functional activity:* combing the hair on the right side of the head with the right hand, lifting a racquet in a tennis serve, and backstroke in swimming.

- UE D_2 extension (shoulder extension–adduction–internal rotation) = scapular depression, abduction, and rotation; shoulder extension, adduction, and internal rotation; elbow in flexion or extension; forearm pronation; wrist extension to the ulnar side; finger flexion and adduction; and thumb opposition (Sabari et al., 2014; Schultz-Krohn et al., 2013). *Examples of functional activity:* pitching a baseball, hitting a ball during a tennis serve, and buttoning pants on the left side with the right hand.

- Lower extremity (LE) D_1 flexion (hip flexion–adduction–external rotation): hip flexion, adduction, and external rotation; knee in flexion or extension; and ankle and foot dorsiflexion with inversion and toe extension (Sabari et al., 2014; Schultz-Krohn et al., 2013). *Examples of functional activity:* kicking a soccer ball, rolling from supine to prone, and putting on a shoe with legs crossed.

- LE D_1 extension (hip extension–abduction–internal rotation): hip extension, abduction, and internal rotation; knee in flexion or extension; and ankle and foot plantar flexion with eversion and toe flexion (Sabari et al., 2014; Schultz-Krohn et al., 2013). *Examples of functional activity:* putting a leg into pants and rolling from prone to supine.

- LE D_2 flexion (hip flexion–abduction–internal rotation): hip flexion, abduction, and internal rotation; knee in flexion or extension; and ankle and foot dorsiflexion with eversion and toe extension (Sabari et al., 2014; Schultz-Krohn et al., 2013). *Examples of functional activity:* karate kick and drawing the heels up during breaststroke when swimming.

- LE D_2 extension (hip extension–adduction–external rotation): hip extension, adduction, and external rotation; knee in flexion or extension; and ankle and foot plantar flexion with inversion and toe flexion (Sabari et al., 2014; Schultz-Krohn et al., 2013). *Examples of functional activity:* push off in gait, the kick during breaststroke in swimming, and long sitting with the legs crossed.

Bilateral Patterns

- Bilateral symmetric UE patterns facilitate trunk flexion and extension. Symmetric patterns occur when paired extremities perform similar movements at the same time (Sabari et al., 2014; Schultz-Krohn et al., 2013). Examples: bilateral symmetric D_1 extension, such as pushing off a chair to stand; bilateral symmetric D_2 extension, such as starting to take off a sweater; and bilateral symmetric D_2 flexion, such as reaching to lift a large item off a high shelf.

- Bilateral asymmetric UE paired movements perform movements toward one side of the body at the same time, which facilitates trunk rotation. Asymmetric patterns can be performed with the arms in contact, such as chopping and lifting patterns in which greater trunk rotation is seen.

- With the arms in contact, self-touching occurs that has been assumed to provide greater control or power. This is seen in a tennis player who uses a two-handed backhand to increase control and power. Examples: bilateral asymmetric flexion to the left with the left arm in D_2 flexion and the right arm in D_1 flexion such as when putting on a left earring, and bilateral asymmetric extension to the left with the right arm in D_2 extension and the left arm in D_1 extension such as when zipping a left-sided zipper.

- Reciprocal UE paired movements move in opposite directions simultaneously, either in the same diagonal or in combined diagonals.

If paired extremities perform movements in combined diagonals, a stabilizing effect occurs on the head, neck, and trunk because movement of the extremities is in the opposite direction, while the head and neck remain in midline. Examples: pitching in baseball, sidestroke in swimming, and walking a balance beam with one extremity in a diagonal flexion pattern and the other in a diagonal extension pattern.

Combined Movements of the UE and LE

Ipsilateral movements are more primitive than contralateral and diagonal reciprocal (Schultz-Krohn et al., 2013). A goal of therapy is to progress from ipsilateral–contralateral–diagonal reciprocal movements. Movements include the following (Sabari et al., 2014; Schultz-Krohn et al., 2013):

- Ipsilateral patterns when the extremities move in the same direction and at the same time on the same side of the body;
- Contralateral patterns when the extremities on the opposite sides of the body move in the same direction and at the same time;
- Diagonal reciprocal when the contralateral extremities move in the same direction at the same time, while the opposite contralateral extremities move in the opposite direction.

Screening and Assessment When Using PNF Techniques

Assessment is an ongoing process that includes observation skills and knowledge about normal movements. The following developmental activities and postures should include these types of questions (Schultz-Krohn et al., 2013):

- Is more stability or mobility needed?
- Is there balance between the flexors and extensors?
- Is the client able to move in all directions?
- To what extent does sensory input help to direct movements?

Intervention Implementations

Recall that diagonal and unilateral repeated patterns of movement may include flexion, extension, abduction, and adduction of upper and lower body patterns. Movements may be symmetrical or asymmetrical/diagonal and reciprocal. The following specific techniques are used to guide movement patterns (Schultz-Krohn et al., 2013):

1. *Techniques directed to the agonists*: Voluntary movements are facilitated with stretch and resistance by performing isometric and isotonic contractions in combination with rhythmic initiations. Rhythmic initiations include voluntary relaxation, passive movement, and repeated isotonic contractions of the agonistic pattern.

2. *Techniques involving reversal of antagonists*: Techniques involving reversal of antagonists and relaxation may also be implemented. These techniques are based on Sherrington's principle of successive induction, according to which the stronger antagonist facilitates the weaker agonist (Sherrington, 1961) and whereby the contraction of the antagonist can be isotonic, isometric, or both. Slow reversal is an isotonic contraction of the antagonist followed by an isotonic contraction of the agonist. For example, the instructions to use a slow-reversal procedure for a client who has difficulty reaching his mouth to brush his teeth because of weakness in the D_1 flexion (shoulder flexion–adduction–external rotation) pattern would be the following: "Push down and out" followed by an isotonic contraction of D_1 flexion against resistance with the verbal command "pull up and across." This contributes to a buildup of power in the agonist that, in turn, facilitates the movement. Rhythmic stabilization is used to increase stability by eliciting isometric contractions of the antagonist muscles at the same time.

3. *Relaxation techniques*: Relaxation techniques are an effective means to increase range of motion (ROM) and include passive stretch. Techniques include contract–relax movements to the point of limitation; hold relax (slow reversal–hold relax), which may be useful for a client with complex regional pain syndrome (CRPD) during self-care activities such as shampooing the hair; and using rhythmic rotation, which may be useful for a client with paraplegia who has LE spasticity and put on a pair of pants.

Overall, the PNF approach emphasizes the client's ability to use their strengths to assist weaker components of movements. PNF uses multisensory input and follows the developmental sequence of normal movements. Use of diagonal patterns that match performance of ADL tasks includes both muscle facilitation and relaxation techniques that are well timed and allow for the production of coordinated movement patterns.

Rood Approach

This approach was based heavily on reflex and hierarchic models in designing interventions. The key components are the use of sensory stimulation, which is applied to muscles and joints in an effort to elicit a specific motor response. Stimulation may provide a facilitatory or inhibitory response. Sensory stimulation may include slow rolling, neutral warmth, deep pressure, tapping, and prolonged stretch. The use of specific developmental sequences was also used (proximal to distal; cephalocaudal) (Schultz-Krohn et al., 2013).

Evaluation and Assessment of Motor Function

Motor function may be assessed using various types of evaluations. Evaluations may be self-report questionnaires and/or surveys, performance-based assessments tested against a known criterion or reported by a trained evaluator. Some assessments are geared to more general functions (e.g., functional assessment); yet to perform them may require some degree of motor skill. Assessments to test function for performing self-care tasks may include basic ADL including eating, toileting, bathing, ambulation, transfers, feeding, grooming, and dressing, and instrumental activities of daily living (IADL) including balancing a checkbook, driving, cooking, shopping, and medication management.

- *Self-reports*: Self-reports allow clients to report a specific level of motor function typically within a numerical range and assigned a verbal descriptor. These may include the DASH, Motor Activity Log, and the Pediatric Motor Activity Log. The 36-item Manual Ability Measure (MAM-36) is a self-report survey that measures the ease associated with completing several everyday tasks.

The following are evaluations of motor function (Gillen, 2014).

- *DASH*: The Disabilities of the Arm, Shoulder, and Hand Questionnaire, known as the DASH, is a 30-item assessment that is used to measure function at each respective joint in the UE. This self-reported questionnaire is used primarily for adults that exhibit various UE musculoskeletal deficits. The questionnaire asks about various symptoms that people with UE deficits may have while also assessing pain and ability to perform certain basic and IADL.
- *Motor Activity Log*: The Motor Activity Log requires individuals to rate the quality and amount of movement during a set of 30, 28, or 14 daily functional tasks. Some examples include fine motor manipulation such as using a pen, fork, or comb, and gross motor activities such as transfers.
- *Pediatric Motor Activity Log*: The Pediatric Motor Activity Log is an assessment that asks caregivers to examine the amount of movement and the quality of movement in their child's UEs during performance of ADL. This assessment is used for caregivers of children that exhibit potential UE functional deficits.

Gillen (2014) discusses assessments of postural control as follows:

- The Trunk Control Test examines four functional movements: rolling from supine to the weak side, rolling from supine to the strong side, sitting up from a lying down position, and sitting on the edge of the bed for 30 seconds. Performance of each task is scored using a number that corresponds to a verbal descriptor.
- The Postural Assessment Scale for Stroke Patients contains 12 four-point items that are scored based on sitting and standing performance.
- The Berg Balance Scale measures balance ability in older individuals. This assessment includes items such as sit–stand, transfers, and retrieving an object from the floor.
- Assessments of limb function are typically composed of items that are best described as simulated ADL movements.
- The Arm Motor Ability Test determines the effectiveness of interventions and includes 13 unilateral and bilateral tasks.

- The Wolf Motor Function Test determines the effectiveness of CI therapy and assesses various UE bimanual tasks following a stroke.
- The Jebsen Test of Hand Function includes the performance of seven activities; writing, picking up small objects, using various grasp and release patterns for object manipulations.

Screening and Assessments to Test for Muscle Tone

The degree of muscle tone relies on normal functioning of the cerebellum, motor cortex, basal ganglia, midbrain, vestibular system, spinal cord, and the stretch reflex. The progression of a disease and/or sustaining an injury to any of these regions may lead to alterations in muscle tone and subsequently to movement disorders. The following terms have been used to describe the degree of muscle tone (Schultz-Krohn et al., 2013):

- *Flaccidity*: Absence of tone.
- *Hypotonus*: A decrease in normal muscle tone.
- *Hypertonus*: An increase in muscle tone.
  - *Cerebral hypertonia*: Increased muscle tone due to TBI, stroke, anoxia, neoplasm, metabolic disorders, CP, and diseases of the brain.
  - *Spinal hypertonia*: Increased muscle tone due to injuries and diseases of the spinal cord.
- *Spasticity*: A motor disorder characterized by a velocity-dependent increase in tonic stretch reflexes (muscle tone) with exaggerated tendon jerks resulting from hyperexcitability of the stretch reflex as one component of the UMN syndrome.
  - *Clonus*: A specific type of spasticity. Repetitive contractions in the antagonistic muscles in response to rapid stretch.
- *Rigidity*: A simultaneous increase in muscle tone of agonist and antagonist muscles (i.e., muscles on both sides of the joint).
  - *Lead pipe rigidity*: Constant resistance is felt throughout the ROM when the part is moved slowly and passively in any direction.
  - *Cogwheel rigidity*: A rhythmic give in resistance occurs throughout the ROM, much like the feeling of turning a cogwheel.
  - *Decorticate rigidity*: Flexion hypertonus in the UEs and extension in the LEs.
  - *Decerebrate rigidity*: Rigid extension of all limbs and neck.

There are specific assessments to test for the degree of muscle tone. These may include the following (Schultz-Krohn et al., 2013):

- Modified Ashworth Scale.
- Mild-to-Moderate–Severe Spasticity Scale.
- Preston's Hypertonicity Scale.
  - Muscle tone or the degree to which it resists slow passive movement is graded on a scale of 0–3 (i.e., no tone, mild, moderate, severe) (Schultz-Krohn et al., 2013).
- EMGs—surface pad or indwelling needles record muscle activity.

Screening and Assessments to Test for Sensation

- *Static two-point discrimination*: Static two-point discrimination is the ability to discriminate one stimulus from two stimuli. To test static two-point discrimination, an OT practitioner uses a two-point discriminator or a discriminator wheel tool on the participant's hand. The participant is asked to close his or her eyes and discriminate between one or two stimuli. The ability to complete this task successfully determines the amount of stimuli often compromised in hand injuries.
- *Kinesthesia*: Kinesthesia is the awareness of the movement of the parts of the body by means of sensory organs, called proprioceptors, in the body's muscles and joints.
- *Proprioception*: Proprioception is the awareness of the position and balance of the parts of the body by means of sensory organs, called proprioceptors, in the body's muscles and joints.
- *Pain*: Pain is a subjective response to distress. OT practitioners assess pain by requesting that the patient or client closes his or her eyes while the therapist uses a sharp and dull point on various areas of the UE. The person participating in the assessment is asked to discriminate between the sharp or dull point.

- *Light touch*: Using an assessment that measures light touch is a way to test a person's ability to detect sensation in various areas of the UEs. While assessing light touch, an OT practitioner uses a cotton ball on various areas of a UE, brushing the cotton ball on the participant's skin in a random, nonpatterned manner. The participant is then asked to voice when he or she feels the cotton ball.

Examples of Evidence-Based Interventions

Constraint-induced movement therapy: Although CIMT is used in a variety of adult therapy interventions, it has been suggested that children may also benefit from CIMT. While in theory this may be the case, one study suggests that the restrictive nature of the constraint (i.e., 90% of waking hours) and the intensity of the structured training (i.e., shaping and repetitive task practice during a six-hour program) used for adults may be too intrusive for children. The corticospinal tract connections continue to develop during the first years of life, and restricting movement of the noninvolved limb for long periods could potentially have permanent repercussions for the development of motor skills in that limb. Therefore, extreme caution should be exercised in restraining children at too young an age (Charles & Gordon, 2005). With any therapeutic intervention for children or adults, such as CIMT, the therapist and therapy assistant should always exercise good clinical judgment before implementing the technique into treatment along with adaptation when indicated.

CIMT as described by Gillen (2011):
- Involves restricting the use of the unaffected limb following a stroke or other neurological event to force the use of the more affected limb; mass practice and shaping of the affected limb during repetitive functional activities appears to be the therapeutic change agent.
- Based on the available evidence, CIMT appears to be an effective intervention for those who have learned nonuse and who fit the motor inclusion criteria.
- CIMT is an intervention developed to reverse the effects of learned nonuse.
- It has been used in pediatric populations for children with CP.

Bilateral arm training:
- Involves the integration of treatment activities that require the bilateral and simultaneous use of the UEs poststroke (Stoykov, Lewis, & Corcos, 2009), particularly chronic stroke; bilateral training may be more advantageous for proximal than distal arm function.
- Examples include opening and closing of two identical drawers, wiping a table with both arms symmetrically, and bilateral reaching toward objects.

Hand–arm bimanual intensive therapy:
- Aimed treatment of UE impairments in congenital hemiplegia. This focuses on functional training and uses the principles of neuroplasticity and motor learning to promote recovery. Principles of neuroplasticity include practice-induced brain changes arising from repetition, increasing movement complexity, motivation, and reward. Principles of motor learning include practice specificity, types of practice, and feedback.

Chapter 9 Self-Study Activities (Answers Are Provided at the End of the Chapter)

1. OT practitioners often use one or more of the four different approaches when treating patients with motor control dysfunction. Match each approach with its appropriate description.

Approach		Definition
A. PNF	1.	This approach involves the use of sensory stimulation, which is applied to muscles and joints in an effort to facilitate or inhibit a specific motor response
B. NDT or Bobath	2.	Emphasis is placed on the developmental sequencing of movement and the interplay between agonist and antagonist in producing volitional movement. This approach uses diagonal motor movement patterns and sensory stimulation to promote a motor response

Approach		Definition
C. Task oriented	3.	This approach is often described as a goal-directed training; the approach involves performing specific activities in order to meet certain goals
D. Rood	4.	This approach is based on restoring normal movement and postural control. The approach uses specific handling techniques, encourages weight bearing on affected limb(s) and bilateral use of the body, and avoids sensory input that adversely affects muscle tone

2. Case study. Choose the correct italicized word in the following case study:

Kathy is a 55-year-old woman who has been referred to outpatient OT services after a right-sided ischemic CVA six months ago. Upon her arrival at the clinic, the therapist noticed that her left elbow, wrist, and fingers are flexed, while her arm was in a resting position. The therapist observed (1) *hypertonia/hypotonia* of her left UE. First, the therapist decides to evaluate Kathy's UE function. To do this, the therapist uses the (2) *Jebsen Test of Hand Function/Motor Activity Log*, an assessment that asks individuals to perform either 30, 28, or 14 daily functional tasks that require both fine and gross motor skills. After the assessment, the therapist performed manual therapy with the patient to increase the ROM and decrease muscle tone in the patient's left UE. The occupational therapist moved the patient's left arm in repeated, diagonal patterns, utilizing the (3) *NDT/PNF* approach. The therapist wanted to conclude the treatment session with a meaningful and purposeful task. The patient expressed interest in cooking, so the therapist showed Kathy the kitchen and asked if she wanted to prepare scrambled eggs. Through introducing the patient to this particular intervention, the therapist is using the (4) *TOA/Rood* approach.

1.	
2.	
3.	
4.	

3. Copy each of the italicized terms that you DID NOT choose in the previous case study and then define each term in the following worksheet. In addition, for numbers 3 and 4, give an example of an OT intervention you could use with Kathy that follows that specific approach.

Question 3: Worksheet

Term	Definition
1.	
Term	**Definition**
2.	
Term	**Definition and OT Intervention**
3.	
Term	**Definition and OT Intervention**
4.	

Chapter 9 Self-Study Answers

Question 1: Matching answers

1. D
2. A
3. C
4. B

Question 2: Case study answers

1. Hypertonia
2. Motor Activity Log
3. PNF
4. Task oriented

Question 3: Worksheet answers

Term	Definition
1. Hypotonia	A decrease in normal muscle tone
Term	**Definition**
2. Jebsen Test of Hand Function	The Jebsen Test of Hand Function includes the performance of seven activities; writing, picking up small objects, using various grasp and release patterns for object manipulations

Term	Definition and OT Intervention
3. PNF	Emphasis is placed on the developmental sequencing of movement and the balanced interplay between agonist and antagonist in producing volitional movement. This approach uses diagonal motor movement patterns and sensory stimulation to promote a motor response. OT intervention will vary

Term	Definition and OT Intervention
4. Rood	This approach involves the use of sensory stimulation, which is applied to muscles and joints in an effort to facilitate or inhibit a specific motor response. OT intervention will vary

References

Carr, J. H., & Shepherd, R. B. (1987). *A motor relearning programme for stroke.* New York, NY: Aspen Publishers.

Charles, J., & Gordon, A. M. (2005). A critical review of constraint-induced movement therapy and forced use in children with hemiplegia. *Neural Plasticity, 12*(2–3), 245–261. doi:10.1155/np.2005.245

Gillen, G. (2011). *Stroke rehabilitation: A function-based approach* (3rd ed.). St. Louis, MO: Elsevier/Mosby.

Gillen, G. (2014). Motor and function and occupational performance. In B. A. B. Schell, G. Gillen, & M. E. Scaffa (Eds.), *Willard & Spackman's occupational therapy* (12th ed., pp. 750–778). Philadelphia, PA: Wolters Kluwer Health/Lippincott Williams & Wilkins.

Kollen, B. J., Lennon, S., Lyons, B., Wheatley-Smith, L., Scheper, M., Buurke, J. H., . . . Kwakkel, G. (2009). The effectiveness of the Bobath concept in stroke rehabilitation: What is the evidence? *Stroke, 40*(4), e89–e97. doi:10.1161/strokeaha.108.533828

Mathiowitz, V. (2010). Task-oriented approach to stroke rehabilitation. In G. Gillen (Ed.), *Stroke rehabilitation: A function-based approach* (4th ed., pp. 80–99). St. Louis, MO: Elsevier Health Sciences.

Nudo, R. J., Wise, B. M., SiFuentes, F., & Milliken, G. W. (1996). Neural substrates for the effects of rehabilitative training on motor recovery after ischemic infarct. *Science, 272*(5269), 1791–1794.

Sabari, J. S., Capasso, N., & Feld-Glazman, R. (2014). Optimizing motor planning and performance in clients with neurological disorders. In M. V. Radomski & C. A. T. Latham (Eds.), *Occupational therapy for physical dysfunction* (7th ed., pp. 614–680). Philadelphia, PA: Wolters Kluwer Health/Lippincott Williams & Wilkins.

Schmidt, R. A., & Lee, T. (2011). Motor learning concepts and research concepts. In M. J. Zavala (Ed.), *Motor control and learning* (5th ed., p. 327). Champaign, IL: Human Kinetics.

Schultz-Krohn, W., Pope-Davis, S. A., Jourdan, J. M., & McLaughlin-Gray, J. (2013). Traditional sensorimotor approaches to intervention. In H. M. Pendleton & W. Schultz-Krohn (Eds.), *Pedretti's occupational therapy: Practice skills for physical dysfunction* (7th ed., pp. 796–830). St. Louis, MO: Elsevier.

Sherrington, C. (1961). *The integrative action of the nervous system* (2nd ed.). New Haven, CT: Yale University Press.

Shumway-Cook, A., & Woollacott, M. H. (2012). *Motor control: Translating research into clinical practice* (4th ed.). Philadelphia, PA: Wolters Kluwer Health/Lippincott Williams & Wilkins.

Stoykov, M. E., Lewis, G. N., & Corcos, D. M. (2009). Comparison of bilateral and unilateral training for upper extremity hemiparesis in stroke. *Neurorehabilitation and Neural Repair, 23*(9), 945–953. doi:10.1177/1545968309338190

Timmermans, A. A. A., Spooren, A. I. F., Kingma, H., & Seelen, H. A. M. (2010). Influence of task-oriented training content on skilled arm-hand performance in stroke: A systematic review. *Neurorehabilitation and Neural Repair, 24*(9), 858–870. doi:10.1177/1545968310368963

Umphred, D. A. (1995). *Neurological rehabilitation* (3rd ed.). St. Louis, MO: Mosby-Year Book.

Wolf, S. L., Winstein, C. J., Miller, J. P., Taub, E., Uswatte, G., Morris, D., . . . Nichols-Larsen, D. (2006). Effect of constraint-induced movement therapy on upper extremity function 3 to 9 months after stroke: The EXCITE randomized clinical trial. *JAMA, 296*(17), 2095–2104. doi:10.1001/jama.296.17.2095

Occupational Functioning: Physical Disabilities (Neuro) Days 6-9

Cerebrovascular Accident

Lori Bravi

Learning Objectives

- Identify and define the two primary etiologies of stroke or cerebrovascular accident.
- Identify two arteries that are included in anterior circulation syndromes and describe the associated clinical presentation of each.
- Identify three arteries that are included in posterior circulation syndromes and describe the associated clinical presentation of each.
- List five examples of preparatory methods and tasks considered when treating stroke.
- Identify and describe standardized assessments and therapeutic interventions that specifically address activities of daily living (ADLs), instrumental activities of daily living (IADLs), upper extremity facilitation and management, functional mobility, vision and perception, cognition, and communication and language.

Key Terms

- *Aphasia:* Characterized as either expressive or receptive aphasia and refers to a diminished ability to verbally express or understand speech
- *Hemorrhage:* Bleeding from a damaged or ruptured blood vessel 13%
- *Ischemia:* A diminished blood supply to a specific part of the body 87%
- *Subluxation:* A partial dislocation or misalignment of a joint
- *Transient ischemic attacks:* Disruption of the blood supply that typically supplies the brain, resulting from neurological dysfunction

Description

Stroke, or cerebrovascular accident (CVA), is a life-threatening vascular disease that results in loss of blood flow to the brain as a result of either ischemia or hemorrhage blockage. Side effects of stroke vary greatly depending on the size and location of the infarct and may result in reduced participation in occupation-based activities. Impaired motor and process performance skills such as organization, reaching, coordination, and walking together with client factors such as attention, emotion, orientation, vision, neuromuscular functions, voluntary movement, and speech affect independence in basic occupations. Stroke is the fourth leading cause of death and the leading cause of disability in adults (Go et al., 2014).

Etiology and Pathology

Stroke affects 795,000 Americans every year, every 40 seconds on average with 185,000 considered recurrent, and 137,000 of these people do not survive (Centers for Disease Control and Prevention, 2015). Hypertension is associated with 77% of first-time strokes. Ischemic strokes account for 87% of events, whereas hemorrhagic stroke accounts for 13%. Stroke prevalence is higher in women, African Americans, and persons from lower socioeconomic backgrounds. Cardiovascular disease, including hypertension, is the highest risk factor (Go et al., 2014). Hypertension management significantly reduces the risk for stroke in diabetic hypertensive adults. Systolic blood pressure is a strong indicator for stroke risk in African Americans compared to Caucasian adults with a 3:1 increased risk for every 10 mmHg increase above the normal range. Other risk factors for stroke include history of diabetes mellitus, smoking, atrial fibrillation, obesity, hyperlipidemia, and deep vein thrombosis (DVT). Symptoms include dizziness, paresthesia, severe headache, and double vision. Hemiplegia, facial paralysis, and impaired communication are three of the most recognizable signs of stroke. Lesions occurring above the brainstem result in contralateral hemiplegia, whereas ipsilateral hemiplegia occurs from lesions within or below the brainstem, including the spinal cord after the motor tracks have crossed. The length of time circulation affected in any of these scenarios is proportionate to the degree of side effects.

Ischemic stroke occurs when a blood clot blocks normal cerebral blood flow causing ischemia or loss of oxygen from impaired blood flow. These clots form as a result of atherosclerosis, or narrowing of the arteries, from fatty plaque buildup such as cholesterol. Blood clots that develop in the arteries of the brain affecting local cerebral circulation are referred to as cerebral thrombi. When a blood clot originates in another major vessel throughout the body, breaks loose, and then travels to the brain eventually occluding circulation when its size can no longer be accommodated, it is referred to as a cerebral embolism. An irregular heartbeat caused by atrial fibrillation decreases normal blood flow out of the heart thus increasing chances of clots forming in pooled blood and is another cause of embolic ischemic stroke. Depending on the size of the blood clot, the force of normal blood flow may dislodge the clot and circulation may resume. This is especially true in transient ischemic attacks (TIA), which create symptoms similar to stroke but resolve in no more than 24 hours. If symptoms are identified within three hours, nonsurgical medical intervention may include the use of tissue plasminogen activator (tPA) to reduce the size of the blood clot (Go et al., 2014). Surgical intervention may be necessary to remove the blood clot in severe cases.

Hemorrhagic stroke occurs when a weakened blood vessel ruptures, or hemorrhages, in the cranium thus creating pooling of blood that interferes with normal cerebral blood flow. Intracranial hemorrhage is further categorized by location and etiology of the bleed. Intracerebral hemorrhage refers to bleeding in the brain tissue itself and may be the result of leaking or ruptured blood vessels or tissue. Aneurysms and arteriovenous malformations are included in this category. Subarachnoid hemorrhage refers to a bleed in the area between the arachnoid membrane and the pia mater. The size of the hemorrhage will determine if the cerebral tissue will naturally absorb the blood or if surgical intervention is required to remove the blood and/or stop the bleeding.

Clinical Presentations

The clinical presentation of stroke is largely determined by the location and size of the ischemic or hemorrhagic infarct. Furthermore, stroke is often classified according to the affected hemisphere, right or left, respectively. The two major arteries creating cerebral blood flow are the carotid artery, supplying blood flow to the anterior cerebrum, and the vertebral-basilar artery, creating the posterior circulation of the brain.

Anterior Circulation Syndromes

Anterior circulation of the brain arises from the internal carotid arteries, providing blood flow to the anterior cerebral artery, middle cerebral artery, anterior communicating artery, and posterior communicating artery. The most common clinical presentations for anterior circulation syndromes are summarized in **Table 10-1**.

Posterior Circulation Syndromes

Posterior circulation of the brain is provided by the vertebral arteries, which combine to form the basilar artery. The vertebral arteries give rise to the posterior inferior cerebellar arteries, anterior spinal arteries, and posterior spinal arteries. The basilar artery gives rise to the posterior cerebral arteries, superior cerebellar arteries, anterior inferior cerebellar arteries, and pontine arteries. The most common clinical presentations for posterior circulation syndromes are summarized in **Table 10-2**.

Diagnostic Tests and Medical Imaging

A variety of medical imaging diagnostic tests are used to formally diagnose the location and size of the infarct (**Table 10-3**).

Table 10-1 Anterior Circulation Syndromes

Blood Supply	Clinical Presentation
Anterior cerebral artery • Medial and superior surfaces of the frontal lobe • Medial surface of the parietal lobe	• Contralateral hemiparesis and sensory loss: lower extremity more involved than the UE and face • Executive dysfunction (planning, organization, judgment, flexibility, reasoning) • Cognitive impairments (sustained attention, alternating attention, memory, following directions) • Behavioral changes (flat affect) • Agraphia (difficulty in producing written language) • Apraxia (reduced motor control) • Urinary incontinence
Middle cerebral artery • Largest branch of the internal carotid artery • Supplies entire lateral surface of the hemisphere including the frontal, parietal, and temporal lobes	• Contralateral hemiplegia and sensory loss: UE more involved than lower extremity, face, and tongue • Executive dysfunction (planning, organization, judgment, flexibility, reasoning) • Cognitive impairments (sustained attention, alternating attention, memory, following directions) • Contralateral homonymous hemianopia (visual field loss) • Ideomotor, ideational, and constructional apraxia • Spatial inattention (left neglect, right inattention) • Aphasia, fluent, or nonfluent (left hemisphere affected) • Dysarthria (reduced motor coordination of speech)

Data from Duncan, P. W., Zorowitz, R., Bates, B., Choi, J. Y., Glasberg, J. J., Graham, G. D., . . . Reker, D. (2005). Management of Adult Stroke Rehabilitation Care: a clinical practice guideline. Stroke, 36(9), e100-143. doi:10.1161/01.str.0000180861.54180.ff; Gillen, G. (2013). Cerebrovascular Accident/Stroke. In L. W. Pedretti, H. M. Pendleton, & W. Schultz-Krohn (Eds.), Pedretti's occupational therapy: practice skills for physical dysfunction (7th ed., pp. 844-857). St. Louis, Mo.: Elsevier.)

Table 10-2 Posterior Circulation Syndromes

Blood Supply	Clinical Presentation
Posterior cerebral artery • Medial surface of the temporal lobes • Medial and lateral surfaces of the occipital lobes • Visual cortex	• Homonymous hemianopia (visual field loss on the same side of each eye) • Memory impairment (verbal or visual) • Alexia (reduced comprehension of written language) • Agraphia (difficulty producing written language) • Acalculia (difficulty with mathematical calculations) • Visual agnosia (impaired object recognition) • Prosopagnosia (impaired familiar facial recognition) • Achromatopsia (loss of color vision) • Anton's syndrome (cortical blindness with lack of awareness of blindness)
Cerebellar artery • Cerebellum	• Ipsilateral ataxia (impaired coordination of movement) • Nystagmus (involuntary eye movement) • Dizziness • Vomiting • Contralateral facial paralysis • Decreased contralateral pain and temperature • Decreased touch, vibration, and position sense • Lower extremity more involved than the UE

(continues)

Table 10-2 Posterior Circulation Syndromes (*continued*)

Blood Supply	Clinical Presentation
Vertebrobasilar artery • Pons • Midbrain • Thalamus • Lateral medulla • Cranial nerves III–XII	• Quadriparesis • Ptosis (drooping eyelid) • Diplopia (double vision) • Esotropia (convergent eye misalignment) • Exotropia (divergent eye misalignment) • Memory loss • Dysarthria (impaired motor coordination of speech) • Dysphagia (difficulty swallowing) • Coma • Tachycardia • Locked-in syndrome

Data from Duncan, P. W., Zorowitz, R., Bates, B., Choi, J. Y., Glasberg, J. J., Graham, G. D., . . . Reker, D. (2005). Management of Adult Stroke Rehabilitation Care: a clinical practice guideline. Stroke, 36(9), e100-143. doi:10.1161/01.str.0000180861.54180.ff; Gillen, G. (2013). Cerebrovascular Accident/Stroke. In L. W. Pedretti, H. M. Pendleton, & W. Schultz-Krohn (Eds.), Pedretti's occupational therapy : practice skills for physical dysfunction (7th ed., pp. 844–857). St. Louis, Mo.: Elsevier.)

Table 10-3 Diagnostic Tests and Medical Imaging

Test	Description
CT	Computed tomography provides efficient cross-sectional x-ray images, with or without the use of iodine contrast dye, of the internal body structure in as few as 10 minutes, including acute and chronic bleeding
MRI	Magnetic resonance imaging requires more time for processing, but produces a more detailed picture of acute and chronic injury using magnets, with or without the use of noniodine dye, and is especially useful in detecting more finite changes; however, it is contraindicated for persons with metal in their bodies
PET	Positron emission tomography is not usually indicated for acute stroke due to time required for the radioactive venous tracer to detect disease processes and structural changes reflected as 3D images
SPECT	Single-photon emission computed tomography is a newer type of 3D scans that also uses a radioactive tracer to detect changes in blood flow through increased absorption in more active areas of insult

Data from: Duncan et al. (2005); Knesek (2009).

Medical and Surgical Procedures

Medical management of acute stroke prioritizes determining the location, cause, and size of the infarct. Blood flow is most commonly restored using medications; however, more invasive procedures to control intracranial pressure and cerebral edema are also initiated when necessary, which will impact the severity of deficits (**Table 10-4**). Prevention of secondary medical complications including DVT and pneumonia is initiated and may include the use of compression stockings to improve blood flow or aspiration precautions for clients who are unable to manage secretions due to impaired swallowing.

Screening and Assessments

A large variety of screening tools and assessments are used to determine potential goal areas for clients. Standardized assessments are preferred over nonstandardized assessments because they have stronger psychometric properties and require the occupational therapist to administer the test items in a consistent manner. The occupational therapist chooses a combination of both formal standardized assessments and informal interview questions that will most closely represent client factors, performance and process skills, and level of independence in occupation-based activities to be considered in the intervention planning and goal-setting process.

Standardized Assessments

• Activity Card Sort requires the client to choose from a variety of picture cards to represent daily activities that he/she finds most valuable.

Table 10-4 Medical Intervention for Ischemic and Hemorrhagic Stroke

Medical Intervention	Ischemic Stroke	Hemorrhagic Stroke
Nonsurgical		
Thrombolytics, including tPA, to dissolve clots only if symptoms are identified within three hours of onset	✓	Contraindicated due to bleeding
Anticoagulants and antiplatelet medications, including aspirin, heparin, Coumadin, Lovenox, Plavix to inhibit growth of hematoma and/or prevent platelets from forming new clots	✓	Contraindicated due to bleeding
Antihypertensive medications to restore normal blood pressure	✓	✓
Surgical		
Craniotomy with hematoma evacuation to remove excess blood or blood clot	✓	
Clipping or coiling to isolate weakened area of vessel and prevent further bleeding		✓
Endovascular procedures, including carotid endarterectomy, to clear plaque from arteries, reducing the risk of future stroke	✓	
Carotid stenting/angioplasty to improve blood flow	✓	
Decompressive craniotomy to reduce pressure	✓	
Precautions		
• Activity precautions may include no jumping, running, lifting, or bending with any of the above medical interventions • A helmet may be required after a craniotomy until the cerebral edema is under control and the bone flap is replaced • Blood pressure parameters may be implemented		

Data from: Duncan et al. (2005).

- Arm Motor Ability Test evaluates gross and fine motor control through the performance of various reach, grasp, and release test items.
- Arnadottir Occupational Therapy Neurobehavioral Evaluation (A-ONE) measures neurobehavioral dysfunction through the performance of activities of daily living (ADLs).
- Assessment of Motor Process Skills (AMPS) is a performance-based assessment of the quality of a person's ADL and instrumental activity of daily living (IADL) performance in a familiar environment.
- Beck Depression Inventory is a self-report questionnaire that quantifies depression.
- Berg Balance Scale is a performance-based assessment that measures balance and fall risk.
- Boston Diagnostic Aphasia Examination measures speech and language skills.
- Canadian Neurological Scale is a brief assessment of cognitive and motor function after stroke.
- Dynamometry measures numerical grip using a handheld gauge.
- Executive Function Performance Test evaluates mental process skills while the client performs structured meal preparation, bill management, placing a phone call, and medication management.
- Frenchay Activities Index (self-report tool) is an assessment of ADL function after stroke.
- Fugl-Meyer Assessment of Motor Function measures a person's ability to move in and out of synergistic gross and fine motor control patterns.
- Functional Reach Test measures the maximum reach of a person in standing.
- Functional Test for the Hemiplegic/Paretic Upper Extremity measures functional use of the hemiparetic upper extremity (UE) after stroke.
- Geriatric Depression Scale assesses depression in the elderly.
- Glasgow Coma Scale is a measure of consciousness after neurological injury.
- Jebsen Test of Hand Function measures hand function through the performance of various reaching, grasp, and release tasks.

- Kohlman Evaluation of Living Skills measures functional independence in ADLs.
- Mini-Mental State Examination is a brief screen of cognitive impairment.
- Montreal Cognitive Assessment screens for changes in visual perceptual skills, attention, memory, and orientation.
- Motor Assessment Scale measures motor function poststroke.
- Motor-Free Visual Perceptual Test is an assessment of visual perceptual skills.
- Motricity Index measures strength in the upper and lower extremities after stroke.
- National Institutes of Health Stroke Scale measures the severity of stroke deficits.
- Nine Hole Peg Test is a timed measurement of finger dexterity.
- Neurobehavioral Cognitive Status Examination quantifies cognitive functioning in the areas of language, constructions, memory, calculations, and memory.
- PCG Instrumental Activities of Daily Living measures IADL performance and independence.
- Pinch Strength uses a handheld gauge to measure lateral and palmar pinch strength.
- Rankin Scale (global disability scale) is a clinician-reported measure of disability.
- Rivermead Mobility Index measures gait, balance, and transfers after stroke.
- Stroke Impact Scale measures health status after stroke.
- Test Evaluant les Membres supérieurs des Personnes Agées (TEMPA) measures UE function.
- Tinetti Test assesses the perception and fear of falling during ADLs.
- Wolf Motor Function Test is a timed, performance-based assessment of gross and fine motor control skills.

Semistandardized Assessments

- Brain Injury Visual Assessment Battery for Adults screens for changes in visual perceptual skills.
- Canadian Occupational Performance Measure measures the importance and performance of client-selected daily activities.
- Goniometry uses a goniometer to objectively measure joint range of motion.

- Functional Independence Measure is a performance-based assessment of ADL independence.
- Manual Muscle Testing measures the strength of each muscle group in both gravity and gravity-eliminated positions.
- Modified Ashworth Scale is a measurement of spasticity in the extremities.

Nonstandardized Assessments

- Formal and informal interview
- Shoulder subluxation palpation

Criterion-Referenced Assessments

- AMPS

Interventions

Occupational therapy (OT) practitioners use detailed activity analysis for intervention planning, implementation of skilled occupation-based activities, and ongoing review of progress and care for clients recovering from stroke throughout multiple levels of care. Preparatory methods and tasks, including assistive devices and adapted equipment that complement intervention planning, are also provided in this section. While the impact of stroke on occupational performance varies greatly depending on the severity of impairment, occupational therapists are skilled at incorporating therapeutic use of personalized occupations into treatment. It is essential that the occupational therapists and therapy assistants provide ongoing education and training for the client and family to ensure carryover of new learning for increased independence and safety. Outcome measures and goals are used to help ensure an evolving treatment plan is being used to maximize the client's participation in occupation-based activities and the most appropriate discharge plan is carried out.

Continuum of Care

The complexity of poststroke management requires multiple stages of medical care and OT intervention throughout a continuum of care that may be classified as the acute phase (Intensive Care and Acute Care) and the poststroke rehabilitation phase (Subacute

Care, Inpatient Rehabilitation, DayRehab, Outpatient Therapy, and Home Health Care) (Duncan et al., 2005). Motor recovery may occur in either phase without limit; however, intense therapy encourages the greatest period of neuroplasticity in the first 12 months poststroke.

The flowchart in **Figure 10-1** provides a continuum of care overview with possible progressions through each level of care. Clients who respond successfully to skilled therapy would most likely follow the central pathway, reflecting the greatest amount of rehabilitation. Access to each level of care may not be possible in every community and, therefore, clients may default to home health or outpatient therapy. The skilled nursing facility level of care is reserved for patients who do not regain sufficient mobility or independence to return home alone or with a caregiver. Minimal therapy is provided at these facilities. Home health therapy is recommended for clients who are medically stable to return home with a responsible caregiver, continue to progress with goals, and remain future candidates for more intense therapy at the day rehabilitation or outpatient therapy levels of care.

The occupational therapist considers evaluation results and client collaboration when determining short- and long-term goals for the intervention plan and upgrades the goals regularly. While short-term goals are set to reflect progress that is attainable within days during the acute phase and up to two weeks during the poststroke rehabilitation phase, long-term goals represent the anticipated level of functioning at discharge from each level of care.

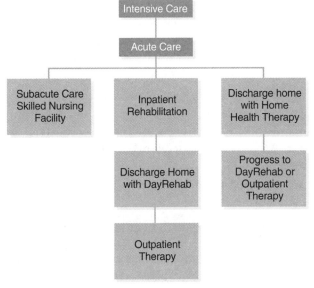

Figure 10-1 Continuum of care.

Expected Functional Outcomes

Acute phase: The acute phase of stroke recovery begins in the Intensive Care Unit (ICU) where OT practitioners are responsible for addressing basic client factors such as mental functions, sensory functions, neuromusculoskeletal functions, and multisystem regulatory functions for organ and speech function in their treatment plans. UE range of motion, sitting balance, alertness, orientation, and visual tracking are included in treatment planning. The OT practitioner documents response to treatment and monitors vitals regularly including blood pressure, heart rate, and oxygen saturation. The OT practitioner is also competent with managing intravenous lines, respiratory care equipment, tracheostomy care, nasogastric and gastrostomy tubes, aspiration and swallowing precautions. Postsurgical clients will have a longer length of stay in the ICU than the client who did not require surgical intervention.

Medically stable clients are transferred from the ICU to Acute Care in the hospital setting to further address medical stability, motor control, cognition, visual perception, communication, and swallowing. Occupational therapists expand treatment plan goals to include ADLs, functional mobility for transfers, and UE function. Adaptive equipment for ADL performance is introduced at this level of care to expedite a client's level of independence and participation in occupational performance. Occupational grooming and dressing tasks may be graded from sitting to standing with assistive devices used for balance as needed. Occupational therapists and OTAs continue client and family education on the importance of incorporating the affected extremities and core trunk control into all functional tasks to improve component skills of strength and coordination. Sensorimotor deficits may emerge at this stage as the activity level of the client is increased including ideational and ideomotor apraxia during ADLs, reduced proprioception and light touch, shoulder pain, and spasticity. The OT or Occupational therapy assistant (OTA) provides tactile or verbal cues or both to aide in motor learning and continues education for proper UE awareness and positioning. Visual perceptual strategies for scanning across the entire visual field improve the client's awareness of the environment. The length of stay in Acute Care varies from days to weeks and may include a transition to Subacute Care while discharge planning is finalized.

The client's level of independence and access to a support system determines if discharge home is appropriate or if admission to a subacute nursing facility or assisted living is warranted. If further progress is anticipated, the client will progress through to the poststroke rehabilitation phase on the Inpatient Rehabilitation Unit within the hospital or at an independent rehabilitation facility.

Poststroke rehabilitation phase: The poststroke rehabilitation phase begins when a client continues to show potential for increasing motor control, cognition, visual perceptual skills, language, and overall independence in daily occupations. Clients may begin this stage when transferred to an Inpatient Rehabilitation Unit that provides a minimum of three skilled therapy hours five days per week. If the client shows potential as a rehabilitation candidate but does not have access to inpatient rehabilitation, the client may begin the rehabilitation stage at the subacute level of care such as skilled nursing facility. When the client demonstrates sufficient strength, cognition, and independence to return home with a responsible caregiver, the client may continue the rehabilitation stage at the DayRehab level of care, which provides up to six intensive hours of skilled therapy per day. DayRehab is becoming more prevalent due to the benefits of intense rehabilitation and is very useful in progressing endurance for clients preparing for return to work or school. When sufficient gains in ADLs and IADLs have been made, clients may use the outpatient therapy level of care to fine-tune residual neurological deficits. Home Health Care is reserved for clients who are unable to attend outside therapy due to personal or environmental factors.

While ADL independence may continue to be a goal area in the poststroke rehabilitation phase, OT also addresses performance in IADLs including, but not limited to, meal preparation, medication management, bill paying, computer use, handwriting, home management, parenting, community reentry, and return to work or school goals. Therapeutic interventions to improve UE motor control and balance should reflect high repetitions of graded tasks that incorporate the affected muscles into functional activities to facilitate neuroplasticity (Winstein et al., 2004). Interdisciplinary team management of a client's rehabilitation ensures that the best comprehensive care is provided. Streamlined communication, team rounds, and goal carryover across disciplines give the interdisciplinary team model an advantage over other models.

Primary team members include physiatry, nursing, OT, physical therapy, speech therapy, psychology, and vocational rehabilitation specialists. Additional referrals may include, but are not limited to, assistive technology specialists, wheelchair seating and positioning, driving rehabilitation, social work, and case management.

Impact on Occupational Performance

Preparatory Methods and Tasks

The level of impairment and subsequent disability also determines if any preparatory methods or tasks are needed to improve participation and positioning in occupation-based activities, including massage, manual therapy, splints, environmental modifications, assistive technology, or assistive devices (**Table 10-5**).

OT practitioners will use range of motion and soft tissue mobilization to prepare a client's UE for functional use if spasticity impedes movement. Other preparatory methods may include moving the placement of activity items to a space that is more noticeable or accessible to improve performance.

The effects of stroke on occupational performance vary greatly and are primarily determined by severity and location of the stroke. Client evaluation may occur using a top-down approach (Gillen, 2013) through the use of occupational performance to determine functional goal areas including increased independence with basic dressing, or using the affected hand to open containers, reach for and grasp light switches, or feed self independently with the affected hand. Therapists may also implement a bottom-up approach to evaluate affected performance skills such as balance, strength, coordination, vision, and cognitive skills. Results from these skilled assessments are used to guide each phase of treatment to ultimately improve independence in client-centered occupations after stroke. Since various levels of care are usually involved in comprehensive stroke rehabilitation, overlap may exist across each phase of recovery.

Therapeutic Use of Occupations

OT practitioners use ongoing activity analysis to determine and implement occupation-based activities to promote

Table 10-5 Preparatory Methods and Tasks

Mobility	• Wheelchair (power, manual, tilt-in-space, transport) • Walker (standard, rolling, hemi-walker) with basket or tray • Cane (large-base quad cane, small-base quad cane, straight cane) • Gait belt	
ADL	• Bedside drop-arm commode • Shower transfer bench • Shower chair • Long-handled reacher • Dressing stick • Zipper pull • Button hook • Foam toothbrush handle • Foam handles for silverware • Scoop dish • Plate guard	• Raised toilet seat • Handheld shower • Grab bars • Long-handled shoe horn • Elastic shoelaces • Sock aide • Heel slide • Wash mitt • Dycem • Rocker knife
IADL	• Walker tray • Walker basket • Foam handle for pen/pencil	• Adapted cutting board • Pot holder
Vision	• Prism glasses • Line guide	• Partial occlusion glasses
Communication	• Communication boards • Phone/computer apps	• Dragon naturally speaking
Orthotics	• Resting hand splint • Antispasticity splint • Thumb strap	• Ankle–foot orthosis • Knee–ankle–foot orthosis

Data from: Duncan et al. (2005); Gillen (2013).

recovery and independence. **Table 10-6** provides examples of multidimensional graded activities that may be incorporated into skilled OT sessions to enable improved client factors and performance skills using motor control, cognitive training, compensatory, and group therapy techniques.

Education and Training

Client and family education begins on the first day of treatment with an introduction to the role and purpose of OT in the rehabilitation process. Education in the acute phase of treatment focuses on safe bed mobility, handling and positioning of the hemiparetic UE, proper use of assistive mobility devices, home exercise programs to promote healthy joint integrity and muscle length, and strategies to improve visual attention and awareness. As the client transitions throughout each level of care, education for the client and family reflects progress made and activity suggestions from the OT practitioner to increase functional use of the affected extremities, safe functional mobility, cognition and visual perceptual skills throughout all ADLs and IADLs. Occupational therapists and OTAs are responsible for educating the client and family in strategies to increase attention and awareness to the complete visual field, use of partial occlusion glasses for diplopia, safe ADL transfers, splint use and care, and pertinent home exercise programs.

Table 10-6 Therapeutic Interventions

Activities of daily living	• **Motor control techniques** include incorporating the hemiplegic UE as a functional assist (e.g., stabilizing toiletry items when opening and stabilizing clothes when managing fasteners), for gross grasp and reaching (e.g., brushing teeth, pumping soap, managing faucets, brushing hair, holding adapted or standard silverware for hand to mouth, sliding jacket off or pulling onto shoulder, and pulling up pants) and for fine motor control (e.g., cutting food, zippering, buttoning, donning socks, and tying shoes). Visual cues, tactile cues, or physical assistance may be provided to facilitate success. Functional mobility may be addressed concurrently by grading the activity from sitting to standing while incorporating safe use of necessary assistive devices • **Cognitive training techniques** incorporate sequencing steps for each task, visually locating required items, attending to the client's complete personal environment and safety awareness • **Compensatory techniques** include donning clothes over the hemiplegic extremities first, using elastic shoelaces, incorporating one-handed strategies for dressing, and incorporating use of assistive devices such as a sock aid, reacher, and long-handled shoe horn to increase overall independence and reduce disability as a result of motor, cognitive, and visual perceptual deficits • **Group therapy** is useful for clients working on improved independence in ADLs including attending to food on their entire plate or learning and practicing the steps of donning a shirt using hemi-techniques as part of eating or dressing groups, respectively
Instrumental activities of daily living	• **Motor control techniques** encourage the client to begin incorporating their affected UE into a greater variety of daily tasks as a functional assist (e.g., gross grasp to stabilize everyday containers when opening, stabilizing paper when writing, carrying items or light bags), for refined grasp and reaching (opening doorway, appliance and cabinet doors, managing light switches, item retrieval, cleaning, and holding onto treadmill), and in fully integrated movement (e.g., feeding a child, handwriting, in-hand manipulation of money, pouring and cutting during meal preparation, folding laundry, zippering a purse, computer use, and dialing a phone). Functional mobility may be addressed concurrently by grading the activity from sitting to standing while incorporating safe use of necessary assistive devices • **Cognitive training techniques** address the process skills contributing to successful performance of meal preparation, medication management, money management, shopping, home maintenance, child care, and leisure skills including attention (e.g., sustained, alternating, divided, and visual), planning, sequencing, organization, short- and long-term memory, reasoning, and problem solving • **Compensatory techniques** improve awareness of the hemiplegic side through the use of positioning (e.g., resting the arm on the table during meal prep or desk work, and supporting the arm in a hand-based sling during functional mobility) and the use of adaptive equipment (adaptive cutting board to stabilize food items during meal preparation) • **Group therapy** may involve clients working together to learn and prepare a multistep meal based on their respective abilities in nutrition and meal planning group, enjoy leisure activities including Wii games, board games, or adaptive bowling, and plan and execute community outings using public transportation
Upper extremity facilitation and management	• **Motor control techniques** including task-oriented training (Winstein et al., 2004) and constraint-induced movement therapy (Dromerick, Edwards, & Hahn, 2000; Taub et al., 1993; Wolf et al., 2006, 2008) facilitate the greatest amount of neuroplasticity when function is the foundation of each activity, and may address proximal, distal, or concurrent proximodistal motor control (e.g., sweeping cotton balls off the edge of the table to encourage shoulder control, prehension of poker chips to place into slotted container for translation and reaching, turning a key for lateral pinch, pouring beans for controlled grasp and forearm control then release for active finger extension, and shuffling cards or folding laundry for bilateral integration). Activities are constantly graded based on client's performance to steadily increase difficulty and number of repetitions to provide the just right challenge. Shoulder strapping is recommended for clients that have the strength and awareness to respond to the taping as tactile feedback and is contraindicated for clients without volitional motor control. Botox may be recommended to reduce spasticity in affected muscle groups for improved positioning and function of the UE. A skilled occupational therapy practitioner appreciates biomechanics, as well as the effects gravity has on emerging movement, and designs a treatment plan that appropriately facilitates improved motor control

Table 10-6 Therapeutic Interventions (*continued*)

	• **Compensatory techniques** include education of passive and self-range of motion to maintain joint and muscle integrity, positioning at rest and positioning during functional mobility using a hand-based sling. Traditional hemi-slings are strongly discouraged as they promote soft tissue shortening of the shoulder internal rotators and elbow flexors • **Group therapy** includes clients at various stages of recovery working together on common goals for improved function and may focus on hand coordination, UE strengthening, and endurance using dowel rods or Thera-Band, and game group (e.g., Wii, balloon volleyball, bean bag toss, and board games requiring management of small pieces or cards)
Functional mobility	• **Motor control techniques** incorporate active participation of the client with assistive devices as needed in bed mobility (e.g., rolling, bridging, supine to sit, and sit to stand), transfers (e.g., bed, toilet, shower, chair, floor, and car), sitting, and standing balance (e.g., static and dynamic ADLs and IADLs) • **Cognitive training techniques** add another level of performance to the activity by engaging the client in attention or visual scanning tasks while engaged in functional mobility activities • **Compensatory techniques** include passively changing the position of the client in bed and during transfers, and relying on a wheelchair for functional mobility when the client has the necessary strength and coordination for higher-level functional mobility using an alternative assistive device that provides less support (e.g., walker, quad cane, and straight cane) • **Group therapy** incorporates functional activities through the use of standing groups (e.g., Wii, balloon volleyball, bean bags, community outings, yoga, and Pilates)
Vision and perception	• **Motor control techniques** encourage extraocular muscle strengthening to improve diplopia, or double vision, as the weaker eye learns to coordinate again with the unaffected eye through the implementation of pen/cap or Brock String exercises. The stronger eye may be patched for intermittent periods to force the use of the weaker eye muscles, including keeping the eye open when ptosis is present • **Cognitive training techniques** include implementation of the lighthouse strategy, or head turning during occupational performance to improve amount of visual input the client processes, if a visual field cut such as homonymous hemianopia is detected (Niemeier, Cifu, & Kishore, 2001) • **Compensatory techniques** reduce the effects of disabling diplopia through the preferred use of partial occlusion glasses over eye patches to preserve peripheral vision while increasing light perception to the eye • **Group therapy** may involve clients working on board games to address visual attention, visual scanning, and visual fields
Cognition	• **Cognitive training techniques** address a large variety of skills including basic orientation, awareness, categorization, money management (e.g., identifying correct coins, collecting, and making change), memory, attention (e.g., sustained, alternating, and divided), executive functions (e.g., planning, organization, problem solving, and reasoning), and safety awareness in the context of functional bill management, meal planning, homemaking tasks, deductive reasoning puzzles, computer use, medication management, and time management • **Compensatory techniques** include using a memory book or notes section in a cell phone to record daily activities, setting alarms in a cell phone for prospective memory • **Group therapy** may address attention levels, problem solving, and following directions while clients are engaged in board games
Communication and language	• **Motor control techniques** may include Supported Conversation for Aphasia, a technique that involves the occupational therapy practitioner or trained conversation partner to anticipate and confirm what the client with reduced expression is saying throughout the conversation using a black marker on white paper to write simple phrases, which encourage and assist the client to express their thoughts purposefully (Kagan, Black, Duchan, Simmons-Mackie, & Square, 2001) • **Compensatory techniques** may include the use of communication boards or personal communication devices that produce a person's voice through prerecorded phrases in the case of reduced verbal expression • **Group therapy** may include conversation groups and book clubs

Data from: Duncan et al. (2005); Gillen (2013); Knesek (2009); Woodson (2014).

Referrals and Discharge Considerations

Clients are continuously reevaluated throughout each level of care using short-term and long-term goals. These goals are established as part of the initial evaluation and are used to guide intervention planning. Short-term goals are modified to reflect progress made. Long-term goals reflect the occupational therapist's best clinical judgment for a client's anticipated status at discharge from the respective level of care.

Discharge planning varies greatly depending on the levels of impairment. Many clients are discharged home with a trained responsible caregiver for a period of time, or permanently, with the necessary assistive devices and adaptive equipment to ensure a safe transition home. The ultimate goal reflects discharge home with increased independence in occupational roles and return to work or school activities on a reduced or full-time schedule. Additional referrals may be made to a fitness center, vocational rehabilitation, psychology, and driver's rehabilitation.

Advocacy efforts are made by the OT team through recommendation of peer support groups, providing helpful documentation to property management companies regarding environmental modifications, assisting with vehicle placard applications for disabled parking permits, and overseeing successful transitions for return to work or school. It is common for the occupational therapist to create a detailed list of recommended accommodations to an employer or school, or revised schedules for a gradual return to work or school trial to enable successful reintegration.

Management and Standards of Practice

Occupational therapists and OT assistants are an integral part of the interdisciplinary team directing the care of clients who are regaining their independence after stroke. Early evaluation and intervention allows the occupational therapist to develop a client-centered intervention plan that incorporates goals of the client and family that address client factors, performance skills, occupations, performance patterns, contexts, and environments that contribute to independence. The occupational therapist and OT assistant collaborate together using clinical reasoning, activity analysis, and outcome measures to implement the most effective and comprehensive intervention plan to ultimately promote independence in daily occupations. While the occupational therapist provides any necessary clarification of evaluation results and goal setting, the OT assistant has the autonomy to create daily treatment plans, direct patient and family education, recommend necessary durable medical equipment and assistive devices and status ongoing short- and long-term goals.

Ethical considerations in the treatment of stroke reflect the importance of maintaining the client's participation in decision making, ADLs, and IADLs. While each client may present with a certain set of deficits that are addressed as part of the rehabilitation plan, each client also presents with certain motor and cognitive skills that remain intact. Emphasizing these strengths may enable the interdisciplinary team to preserve some level of independence for the client during difficult decisions regarding caregiving needs. Concerns may also arise during discharge planning if a client requires ongoing supervision or assistance yet the client and/or family is not in agreement with each other or with recommendations for ongoing assistance. The client's safety is of utmost importance, and every effort should be made to provide sufficient training and education to facilitate a successful discharge. If the family is unable to provide support for the client at discharge, a referral to social work or case management is necessary.

Chapter 10 Self-Study Activities (Answers Are Provided at the End of the Chapter)

Correctly answer the following multiple choice questions:

1. This is the leading cause of disability in adults:
   A. Gunshot wounds
   B. Stroke
   C. Cancer
   D. Diabetes
2. Which of the following conditions contribute to increased stroke risk?
   A. Hypertension
   B. Smoking
   C. Atrial fibrillation
   D. All of the above

3. CVA is an abbreviation for:
   A. Cardiovascular accident
   B. Cerebrovascular accident
   C. Cerebrovascular arrest
   D. None of the above

4. Which of the following are the most recognizable signs of stroke?
   A. Weight loss, hypertension, and hemiplegia
   B. Incontinence, hypertension, and hemiplegia
   C. Hemiplegia, facial paralysis, and impaired communication
   D. All of the above

5. This type of stroke occurs when a blood clot blocks normal cerebral flow causing a lack of oxygen to the brain:
   A. Ischemic
   B. Hemorrhagic
   C. Aortic
   D. None of the above

6. This type of stroke causes pooling of blood in the brain, interrupting normal blood flow:
   A. Ischemic
   B. Hemorrhagic
   C. Aortic
   D. None of the above

7. TIA is an abbreviation for:
   A. Temporary ischemic attack
   B. Transient ischemic attack
   C. Temporary ischemic arrest
   D. None of the above

8. Which of the following are considered to be levels of care in the management of stroke?
   A. Acute Care
   B. Inpatient Rehabilitation
   C. DayRehab
   D. All of the above

9. Which of the following blood supplies are included in anterior circulation syndromes?
   A. Anterior cerebral artery
   B. Middle cerebral artery
   C. A and B
   D. None of the above

10. Which of the following blood supplies are included in posterior circulation syndromes?
    A. Posterior cerebral artery
    B. Cerebellar artery
    C. Vertebrobasilar artery
    D. All of the above

11. Answer the following short-answer question: You evaluated a client in Acute Care who was found to have a middle cerebral artery stroke two weeks ago. Goals include independent sitting at the edge of the bed for grooming and dressing, moderate assistance for standing balance during transfers for toileting and functional mobility, and moderate cues to consistently locate items on the left side. Describe three different skilled therapy sessions that you would include in your intervention plan.

Chapter 10 Self-Study Answers

1. B
2. D
3. B
4. C
5. A
6. B
7. B
8. D
9. C
10. D
11. There are many acceptable examples of skilled therapy sessions for treating middle cerebral artery stroke. One example could include sitting at the edge of the bed with support as needed to address sitting balance while visually scanning for various food items on the left side of the plate during feeding. Other examples may include visually scanning for grooming items on the sink or using visual perceptual skills to don a shirt correctly. Standing may also be incorporated into the grooming routine in the bathroom or while transferring to a bedside commode.

References

Centers for Disease Control and Prevention. (2015). *Stroke in the United States.* Retrieved from http://www.cdc.gov/stroke/facts.htm

Dromerick, A. W., Edwards, D. F., & Hahn, M. (2000). Does the application of constraint-induced movement therapy during acute rehabilitation reduce arm impairment after ischemic stroke? *Stroke, 31*(12), 2984–2988.

Duncan, P. W., Zorowitz, R., Bates, B., Choi, J. Y., Glasberg, J. J., Graham, G. D., . . . Reker, D. (2005). Management of adult stroke rehabilitation care: A clinical practice guideline. *Stroke, 36*(9), e100–e143. doi:10.1161/01.str.0000180861.54180.ff

Gillen, G. (2013). Cerebrovascular accident/stroke. In L. W. Pedretti, H. M. Pendleton, & W. Schultz-Krohn (Eds.), *Pedretti's occupational therapy: Practice skills for physical dysfunction* (7th ed., pp. 844–857). St. Louis, MO: Elsevier.

Go, A. S., Mozaffarian, D., Roger, V. L., Benjamin, E. J., Berry, J. D., Blaha, M. J., . . . Turner, M. B. (2014). Heart disease and stroke statistics—2014 update: A report from the American Heart Association. *Circulation, 129*(3), e28–e292. doi:10.1161/01.cir.0000441139.02102.80

Kagan, A., Black, S. E., Duchan, F. J., Simmons-Mackie, N., & Square, P. (2001). Training volunteers as conversation partners using "Supported Conversation for Adults with Aphasia" (SCA): A controlled trial. *Journal of Speech, Language, and Hearing Research, 44*(3), 624–638.

Knesek, K. (2009). Cerebrovascular accident. In E. B. Crepeau, E. S. Cohn, & B. A. B. Schell (Eds.), *Willard & Spackman's occupational therapy* (11th ed., pp. 1001–1005). Philadelphia, PA: Wolters Kluwer Health/Lippincott Williams & Wilkins.

Niemeier, J. P., Cifu, D. X., & Kishore, R. (2001). The lighthouse strategy: Improving the functional status of patients with unilateral neglect after stroke and brain injury using a visual imagery intervention. *Top Stroke Rehabilitation, 8*(2), 10–18. doi:10.1310/7ukk-hj0f-gdwf-hhm8

Taub, E., Miller, N. E., Novack, T. A., Cook, E. W., III, Fleming, W. C., Nepomuceno, C. S., . . . Crago, J. E. (1993). Technique to improve chronic motor deficit after stroke. *Archives of Physical Medicine and Rehabilitation, 74*(4), 347–354.

Winstein, C. J., Rose, D. K., Tan, S. M., Lewthwaite, R., Chui, H. C., & Azen, S. P. (2004). A randomized controlled comparison of upper-extremity rehabilitation strategies in acute stroke: A pilot study of immediate and long-term outcomes. *Archives of Physical Medicine and Rehabilitation, 85*(4), 620–628.

Wolf, S. L., Winstein, C. J., Miller, J. P., Taub, E., Uswatte, G., Morris, D., . . . Nichols-Larsen, D. (2006). Effect of constraint-induced movement therapy on upper extremity function 3 to 9 months after stroke: The EXCITE randomized clinical trial. *JAMA, 296*(17), 2095–2104. doi:10.1001/jama.296.17.2095

Wolf, S. L., Winstein, C. J., Miller, J. P., Thompson, P. A., Taub, E., Uswatte, G., . . . Clark, P. C. (2008). Retention of upper limb function in stroke survivors who have received constraint-induced movement therapy: The EXCITE randomized trial. *Lancet Neurology, 7*(1), 33–40. doi:10.1016/s1474-4422(07)70294-6

Woodson, A. (2014). Stroke. In M. V. Radomski & C. A. T. Latham (Eds.), *Occupational therapy for physical dysfunction* (7th ed., pp. 1000–1037). Philadelphia, PA: Wolters Kluwer Health/Lippincott Williams & Wilkins.

Traumatic Brain Injury

Lori Bravi

Learning Objectives

- Identify and define the various levels of traumatic brain injury.
- Classify the appropriate assessments based on their overall goal of impairment, activity, and/or participation.
- Compare and contrast between the appropriate interventions based on the level of injury.
- Identify appropriate circumstances for referrals and discharge considerations.

Key Terms

- *Aphasia*: Characterized as either expressive or receptive aphasia and refers to a diminished ability to verbally express or understand speech
- *Apraxia*: Characterized by difficulty or inability to complete precise motor movements secondary to difficulty with understanding sensory input
- *Ataxia*: Characterized by difficulty or inability to perform activities of daily living (ADLs) secondary to muscle incoordination
- *Bimanual integration*: Coordinated use of both sides of the body
- *Perception*: The ability to understand, interpret, and appropriately respond to sensory input related to vision, hearing, touch, taste, and smell

Description

Traumatic brain injury (TBI) is the result of a sudden, forceful impact to the skull that creates a primary focal point of injury, closed or open, with resultant secondary bruising, bleeding, and edema causing damage to the primary tissue and surrounding areas (Tipton-Burton, McLaughlin, & Englander, 2013). Diffuse axonal injury (DAI), a less focal type of TBI, is equally traumatic to the brain because of the shearing that occurs throughout the deep brain structures as a result of sudden forceful shaking or coup–contrecoup injuries or both. TBIs range from mild to severe and are associated with a wide spectrum of physical, cognitive, perceptual, visual, neuroendocrine, and psychological impairments that may impact the client and family for months, years, or a lifetime. In 2010, over 2 million Americans were treated in an emergency room department for TBI resulting in 280,000 hospitalizations and 50,000 deaths. Between 2006 and 2010, men were more likely to be seen in an emergency department and subsequently hospitalized, and three times more likely to die from TBI, compared to women. The rate of occurrence for TBI is highest in persons older than 65 years of age (Centers for Disease Control and Prevention [CDC], 2011; Faul, Xu, Wald, & Coronado, 2010).

Etiology and Pathology

Falls are the most common cause of TBI across all age groups; however, they account for as many as 55 and 81% of TBIs in children younger than 15 years of age and adults older than 65 years of age, respectively. Motor vehicle accidents and motorcycle accidents are the most common causes of TBI in persons between 15 and 40 years of age (CDC, 2014). Alcohol is associated with approximately one-third of persons sustaining a TBI (Corrigan, 1995) and the risk of recurrent TBI increases up to three times that of persons without a history of TBI (Annegers, Grabow, Kurland, & Laws, 1980).

The etiology of TBI includes, but is not limited to, falls, motor vehicle accidents, sports injuries, weapon injuries, violent physical assaults, motorcycle accidents, and blasts. Open head injuries are considered penetrating if an object enters then remains inside the skull, or perforating if the object enters and subsequently exits the skull. Closed head injuries are considered static in the case of a crush injury or dynamic if the brain injury is a result of violent acceleration and deceleration resulting in coup–contrecoup injuries. While body armor may be credited for saving lives, it does not always prevent injuries to the face, brain, or extremities. Blast injuries, open or closed, are considered a new category of TBI due to the increase in injuries from explosives in recent years (Maas et al., 2010).

TBI is further identified by the primary tissue location affected with respect to the cranium. Examples include intracerebral hemorrhage (ICH), epidural hematoma (EDH), subdural hematoma (SDH), intraventricular hemorrhage (IVH), and DAI. While the aforementioned etiologies of TBI are responsible for the primary, or focal, point of injury, secondary injury such as bruising, swelling, changes in intracranial pressure, ischemia, anoxia, seizure, and neuroendocrine and metabolic dysfunction equally contributes to impairment. Early intervention to reduce the effects of these secondary incidents is crucial to reducing severity of side effects.

Clinical Presentation

Classification of TBI (**Table 11-1**) ranges from mild, moderate, to severe, which is initially documented by the emergency medical responders on scene using the Glasgow Coma Scale (GCS). This scale rates motor responses, sensory responses, and eye opening using an ordinal scale, classifying a total point score of 3–8 as

severe TBI, 9–12 as moderate TBI, and 13–15 as mild TBI (Teasdale & Jennett, 1974). Severe TBI may result in a coma, a state of unresponsiveness, which is characterized by an inability to open one's eyes, respond to stimuli, or communicate. Once the eyes open, a person emerges from a coma to a vegetative state; however, there is no purposeful awareness, interaction with others in the environment, or nonreflexive movement present. Typically, a person who remains at this level for one month is considered to be in a persistent vegetative state (Tipton-Burton et al., 2013). Giacino et al. (2002) determined a set of key responses that must be made in order to formally document that a person has progressed from a vegetative state to a minimally conscious state, which is characterized by any sustained interaction with other persons or the environment including following simple commands, performing purposeful motor control, or both.

Giacino et al. (2002) also describe a protocol used by skilled therapists and other medical team members to determine when a client emerges out of the minimally conscious state of severe TBI into moderate TBI. Key behaviors include consistent functional yes-and-no communication and consistent functional object use, with both behaviors reproducible in two consecutive sessions. When a person presents at the moderate level of TBI, it is common for increased awareness and alertness to be accompanied by confusion and agitation due to persistent physical, cognitive, communicative, and visual perceptual impairments. The Rancho Los Amigos Levels of Cognitive Functioning (Hagen 1998; Hagen, Malkmus, & Durhman, 1979) is a spectrum that describes emerging cognitive behavioral patterns used to stage a client at a particular time in recovery. While these levels provide a defined continuum of emerging cognition and awareness, persons with TBI may skip levels based on progress

Table 11-1 Levels of Consciousness for Severe, Moderate, and Mild TBI

	Severe TBI	Moderate TBI	Mild TBI
GCS	3–7	8–12	13–15
Rancho Los Amigos Levels	1–3	4–8	9–10
Loss of consciousness	>30 min	>30 min	<30 min
Key signs	• Coma • Vegetative state • Minimally conscious state	• Agitated • Confused • Automatic • Purposeful	• Purposeful • Appropriate • Potentially undiagnosed

Data from (Hagen, 1998; Powell, 2014; Teasdale & Jennett, 1974; Tipton-Burton, McLaughlin, & Englander, 2013)

made or because initial staging is a higher level. Moderate TBI has the greatest representation in this scale covering five levels (i.e., 4–8) with cognitive behavioral patterns emerging as confused, agitated, and then automatic. Rancho IV is the hallmark level that indicates a person has emerged from a minimally conscious state to a confused and agitated state. See Table 11-1 for levels of consciousness for severe, moderate, and mild TBI.

Mild TBI, including concussion, is on the far end of the spectrum because the side effects generally are not life threatening, loss of consciousness usually does not persist beyond 30 minutes, and an eventual return to one's occupational roles is more likely (National Center for Injury Prevention and Control, 2003). Mild TBI may result in subtle cognitive and physical impairments that are not noticeable in the days and weeks following injury; however, delayed processing, mild memory deficits, or fatigue may persist for months after the event without formal identification by the victim. These clients demonstrate purposeful and appropriate cognitive functioning and are often working toward a successful return to occupational roles and habits as facilitated by skilled therapy interventions.

Prevention measures for TBI recommended by the CDC (2013) include the use of proper seating systems and safety belts for children and adults every time one rides in a motor vehicle. Helmets should be worn when riding bicycles, motorcycles, all-terrain vehicles, horses, skateboards, rollerblades, ice-skating, and while engaged in similar sports activities such as contact sports and climbing. Playgrounds should be designed with natural or rubberized mulch or similar materials that absorb potential impact from high-velocity contact. Simple environmental changes including removing trip hazards (e.g., throw rugs and other obstacles) aid in the prevention of falls for seniors and others at risk groups (CDC, 2013).

Diagnostic Tests

There are a variety of diagnostic tests used after a person acquires a TBI. **Table 11-2** provides a summary of commonly used diagnostic tests and imaging for TBI.

Medical Procedures and Postsurgical Precautions/Contraindications

There are also common medical procedures, both surgical and nonsurgical, that are used to treat TBI. **Table 11-3** provides a summary of these procedures, along with a list of precautions and contraindications that occupational therapy practitioners should consider.

Table 11-2 Diagnostic Tests and Medical Imaging for TBI

CT	Computed tomography provides efficient cross-sectional x-ray images, with or without the use of iodine contrast dye, of the internal body structure in as few as 10 min, including acute and chronic bleeding
MRI	Magnetic resonance imaging requires more time for processing, but produces a more detailed picture of acute and chronic injury using magnets with or without the use of noniodine dye, and is especially useful in detecting more finite changes; however, it is contraindicated for persons with metal in their bodies
PET	Positron emission tomography is not usually indicated for acute stroke due to time required for the radioactive venous tracer to detect disease processes and structural changes reflected as 3D images
SPECT	Single-photon emission computed tomography is a newer type of 3D scans that also uses a radioactive tracer to detect changes in blood flow through increased absorption in more active areas of insult
GCS	The Glasgow Coma Scale, the standard assessment immediately following TBI, is commonly used to status a person's level of consciousness using a 15-point scale through the assessment of motor responses, sensory responses, and eye opening
Rancho Los Amigos Levels of Cognitive Functioning	The Rancho Los Amigos Scale is a descriptive scale that uses cognitive and behavioral interactions of a person within their environment after TBI to provide staging on 1 of 10 levels
Neuropsychological testing	Neuropsychological testing, a battery of performance-based assessments, provides valuable information on the level of cognitive functioning and may be used to determine readiness for return to occupational roles

Data from Powell, 2014; Tipton-Burton, McLaughlin, and Englander, 2013.

Table 11-3 Medical Procedures for TBI

Nonsurgical medical intervention	• Medications are used to regulate neuroendocrine function, sleep, appetite, seizure activity, and attention
	• Drug-induced coma may be initiated in severe TBI to allow the brain to rest
	• Mechanical ventilation using noninvasive measures assists respiration
Surgical medical intervention	• Craniotomy with hematoma evacuation is used to remove excess blood or blood clot
	• Decompressive craniotomy is used to reduce severe intracranial pressure and edema
	• Ventriculoperitoneal shunt placement to drain excess cerebrospinal fluid and manage hydrocephalus reduces intracranial pressure on the brain
	• Mechanical ventilation with endotracheal intubation is used with clients in respiratory failure

Precautions and contraindications:

• Activity restrictions may include no jumping, running, lifting, or bending with any of the above medical interventions

• A helmet may be required after a craniotomy until the cerebral edema is under control and the bone flap is replaced

• Blood pressure parameters may be implemented

Data from Powell, 2014; Tipton-Burton, McLaughlin, and Englander, 2013.

Screening and Assessments

Occupational therapy evaluation of clients with TBI includes completing an occupational profile to determine strengths and weaknesses affecting the client's occupational performance. This portion of the evaluation may involve informal interview, discussion, and clinical observation of the client to provide valuable information regarding the client's goals. Key family members are also included in this part of the evaluation if the client is unable to communicate due to severity of injury or reduced language skills from the injury or both. Establishing a personalized occupational profile at the onset of intervention planning allows the occupational therapist (OT) to identify goal areas and prioritize subsequent occupational performance analyses. For example, if the client is able to express a strong desire to improve hand strength, coordination, and reaching in order to perform drinking, lifting an upper extremity (UE) for dressing, or picking

up a pencil to write, occupational performance analysis may include the standardized Wolf Motor Function Test (WMFT).

Components of the occupational therapy evaluation are often categorized as nonstandardized, standardized, semistandardized, or criterion referenced. Nonstandardized screening and assessment procedures include an initial informal and formal interview, direct observation of occupational performance in the naturalistic environment, and client and/or family report. Documentation may include observed or reported changes in sensation, kinesthesia, proprioception, posture, gross and fine motor control, cognition, vision, and psychological status not otherwise reflected in objective assessments conducted by the OT.

Standardized assessments are the gold standard because they include specific instructions for the setup of the assessment; specific language used while offering verbal directions to a patient; language employed while providing verbal cueing; and scoring and cutoff times if indicated, which reduce measurement error and increase the validity and reliability of the assessment tool. Standardized assessments also have established psychometric properties for reliability and validity. A variety of standardized assessments now have established minimal detectable change values and standard errors of measurement that are useful in goal setting to demonstrate real changes in functioning are occurring. Examples of standardized assessments include the WMFT, the Action Research Arm Test (ARAT), the Assessment of Motor and Process Skills (AMPS), and the Arnadottir Occupational Therapy Activities of Daily Living Neurobehavioral Evaluation (A-ONE). The AMPS and the A-ONE are especially useful standardized assessments because they allow for scoring occupational performance in the naturalistic setting (Golisz, 2009).

Standardized assessments are considered criterion referenced if test items measure a body function or performance skill and allow for comparison of performance for what the person can do over time. Examples of criterion-referenced assessments include the AMPS, Fugl-Meyer Assessment (FMA), Barthel Index, and the Motor-Free Visual Perceptual Test.

Assessments are also categorized according to the World Health Organization's International Classification of Functioning, Disability, and Health (ICF). This framework is used internationally to guide health and disability outcomes with consideration for three domains: impairment, activity, and participation. These domains compliment the Occupational Therapy Practice Framework III when considering appropriate assessments to include as part of the occupational profile and occupational performance evaluation (American Occupational Therapy Association, 2014; World Health Organization, 2002). **Table 11-4** provides a basic list of standardized assessments in reference to the ICF domains that are used in evaluating TBI.

Interventions

Expected Functional Outcomes

Occupational therapy interventions for TBI are targeted to meet the needs of the client based on the level of injury and presentation upon evaluation. While the overall goal of improving a person's level of occupational

Table 11-4 Standardized Assessments with ICF Classifications

Standardized Assessment	Impairment	Activity	Participation
ARAT	x	x	
Activity Card Sort		x	x
ABS	x		
A-ONE		x	x
AMPS	x	x	
Barthel Index			x
biVABA	x		
COPM		x	x
CHART		x	x
CNC	x		
Dynamometry	x		
FMA	x	x	
FIM		x	
GOAT	x		
Goniometry	x		
GCS	x		
KELS		x	
LOTCA	x		
Manual Muscle Testing	x		
Modified Ashworth Scale	x		
MAS		x	x
MVPT-3	x		
MET		x	x
RMBT-E		x	
Role Checklist			x
SIP	x	x	x
WNSSP	x		

ARAT, Action Research Arm Test; ABS, Agitated Behavior Scale; A-ONE, Arnadottir Occupational Therapy Activities of Daily Living Neurobehavioral Evaluation; AMPS, Assessment of Motor and Process Skills; biVABA, Brain Injury Visual Assessment Battery for Adults; COPM, Canadian Occupational Performance Measure; CHART, Craig Handicap Assessment and Reporting Technique; CNC, Coma/Near Coma Scale; FIM, Functional Independence Measure; GOAT, Galveston Orientation and Amnesia Test; KELS, Kohlman Evaluation of Living Skills; LOTCA, Lowenstein Occupational Therapy Cognitive Assessment; MAS, Motor Assessment Scale; MVPT-3, Motor-Free Visual Perception Test; MET, Multiple Errands Test; RMBT-E, Rivermead Behavioral Memory Test—Extended Version; SIP, Sickness Impact Profile; WNSSP, Western Neurosensory Stimulation Profile. Data from Golisz, 2009; Powell, 2014; Tipton-Burton, McLaughlin, and Englander, 2013.

performance is paramount, certain interventions are more appropriate than other methods at each respective level of injury. Intervention plans are dynamic and reflect a client's ongoing progress.

Preparatory Tasks

Examples of preparatory tasks for each level of TBI include the following: (1) employing strategies that help to ensure the environment optimizes a client's ability to focus on the task at hand while minimizing environmental distractions; (2) utilizing range of motion (ROM) or stretching or both to prime muscles for functional use and strengthening; (3) positioning to ensure proper body alignment and to prepare the trunk and limbs for engagement in functional activities; (4) using partial occlusion glasses or prism glasses to reduce diplopia; (5) incorporating adaptive equipment to improve independence in ADLs and IADLs; and (6) using a communication board to facilitate a client's ability to express wants and needs.

Impact on Occupational Performance

Occupational performance is clearly impacted on all levels for moderate and severe injuries; however, it can be less apparent in mild TBI cases. Client factors such as body functions and body structures, in addition to motor, process, and social interaction performance skills, are foundational because they enable a client to engage in performance patterns. Intervention planning for clients with severe TBI focuses more on body structures necessary for performance skills; for example, serial casting for UE spasticity management and implementation of sensory integration to activate the reticular activating system are common occupational therapy interventions with this population (Tipton-Burton et al., 2013).

Intervention planning for moderate TBI continues to address foundational body functions while expanding to include motor, process, and social interaction performance skills. Functional activities in skilled therapy sessions may include trunk stabilization in sitting or standing (e.g., to enable a client to reach for utensils while self-feeding), initiating organized scanning patterns (e.g., while choosing clothes to wear), and regulating behavior (e.g., recognizing and controlling one's anger or frustration during a group activity or challenging financial management task). Specific roles, habits, and routines typically are incorporated into client-specific interventions at this level of functioning.

Occupational performance for a client recovering from a mild TBI may be preserved on many levels; however, intervention planning to address residual endurance or coordination deficits or both is important to help ensure the best recovery. Skilled therapy sessions often focus on reintegration of purposeful performance patterns of the individual and performance patterns of the individual within a larger group or population. Activities may address return to parenting, work, school, volunteer, and driving roles. The tables below reflect typical interventions for each level of injury and may be modified for or applied to the other levels of TBI as seen relevant.

Severe TBI: Intervention planning for severe TBI (**Table 11-5**) is aimed at body functions and includes increasing stimulation, arousal, alertness, protective extension reactions, ROM, and localized responses. Clients are closely monitored for progression through the stages of consciousness from coma, vegetative state, and minimally conscious state. A quiet room provides the best environment to gauge the client's responses to stimuli.

Moderate TBI: Intervention planning for moderate TBI continues to address client factors including body functions, but also expands to include performance skills that reflect motor skills, process skills, and social interaction skills, and performance patterns that define the client's habits, routines, rituals, and roles both as an individual and as part of a larger group or population. As participation increases, interventions engage the client in ADLs and IADLs and may include behavioral modification if agitation is present. **Table 11-6** provides a summary of interventions appropriate for people with moderate TBI.

Mild TBI: Intervention planning for mild TBI most commonly reflects reintegration of the client into premorbid habits, routines, rituals, and roles as part of individual or group performance patterns. While motor, process, and social interaction performance skills may be included as noted above, intervention planning expands to include return to work, school, family, and community activities. **Table 11-7** provides a summary of interventions appropriate for people with mild TBI.

Reevaluation and Plan Modification

Intervention plans are considered a dynamic component of the rehabilitation program and are reevaluated on an ongoing basis. Short- and long-term goals are established

Table 11-5 Severe TBI Intervention Planning

Intervention Planning

Physical	**Positioning** • **Cervical ROM** is indicated to preserve integrity of the neck muscles that are used for head control, communication, and swallowing • **Head control** is continuously assessed for potential motor control and communication of yes/no while the client is in bed, supported at the edge of the bed, prone on a wedge, or in a wheelchair • **Trunk control** at the edge of the bed or mat is used to assess emerging protective extension reactions and balance, provide beneficial stimulation to the pulmonary and cardiovascular systems, and encourage alertness and arousal • **Bed positioning** techniques are followed to reduce pressure areas on bony prominences (e.g., head, elbows, hips, and heels), reduce chances for aspiration, and incorporate frequent change of position to prevent skin breakdown • **Prone positioning** is a useful intervention to increase thoracic and lumbar ROM and for increased overall stimulation to the pulmonary and cardiovascular systems in response to change in positioning • **Seating and positioning** using advanced tilt-in-space wheelchair systems ensures that the head, neck, trunk, extremities, and pelvis are aligned with the proper support and seat cushioning **UE Management** • **Scapular mobilization** is performed prior to UE PROM to ensure sufficient scapular–humeral gliding occurs • **PROM** is performed daily to preserve ROM throughout the UEs, prevent heterotopic ossification, and provide stimulation to the client • **Casting and/or splinting** is implemented to reduce or prevent soft tissue contractures of muscles and tendons that may occur as a result of spasticity or more severe rigidity and may include short arm casts to improve ROM at a single joint, long arm casts to improve ROM at two joints (e.g., elbow and wrist or wrist and hand), bivalve casts, dropout elbow casts, custom resting hand splints, prefabricated antispasticity hand splints, or more elaborate dynamic orthotics • **Localized responses** may include withdrawal from noxious stimuli or squeezing a hand on command
Cognitive	• **Facilitation of alertness and awareness** is performed throughout the treatment session and any response is documented to determine if reactions are purposeful, including opening the eyes in response to sensory stimuli • **Simple commands** are used to encourage awareness and comprehension and may include "close/open your eyes," "squeeze/release my hand," and "turn your head" • **Reliable yes/no systems** are implemented, for example, the use of a simple communication board, head nods, or eye blinking, and are used consistently by all members of the medical team • **Oral medications** may be part of the medical treatment plan to stimulate arousal and alertness
Visual	• **Facilitation of eye opening** is initiated to encourage transition from a coma to a vegetative state and may include playing familiar music or noxious stimuli such as clapping or ringing a bell • **Visual tracking** of familiar people, a flashlight, or meaningful items or photos is used to improve oculomotor control
Sensory integration	• **Olfactory stimuli** include the use of common food extracts (e.g., vanilla, almond, and lemon), familiar grooming products (shaving cream, soap), and familiar lotions or perfumes to stimulate the sense of smell • **Auditory stimuli** include the use of familiar music, conversation, and also noxious stimuli (e.g., bell, horn, and clapping) to elicit reactions including eye opening or head turning • **Visual stimuli** include presentation of familiar faces or items (e.g., movies or favorite magazines) and may involve using a flashlight to encourage visual tracking or noxious visual stimuli (e.g., unexpected gesture close to the face) to elicit blink response • **Tactile stimuli** include the use of light and deep manual touch in addition to various textures to discriminate responses between soft chamois fabric and noxious fine grit sandpaper • **Gustatory stimuli** include pleasure feeds of pudding tastes on the lips when allowed or more noxious stimuli such as a cold spoon to elicit a swallow response

(continues)

Table 11-5 Severe TBI Intervention Planning (*continued*)

Intervention Planning	
Rest and sleep	• **Rest and sleep** are critical components of recovery in every stage and may be managed using oral medications, especially if restlessness is noted
Education	• **Family education** begins as soon as possible and addresses a wide variety of topics such as skin integrity, UE and cervical ROM, bed and wheelchair positioning, sensory integration for arousal, benefits of ongoing interaction with the client, and management of orthotics

PROM, passive range of motion.
Data from Golisz, 2009; Tipton-Burton, McLaughlin, and Englander, 2013.

Table 11-6 Moderate TBI Intervention Planning

Intervention Planning	
Physical	• **Balance activities** in unsupported and supported sitting and standing, tall kneeling, and quadruped become part of the daily intervention plan to improve static and dynamic trunk control, gross motor control of the extremities, vestibular reactions, kinesthetic processing, and overall participation within the environment. Mirrors are used for biofeedback, foam cushions challenge balance in sitting and standing, and interactive computer games are used to challenge multiple systems simultaneously
	• **UE strengthening and coordination** of the affected limbs include bimanual integration, functional object use, weight bearing, reaching, grasp, prehension, pinch, release, and in-hand manipulation through graded functional activities to improve strength, coordination, sensation, apraxia, and ataxia. Catch and release activities, clothing management, and cutting activities are used to encourage bimanual integration while graded object translation improves in-hand manipulation
	• **ROM and stretching** of the scapulae and UEs is used to promote normal tissue length and maintain integrity of joints for functional use
	• **Casting and splinting** continue to be used to reduce spasticity, increase ROM, and prepare soft tissue for functional use. Adjuncts include oral medications, neuromuscular injections, or nerve blocks to reduce hypertonicity
	• **Dysphagia strategies** prevent aspiration and increase success with oral motor control and include proper elevation at rest, implementing chin tucks when swallowing, following appropriate food and drink consistencies, and actively involving client in management of secretions
Cognitive	• **Self-awareness and self-monitoring** are encouraged through verbal and tactile cueing for appropriate behaviors as the client increases interactions with self, others, and surroundings
	• **Orientation methods** include the use of calendars, memory books, newspapers, and familiar photographs in albums
	• **Attention** activities are graded for performance in closed or open environments to manage levels of distraction and may be measured using units of times in minutes for sustained, alternating, and divided attention. Functional pen and paper tasks, games, and interactive ADL and IADL routines may be used in intervention planning
	• **Sequencing and procedural memory** activities are used to improve comprehension of steps in correct order required to complete both familiar and novel functional activities and include ADL routines, games, and following multistep directions
	• **Short- and long-term memory** activities may include the use of memory books, current events, family relationships, and frequent errorless cueing to improve carryover. Attention is a prerequisite to encoding new memories

Table 11-6 Moderate TBI Intervention Planning (*continued*)

Intervention Planning

	• **Visual perception** activities may include parquetry puzzles using parts to make a whole or more complex skills involving telling time on a watch or standard clock
	• **Perception** activities may include both motor and sensory skills that focus on the right (e.g., holistic thinking) and left (e.g., attention to details) hemisphere's of the brain
	• **Language comprehension and expression** interventions are integrated throughout all treatment sessions to improve communication and include the use of communication boards, Supported Conversation for Aphasia, computer programs, gestures, and graded written and verbal language to increase total communication
	• **Planning and problem-solving** activities range from simple to complex and require the client to use reasoning and judgment to determine the best solution to daily living situations including time management, safety awareness, and financial management
Visual	• **Oculomotor control exercises** using a pen and cap or the Brock string are used to strengthen eye muscles to improve smooth pursuits, saccades, convergence, and divergence, and reduce diplopia that limits occupational performance
	• **Prism glasses and partial occlusion glasses** are used as either a temporary or permanent strategy to reduce the effect of diplopia and may be used intermittently throughout the day or during all waking hours
	• **Visual scanning** using organized patterns is implemented to increase visual attention and visual fields to locate food, ADL or IADL items, obstacles, and pathways in the client's personal or extra-personal space
ADL	• **Eating** addresses head control, trunk control, swallowing, functional object use, bimanual integration, fine and gross motor control, initiation, attention, and vision and may include the use of foam handles, plate guards, or arm supports
	• **Grooming, dressing, and bathing activities** are implemented at bedside, from the wheelchair or in standing as appropriate and address functional mobility, balance, strength, coordination, motor control, bimanual integration, sequencing, attention, and vision
	• **Toileting programs** may be implemented to increase self-awareness of continence and also improve balance, strength, coordination, sequencing, attention, and vision
IADL	• **Instrumental activities of daily living**, including financial management, home management, medication management, safety awareness, and shopping, are used in skilled therapy sessions to improve body functions and structures in addition to motor, process, and social interaction performance skills. Tasks are continuously graded from simple (e.g., identifying coins) to complex (e.g., managing monthly checkbook balance) to address the current level of processing and functioning
Rest and sleep	• **Rest and sleep** continue to be emphasized in order to facilitate healing, recovery, and improved overall attention when awake. Oral medications may be used to regulate sleep cycles
Education and work	• **Education and work activities** are considered and gradually integrated into skilled therapy sessions as other process performance skills improve
Play, leisure, and social participation	• **Purposeful leisure activities** incorporate computer or board games, musical instruments, or sports into skilled interventions to facilitate occupational performance in premorbid play, leisure, and social activities while improving body functions and process performance skills
Psychosocial	• **Psychological support** in the form of individual, couple, family, or group treatment is essential to assisting clients and family members with coping mechanisms as they begin to process changes in premorbid occupational performance and roles
Group	• **Group activities** are gradually introduced to address attention, social interaction, strengthening, coordination, standing endurance, balance, and community reintegration

ADL, activities of daily living; IADL, instrumental activities of daily living.
Data from Golisz, 2009; Tipton-Burton, McLaughlin, and Englander, 2013.

Table 11-7 Mild TBI Intervention Planning

Intervention Planning	
Physical	• **Refinement of body functions** continues through balance, strengthening, and coordination activities as performance approaches premorbid levels
Cognitive	• **Process and social interaction skills** address executive functions and complex reasoning skills necessary for independence in one's daily routine and may include expectations for normal processing speed and accuracy in all cognitive tasks if return to driving, work, or school is the goal
Visual	• **Oculomotor control exercises** using a pen and cap or the Brock string are used to strengthen eye muscles to improve smooth pursuits, saccades, convergence, and divergence and to reduce diplopia that limits occupational performance and include the expectation that the client may initiate and perform exercises independently
	• **Prism glasses and partial occlusion glasses** are used as either a temporary or a permanent strategy to reduce the effects of diplopia and may be used intermittently throughout the day or during all waking hours
	• **Visual scanning** using organized patterns is implemented to increase visual attention and visual fields to locate food, ADL or IADL items, obstacles, and pathways in the client's personal or extra-personal space
ADL	• **Activities of daily living independence** is the goal at this level and may include the use of adaptive equipment as needed for balance, coordination, or object manipulation
IADL	• **Instrumental activities of daily living** are included in treatment planning as indicated based on isolated needs and often focus on independence, accuracy, and client initiation of strategies for memory or attention, including pacing and managing distractions as needed
Rest and sleep	• **Rest and sleep** continue to be emphasized in order to facilitate healing, recovery, and improved overall attention when awake. Oral medications may be used to regulate sleep cycles
Education and work	• **Education and work trials** are considered and gradually integrated into skilled therapy sessions as other process performance skills improve, and accommodations may be recommended to increase success
Play, leisure, and social participation	• **Purposeful leisure activities** incorporate computer or board games, musical instruments, or sports into skilled interventions to facilitate occupational performance in premorbid play, leisure, and social activities while improving body functions and process performance skills
Education	• **Client and family education** continues to include goal setting, home exercise programs, visual scanning and memory strategies, return to work and school trials, ongoing supervision needs, and discharge planning

ADL, activities of daily living; IADL, instrumental activities of daily living.
Data from Golisz, 2009; Tipton-Burton, McLaughlin, and Englander, 2013.

as part of the initial evaluation and guide daily intervention planning that targets the client's current level of occupational performance as an individual and within the environment. These goals are reevaluated on a weekly or biweekly schedule with the expectation that goals are marked as progressing, revised, or met, and new goals are created allowing the intervention plan to continue progressing the client toward increased independence.

Medical complications associated with TBI include recurrent cerebral edema, infection, and shunt revisions, which often result in physical and cognitive changes. If significant status changes occur, or if surgical intervention is necessary, formal reevaluation of the client is indicated. Skilled occupational therapy practitioners appreciate fluctuations in performance and modify the intervention plan as necessary to provide the most appropriate challenge for each individual client.

Referrals and Discharge Considerations

The highly complex nature of TBI results in a wide spectrum of referral and discharge planning options. Clients diagnosed initially with moderate or severe TBIs require months of hospitalization and rehabilitation beginning in the intensive care unit and progressing through acute care, inpatient rehabilitation, day rehabilitation, and outpatient rehabilitation. However, if aggressive rehabilitation is not indicated or available, clients may be discharged to skilled nursing facilities or residential treatment centers that specialize in the long-term care of clients with TBIs. Clients may be discharged to home if sufficient support from trained caregivers is available. Consideration and planning must also occur for managing the client's medical status, securing durable medical equipment (DME), and completing home modifications to help ensure a smooth transition and optimal safety and functioning at home.

Length of stay and discharge planning for clients diagnosed with mild TBI may be less complicated from a medical status perspective; however, changes in occupational performance affecting roles, routines, and habits may require weeks to months of day rehabilitation or outpatient therapy to ensure the most successful recovery possible. These clients benefit from work trials facilitated through collaboration with occupational therapy, vocational rehabilitation, and the client's employer or school. Additional supportive referrals to aid in discharge planning may be made to vocational rehabilitation, driving rehabilitation, assistive technology, outpatient psychology, social work, and community support groups, to name a few.

Management and Standards of Practice

OTs and occupational therapy assistants (OTAs) provide valuable insight into the interdisciplinary team members about the client's occupational profile and roles at each stage of rehabilitation for TBI. This ongoing communication helps ensure that each discipline is aware of and has the opportunity to incorporate meaningful activities into daily interventions with the client and family. The role of occupational therapy within the team may also include oversight for transfer training with family and interdisciplinary team members, integration of visual perceptual strategies through the client's daily routine to increase personal and environmental awareness, and use of UE supportive devices when the client is at rest or engaged in a functional activity. Depending on each facility, OTs and OTAs may be responsible for identifying and ordering DME such as mobility and seating and positioning systems, bathroom transfer equipment, and hospital beds. OTs and OTAs report ongoing progress in daily or weekly rounds and maintain an open dialogue with the client, family members, and interdisciplinary team members (e.g., physical therapy, speech and language pathology, nursing, vocational rehabilitation, psychology, social work, case management, driver rehabilitation, orthotics, seating and positioning, assistive technology, research, and physiatry).

The working relationship between OTs and OTAs involves ongoing collaboration during the evaluation, intervention planning, and discharge stages of the client's admission, with supervision guidelines varying by state. It is common for the OT to complete the standardized assessment portions of the evaluation, approve intervention planning suggested by the OTA, authorize progress notes, and update goals as needed. OTAs make significant contributions to these components of the occupational therapy plan and collaborate with the interdisciplinary team to order DME, complete family education and training, and help ensure carryover of any home exercise program.

Scenarios that pose ethical concerns are presented at any stage of recovery. Examples of these scenarios may include the treatment team recommending that the client receive 24-hour supervision, implementation of a behavioral modification plan, or discontinuing therapy services if measureable progress does not occur over multiple reevaluation periods. The OTs and OTAs are under an ethical obligation to recommend discontinuation of skilled occupational therapy services in the absence of functional progress despite pleas for continued care from the client or family members. Understanding the complex and sensitive nature of TBI enables OTs and OTAs to educate and prepare clients and families for each stage of rehabilitation including discharge. While OTs and OTAs are skilled at managing the physical and cognitive components associated with brain injury, they are also skilled in identifying psychological and emotional needs of the client and family and provide support and referrals for additional services as needed.

Chapter 11 Self-Study Activities (Answers Are Provided at the End of the Chapter)

Write out the complete term for each of the following acronyms:

1. ICH
2. EDH
3. SDH
4. IVH
5. DAI
6. TBI
7. GCS

8. ROM
9. MRI

Answer the following multiple choice and true and false questions.

10. TBI may result in the following deficits:
    A. Physical
    B. Cognitive
    C. Psychological
    D. All of the above

11. The most common cause of TBI across all age groups is:
    A. Car accidents
    B. Violent physical assaults
    C. Falls
    D. None of the above

12. Closed coup–contrecoup injuries are the result of sudden:
    A. Acceleration
    B. Deceleration
    C. Acceleration and deceleration
    D. None of the above

13. The following assessment is used immediately following TBI to determine the level of consciousness:
    A. GCS
    B. Functional Independence Measure (FIM)
    C. Rancho Los Amigos Scale
    D. None of the above

14. The following scale quantifies cognitive and behavioral interactions of persons with TBI on 1 of 10 levels:
    A. Magnetic resonance imaging
    B. Rancho Los Amigos Scale
    C. GCS
    D. None of the above

15. The Activity Card Sort, Barthel Index, and Canadian Occupational Performance Measure (COPM) are standardized assessments that evaluate clients within the domain of participation.
    A. True
    B. False

16. Dynamometry and goniometry evaluate the activity level of a client in their daily routine.
    A. True
    B. False

17. While there may be some overlap, intervention planning is specific to mild, moderate, and severe TBI.
    A. True
    B. False

18. Rest and sleep are only needed for severe TBI.
    A. True
    B. False

19. Group activities are used in intervention planning for severe TBI.
    A. True
    B. False

Chapter 11 Self-Study Answers

1. Intracerebral hemorrhage
2. Epidural hematoma
3. Subdural hematoma
4. Intraventricular hemorrhage
5. Diffuse axonal injury
6. Traumatic brain injury
7. Glasgow Coma Scale
8. Range of motion
9. Magnetic resonance imaging
10. D
11. C
12. C
13. A
14. B
15. T
16. F
17. T
18. F
19. F

References

American Occupational Therapy Association. (2014). Occupational therapy practice framework: Domain and process (3rd edition). *American Journal of Occupational Therapy, 68*(Suppl. 1), S1–S48. doi:10.5014/ajot.2014.682006

Annegers, J. F., Grabow, J. D., Kurland, L. T., & Laws, E. R., Jr. (1980). The incidence, causes, and secular trends of head trauma in Olmsted County, Minnesota, 1935–1974. *Neurology, 30*(9), 912–919.

Centers for Disease Control and Prevention. (2013). *Injury prevention and control: Traumatic brain injury*. Retrieved from http://www.cdc.gov/traumatic braininjury/prevention.html

Centers for Disease Control and Prevention. (2014). *Traumatic brain injury in the United States: Fact sheet*. Washington, DC: Author. Retrieved from http://www.cdc.gov/traumaticbraininjury/get_the_facts.html

Corrigan, J. D. (1995). Substance abuse as a mediating factor in outcome from traumatic brain injury. *Archives of Physical Medicine and Rehabilitation, 76*(4), 302–309.

Faul, M., Xu, L., Wald, M. M., & Coronado, V. G. (2010). *Traumatic brain injury in the United States: Emergency department visits, hospitalizations, and deaths 2002–2006.* Atlanta, GA: Centers for Disease Control and Prevention, National Center for Injury Prevention and Control.

Giacino, J. T., Ashwal, S., Childs, N., Cranford, R., Jennett, B., Katz, D. I., . . . Zasler, N. D. (2002). The minimally conscious state: Definition and diagnostic criteria. *Neurology, 58*(3), 349–353.

Golisz, K. (2009). *Occupational therapy practice guidelines for adults with traumatic brain injury.* Bethesda, MD: AOTA Press.

Hagen, C. (1998). *Rancho levels of cognitive functioning: The revised levels* (3rd ed.). Downey, CA: Rancho Los Amigos Medical Center.

Hagen, C., Malkmus, D., & Durhman, P. (1979). *Levels of cognitive functioning, rehabilitation of the brain-injured adult: Comprehensive physical management* (3rd ed.). Downey, CA: Professional Staff Association of Rancho Los Amigos Hospital.

Maas, A. I., Harrison-Felix, C. L., Menon, D., Adelson, P. D., Balkin, T., Bullock, R., . . . Schwab, K. (2010). Common data elements for traumatic brain injury: Recommendations from the interagency working group on demographics and clinical assessment. *Archives of Physical Medicine and Rehabilitation, 91*(11), 1641–1649. doi:10.1016/j.apmr.2010.07.232

National Center for Injury Prevention and Control. (2003). *Report to Congress on mild traumatic brain injury in the United States: Steps to prevent a serious public health problem.* Atlanta, GA: Centers for Disease Control and Prevention.

Powell, J. (2014). Traumatic brain injury. In M. V. Radomski & C. A. T. Latham (Eds.), *Occupational therapy for physical dysfunction* (7th ed., pp. 1042–1075). Philadelphia, PA: Wolters Kluwer Health/Lippincott Williams & Wilkins.

Teasdale, G., & Jennett, B. (1974). Assessment of coma and impaired consciousness. A practical scale. *Lancet, 2*(7872), 81–84.

Tipton-Burton, M., McLaughlin, R., & Englander, J. (2013). Traumatic brain injury. In L. W. Pedretti, H. M. Pendleton, & W. Schultz-Krohn (Eds.), *Pedretti's occupational therapy: Practice skills for physical dysfunction* (7th ed., pp. 881–915). St. Louis, MO: Elsevier.

World Health Organization. (2002). *Towards a common language for functioning, disability, and health: ICP.* Retrieved from http://www.who.int/classifications/icf/icfbeginnersguide.pdf?ua=1

Spinal Cord Injury

Piper Hansen

Learning Objectives

- Define spinal cord injury (SCI).
- Describe spinal cord injury pathology incidence, pathogenesis, and risk factors.
- Define the diagnostic categories of spinal cord injury determined by the International Standards for Neurological Classification of Spinal Cord Injury.
- Describe the most common clinical presentations of spinal cord injury.
- Describe the most common diagnostic tests for spinal cord injury.
- Describe the most common medical and surgical procedures for spinal cord injury.
- Describe common surgical and nonsurgical precautions and contraindications for spinal cord injury rehabilitation.
- Describe associated and secondary complications of spinal cord injury.
- Identify the assessment areas for comprehensive spinal cord injury rehabilitation.
- Describe the primary areas of intervention and expected functional outcomes for cervical, thoracic, and lumbar spinal cord injury rehabilitation.
- Describe individual and group interventions for spinal cord injury rehabilitation.
- Describe referral, discharge standards, management, and ethical considerations for spinal cord injury rehabilitation.

Key Terms

- *Durable medical equipment*: A piece of medically necessary equipment prescribed by a medical professional that can be used in the home (i.e., commodes, walker, and wheelchair).
- *Injury level*: Level of the spinal cord most impacted by injury or area where trauma occurred.
- *Key muscles*: Primary muscle group associated with innervation from each dermatome level.
- *Nontraumatic*: An injury not caused by an associated traumatic event.
- *Orthotic*: A support device, brace, or splint fabricated to support joints and promote function.
- *Paralysis*: A condition or state when one is unable to move or feel a part of the body.
- *Traumatic*: A serious and unexpected injury to the body due to an external mechanism.

Description

Spinal cord injury (SCI) is a loss of sensory and/or motor functions due to damage to the spinal cord. SCI can lead to decreased physical capacity, disruption of daily routines, loss of community roles, and psychological distress after diagnosis (Atkins, 2014). SCI impacts all aspects of one's life (Atkins, 2014). SCI symptoms can include paralysis, spasticity, sensory deficits, loss of bowel and bladder control, sexual dysfunction, difficulties with body temperature regulation, and decreased respiratory function (Adler, 2013; Atkins, 2014).

Etiology and Pathology

Approximately 12,000 individuals experience an SCI in the United States each year (Atkins, 2014). There are between 236,000 and 327,000 people living in the United States with SCI (Atkins, 2014). Studies have reported a male/female ratio of 4:1 (Atkins, 2014). Age groups most affected by SCI are young adults, 15–29 years of age, and older adults aged 65 and above (Atkins, 2014). SCI can be classified as traumatic and nontraumatic. The most common causes of traumatic injuries are motor vehicle accidents, violence, sporting accidents, and falls (Atkins, 2014). The most common causes of nontraumatic SCI include arthritis, cancer, spinal cord inflammation or infection, and disk degeneration (Sachs, 2014). An SCI diagnosis is expressed using the ASIA impairment scale (AIS). The AIS is determined by the International Standards for Neurological Classification of Spinal Cord Injury (ISNCSCI) for accurate neurological classification as described in **Table 12-1** (Atkins, 2014; Kirshblum & Waring, 2014; Kirshblum et al., 2011). Common clinical presentations, medical and surgical procedures, and diagnostic tests for SCI are described in **Tables 12-2**, **12-3**, and **12-4**, respectively.

Table 12-1 AIS Levels for Spinal Cord Injury

Level	Clinical Presentation
AIS A	No motor or sensory function is preserved below the level of spinal injury.
AIS B	Only sensory function is preserved below the level of injury, including at the S4 and S5 sacral levels.
AIS C	Both motor and sensory functions are preserved below the level of injury. More than half of the key muscles below injury level present with a muscle grade less than 3/5 or fair muscle grade.
AIS D	Both motor and sensory functions are preserved below the level of injury. More than half of the key muscles below injury level present with a muscle grade of more than 3/5 or more.
AIS E	Both motor and sensory functions are intact.
Complete	Absence of sensory and motor function in the lowest sacral segments of the spinal cord.
Incomplete	Preservation of sensory and motor function in the lowest sacral segments of the spinal cord.

Data from: Atkins (2014); Kirshblum and Waring (2014); Kirshblum et al. (2011).

Table 12-2 Most Common Clinical Presentations of SCI

Type of SCI	Description	Main Signs and Symptoms
Tetraplegia	Motor and/or sensory impairment that involves all four limbs and trunk.	Paralysis of the lower extremities and trunk and paralysis or partial paralysis of the upper extremities.
Paraplegia	Motor and/or sensory impairment of the lower extremities and/or trunk.	Paralysis of the lower extremities with potential involvement of the hips and/or trunk.
Central cord syndrome	Greater weakness of the upper extremities than the lower extremities.	Individual may be ambulatory but present with significant upper extremity weakness, especially proximally. Common mechanism of injury is due to severe cervical hyperextension.
Brown–Sequard syndrome	Incomplete injury resulting in ipsilateral proprioceptive and motor loss and contralateral loss of pain and temperature sensation.	Most often associated with violently acquired SCI, such as a stab or gunshot wound, resulting in damage to one half of the spinal cord. Presentation occurs when the dorsal column-medial lemniscus tract and corticospinal tract are affected on the ipsilateral side of the spinal injury and the spinothalamic tract contralaterally.
Cauda equina syndrome	Lower motor neuron injury of the lumbosacral nerve roots.	Because only peripheral nerves are impacted, not the spinal cord itself, prognosis is greater. Common presentation is asymmetric and results initially in a flaccid-like muscle presentation of the lower extremities.
ZPP, Zone of partial preservation.	Dermatomes and myotomes below the sensory and motor levels that remain partially innervated.	This area of partial innervation can differ for the left and right side of the body in addition to differences between the motor and sensory ZPPs. The ZPP can have significant impact on the potential for function depending on the ZPP.

Data from: Adler (2013); Atkins (2014); Kirshblum and Waring (2014); Kirshblum et al. (2011).

Table 12-3 Common Medical and Surgical Procedures for SCI

Procedure	Description
Bony realignment and stabilization	Use of skeletal traction and immobilization or orthotic intervention is utilized to prevent further damage and promote healing.
Decompression or laminectomy	Surgical procedure is used to decrease pressure within the spinal column.
Fusion	Bone tissue is used to fuse the vertebrae to improve stability.

Data from Adler, 2013.

Table 12-4 Common Diagnostic Tests for SCI

Test	Possible Findings
ASI testing	Motor and sensory level diagnosis (complete vs. incomplete injury and spinal level of injury)
Imaging	X-ray, CT, and/or MRI may be used to determine the type of spinal injury and the alignment of the spine to determine medical treatment

ASI, American Spinal Association; CT, computed tomography; MRI, magnetic resonance imaging.
Data from Adler, 2013; Atkins, 2014; Kirshblum and Waring, 2014; Kirshblum et al., 2011.

Precautions and Contraindications

After undergoing a surgical procedure or to promote bony realignment and stabilization, specific precautions may be indicated by the surgeon. These include spinal precautions such as no twisting, excessive bending, and a restriction on the number of pounds someone can lift (Adler, 2013). After undergoing a surgical procedure or to promote bony realignment and stabilization, spinal orthoses bracing may be indicated. These may include a cervical collar, Halo vest orthotic, or a thoracic lumbar sacral orthotic. Individuals prescribed a spinal orthosis will commonly also follow spinal precautions during the acute stage of an SCI (Adler, 2013).

Complications of SCI

1. *Autonomic dysreflexia (AD)*: AD is an associated condition of SCI for injuries that are above the T6 spinal level. AD is an increase in blood pressure caused by a reflexive action of the autonomic nervous system. It is a medical emergency and quick action should be taken to resolve this complication (Adler, 2013; Atkins, 2014). Causes of AD can be related to bowel or bladder function or irritation, pain, skin-related disorders, or other medical irregularities (Field-Fote, 2009). In addition to presenting with increased blood pressure, other symptoms that may occur are a pounding headache, sweating, chills, nasal congestion, and a slowing of heart rate (Adler, 2013; Atkins, 2014; Field-Fote, 2009).

   To treat AD, make the person sit upright and remove or address any irritating condition; for example, draining the bladder and removing tight clothing, shoes, elastic garments, or abdominal binders. In persistent AD, a fast-acting vasodilator may be administered (Field-Fote, 2009).

2. *Orthostatic hypotension (OH)*: OH can occur after an SCI at any injury level. It features a sudden drop in blood pressure typically related to the lack of venous blood return from the abdomen or lower extremities (Adler, 2013; Atkins, 2014). If not treated, the individual may lose consciousness. Other symptoms of OH include a sudden onset of nausea or dizziness (Adler, 2013; Atkins, 2014).

   To treat OH, lay the person back or have the person sit down immediately. Elevate the legs as needed to restore a normal blood pressure level (Adler, 2013; Atkins, 2014). To prevent OH, medication can be used in addition to elastic stockings or abdominal binders or both to improve venous blood return.

3. *Heterotopic ossification (HO)*: HO is the development of ectopic bone below the neurological injury level. The most common areas of occurrence include the hips, knees, and elbows (Adler, 2013; Atkins, 2014). Symptoms of HO include swelling, warmth, and decreased range of motion (ROM) in the area of the affected joint. Swelling, tightness, and warmth may also be present in the surrounding muscles of the joint.

   To treat HO, early detection is preferred to prevent the progression of the condition (Field-Fote, 2009). Early ROM exercises are important to maintain joint mobility, and medication may also be beneficial (Field-Fote, 2009). Passive ROM exercises should be completed to the available end range regularly. When available, active ROM is indicated if the HO is outside an acute stage of inflammation and as determined by experienced pain. Surgical intervention may be indicated once the HO bone skeletal genesis in the affected joint has stabilized and outside acute inflammation, which commonly occurs between 12 and 18 months after onset (Field-Fote, 2009).

4. *Skin integrity*: Sensory loss increases the risk of experiencing skin breakdown and the development of pressure ulcers (Adler, 2013; Field-Fote, 2009). Risk factors for developing pressure ulcers include pressure to an area of the skin that results in decreased blood flow to the area, heat, friction, and moisture (e.g., incontinence). The most common areas for skin breakdown after SCI include the sacrum, bilateral greater trochanters, ischial tuberosities, elbows, heels, and other bony prominences where sensation is decreased such as the scapulae and heels (Adler, 2013; Field-Fote, 2009).

   The treatment and prevention of pressure ulcers includes reducing pressure or restricting weight bearing to the involved area or areas, employing a clean catheterization technique, and educating the patient about hydration, dysreflexia, and transfer and mobility techniques that decrease friction and shear forces (Field-Fote, 2009).

5. *Pain*: The most common types of pain experienced after SCI are nociceptive and neuropathic (Field-Fote, 2009). Nociceptive pain is categorized as musculoskeletal pain or visceral pain (Field-Fote, 2009). Neuropathic pain is described as a sharp, shooting, burning, or electric feeling of pain (Field-Fote, 2009). Neuropathic pain can be experienced above, at, and below the neurological level of injury (Field-Fote, 2009). Thorough pain assessment is necessary to implement effective pain management strategies, including if the experienced pain is in an acute or chronic stage (Field-Fote, 2009).

Screening and Assessments

6. *Screenings*: There are a variety of screening tools that are applicable to SCI that help to ensure an accurate diagnosis as well as the formulation of a comprehensive treatment plan. One primary area to screen is for a dual diagnosis of traumatic brain injury (TBI). The incidence of mild to moderate TBI with SCI is between 24 and 59% and as high as 60% (Kushner & Alvarez, 2014; Sommer & Witkiewicz, 2004). Determining

whether a dual diagnosis is present is important because it can significantly impact the rehabilitation process and the functional recovery after the initial SCI. Individuals presenting a dual diagnosis of SCI and TBI may respond to medications differently, experience difficulty with new learning and the use of adaptive techniques, and demonstrate decreased motivation (Kushner & Alvarez, 2014; Sommer & Witkiewicz, 2004).

7. *Assessments*: Both top-down and bottom-up assessments are required to fully assess the patient after SCI to better understand the medical and social history. It is important to include assessment at the body function, activity, and participation levels for a more comprehensive assessment of current strengths and areas to address during occupational therapy.

Top-Down Assessments

1. A semistandardized interview can be used to determine functional limitations and goals for therapy interventions such as the Canadian Occupational Performance Measure.

2. A daily record log such as the Occupational Performance History Index II can be used to better understand daily routines and tasks (Kielhofner, Mallinson, Forsyth, & Lai, 2001).

3. Leisure or vocational interest questionnaires can be used to determine limitations on leisure and productivity tasks.

4. Standardized assessments that focus on activities of daily living (ADLs) such as the functional independence measure, Barthel index, and Lawton instrumental activities of daily living (IADL) scale can establish outcome data on functional performance of activities (Field-Fote, 2009).

5. SCI-specific measures may provide a more comprehensive and sensitive assessment of activity after SCI. These standardized assessments can include the Spinal Cord Independence Measure, Quadriplegia Index of Function, and the Wheelchair Skill Test (Field-Fote, 2009).

Bottom-Up Assessments

1. Assessment of passive ROM is used to determine joint mobility limitations.

2. Assess pain using a standardized scale such as the Numeric Pain Intensity Scale (Atkins, 2014).

3. Complete specific manual muscle testing for full appreciation of current areas of strength and weakness to address for maximized function and compensatory training.

4. Complete grip and pinch strength testing (key and palmar pinch) using a dynamometer to determine current strength compared to age- and gender-based normative values.

5. A postural assessment to determine proper spinal and scapular alignment is required for determining individualized seating system (Field-Fote, 2009).

6. Complete standardized sensation testing using monofilaments for additional sensation information for the hand beyond the ISNCSCI results.

Interventions

SCI treatment includes four primary areas of practice to address. These are biomechanical, skill acquisition, adaptive or compensatory techniques, and training, education, and psychosocial support (Sachs, 2014). Central to treatment is occupation as means or purposeful activity, as it is important when composing a meaningful and purposeful treatment plan (Atkins, 2014). When determining areas of occupation and treatment, it is important to consider the functional outcomes for each neurological level for optimal intervention.

Expected Functional Outcomes

Functional outcomes are those individuals with complete SCI. Functional outcomes can vary greatly with an incomplete SCI. The projected functional outcomes for each spinal level build upon the previous interventions and capabilities; expected SCI functional outcomes are described in **Table 12-5** by spinal level, primary key muscles, and functional outcomes and interventions (Adler, 2013; Atkins, 2014).

Table 12-5 Expected SCI Functional Outcomes

Spinal Level	Primary Key Muscles	Functional Outcomes and Interventions
C1–C3	Cervical muscles	• Requires respiratory support and total assistance with ADLs. • Focus of interventions on use of environmental controls, adaptive devices and computer control, orthotics, and direction of care.
C4	Upper trapezius and diaphragm	• Requires assistance with ADLs but can progress to independence with use of adaptive equipment and techniques. • Focus of interventions on the use of adaptive devices, assistive technology, and direction of care.
C5	Deltoids and biceps	• Requires some assistance with the majority of ADLs, but can be set up assistance with self-feeding and some grooming activities. • Focus of interventions on increasing strengthening to maximize ADL and IADL participation, orthotics, adaptive equipment, assistive technology, functional and bed mobility, and direction of care.
C6	Wrist extensors	• May be able to complete the majority of ADL with modified independence for increased time or use of adaptive equipment. • Focus of interventions on functional mobility and transfers, adapted dressing techniques, orthotics, bladder and bowel care, and the progression of power to manual wheelchair propulsion.
C7	Triceps, increased wrist control, and emerging thumb muscles	• Will be independent with all basic ADL activities with limited use of adaptive equipment or orthotics. • Focus of interventions on improving manual wheelchair skills, shoulder preservation, dressing, bathing and toileting efficiency and independence, increased challenging transfers and mobility skills, and increased participation in complex IADLs.

(continues)

Table 12-5 Expected SCI Functional Outcomes (*continued*)

Spinal Level	Primary Key Muscles	Functional Outcomes and Interventions
C8	Additional finger flexion/extension and lumbricals	• Will be independent with all basic ADL activities without the need of adaptive equipment. • Focus of interventions on efficiency with bowel and bladder care, IADLs, wheelchair skills, lateral transfers and push-up pressure reliefs, and shoulder preservation. Driving can now be achieved with only basic hand controls.
TI	Hand intrinsics, emerging intercostals, remaining upper extremity muscles, including the opponens pollicis	• Will be independent with all basic ADL activities. • Focus of interventions on efficiency with bowel and bladder care, IADLs, wheelchair skills, lateral transfers and push-up pressure reliefs, and shoulder preservation.
T2 to T9	Erector spinae	• Will be independent with all basic ADL activities at a wheelchair level. • Focus of interventions on efficiency with bowel and bladder care, IADLs, wheelchair skills, lateral transfers and push-up pressure reliefs, and shoulder preservation. May try standing with the use of KAFOs.
T10 to T12	Oblique and rectus abdominals	• Will be independent with all basic ADL activities at a wheelchair level and can complete ADLs seated with improved balance or need for seated support. • Focus of interventions on efficiency with bowel and bladder care, IADLs, and shoulder preservation. May begin to incorporate standing with the use of KAFOs into ADLs.
L1	Additional abdominals	• Will be independent with all basic ADL activities at a wheelchair level and may begin to incorporate standing with ADLs using KAFOs. • Focus of interventions on efficiency with bowel and bladder care, IADLs, and shoulder preservation. May initiate learning ambulation skills.
L2	Hip flexors	• Will be independent with all basic ADL activities at a wheelchair level and may incorporate standing with ADLs using KAFOs. • Focus of interventions on efficiency with bowel and bladder care, IADLs, and shoulder preservation. May initiate minimal ambulation skills with KAFOs into ADL routines.
L3	Knee extensors	• Will be independent with all basic ADL activities with standing incorporated as appropriate. • Continue to improve ADL and IADL efficiency. May incorporate ambulation with assistive devices and orthotics with ADLs.
L4	Ankle dorsiflexors	• Will be independent with all basic ADL activities at a wheelchair level and may begin to incorporate standing with ADLs using AFOs as appropriate. • Continue to improve ADL and IADL efficiency and increased standing and ambulation with ADLs and IADLs. Progressing to decrease assistive devices and orthotics required.
L5	Long toe extensors	• Will be independent with all basic ADL activities at a wheelchair level and may begin to incorporate standing with ADLs using AFOs as appropriate. • Continue to improve ADL and IADL efficiency and increased standing and ambulation with ADLs and IADLs. Progressing to decrease assistive devices and orthotics required.
Sacral	Plantar flexors and lower extremity adduction	• Will be independent with all basic ADL activities and incorporating standing and ambulation with ADLs. • Continue to improve ADL and IADL efficiency and increased standing and ambulation with ADLs and IADLs. Progressing to decrease assistive devices and orthotics required.

AFOs, ankle foot orthosis; KAFOs, knee ankle foot orthosis.
Data from Adler, 2013; Atkins, 2014.

Impact on Occupational Performance

Examples of Remedial Methods

1. Integrate evidence-based strengthening protocols to maximize strength required to complete ADLs, functional mobility, and transfers.
2. Use principles of neuroplasticity to structure task-specific training and high repetition training to promote improved participation in functional activities and increased strength.
3. Integrate functional electrical stimulation to promote task participation and strength.
4. As appropriate, incorporate standing or ambulation, with and without orthotics as required, into ADL routines.

Examples of Compensatory Methods

1. Match compensatory methods to the client's neurological SCI level and modify adaptive techniques with functional skill progression.
2. Train the individual how to perform adaptive functional mobility techniques to increase independence with transfers and completing bed mobility.
3. Complete patient and family education on the client's condition and functional limitations, as well as facilitating appropriate compensatory approaches.
4. Recommend and train the client in the use of adaptive equipment to facilitate reaching, activity performance, and environmental modifications that may be necessary to promote maximal participation in ADLs.
5. Educate on available assistive technology and environmental controls and integrate into interventions as appropriate.
6. Trial and provide recommendations for wheeled mobility, and seating and positioning to support participation.
7. Educate the patient in how to effectively communicate their needs and instruct others in the direction of their care.

Therapeutic Interventions

Therapeutic interventions can include both individual and group treatment. The use of occupations and activities should include the use of compensatory methods, such as adaptive equipment and techniques, as needed to maximize occupational performance.

Examples of Preparatory Exercises for SCI

1. *ROM and strengthening*: Preparatory methods are important to support occupational performance. Participation in a ROM and stretching program can maintain joint mobility and improve positioning and cosmesis. Exercise can be integrated into either individual or group interventions. A progressive strengthening program should be implemented to improve functional reaching during activities and increase participation in functional mobility skills and transfers.
   - Shoulder active ROM.
   - Isometric strengthening.
   - Shoulder preservation strengthening and stretching program.
2. *Orthotics*: Occupational therapists can recommend or fabricate orthotic devices to promote functional positioning and prevent contractures. These can include a short or long opponens, resting hand splint, wrist support, or elbow extension orthotic. Orthotic management education includes care of the orthotic material, wearing schedule for optimal outcome, donning and doffing techniques, and skin care precautions.
3. *Physical agent modalities*: Neuromuscular electrical stimulation (NMES) for muscle strengthening and neuromuscular reeducation is commonly integrated into SCI rehabilitation (Protos, Stone, & Grinnell, 2009). NMES can assist to restore useful movement during grasp and gait training with consistent use (Protos et al., 2009).
4. *Education and training*: Education is a central component to SCI rehabilitation. Comprehensive education can prevent secondary conditions and maximize independence and occupational performance.

Training should occur with the client and their caregiver when it is appropriate. Training on shared problem-solving strategies with the caregiver included can decrease depression and anxiety (Protos et al., 2009). It is estimated that 40–45% of all individuals with SCI will require assistance performing ADLs (Sachs, 2014). Clients and caregivers need to be educated on how to safely and effectively perform these activities.

Other areas of education to include in SCI rehabilitation are sexual function, bladder and bowel function, skin care and the timely performance of timely and effective pressure reliefs, and shoulder preservation and pain management strategies.

Referrals and Discharge Considerations

Patients are typically ready for discharge when a safe home environment has been established and home modification recommendations have been implemented. In preparation for discharge, education on adaptive equipment and compensatory techniques should be completed to maximize independence with ADLs and/or the individual is independent to direct their care. Other discharge considerations include ensuring that the appropriate wheelchair has been prescribed and required durable medical equipment has also been prescribed to promote safety with bathing and toileting tasks. An effective plan for skin management and performance of pressure relief is necessary in preparation for discharge to prevent complications to skin integrity.

Referrals to vocational rehabilitation services, technology specialist, adaptive sports and fitness programs, community and support groups, and/or a certified seating specialist or assistive technology practitioner may be appropriate to continue to address continuing needs.

Management and Standards of Practice

In the neurological area of practice, occupational therapy practitioners need to ensure that they are working very closely with the physician and other members of the interdisciplinary rehabilitation team. This will ensure safe and appropriate therapeutic recommendations and treatment, as well as encouraging an open line of communication within the treatment team. This will also facilitate communication with the occupational therapy assistant (OTA), who, if involved, will carry out specific interventions. The OTA role in SCI rehabilitation includes education on compensatory techniques, including the use of adaptive equipment and assistive technology prescribed, ensuring the client and/or their caregiver's independence to carry out the prescribed home exercise program and orthotic management, and educating the client and/or their caregiver on the prevention of secondary conditions associated with SCI.

There are specific considerations associated with SCI rehabilitation. One is the importance of educating your clients with SCI about aging with a spinal injury. Life expectancy continues to increase with the advancement of medicine and the rehabilitative field. Maintaining wellness and preventing secondary conditions after initial injury are important considerations.

The exploration for a cure for SCI continues to evolve. Clients will be interested in learning about and potentially participating in clinical trials, experiential medicine, and surgical procedures occurring in the United States and internationally. It is imperative that occupational therapy practitioners and healthcare professionals educate clients on what to look for when reviewing research they encounter and learn how to determine the credibility of the claims made by stem cell companies or other organizations promising regeneration of the spinal cord.

In today's healthcare market, there is not a shortage of technological devices to aid individuals with SCI to ambulate. As an occupational therapy practitioner, it will be important to solve problems with the consumer about how any device or advanced technology will fit into their lifestyle and promote advanced participation. It will be important to address any orthopedic or skin integrity concerns to ensure an optimal fit of technology and functional performance.

Chapter 12 Self-Study Activities (Answers Are Provided at the End of the Chapter)

1. Match the primary emerging muscle group (left column) with the corresponding spinal cord level (right column) by drawing lines.

Definition	Term
1. Long toe extensors	A. T1
2. Upper trapezius	B. C8
3. Biceps	C. L5

4. Ankle dorsiflexors	D. C6
5. Wrist extensors	E. T2
6. Erector spinae	F. C4
7. Lumbricals	G. C5

8. Knee extensors	H. L4
9. Triceps	I. C7
10. Hand intrinsics	J. L2
11. Hip flexors	K. L3

2. Solve the spinal cord injury crossword puzzle by properly entering the correct terms for the provided questions:

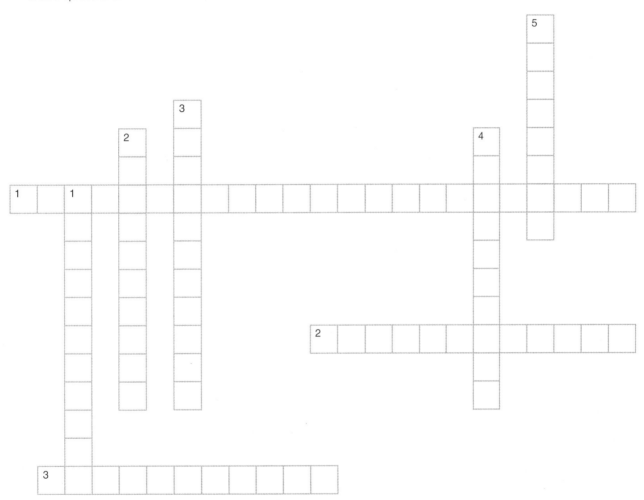

Across

1. The development of ectopic bone below the neurological injury level.
2. Incomplete injury resulting in ipsilateral proprioceptive and motor loss and contralateral loss of pain and temperature sensation.
3. Preservation of sensory and motor function in the lowest sacral segments of the spinal cord.

Down

1. Motor and/or sensory impairment that involves all four limbs and trunk.
2. Motor and/or sensory impairment of the lower extremities and/or trunk.
3. Greater weakness of the upper extremities than the lower extremities.
4. Lower motor neuron injury of the lumbosacral nerve roots.
5. Absence of sensory and motor function in the lowest sacral segments of the spinal cord.

3. Describe the missing SCI medical and surgical procedures in the following table.

Procedure	Description
Bony realignment and stabilization	
Decompression or laminectomy	
Fusion	

4. Answer the following multiple-choice question: Alex is a 55-year-old female who sustained a C6 AIS B SCI after a motor vehicle accident resulting in tetraplegia. She is currently receiving inpatient rehabilitation services. Alex is currently requiring maximal assistance with ADLs such as dressing, bathing, and transfers but is gaining upper extremity strength. She is significantly limited in her ability to complete functional activities due to limited hand function. Alex is working to improve her independence with functional mobility and has verbalized this as a priority goal area. What type of transfer should the OTA initially focus on training with Alex to increase her independence with transfers and to address this goal?
   A. Mechanical lift transfer
   B. Stand-pivot transfer
   C. Squat-pivot transfer
   D. Slideboard transfer

5. Fill out the correct SCI level for each of the following interventions.

Interventions	Level
A. The focus of intervention is on increasing strengthening to maximize ADL and IADL participation, orthotics, adaptive equipment, assistive technology, functional and bed mobility, and direction of care.	
B. The focus of intervention is on use of environmental controls, adaptive devices and computer control, orthotics, and direction of care.	
C. The focus of intervention is on efficiency with bowel and bladder care, IADLs, and shoulder preservation. May initiate learning ambulation skills.	
D. The focus of intervention is on efficiency with bowel and bladder care, IADLs, wheelchair skills, lateral transfers and push-up pressure reliefs, and shoulder preservation. Driving can now be achieved with only basic hand controls.	
E. The focus of intervention is on tenodesis training, functional mobility and transfers, adapted dressing techniques, orthotics, bladder and bowel care, and the progression of power to manual wheelchair propulsion.	

Chapter 12 Self-Study Answers

Question 1

1. C
2. F
3. G
4. H
5. D
6. E
7. B
8. K
9. I
10. A
11. J

Question 2

Across
1. Heterotopic ossification
2. Brown–Sequard
3. Cauda equina

Down
1. Tetraplegia
2. Paraplegia
3. Central cord
4. Incomplete
5. Complete

Question 3

- Please see Table 12-4. Common Medical and Surgical Procedures for SCI

Question 4

- Slideboard transfer

Question 5

A. C5
B. C1–C3
C. L1
D. C8
E. C6

References

Adler, C. (2013). Spinal cord injury. In L. W. Pedretti, H. M. Pendleton, & W. Schultz-Krohn (Eds.), *Pedretti's occupational therapy: Practice skills for physical dysfunction* (7th ed., pp. 954–982). St. Louis, MO: Elsevier.

Atkins, M. S. (2014). Spinal cord injury. In M. V. Radomski & C. A. T. Latham (Eds.), *Occupational therapy for physical dysfunction* (7th ed., pp. 1168–1214). Philadelphia, PA: Wolters Kluwer Health/Lippincott Williams & Wilkins.

Field-Fote, E. C. (2009). *Spinal cord injury rehabilitation.* Philadelphia, PA: F. A. Davis.

Kielhofner, G., Mallinson, T., Forsyth, K., & Lai, J.-S. (2001). Psychometric Properties of the Second Version of the Occupational Performance History Interview (OPHI-II). *American Journal of Occupational Therapy, 55*(3), 260–267. doi:10.5014/ajot.55.3.260

Kirshblum, S. C., Burns, S. P., Biering-Sorensen, F., Donovan, W., Graves, D. E., Jha, A., . . . Waring, W. (2011). International standards for neurological classification of spinal cord injury (Revised 2011). *Journal of Spinal Cord Medicine, 34*(6), 535–546. doi:10.1179/204577211X13207446293695

Kirshblum, S., & Waring, W., III. (2014). Updates for the international standards for neurological classification of spinal cord injury. *Physical Medicine and Rehabilitation Clinics of North America, 25*(3), 505–517, vii. doi:10.1016/j.pmr.2014.04.001

Kushner, D. S., & Alvarez, G. (2014). Dual diagnosis: Traumatic brain injury with spinal cord injury. *Physical Medicine and Rehabilitation Clinics of North America, 25*(3), 681–696, ix–x. doi:10.1016/j.pmr.2014.04.005

Protos, K. M., Stone, K.-L., & Grinnell, M. (2009). Spinal cord injury. In H. S. Willard, E. B. Crepeau, E. S. Cohn, & B. A. B. Schell (Eds.), *Willard & Spackman's occupational therapy* (11th ed., pp. 1065–1069). Philadelphia, PA: Wolters Kluwer Health/Lippincott Williams & Wilkins.

Sachs, L. (2014). Appendix 1: Common conditions, resources, and evidence. In H. S. Willard & B. A. B. Schell (Eds.), *Willard & Spackman's occupational therapy* (12th ed., pp. 1179–1182). Philadelphia, PA: Wolters Kluwer Health/Lippincott Williams & Wilkins.

Sommer, J. L., & Witkiewicz, P. M. (2004). The therapeutic challenges of dual diagnosis: TBI/SCI. *Brain Injury, 18*(12), 1297–1308. Retrieved from http://www.ncbi.nlm.nih.gov/pubmed/15666572

Neurodegenerative and Productive Aging

Lori Bravi

Learning Objectives

- Identify and define five examples of neurodegenerative disease that are commonly treated by occupational therapists and occupational therapy assistants.
- Determine one similarity and one difference in pathology and medical management across each of the five diagnoses described in this chapter.
- Describe three examples of skilled occupational therapy interventions for each of the five diagnoses described in this chapter.

Key Terms

- *Akinesia*: Impaired ability or loss of ability to initiate voluntary movement.
- *Bradykinesia*: Slow or diminished body movement.
- *Cogwheel rigidity*: A combination of catch and release resistance to movement as muscles contract and relax.
- *Demyelination*: Damage to the myelin sheath surrounding neurons affecting the conduction of nerve signals.
- *Festinating gait*: Involuntary movement including short and accelerated steps characterized along with forward flexion of the trunk, and stiffly flexed hips and knees.
- *Myelin*: The sheath surrounding nerve fibers that aids in the conduction of impulses.
- *Rigidity*: Increased stiffness or inflexibility often as a result of hypertonicity of both agonist and antagonist muscles.

Description

Neurodegenerative disease includes diagnoses characterized by an evolving disease process with progression of debilitating effects on the nervous system. Amyotrophic lateral sclerosis (ALS), multiple sclerosis (MS), Parkinson's disease, Alzheimer's disease, and Guillain–Barré syndrome (GBS) are examples of neurodegenerative disease. While the etiologies, pathogeneses, and prognoses are unique to each specific diagnosis, the impact on occupational performance is similar. Over time, neurodegenerative disease manifests as deterioration in motor and process performance skills often leading to reduced independence and participation in occupational performance patterns. The pathogenesis of each diagnosis determines the onset of signs and symptoms, pattern of deterioration, and if periods of remission are expected.

Skilled occupational therapy (OT) plays a critical role in improving the occupational performance of persons with neurodegenerative disease (Forwell, Hugos, Copperman, & Ghahari, 2014; Schultz-Krohn, Foti, & Glogoski, 2013). Intervention is not only initiated at the onset of acute symptoms, but also incorporated during periods of relapse and active maintenance periods to maximize restoration of functional independence throughout the disease process. OT practitioners also play an important role in preserving even the slightest amount of ongoing participation in occupational performance for persons facing a potentially fatal prognosis associated with a disease such as ALS.

Section One: Etiology, Pathology, and Medical Management of Neurodegenerative Conditions

The pathology and medical management are presented in the first section of this chapter with respect to each specific diagnosis. Skilled OT intervention planning, implementation, and standards of practice for these diagnoses have considerable overlap; therefore, these areas of practice are discussed within the context of neurodegenerative disease as a whole in the second section of this chapter.

ALS Etiology and Pathology

ALS, commonly known as Lou Gehrig's disease, is an aggressive neurodegenerative disease of unknown etiology that destroys the motor neurons associated with voluntary muscle contraction. Upper motor neurons controlling signals from the brain to the spinal cord and lower motor neurons controlling signals from the spinal cord to peripheral muscles slowly lose the ability to conduct voluntary muscle contraction. Muscle weakness progresses to atrophy until nerve signal conduction ceases completely. Peripheral muscles of the extremities controlled by the corticospinal tracts and anterior horn cells, and bulbar muscles for swallowing, speech production, and respiration controlled by the brainstem, are most commonly affected (Fleming, Stone, & Grimell, 2009; Schultz-Krohn et al., 2013).

Signs and symptoms include peripheral muscle weakness, dysphagia, dysarthria, shortness of breath, and general fatigue, and may progress at a variable rate depending on the individual. Muscle cramping, twitching (i.e., fasciculation), and general weakness are examples of early signs and symptoms that generally emerge in a person's fifties or early sixties (Genetics Home Reference, 2012). Sporadic ALS, the most common type of the disease, is associated with 90–95% of cases, and is not hereditary. Familial ALS affects the remaining 5–10% of ALS diagnoses, and has a clear genetic association. Approximately 2 in 100,000 adults are diagnosed every year with ALS with approximately 5,000 new cases annually in the United States (National Institute of Neurological Disorders and Stroke [NINDS], 2013). Men are more often affected than women (Amyotrophic Lateral Sclerosis Association [ALSA], 2010).

Medical Management

The diagnosis of ALS is one of exclusion. A series of diagnostic tests and clinical examination are used to rule out other disorders that are known to cause signs and symptoms similar to ALS. **Table 13-1** provides a summary of these tests and associated differential diagnoses considered prior to determining if an individual's progression is most consistent with ALS. Respiratory failure is the most common cause of death in individuals with ALS. Prognosis is poor with a life expectancy of 3–5 years from symptom onset for most individuals, with approximately 10% living as long as 10 years or more (NINDS, 2013). See **Figure 13-1** for a comparison of normal and atrophied muscle cells due to ALS.

Medical management begins with introducing medications to reduce the burden of common side effects of the disease process. Oral medications may be prescribed to reduce pain, spasticity, and excess saliva production as well as to improve sleep and mood (NINDS, 2013). There is no known cure for ALS. The only drug approved by the Food and Drug Administration identified to slow the disease progression is riluzole, which inhibits the excess

Table 13-1 Common Diagnostic Tests and Differential Diagnoses for ALS

Diagnostic Test	Differential Diagnosis
Electromyography	Polyneuropathy
Nerve conduction velocity tests	Peripheral nerve injury
	Myopathy
Magnetic resonance imaging	Tumor of the brain or spine
	Herniated disk
	Cervical spondylosis
Blood and urine studies	Blood cancers
High-resolution serum protein studies	HIV
Thyroid and parathyroid hormone levels	Viral infections (Lyme disease, West Nile virus)
Spinal tap	
Muscle and/or nerve biopsy	Myopathy
	Polyneuropathy

HIV, human immunodeficiency virus.
Data from: NINDS (2013).

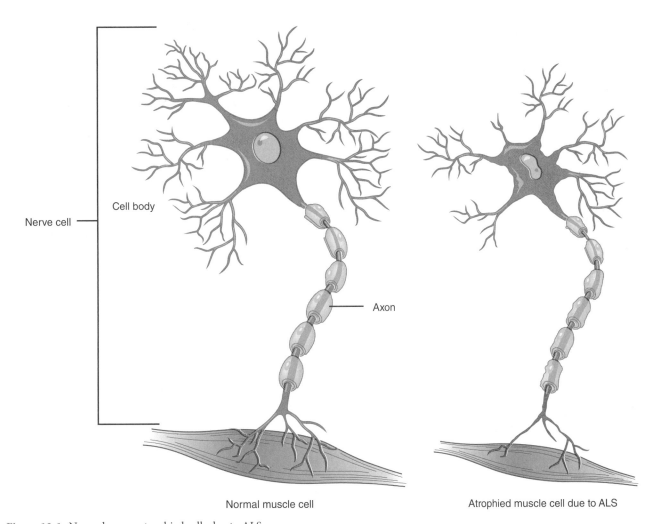

Figure 13-1 Normal versus atrophied cells due to ALS.

release of glutamate that contributes to motor neuron death (Robberecht & Brown, 1996). Supportive medical services are implemented to ensure that the client maintains the highest level of functioning despite progressive deterioration. Examples of these services include skilled OT, physical therapy, speech therapy, psychology, nutritional counseling, case management, wheelchair seating and positioning, assistive technology, home modifications, and home health services. As the disease progresses, medical management includes implementation of feeding tubes and respiratory aides, including ventilator support (ALSA, 2010; Fleming et al., 2009; Forwell et al., 2014; NINDS, 2013; Schultz-Krohn et al., 2013).

MS Etiology and Pathology

MS is the most prevalent neurological disease afflicting an estimated 400,000 young adults in the United States (National Multiple Sclerosis Society [NMSS], 2015) and

2.5 million adults worldwide (Multiple Sclerosis Trust, 2013). While it is usually diagnosed in persons between 15 and 50 years of age, childhood cases have also been documented (Krupp & Macallister, 2005). MS is most common in persons of Caucasian descent, especially Northern Europeans, living further away from the equator. Women are two to three times more likely to have the diagnosis compared to men. While there may be a genetic association, MS is likely triggered by environmental factors or acute infection (NMSS, 2015; Trapp et al., 1998).

While the clinical presentation of chronic and progressive neurological deficits associated with MS is consistent with neurodegenerative disease, the pathology is widely accepted as an autoimmune disease because of its inflammatory effect on the central nervous system (Trapp & Nave, 2008). The disease process attacks the protective myelin sheath of nerves in the white matter. The axons, which are most critical in nerve conduction synapses, are preserved in less severe cases. Over time, the demyelinating nerves develop hardening plaques, becoming sclerotic in multiple areas of the central nervous system including the spinal cord, optic nerve, and periventricular white matter. This progression of demyelination results in slower nerve impulses manifested as muscle weakness, visual deficits, incoordination, hyperreflexia, nystagmus, and impaired proprioception (Schultz-Krohn et al., 2013).

Medical Management

A variety of criteria are used to diagnose each pattern of disease progression for MS, which are outlined in detail as the 2010 McDonald Criteria for Diagnosis of Multiple Sclerosis (Polman et al., 2011). These criteria include a comprehensive medical history, neurological evaluation for specific signs and symptoms of the disease, magnetic resonance imaging (MRI) results positive for central nervous system demyelination and sclerotic plaques, delayed visual evoked potential response, and cerebrospinal fluid positive for oligoclonal bands and/or elevated immunoglobulin G. Fulfillment of these criteria ensures a definitive diagnosis of MS when another neurodegenerative disease or neuromyelitis optica may be in question.

There are four primary patterns of MS described in the literature, each characterized by a specific disease progression and managed by respective disease-modifying therapies as summarized in **Table 13-2** (American Occupational Therapy Association [AOTA], 1999; Hugos & Copperman, 1999; NMSS, 2015; Noseworthy, Lucchinetti, Rodriguez, & Weinshenker, 2000; Schultz-Krohn et al., 2013; Trapp et al., 1998). While all patterns of MS are partially managed with anti-inflammatory medications, injectable disease-modifying therapies are only effective for slowing progression of relapsing–remitting MS (Noseworthy et al., 2000). Individuals with MS experience fluctuations in symptoms throughout

Table 13-2 Primary Patterns of Multiple Sclerosis	
Relapsing and Remitting	Disease progression:
	• Accounts for 85% of the multiple sclerosis population
	• Characterized by periods of exacerbation and remission with a gradual accumulation of deficits
	Disease-modifying therapies:
	• Anti-inflammatory medications (prednisone and methylprednisolone)
	• Interferon beta-1b (Betaseron, Extavia)
	• Interferon beta-1a (Avonex, Rebif)
	• Glatiramer acetate (Copaxone)
	• Natalizumab (Tysabri)
Secondary Progressive	Disease progression:
	• Begins with periods of exacerbation and remission
	• Eventually evolves into progressive form of multiple sclerosis after 10–15 years of initial diagnosis
	Disease-modifying therapies:
	• Anti-inflammatory medications (prednisone and methylprednisolone)
	• Mitoxantrone (Novantrone)
Primary Progressive	Disease progression:
	• Accounts for 10% of the multiple sclerosis population
	• Characterized by steady decline of motor control without periods of significant recovery
	• Anti-inflammatory medications (prednisone and methylprednisolone)
Progressive and Remitting	Disease progression:
	• Accounts for 5% of the multiple sclerosis population
	• Characterized by steady decline with intermittent periods of relapse
	• Anti-inflammatory medications (prednisone and methylprednisolone)

Data from Forwell et al., 2014; Schultz-Krohn, Foti, and Glogoski, 2013.

the course of the disease progression. Each pattern of symptom manifestation clarifies the pattern of each individual's disease progression as described below.

In addition to the use of anti-inflammatory medications, alternative interventions are used to manage the symptoms of disease progression, especially during periods of relapse or exacerbation (Forwell et al., 2014; Hugos & Copperman, 1999; Schultz-Krohn et al., 2013). Specifically, antispasticity medications are used to control hypertonic muscles in the upper and lower extremities; however, they may also increase fatigue through a systemic effect. A neurogenic bladder may be managed through catheterization to prevent infection from insufficient voiding. Energy conservation, nutrition planning, and incorporation of skilled therapy to increase strength and endurance reduce symptoms of fatigue and cognitive changes. Furthermore, elevated body temperature may intensify symptoms of muscle weakness, incoordination, and overall fatigue, and may be regulated using cooling vests or limiting exposure to activities or environments involving prolonged heat exposure. Reports of primary pain are managed by medication, whereas secondary pain is most often improved with proper positioning techniques. Individuals with MS may also develop depression as a psychological or physiological response to the disease process, which should be addressed with medication and support groups.

Parkinson's Disease, Etiology, and Pathology

Parkinson's disease is a nonfatal, neurodegenerative disease characterized by a gradual onset of four cardinal signs including tremor, rigidity or stiffness, bradykinesia or slowness of movement, cogwheel rigidity, festinating gait, and postural instability in the absence of other neurological diagnoses (Conley & Kirchner, 1999; Jankovic, 2008). Parkinson's disease is the second most common adult-onset neurodegenerative disease and is diagnosed in 1% of the population over 60 years of age (Bertram & Tanzi, 2005; de Lau & Breteler, 2006). Prevalence is greater in men between the ages of 55 and 74 years, a trend that reverses with prevalence greater in women older than 75 years of age (Schultz-Krohn et al., 2013). While the exact cause is unknown, genetic and environmental risk factors are associated with the development of Parkinson's disease including chromosome 4 abnormalities and exposure to both well water and pesticides,

respectively (Conley & Kirchner, 1999; Forwell et al., 2014; Marder et al., 1998).

There is no established biomarker or laboratory test to confirm the diagnosis of Parkinson's disease. Clinical examination and presentation of cardinal signs are the most acceptable criteria for diagnosis (Forwell et al., 2014; NINDS, 2014b). Tremor, rigidity, and bradykinesia indicate that a reduction in dopamine synthesis is occurring in the substantia nigra, resulting in impaired efferent motor planning and smooth movement from the motor cortex on both voluntary and involuntary levels. Similar signs may also occur in the face and are responsible for the characteristic masklike facies (Conley & Kirchner, 1999). Progression of the disease over years and even decades includes shuffling gait, freezing or akinesia during gross and fine motor control, impaired reflexes, and postural instability of the head, neck, shoulders, and trunk. When combined, these impairments contribute to an increase in falls seen in this population due to reduced functional mobility. Executive functioning, visual perceptual skills, and emotional status are also impacted in persons with Parkinson's disease (Forwell et al., 2014; Schultz-Krohn et al., 2013). See **Figure 13-2** for image of common Parkinsonian posturing.

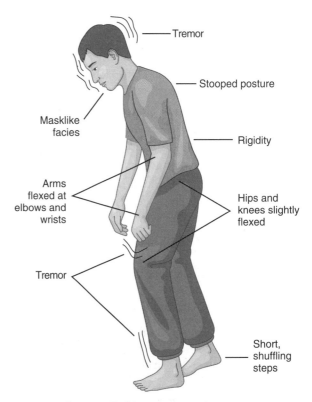

Figure 13-2 Common Parkinsonian posturing.

Medical Management

While there is no cure for Parkinson's disease, certain oral medications are used to manage the signs and symptoms of the disease. Levodopa is generally the first medication prescribed to manage bradykinesia and rigidity because the nerve cells use it to replenish dopamine (NINDS, 2014b). Over time, however, individuals become less responsive to this medication and "on–off" periods of effectiveness occur. Dyskinesia, or involuntary movement, indicates onset of the hallmark "off periods" as the medication dosage is used up in the nervous system. In an effort to extend the conversion of the levodopa into dopamine until it reaches the brain, carbidopa may be prescribed in combination with levodopa (Schultz-Krohn et al., 2013). Oral medications that imitate the effects of dopamine in the brain may also be prescribed and include bromocriptine, pramipexole, and ropinirole (NINDS, 2014b).

The progression of symptoms determines the staging of the disease process as defined by Hoehn and Yahr (1967) and Bradley (1996). Hoehn and Yahr refer to five stages of Parkinson's disease beginning with unilateral symptoms and the presence of a resting tremor in stage one, progressing to bilateral involvement with early trunk and reflex difficulties in stage two. Individuals in stage three begin to show signs of functional decline with postural instability noted while the final stages of the disease process are characterized by significant functional decline and use of a wheelchair, respectively. Bradley (1996) provides a simplified three-step staging process that refers to early, nonfluctuating, and fluctuating symptoms. The earliest stage is characterized by nondisabling symptoms that respond well to medication. Once levodopa is prescribed, the disease is staged as nonfluctuating and disability is quantified as affecting 20% of the individual's level of functioning. The most advanced stage, according to Bradley, is referred to as fluctuating because the symptoms no longer consistently respond to medication.

Alternative surgical interventions are used to reduce signs and symptoms of Parkinson's disease in individuals experiencing reduced effectiveness of medication. Stereotactic surgical procedures create intentional lesions in overactive areas of the pallidum, thalamus, and subthalamus in an effort to reduce the frequency and intensity of movement impairments. Similarly, deep brain stimulation produces similar effects to ablative procedures without irreversible consequences. This alternative therapy approved by the U.S. Food and Drug Administration utilizes a pulse generator to activate electrodes surgically implanted in the overactive regions, thus reducing over activity and involuntary movement symptoms without creating permanent lesions (NINDS, 2014a; Rodriguez-Oroz et al., 2005). These interventions are particularly useful in persons with the effects of Parkinson's disease persisting through multiple decades.

Alzheimer's Disease Etiology and Pathology

Alzheimer's disease is the leading cause of adult-onset neurodegenerative disease affecting 5 million people in the United States, or 13% of adults older than 65 years. After the age of 65, the incidence of Alzheimer's disease doubles every 5 years with up to 50% of persons 85 years and older afflicted by the disease. While one specific cause is unknown, several risk factors have strong associations with the disease. Genetic mutations and protein markers have been connected to both early-onset, or familial Alzheimer's disease, and late-onset Alzheimer's disease. However, environmental factors and lifestyle have been linked to whether or not genetic mutations are actually expressed, or turned on, in late-onset Alzheimer's disease. Reduced activity level, diet, smoking, diabetes mellitus, depression, and previous head trauma are all considered environmental factors that could increase a person's risk for developing the disease (Galvin, Fagan, Holtzman, Mintun, & Morris, 2010; National Institute on Aging [NIA], 2014; Schultz-Krohn et al., 2013).

Alzheimer's disease causes neurodegenerative changes in the cerebral cortex and hippocampus as a result of protein accumulation in the brain. The process starts when beta-amyloid protein deposits, and later tau protein deposits, accumulate in the brain. This sets off an inflammatory response in the tissue that results in disfigurement of neurons in the area. As this microtubular dysfunction increases, neuronal communication and nutrient transport become impaired as the nerve fibers become tangled. Over time, these tangles in combination with other neuronal debris become larger plaques that take up vital space in the cells. Eventually, impaired function of these nerves causes tissue death and brain atrophy. The areas most commonly affected are the temporal and parietal lobes of the cerebral cortex. In addition to the accumulation of protein deposits and subsequent atrophy, individuals with Alzheimer's disease present with a disruption in conversion of choline to the neurotransmitter acetylcholine. This cholinergic dysfunction results in decreased synapses in the frontal lobe, hippocampus, and temporal lobes. Atrophy in these areas manifests as reduced motor planning, executive functioning, new learning, visual spatial skills, mood, and memory (Galvin et al., 2010; Schultz-Krohn et al., 2013).

Medical Management

Alzheimer's disease is considered primary dementia because it is not associated with secondary disease processes (Galvin et al., 2010; NIA, 2014). While computed tomography, MRI, and positron emission tomography may detect enlarged ventricles, these diagnostic tests are more useful in identifying alternative disease processes such as stroke, brain injury, and tumor growth. The most useful asset in identifying signs and symptoms of Alzheimer's disease is a comprehensive medical examination and interview with the primary care physician, patient, and supportive family members. Laboratory tests, a mental status evaluation, and brief neurological examination are tools used during this medical examination to formulate a comprehensive history leading to diagnosis.

Early detection is critical to managing signs and symptoms of Alzheimer's disease. The most common medical intervention consists of building relationships with an interdisciplinary team of professionals including the physician, nurse, social worker, occupational therapist, physical therapist, speech language pathologist, and psychologist (Forwell et al., 2014; Schultz-Krohn et al., 2013; Takahashi & Huang, 2009). This team of medical professionals work together to provide structured support for the patient and family, in addition to skilled therapy interventions used to improve occupational performance. Pharmacological therapy may include the use of galantamine or donepezil, cholinesterase inhibitors, to temporarily improve cognitive performance skills (Galvin et al., 2010; NIA, 2014). Dietician services may be indicated to educate patient and families on the benefits of physical activity and a Mediterranean diet to improve cardiovascular health, which influences metabolic brain function. Finally, it is imperative to manage comorbid diagnoses affecting overall health and wellness to slow the progression of Alzheimer's disease.

GBS Etiology and Pathology

GBS is a neurodegenerative disease of unknown etiology that produces similar signs and symptoms to the other diseases in this chapter. Signs and symptoms include motor paralysis, paresthesia, and impairments of the autonomic nervous system; however, the onset is rapid and acute in nature, and cognition is generally spared. GBS affects 1.2–2 per 100,000, or 0.001% of the U.S. population every year (Centers for Disease Control and Prevention [CDC], 2014). Persons older than the age of 50 years and men are at a greater risk for developing the disease (CDC, 2014; van Doorn, Ruts, & Jacobs, 2008).

While the cause is unknown, a preceding diagnosis of enteritis has been discovered in 41% of cases (Carroll, McDonnell, & Barnes, 2003). Similarly, episodes of diarrhea or respiratory illness are identified in two-thirds of cases. Exposure to specific bacteria and virus strains increases a person's risk, specifically *Campylobacter jejuni* and cytomegalovirus, respectively (CDC, 2014). Despite growing concerns that the influenza vaccine increases a person's risk for developing GBS, the risk of developing GBS within six weeks of contracting the influenza virus is greater than the risk of developing GBS from the influenza vaccine itself (Kwong et al., 2013). GBS is considered sporadic without hereditary risk (Genetics Home Reference, 2011).

The pathogenesis of GBS is rooted in an autoimmune response that attacks the peripheral nervous system. The disease process targets the axons of motor neurons, sensory neurons, and less commonly cranial nerves depending on the type of manifestation. The disease pattern of GBS begins with the acute inflammatory phase, characterized by a sudden onset of peripheral muscle weakness in two or more limbs starting distally in the feet and hands, progressing upward toward the head, and proximally toward the trunk (Forwell et al., 2014; van Doorn et al., 2008). Initially, voluntary muscle contraction is affected with the potential for demyelination of involuntary motor neurons including those for respiration. Mechanical ventilation is necessary in 20–30% of cases (Dematteis, 1996). Signs and symptoms include muscle weakness in the extremities and trunk, paresthesia, pain, ataxia, areflexia, fatigue, oropharyngeal weakness, and ophthalmoplegia. Autonomic dysfunction presents as tachycardia, bradycardia, orthostatic hypotension, and urinary retention. This acute inflammatory phase may persist for days or weeks and often reaches its peak by week 4 in 95% of cases (van Doorn et al., 2008). The disease is considered to be in stage two once the development of new signs and symptoms is stabilized (van Doorn et al., 2008). This second stage is characterized by a plateau phase during which no significant deterioration continues. This plateau stage may last days or weeks before the final stage of spontaneous recovery begins, indicating further disease progression is unlikely.

During the final stage of progressive recovery, remyelination and axonal regeneration occurs proximally to distally and persists between an average of 12 weeks and up to 2 years (van Doorn et al., 2008). Overall recovery varies greatly with 50% of individuals achieving a full recovery, 35% living with residual weakness, and 15% adjusting to permanent disability (Karavatas, 2005; Khan, Pallant, Ng, & Bhasker, 2010). Death occurs in up to 10% of cases (Khan, 2004).

Several types of GBS have been discovered; each one is distinguished by the type of axon, the location along the axon, and the disease targets (Ramachandran, 2012). Furthermore, each subtype of GBS is associated with distinct differences in prevalence for individuals living in North American and European countries compared to those in Asian and Latin American countries. Acute inflammatory demyelinating polyradiculoneuropathy is the most common type of GBS occurring in 90% of cases in North America and Europe. The body's immune system attacks the myelin surrounding the peripheral nerve axons, impeding nerve impulses and subsequent muscle contraction. Acute motor axonal neuropathy (AMAN) and acute motor-sensory axonal neuropathy (AMSAN) attack the actual axons resulting in more significant impairment. While these subtypes account for only 3–5% of cases in North America and Europe, their prevalence in Asian and Latin American countries occurs in 30–50% of cases. Miller Fisher syndrome (MFS), a much less common type of GBS, attacks the cranial nerves in addition to peripheral motor and/or sensory involvement. Similar to the prevalence of AMAN and AMSAN, MFS is far more common in Asian countries as compared to North American and European countries with a representation in 20% of cases compared to less than 5% of cases, respectively (Genetics Home Reference, 2011).

Medical Management

A comprehensive medical history identifies the hallmark signs of rapid ascending symmetrical muscle weakness and absence of deep tendon reflexes. Blood count tests provide valuable information necessary to rule out differential diagnoses associated with infection while a lumbar puncture may be used to detect elevated protein levels in cerebrospinal fluid. Nerve conduction tests with needle electromyography are useful in identifying demyelination of peripheral nerve axons. In extreme cases, nerve biopsy may be indicated to confirm a diagnosis (Ramachandran, 2012).

The most successful medical intervention begins immediately with intravenous immunoglobulin in an effort to boost the immune system and diminish the effects of the disease. Plasmapheresis may also be implemented (Forwell et al., 2014; Ramachandran, 2012; van Doorn et al., 2008). Conventional corticosteroid therapy is only recommended as an adjunct to the aforementioned interventions (Ramachandran, 2012). Additional interventions may be necessary to manage the side effects of the disease process including mechanical ventilation, enteric nutrition supplementation, cardiac management, antithrombolytics, and bowel and bladder management. Skilled OT, physical therapy, and speech therapy provide essential rehabilitation to maximize functional recovery (Ramachandran, 2012).

Section Two: Screening and Assessments, Impact on Occupational Performance, Interventions, Referrals and Discharge Considerations, and Management and Standards of Practice for Neurodegenerative Conditions

OT evaluation and treatment of clients with neurodegenerative disease addresses a broad spectrum of occupations, client factors, performance skills, and performance patterns that may be impacted at various stages of each respective disease process (Forwell et al., 2014; Schultz-Krohn et al., 2013). The pace, at which signs and symptoms evolve for each diagnosis, as well as overall prognosis, guides the evaluation and intervention process. In cases of ALS and GBS, peripheral muscle weakness and decreased functional independence in one's daily routine occurs at a more rapid pace compared to the development of signs and symptoms of MS, Parkinson's disease, and Alzheimer's disease. There is an urgency applied in the former cases for initiating rehabilitation services in an effort to begin managing and preventing further functional decline, whereas the latter diagnoses evolve over the course of months or years and skilled therapy may not be initially indicated.

Similarly, the prognosis and staging of each disease is carefully considered when prioritizing intervention methods, goals, and long-term planning. The pathogenesis that determines the prognosis of ALS and GBS is strikingly different; therefore, very different treatment approaches are utilized. While the deterioration of performance skills is permanent in ALS, there is great potential for motor recovery in the rehabilitation of GBS. An understanding of the pathology for each disease process allows the skilled OT practitioner to prioritize evaluation methods and treatment interventions to guide best practice with each neurodegenerative disease diagnosis covered in this chapter.

Section two of this chapter is designed to provide an overview of the role of OT in treating neurodegenerative disease. The OT screening and assessment tools, preparatory methods, interventions, discharge planning, and ethical scenarios are presented with respect to neurodegenerative disease as a whole. Evaluations and interventions that apply to a specific diagnosis are clearly stated.

Screening and Assessments

All neurodegenerative diseases result in impaired motor and process performance skills and altered levels of independence in daily occupations. OT evaluation focuses on building a cohesive medical history with details regarding onset of signs of symptoms, establishment of client's personal priorities and goals, and objective determination of impaired performance skills. A comprehensive evaluation includes an informal interview, observation, and chart review; performance-based standardized assessments; and client-directed standardized assessments. It is the responsibility of the occupational therapist to consider the overall disease stage and prognosis when choosing and prioritizing the use of specific screening tools and assessments. The pace at which certain diseases progress will also determine the frequency of reassessment to ensure progression or regression is captured and addressed through future intervention. **Table 13-3** provides a list of standardized assessments that may be used when evaluating an individual with neurodegenerative disease (Fleming et al., 2009; Forwell et al., 2014; Kuo, 2009; Schultz-Krohn et al., 2013; Takahashi & Huang, 2009).

Intervention Planning, Implementation, and Review

Skilled OT intervention for neurodegenerative disease addresses all areas of daily occupation with attention to client factors, performance skills, context, and environment. While most intervention plans reflect activities of daily living (ADLs), instrumental activities of daily living (IADLs), body functions, and motor and process performance skills at some point during the progression of each neurodegenerative disease, the implementation approach for each diagnosis is client specific and reflective of the overall prognosis (AOTA, 1999; Forwell et al., 2014; Schultz-Krohn et al., 2013).

Preparatory Methods

Preparatory methods are included in intervention planning to prepare each client for participation in occupational performance during a skilled therapy session and throughout each day (AOTA, 2014). **Table 13-4** provides a list of common preparatory methods that may be introduced to clients with neurodegenerative disease.

Impact on Occupational Performance

Each disease process in this chapter shares the theme of neurological degeneration; however, some progress slowly while others demonstrate a more rapid decline. The pace at which signs and symptoms evolve determines the goals and priorities of the intervention plan for each diagnosis and each individual. The development of signs and symptoms in Parkinson's disease and Alzheimer's disease, respectively, is more gradual and occurs over months or years, whereas GBS and ALS are characterized by more rapid onsets that occur over the course of days or months. The approach to intervention planning with GBS is unique in that there is a clear period of remission and recovery without further decline. The onset of MS is somewhere in between, usually dependent on the pattern, and may progress quickly over months or slowly over years, with periods of remission in between. Each of these scenarios is considered when creating an intervention plan with short- and long-term goals to prepare the client and family for future stages of each disease process.

The specific type of neurological decline and associated impact on occupational performance is also characteristic of each disease. Client factors of neuromusculoskeletal and movement-related functions,

Table 13-3 Standardized Assessments for Neurodegenerative Disease

Standardized Assessment	Description
6MWT	Performance-based assessment of functional mobility and endurance used to establish distance covered in six minutes of ambulation with assistive device as needed.
ACL	Performance-based assessment that measures ability to follow directions and complete various visual perceptual motor tasks.
ALSFRS-R	Objective questionnaire that uses a 5-point ordinal scale to measure levels of participation in 12 areas including communication, oral pharyngeal function, functional mobility, respiratory function, handwriting, dressing, and hygiene in individuals with ALS.
AMPS	Performance-based assessment of motor and process skills through IADLs.
BDI-II	Self-report assessment to determine behavioral characteristics of depression.
BBT	Timed, performance-based assessment that measures unilateral manual dexterity including fine and gross motor control.
biVABA	Performance-based screening of visual perceptual skills used to measure visual acuity, contrast sensitivity function, visual fields, oculomotor function, and visual attention.
COPM	Self-report assessment of occupational performance ability in self-care, productivity, and leisure activities.
CSI	Self-report of caregivers used to measure levels of stress caused by 13 variables related to caregiving including finances, emotional status, sleep, work, and personal life.
Dynamometry	Objective, performance-based assessment that measures the isokinetic strength of grip and pinch strength using an interval scale.
EFPT	Performance-based assessment of cognitive function in four domains of IADL including hot meal preparation, bill management, medication management, and placing a phone call.
GBS Disability Scale	Objective assessment that uses status of ambulation and respiratory function to stage the severity of disability in persons with GBS.
MMT	Performance-based assessment that measures the strength of prime muscle movers in graded planes of movement using an ordinal scale.
MMSE	Brief cognitive screen of orientation, attention, recall, calculation, language, and visual construction used to detect current cognitive status and cognitive changes over time.
MFIS	Self-report assessment of fatigue impact on physical, cognitive, and psychosocial functioning in persons with multiple sclerosis.
MoCa	Performance-based cognitive screen of visual construction skills, naming, memory, attention, abstraction, and orientation.
MSWS-12	Self-report of walking ability in persons with multiple sclerosis using a 5-point scale for 12 variables affecting gait.
Parkinson's Disease Questionniare-39	Self-report assessment of quality of life across eight domains including motor control, functional mobility, ADL, IADL, cognition, sleep, and psychosocial status.
PPBT	Performance-based, timed assessment that measures fine and gross motor control efficiency to place pegs into pegboard and bimanual integration to assemble pins, washers, and collars.
Semmes Weinstein Monofilaments	Objective measurement of cutaneous sensation using a nominal scale that measures detection of touch.
Standard ROM	Objective measurement of passive and active joint range of motion using ratio goniometry.

ACL, Allen Cognitive Level test; ALSFRS-R, ALS Functional Rating Scale; AMPS, Assessment of Motor and Process Skills; BDI-II, Beck Depression Inventory; BBT, Box and Block Test; biVABA, Brain Injury Visual Assessment Battery for Adults; COPM, Canadian Occupational Performance Measure; CSI, Carssessment Battery for Adults; EFPT, Executive Function Performance Test; 6MWT, 6 Minute Walk Test; MMT, Manual Muscle Testing; MMSE, Mini-Mental Status Examination; MFIS, Modified Fatigue Impact Scale; MoCa, Montreal Cognitive Assessment; MSWS-12, Multiple Sclerosis Walking Scale; PPBT, Purdue Pegboard Test; ROM, range of motion.

Data from: Golisz (2009).

Table 13-4 Preparatory Methods for Neurodegenerative Disease

Method	Description
Modalities	Modalities are used to prepare body structures for occupational performance. Passive range of motion and joint mobilization may be used to prepare soft tissue for increased movement. Cooling vests may be used to lower the core temperature of an individual with multiple sclerosis, which improves endurance. • **Range of motion** is performed by the occupational therapy practitioner and/or client to improve muscle lengthening, reduce the potential for contractures, and maintain joint integrity of the extremities. • **Cooling vests** may be worn intermittently by individuals with multiple sclerosis to reduce body temperature while at rest or engaged in a functional activity, ultimately improving occupational performance and endurance. • **Moist heat** may be used to improve circulation in the extremities when natural movement is limited.
Splints	The pathology of neurodegenerative disease often results in abnormal muscle tone including hypertonicity from spasticity and hypotonicity from muscle weakness or atrophy in the extremities. Splints are used for improved functional alignment, joint stability, and preservation of muscle length and joint range of motion. Hand and foot orthotics are commonly used when neuromuscular degeneration limits function or balance. • **Short opponens splints** provide functional thumb and index finger opposition positioning in the presence of thenar and hypothenar atrophy during object manipulation. • **Long opponens splints** provide functional wrist support in addition to thumb and index finger opposition positioning in the presence of thenar, hypothenar, and extrinsic wrist atrophy during object manipulation. • **Resting hand splints** provide functional positioning for the wrist and fingers at rest to prevent contractures in muscles with increased spasticity or atrophy. • **Ankle–foot orthoses** provide stability for the ankle during functional mobility and allow for improved foot clearance necessary to reduce falls when foot drop is present.
Assistive technology and environmental modifications	**Assistive technology** is useful in a variety of applications for neurodegenerative disease. Individuals with ALS may use communication devices, while applications in a smartphone may assist with planning and organization for persons with executive functioning deficits in the case of multiple sclerosis or Alzheimer's disease. • **Speech generating devices** allow individuals with progressive bulbar palsy from ALS to type or use head movements to produce computer-generated speech output. • **Smartphones** provide alarms, calendars, and other useful applications to assist with planning, organization, and memory when process skills are impacted by neurodegenerative disease. • **Computer accessibility options** provide a range of adaptations that may be used to make typing more efficient for persons with reduced coordination or strength. • **Speech recognition software** enables an individual with reduced hand function to speak into a computer or phone-based headphone to generate text instead of typing. **Environmental modifications** enable an individual to maintain a safe and functional level of participation in daily occupations through modification of their current environment at home, work, school, or in the community. For example, durable medical equipment for ADLs may enable individuals with decreased balance and endurance to maintain a respectable level of independence in a modified context without the assistance of another person. • **Durable medical equipment** includes any piece of equipment that is used in a person's home to improve occupational performance including grab bars, shower chairs, transfer benches, sliding boards, raised toilet seats, bedside commodes, hospital beds, walkers, canes, and wheelchairs. • **Adaptive equipment** is used to improve occupational performance when neuromuscular degeneration impacts strength and coordination during daily occupations. Examples include modified utensils, writing devices, foam handles, plate guards, adapted kitchen equipment, and dressing equipment. • **Ramps and lifts** are recommended when stair negotiation is unsafe due to reduced functional mobility, or to reduce the strain of caregiving. Examples include simple ramps and vertical electronic lifts to enter a home or an electric chair lift to access multiple floors inside the home.

(continues)

Table 13-4 Preparatory Methods for Neurodegenerative Disease (*continued*)

Method	Description
	• **Car modifications** are indicated when an individual maintains sufficient motor and process skills to drive a vehicle but with slight modifications for hand controls. Ramps and lifts for power wheelchairs may also be considered to enable transport for either a driver or passenger using a wheelchair. • **Item accessibility** includes moving most commonly used ADL and IADL items to a more accessible location including lower shelves in a closet, cabinet, or refrigerator.
Wheeled seating and mobility	Wheeled mobility is indicated to augment or replace ambulation for individuals with significant lower extremity and trunk weakness. • **Rolling walkers** are used to provide additional support during functional mobility when balance and endurance are compromised. • **Rollator walkers** are rolling walkers with a wider base of support, caster wheels, padded seats, and locking brakes, which provide improved balance, coordination, and safety features. • **Manual wheelchairs** are indicated for use with longer distance, although functional ambulation may still be possible for shorter distances. This includes seating systems to address support of the trunk and all extremities when applicable. • **Power wheelchairs** are indicated when lower extremity weakness prevents functional ambulation over most distances and upper extremity weakness is insufficient for wheelchair propulsion. Decreased trunk support is another indication for power wheelchair use. Distal hand function or head control is preserved for access of joysticks or sip and puff controls. • **Power-assist wheelchairs** are manual wheelchairs with a power-assist attachment to the wheels that may be engaged to provide enhanced propulsion over longer distances, uneven surfaces, or inclines.

Data from: Forwell et al. (2014); Schultz-Krohn, Foti, and Glogoski, (2013).

muscle functions, and movement functions are prioritized in intervention plans for ALS, GBS, MS, and Parkinson's disease. Gross and fine motor control, static and dynamic balance in sitting and standing, and upper and lower extremity strength are represented in most skilled interventions for these individuals.

Mental functions and process skills are often predominant in intervention planning for Alzheimer's disease. As all of these neurodegenerative diseases progress, mental functions and process skills may become a greater focus as independence in daily occupations require cognitive functioning in addition to neuromusculoskeletal functioning. Financial management, meal preparation, daily scheduling, and medication management are examples of common IADLs that are reflected in interventions addressing sustained and alternating attention, prospective memory, planning, problem-solving, organization, reasoning, safety awareness, comprehension, and expression.

Therapeutic Interventions

A skilled occupational therapist considers each unique set of occupations, client factors, performance skills, performance patterns, contexts, and environments when creating a cohesive and comprehensive intervention plan. Intervention planning for a young mother recently diagnosed with relapsing–remitting MS may prioritize energy conservation techniques required for endurance throughout a full day of parenting and homemaking, fine motor control exercises for coordination necessary to dress a toddler, and balance exercises for carrying personal belongings and groceries in the community. Education is provided for using certain strategies over the course of a lifetime. While certain goals may be met during a previous admission, a relapse may require the occupational therapist and client to revisit the same goals during a future admission years later.

In contrast, intervention planning for an individual with ALS reflects occupational performance goals to maintain participation in ADLs, IADLs, and work activities through the use of assistive technology to compensate for a progressive rapid decline of coordination, strength, and speech. Interactive sessions are used to encourage the client to problem solve permanent changes in function that may progress from week to week. Clients with ALS are also encouraged to maintain participation in, and control of, their daily routines through directing others to assist them as needed. Neudert, Wasner, and Borasio (2004) determined that a supportive family and social network enables quality of life to remain stable despite physical decline for persons with ALS.

Table 13-5 provides a summary of skilled OT interventions to consider when planning interventions for each neurodegenerative disease discussed in this chapter. Summary points are included to highlight the overall trend in intervention planning for each diagnosis with respect to occupational performance. While each neurodegenerative disease is presented separately, overlap in skilled interventions is common (AOTA, 1999; Fleming et al., 2009; Forwell et al., 2014; Kuo, 2009; Schultz-Krohn et al., 2013; Takahashi & Huang, 2009).

Reevaluation and Plan Modification

Neurodegenerative disease presents a complex set of factors that are best managed using a dynamic approach. The skilled occupational therapist recognizes physical and mental status changes and responds through reevaluation and plan modification to ensure interventions meet changing needs. Medical complications including respiratory or cardiac insufficiency, worsening dysphagia, or rapid systemic muscle atrophy will affect participation and requires immediate attention to ensure best care.

The rapid degeneration in ALS warrants frequent plan modification to ensure that the client has access to the most appropriate assistive technology or equipment. These plan modifications allow for continued participation in daily occupations despite muscle atrophy progression. Once respiratory function is compromised, an individual's intervention plan may shift to focus on directing care rather than physically performing daily tasks that result in exhaustion or difficulty breathing.

Treatment plan modification for GBS also occurs frequently in response to changing needs. Furthermore, it is common for individuals to modify their participation in daily occupations as time goes on due to progressive recovery and strengthening, as their health is not threatened by potential further decline. An individual who required the use of tub transfer bench for bathing may demonstrate sufficient strength and balance to stand as progressive recovery occurs. The acute inflammatory period may result in reduced extremity and trunk strength that indicates the need for a rolling walker during functional mobility. Through the progressive recovery stage, an individual may develop improved strength to ambulate without a device. A client with MS may experience similar improvements in strength during a period of remission, requiring less assistance for functional mobility or transfers.

Mental status changes associated with MS and Alzheimer's disease is addressed through recommendations for assistance with critical IADLs including driving, medication management, meal preparation, and financial management to ensure safety of the individual. The implementation of heightened supervision levels in the home and community preserves a certain level of autonomy for the client while enabling continued wellness and participation in one's daily routine. These recommendations may not be included during the initial evaluations; however, they may be reflected months or years later in the intervention plan when mental status changes become more severe.

There are unlimited examples to support reevaluation and plan modification for each neurodegenerative disease. A skilled occupational therapist or OT assistant recognizes subtle changes that may persist over the course of days or weeks then responds through reevaluation. Significant changes in client factors or performance patterns should be addressed and discussed as soon as possible to ensure the client, family, and caregivers are enabled to promote ongoing participation in daily occupations.

Referrals and Discharge Considerations

A large variety of referral and discharge planning options are available in the management of neurodegenerative disease. The treatment of these diagnoses is a collaborative effort of an interdisciplinary medical and rehabilitation team that works together to identify and address the complex and dynamic medical, psychosocial, and rehabilitative needs of the client and family.

When acute hospitalization occurs with GBS, there is a more definitive process in place for medical management followed by rehabilitation. The severity of deficits for any neurodegenerative disease determines the levels of care through which each individual progresses. Intensive care, acute care, subacute care, inpatient rehabilitation, day rehabilitation, and outpatient rehabilitation are examples of potential levels of care that address the dynamic needs of these individuals. Contrary to other neurological diagnoses that follow more predictable courses,

Table 13-5 Intervention Planning for Neurodegenerative Disease

Intervention Planning	
Amyotrophic lateral sclerosis	**Ambulatory period**: Participation in daily occupations promotes independence and preservation of a client's roles despite the reality of facing a fatal disease. Social support and psychological support provide a safe environment for the client to accept a potentially rapid functional decline.

- **ADLs and IADLs** provide opportunity for ongoing functional strengthening, coordination, and mobility training. Adaptive equipment or durable medical equipment including foam handles, grab bars, ambulation devices, and/or bathroom devices may be recommended to compensate for progressive muscle atrophy and limit unnecessary exertion while enabling some level of independence. The skilled occupational therapy practitioner incorporates swallowing strategies during eating if bulbar palsy develops. Assistance or activity modifications may be introduced for IADLs including meal preparation, homemaking tasks, and financial management.

- **Rest and sleep** is important as muscles that remain innervated may fatigue quickly. Energy conservation techniques are beneficial. Taking breaks during tasks that utilize weaker muscles prevents exhaustion that may limit continued participation in functional activities. Sitting instead of standing during grooming, meal preparation, and social activities may also conserve energy while encouraging ongoing participation.

- **Patient and family education** regarding progression and prognosis begins immediately to enable swift decision-making for eventual caregiving services. Education is provided for splint and durable medical equipment use, home exercise programs, assistive technology use, and functional transfers.

- **Work activities** enable individuals to maintain a sense of purpose and role identification that has likely been important throughout a lifetime. Accommodations are recommended for a reduced schedule, rest breaks, or assistive technology to promote ongoing participation.

- **Social interaction (play and leisure)** is a valuable component of the intervention plan to enable the client to engage in activities that are enjoyable, fun, and motivating despite physical decline.

- **Client factors and performance skills** for upper and lower extremity strengthening, coordination, and bilateral integration are addressed through participation in functional activities. Technology may be introduced for expression if speech production or computer use is altered. Executive functioning is addressed through functional planning and problem-solving.

Wheelchair-dependent period: Every effort is made to enable ongoing participation in daily occupations to promote independence, encourage muscle strengthening and coordination, and enable quality of life; however, assistance is eventually needed for all daily occupations. The client is encouraged to direct care to maintain autonomy. Respiratory assistance is required either intermittently or ongoing and is a consideration during skilled therapy sessions.

- **ADLs and IADLs** are used to promote functional strengthening and coordination of the extremities, trunk, head, and neck when the client is strong enough to participate. The client is encouraged to direct care verbally when physical participation is no longer possible. Swallowing strategies and tongue sweep movements are incorporated, food and drink consistencies are thickened or modified, and pleasure feeds for eating are indicated on occasion as dysphagia progresses.

- **Rest and sleep** continues to be encouraged and the frequency may increase as endurance decreases.

- **Patient and family education** emphasizes bed and wheelchair positioning techniques, skin care, management of life supporting respiratory and nutrition needs, and use of assistive technology for expression of wants and needs.

- **Work activities** may continue to be possible with a reduced schedule or accommodations fading to permanent disability.

Table 13-5 Intervention Planning for Neurodegenerative Disease (*continued*)

- **Social interaction** (play and leisure) remains valuable even if participation is verbal or passive only. It is strongly encouraged to provide ongoing support and motivation for the client and family as the burden of care increases.
- **Client factors and performance skills** begin to focus on range of motion for the extremities, trunk, and neck as atrophy increases. Balance activities in sitting remain beneficial for total body strengthening, functional mobility, and cardiac and respiratory functioning. Residual head control may be used to perform head nods for yes/no, drive a sip and puff power wheelchair, or activate assistive technology switches. Oculomotor control through blinking or visual scanning is encouraged for nonverbal communication when head and neck musculature is no longer sufficient for nodding or speech production. Sensory integration is used to stimulate vision, touch, smell, hearing, and taste. Respiratory function requires intermittent or permanent ventilation and is considered during treatment. The client is encouraged to communicate pain status and need for medication. If mental functions become impaired, family performs decision-making. Utmost care is given to maintain quality of life.

Intervention Planning

Multiple sclerosis	**Relapsing and remitting**: Participation in daily occupations, including work, is preserved overall with activity, equipment, or environment modifications implemented to promote ongoing independence. Periods of relapse followed by remission often occur many times throughout an individual's lifetime; therefore, skilled therapy interventions of strengthening and coordination through functional activity are implemented during each admission. Mental process skills are included in skilled interventions to improve executive functioning. Ongoing, nurturing relationships are often developed between the client and occupational therapy team as long-term rehabilitation needs are often indicated throughout a lifetime.

- **ADLs and IADLs** are incorporated into short- and long-term goals to facilitate strengthening, coordination, and independence. Adaptive equipment and durable medical equipment is introduced when decreased strength and coordination interfere with function. Energy conservation techniques are encouraged and include performance of daily activities in sitting rather than standing. The use of activity modifications or assistance from a caregiver may be temporary as periods of remission occur with each cycle.
- **Rest and sleep** preserve physical and mental endurance, and ensure muscles have time to recover between daily activities. There may be a greater need for rest and sleep during periods of relapse and less need during periods of remission.
- **Patient and family education** emphasizes the benefits of ongoing occupational performance to increase functional strength, balance, and coordination. Education also includes orthotic and durable medical equipment use, energy conservation techniques, home exercise programs, and recommendations for home modifications.
- **Work activities** may be incorporated into intervention plans to include computer use, executive functions, and functional mobility. Activity or environmental modifications may be recommended to facilitate ongoing gainful employment during periods of relapse.
- **Social interaction (play and leisure)** is encouraged with modifications as necessary. Connections with support groups are helpful to provide ongoing partnerships in the community.
- **Client factors and performance skills** are reflected as coordination, strength, balance, and endurance goals. Handwriting, typing speed, in-hand manipulation, and translation of coins may represent hand function goals. Carrying, dynamic standing balance, and lifting are also incorporated. Mental functions are addressed through financial management, meal planning, and complex daily scheduling tasks. Strategies for prospective memory are included through the use of daily calendars or smartphone applications.

(continues)

Table 13-5 Intervention Planning for Neurodegenerative Disease (*continued*)

Primary progressive, secondary progressive, and progressive-remitting: Participation in daily occupations, including work, is preserved initially with modifications to promote ongoing independence. However, as disease progression occurs and participation in daily occupations becomes increasingly difficult, intervention plans address performance of daily occupations from a wheelchair level and emphasize caregiver training. The specific progressive disease pattern influences goals and expectations for levels of independence in each daily activity. Mental process skills are included in skilled interventions to improve executive functioning. Functional decline occurs over a shorter period of time and without significant improvement associated with remitting and relapsing multiple sclerosis.

- **ADLs and IADLs** are incorporated into short- and long-term goals to facilitate strengthening, coordination, and independence. Adaptive equipment and durable medical equipment is introduced when decreased strength and coordination interfere with function and safety. Energy conservation techniques are encouraged and include performance of daily activities in sitting rather than standing. The use of activity modifications or assistance from a caregiver for ADLs and IADLs is more common with progressive patterns of multiple sclerosis and eventually becomes a necessity.

- **Rest and sleep** preserves physical and mental endurance, and ensures muscles have time to recover between daily activities. The need for rest and sleep may increase with disease progression.

- **Patient and family education** emphasizes the benefits of ongoing occupational performance to increase functional strength, balance, and coordination despite disease progression. Education also includes orthotic and equipment use, energy conservation techniques, and home exercise programs. Recommendations for more permanent wheelchair accessible home modifications are made to emphasize the potential for preserved independence despite physical decline.

- **Work activities** may be incorporated into intervention plans to include computer use, executive functions, and functional mobility. Activity or environmental modifications may be recommended to facilitate ongoing gainful employment while it is still possible. Eventually, the disease progression may interfere with ongoing work activities or modifications may not be granted ongoing.

- **Social interaction (play and leisure)** is encouraged with modifications as necessary. Connections with support groups are helpful to provide ongoing partnerships in the community.

- **Client factors and performance skills** initially focus on goals similar to relapsing–remitting multiple sclerosis; however, a significant improvement in strength and coordination is not as likely as disease progression occurs. Static and dynamic balance activities in sitting and standing are used to improve functional transfers from the wheelchair. Functional reaching activities in a gravity-eliminated position may be used for strengthening to improve dressing independence as a long-term goal. Mental functions are incorporated to encourage participation with daily scheduling, financial management, and medication management.

Intervention Planning

Parkinson's disease	Participation in daily activities generally remains the same and skilled occupational therapy needs are minimal during the early stages of the disease. Eventually, skilled therapy interventions are indicated to improve bilateral integration, strength, and functional mobility, fine and gross motor control, communication, and mental process skills. Lee Silverman Voice Training (LSVT) and LSVT®BIG training are incorporated into multiple treatment areas to improve motor control. Medications to manage dyskinesia are often timed to coincide with scheduled therapy or specific daily activities to maximize participation.

Table 13-5 Intervention Planning for Neurodegenerative Disease *(continued)*

- **ADLs and IADLs** are incorporated into therapy sessions during the later stages of the disease process when fine and gross motor coordination and balance impact performance, independence, and safety. Individuals are trained to perform grooming, dressing, bathing, and meal planning from a seated position if falls and safety awareness are a concern. ADLs and IADLs are also included in goals that address sequencing, initiation, and problem-solving. Adaptive equipment such as weighted silverware and weighted writing utensils encourage activity success despite tremors or dyskinesia. Durable medical equipment is introduced to improve participation in ADLs and IADLs when balance is concerned. Swallowing strategies are implemented during feeding when necessary.

- **Rest and sleep** is encouraged to improve functional endurance. Energy conservation strategies are implemented to improve physical and mental functions throughout the day.

- **Patient and family education** emphasizes ongoing activity performance to increase functional strength, balance, and coordination despite disease progression. Education also includes energy conservation techniques and home exercise programs using high-amplitude movements to improve successful carryover of motor control strategies. Recommendations for more permanent home accessibility options include installation of grab bars and limiting environmental hazards that increase the risk of falls.

- **Work activities** are possible in early stages of the disease; however, permanent disability from physical and cognitive changes is inevitable in most cases.

- **Social interaction (play and leisure)** is encouraged and may be modified to include activity or environmental modifications. Balance, endurance, and information processing speed are considered when exploring accommodations.

- **Client factors and performance skills** are reflected in treatment planning, as changes in body and mental functions occur over the course of years. A gradual decline in fine and gross motor control eventually impacts balance and functional mobility as voluntary movements such as stride length and postural reflexes become characteristically smaller and less responsive. Similarly, volume control in voice is also affected. LSVT, a trademark intervention for Parkinson's disease, encourages exaggerated voice amplitude and facial expressions to compensate for motor control changes caused by dopamine loss. High-amplitude movement is also applied to fine and gross motor control through the performance of LSVT®BIG movement strategies to improve handwriting, dynamic balance, postural control, and multidirectional movement. Mental process skills are incorporated into intervention plans to improve information processing speed, comprehension, expression, memory, attention, initiation, planning, and problem-solving.

Intervention Planning	
Alzheimer's disease	Participation in daily activities is gradually impacted by a cognitive decline manifested as forgetfulness, confusion with changing routines or difficulty with new learning. Eventually, mood changes, unawareness of deficits, visuospatial skills, and willingness to accept caregiver assistance interfere with daily occupations. Physical decline occurs in the later stages of the disease process and results in decreased balance, reflexes, and increased falls. Permanent caregiver support is inevitable.
	• **ADLs and IADLs** may not be affected from a physical perspective in the early stages of the disease; however, gradual decline in mental process skills may impact initiation and sequencing of dressing, bathing, medication management, financial management, and meal planning. The client often notices subtle changes in memory or executive functions that are not immediately reported due to embarrassment or fear of diagnosis. Family and caregivers play an essential role in encouraging independence and initiation of one's daily routine through the use of memory aids, checklists, and consistent routines. Eventually, full caregiver support is necessary to meet the physical and cognitive demands of ADLs and IADLs.

(continues)

Table 13-5 Intervention Planning for Neurodegenerative Disease (*continued*)

- **Rest and sleep** is useful in managing endurance and frustration with mental process skills.
- **Patient and family education** begins with enabling the client to maintain a certain level of autonomy using strategies to compensate for forgetfulness. Supervision from a distance may be indicated in early stages, progressing over the course of years to direct supervision and assistance daily. Caregiver support groups are beneficial to provide resources and assistance for years of potential caregiver assistance.
- **Work activities** are most often impacted in early-onset Alzheimer's disease. Job modifications may be recommended to enable continued employment until cognitive limitations prohibit on-going purposeful work.
- **Social interaction (play and leisure)** is encouraged with family and friends throughout the disease progression to promote ongoing interactions, as individuals are most comfortable with familiar people and routines. Activity modifications to simplify directions improve successful performance.
- **Client factors and performance skills** most often addressed in skilled intervention plans include mental process skills for memory, attention, new learning, comprehension, expression, planning, organization, flexibility of thought, information processing speed, initiation, visual perception, and social interaction. Memory books and familiar photographs serve as purposeful daily reminders. Over time, goals also address motor control, balance, endurance, and safety awareness. Directions are simplified and consistent routines are encouraged to maximize ongoing participation in one's daily routine. Ongoing participation with subtle cues for word finding, topographical orientation, calendar events, medication management, and financial management may minimize frustration while fostering a supportive context for the client to remain engaged. Puzzle books, newspapers/magazines, and websites such as Lumosity serve as adjuncts to stimulate the client's daily routine.

Intervention Planning	
Guillain–Barré syndrome	Participation in daily activities declines at a rapid pace over the course of days or weeks during the acute inflammatory period of peripheral nerve demyelination when initial hospitalization occurs, and persists through the plateau phase of days or weeks until no further decline is noted and progressive recovery begins. The extent of disease progression begins in the extremities and proceeds proximally to impact trunk control, reflexes, and cranial nerve innervation responsible for cardiac and respiratory functioning in severe cases. Intervention planning is unique among other neurodegenerative disease discussed in this chapter because further degeneration no longer occurs once signs of recovery begin. Progressive recovery varies from a full return of function with months of rehabilitation to incomplete recovery that may manifest as residual paraplegia or quadriplegia. • **ADLs and IADLs** are impacted immediately within days of acute symptom onset and are a significant part of the skilled therapy interventions upon initial hospitalization. The extent of disease progression will determine if the individual is able to physically participate in ADLs or if verbally directing care is more realistic in the initial stages of rehabilitation. Activity demands are modified using positioning techniques, adaptive equipment, and durable medical equipment. These accommodations may be temporary until strength returns; however, clients with greater axonal loss may pursue a return to independence with permanent modifications or from the wheelchair level if ambulation does not improve. • **Rest and sleep** is a critical component of progressive recovery as residual fatigue is commonly reported due to reduced innervation of peripheral muscles. Energy conservation techniques are incorporated to extend participation in daily activities. • **Patient and family education** includes caregiver training for home exercise programs to maintain joint integrity and strength, orthotic and equipment use, functional transfers and positioning, and modifications for activity and environmental demands.

Table 13-5 Intervention Planning for Neurodegenerative Disease (*continued*)

- **Work activities** are significantly impacted upon diagnosis and return to work is gradual with accommodation requests for activity and environmental demands as necessary. Job descriptions are useful when incorporating physical requirements into skilled therapy sessions.

- **Social interaction (play and leisure)** is impacted initially but is encouraged as soon as the client is able to tolerate activity. The presence of family and friends provides support during the acute inflammatory period and remains beneficial through the progressive recovery phase. Modifications for activity or environmental demands are incorporated into skilled therapy interventions as strength returns.

- **Client factors and performance skills** are impacted by peripheral nerve dysfunction and are included in skilled intervention plans as fine and gross motor control, upper and lower extremity strengthening, static and dynamic balance in sitting and standing, and transitional movement for functional mobility throughout an individual's daily routine. Functional reaching is addressed in a gravity-eliminated position until strength improves for movement through gravity. In-hand manipulation of coins, buttons, and silverware improves fine motor control and functional coordination for handwriting. Mental process skills are addressed if respiratory or cardiac distress resulted in mental status changes.

Data from: Forwell et al. (2014); NINDS (2013); Schultz-Krohn, Foti, and Glogoski, (2013).

the pathogenesis of each neurodegenerative disease determines referrals and next levels of care. Furthermore, a disease process characterized by cycles of relapse and remission such as MS may indicate the need for multiple episodes of hospitalization or rehabilitation throughout an individual's lifetime.

Additional sources for referral in the management of neurodegenerative disease that complement OT services include physical therapy, speech therapy, psychology, vocational rehabilitation, wheelchair seating and positioning, driver rehabilitation, assistive technology, home health care, nutrition counseling, personal training, support groups, home modification planning, and research study participation. A skilled occupational therapist works to identify and initiate referrals as necessary to ensure ongoing participation in daily occupation and provides educational training as needed.

Management and Standards of Practice

Occupational therapists and OT assistants collaborate to evaluate clients, create intervention plans, and modify priorities and goals in response to the dynamic nature of neurodegenerative disease (AOTA, 1999; Fleming et al., 2009; Forwell et al., 2014; Kuo, 2009; Schultz-Krohn et al., 2013; Takahashi & Huang, 2009). The OT team is responsible for determining upper extremity orthotic needs to support muscles and joints

while promoting function in ADLs and IADLs. They also introduce durable medical equipment used to improve endurance and safety during occupational performance including bathroom equipment, walker accessories, and grab bars.

Team and family members receive education and training in active behavioral strategies for visual scanning, memory, and energy conservation to limit the functional effects of disease progression on independence. The occupational therapist and OT assistant communicate these recommendations to the client, family, and interdisciplinary team to ensure carryover as soon as successful strategies are integrated during skilled therapy sessions. Informative updates may be shared verbally during an informal conversation or more formal training for functional transfers, home exercise programs, or assistive technology may be indicated. Informal written signage may be incorporated to remind the client, family, and team of transfer status, orthotic schedules, or swallowing precautions. Formal documentation in daily notes, progress reports, and discharge plans provides a comprehensive record of evolving needs and progression. This open verbal and written dialogue within the interdisciplinary team ensures that the client has the support needed to maximize independence in all areas of occupational performance.

Neurodegenerative disease presents ethical scenarios that impact the management of OT services. Educating clients and families on the importance of maintaining autonomy through decision-making and directing care when physical participation is no longer possible helps to address quality of life concerns. OT practitioners play an important role in supporting the need for continued skilled therapy services despite gradual muscle atrophy and functional decline with ALS, MS, Parkinson's disease, and Alzheimer's disease. Occupational therapists and assistants are also responsible for representing the client's goals in intervention and discharge planning when they differ from those of the family or other interdisciplinary team members. If the client repeatedly expresses a desire to discontinue skilled therapy in the absence of mental process skill impairments, this request must be considered and respected in an effort to enable autonomy.

On the contrary, clients with decreased executive functioning and awareness of deficits associated with MS, Parkinson's disease, and Alzheimer's disease may insist that participation in certain premorbid activities proceed without modification or restriction despite changes in motor or process skills. The OT team has an ethical responsibility to intervene and discourage activities that present safety hazards including driving, meal preparation, medication management, and work activities even if the client expresses a desire to continue. It is the role of the occupational therapist and assistant to identify accommodations or present supervision alternatives in an effort to maintain participation.

The characteristics of neurodegenerative disease have similarities and differences that the OT team considers during all stages of evaluation, intervention, and discharge planning. The greatest similarity between each disease discussed in this chapter is the presence of neurodegeneration that may affect both mental and process skills. While these degenerative changes occur more rapidly in ALS and GBS, progression occurs slowly over the course of years with MS, Parkinson's disease, and Alzheimer's disease. Similarly, the prognosis of each diagnosis varies greatly and is also reflected throughout a specific plan of care created to address an individual's needs. An ability of the skilled occupational therapist and OT assistant to incorporate this appreciation for each disease pathogenesis and prognosis ultimately ensures the best practice and continuum of care to facilitate ongoing participation in valued daily occupations.

Chapter 13 Self-Study Activities (Answers Are Provided at the End of the Chapter)

Neurodegenerative Disease Worksheet One

Fill in the blanks using the following options:

- A. Amyotrophic lateral sclerosis
- B. Parkinson's disease
- C. Relapsing and remitting multiple sclerosis
- D. Guillain–Barré syndrome
- E. Primary progressive multiple sclerosis
- F. Alzheimer's disease

1. _____ accounts for 85% of the multiple sclerosis population and is characterized by periods of exacerbation and remission with a gradual accumulation of deficits.

2. _____ accounts for 10% of the multiple sclerosis population and is characterized by steady decline of motor control without period of significant recovery.

3. _____ is characterized by a gradual onset of four cardinal signs including tremor, rigidity or stiffness, bradykinesia, and postural instability.

4. _____ is an aggressive and fatal neurodegenerative disease of unknown etiology that destroys the motor neurons associated with voluntary muscle contraction.

5. _____ is the leading cause of adult-onset neurodegenerative disease causing gradual cognitive and physical decline as a result of protein deposits in the cerebral cortex.

6. _____ is characterized by a rapid onset of motor paralysis, paresthesia, and impairments of the autonomic nervous system that targets the peripheral nervous system following by periods of plateau and progressive recovery.

Neurodegenerative Disease Worksheet Two

Complete the following lists relating to preparatory methods associated with neurodegenerative disease:

1. List four types of splints that may be used in the treatment of neurodegenerative disease to improve hand and/or foot positioning and function.

   _____

   _____

   _____

   _____

2. List five examples of wheeled seating and mobility used to improve functional positioning and independence for persons with neurodegenerative disease.

   _____

   _____

   _____

   _____

   _____

Answer the following questions as True or False.

3. _____ Management of neurodegenerative disease may occur over the course of a lifetime after initial diagnosis.

4. _____ Multiple sclerosis is often associated with a fatal prognosis soon after initial diagnosis.

5. _____ It is unnecessary to include the client in goal setting when cognitive deficits are present.

6. _____ Fine and gross motor control is almost always addressed in the treatment planning for neurodegenerative disease.

7. _____ Cognitive deficits may be included in treatment planning for multiple sclerosis and Alzheimer's disease.

8. _____ Periods of exacerbation are common in persons with multiple sclerosis and may warrant a new occupational therapy evaluation even years after initial diagnosis.

9. _____ The symptoms of bradykinesia and rigidity associated with Parkinson's disease are managed with an oral medication, levodopa.

10. _____ The acute inflammatory period of Guillain–Barré syndrome usually persists for 1 year or longer before signs of the plateau phase are present.

11. _____ Respiratory assistance may be indicated during the wheelchair-dependent period of amyotrophic lateral sclerosis.

12. _____ Financial management tasks, meal planning, and complex scheduling tasks may be used to address mental functions in persons with multiple sclerosis.

Chapter 13 Self-Study Answers

Neurodegenerative Disease Worksheet One Answers

1. Relapsing and remitting multiple sclerosis
2. Primary progressive multiple sclerosis
3. Parkinson's disease
4. Amyotrophic lateral sclerosis
5. Alzheimer's disease
6. Guillain–Barré syndrome

Neurodegenerative Disease Worksheet Two Answers

1. List four types of splints that may be used in the treatment of neurodegenerative disease to improve hand and/or foot positioning and function.
   - Short opponens splints
   - Long opponens splints
   - Resting hand splints
   - Ankle–foot orthoses
2. List five examples of wheeled seating and mobility used to improve functional positioning and independence for persons with neurodegenerative disease.
   - Rolling walkers
   - Rollator walkers
   - Manual wheelchairs
   - Power wheelchairs
   - Power-assist wheelchairs
3. True
4. False
5. False
6. True
7. True
8. True
9. True
10. False
11. True
12. True

References

American Occupational Therapy Association. (1999). *Occupational therapy practice guidelines for adults with neurodegenerative diseases: Multiple sclerosis, transverse myelitis, and amyotrophic lateral sclerosis.* Bethesda, MD: AOTA Press.

American Occupational Therapy Association. (2014). Occupational therapy practice framework: Domain and process (3rd ed.). *American Journal of Occupational Therapy, 68*(Suppl. 1), S1–S48. doi:10.5014 /ajot.2014.682006

Amyotrophic Lateral Sclerosis Association. (2010). *What is ALS?* Washington, DC: Author. Retrieved from http:// www.alsa.org/about-als

Bertram, L., & Tanzi, R. E. (2005). The genetic epidemiology of neurodegenerative disease. *Journal of Clinical Investigation, 115*(6), 1449–1457. doi:10.1172 /JCI24761

Bradley, E. (1996). *Neurology in clinical practice* (2nd ed.). Boston, MA: Butterworth-Heinemann.

Carroll, A., McDonnell, G., & Barnes, M. (2003). A review of the management of Guillain-Barre syndrome in a regional neurological rehabilitation unit. *International Journal of Rehabilitation Research, 26*(4), 297–302. doi:10.1097/01.mrr.0000102064.48781.30

Centers for Disease Control and Prevention. (2014). *Guillain-Barre syndrome: Questions and answers.* Retrieved from http://www.cdc.gov/flu/protect /vaccine/guillainbarre.htm

Conley, S. C., & Kirchner, J. T. (1999). Parkinson's disease— the shaking palsy. Underlying factors, diagnostic considerations, and clinical course. *Postgraduate Medicine, 106*(1), 39–42, 45–36, 49–50 passim.

de Lau, L. M., & Breteler, M. M. (2006). Epidemiology of Parkinson's disease. *Lancet Neurology, 5*(6), 525–535. doi:10.1016/s1474-4422(06)70471-9

Dematteis, J. A. (1996). Guillain-Barre syndrome: A team approach to diagnosis and treatment. *American Family Physician, 54*(1), 197–200. Retrieved from http://www.ncbi.nlm.nih.gov/pubmed/8677835

Fleming, R., Stone, K., & Grimell, M. (2009). Amyotrophic lateral sclerosis. In H. S. Willard, E. B. Crepeau, E. S. Cohn, & B. A. B. Schell (Eds.), *Willard & Spackman's occupational therapy* (11th ed., pp. 981–983). Baltimore, MD: Wolters Kluwer Health/Lippincott Williams & Wilkins.

Forwell, S. J., Hugos, L., Copperman, L. F., & Ghahari, S. (2014). Neurodegenerative diseases. In M. V. Radomski &

C. A. T. Latham (Eds.), *Occupational therapy for physical dysfunction* (7th ed., pp. 1077–1102). Baltimore, MD: Wolters Kluwer Health/Lippincott Williams & Wilkins.

Galvin, J. E., Fagan, A. M., Holtzman, D. M., Mintun, M. A., & Morris, J. C. (2010). Relationship of dementia screening tests with biomarkers of Alzheimer's disease. *Brain, 133*(11), 3290–3300. doi:10.1093/brain /awq204

Genetics Home Reference. (2011). *Guillain-Barre syndrome.* Retrieved from http://ghr.nlm.nih.gov/condition /guillain-barre-syndrome

Genetics Home Reference. (2012). *Amyotrophic lateral sclerosis.* Retrieved from http://ghr.nlm.nih.gov /condition/amyotrophic-lateral-sclerosis

Golisz, K. (2009). *Occupational therapy practice guidelines for adults with traumatic brain injury.* Bethesda, MD: AOTA Press.

Hoehn, M. M., & Yahr, M. D. (1967). Parkinsonism: Onset, progression and mortality. *Neurology, 17*(5), 427–442.

Hugos, C., & Copperman, L. (1999). *Workshop: The new multiple sclerosis guidelines, delivering effective comprehensive therapy services.* Monterey, CA.

Jankovic, J. (2008). Parkinson's disease: Clinical features and diagnosis. *Journal of Neurology, Neurosurgery & Psychiatry, 79*(4), 368–376. doi:10.1136/jnnp.2007 .131045

Karavatas, S. G. (2005). The role of neurodevelopmental sequencing in the physical therapy management of a geriatric patient with Guillain-Barré syndrome. *Topics in Geriatric Rehabilitation, 21*(2), 133–135. Retrieved from http://journals.lww.com/topicsingeriatricrehabilitation /Fulltext/2005/04000/The_Role_of_Neurodevelopmental _Sequencing_in_the.8.aspx

Khan, F. (2004). Rehabilitation in Guillian Barre syndrome. *Australian Family Physician, 33*(12), 1013–1017.

Khan, F., Pallant, J. F., Ng, L., & Bhasker, A. (2010). Factors associated with long-term functional outcomes and psychological sequelae in Guillain-Barre syndrome. *Journal of Neurology, 257*(12), 2024–2031. doi:10.1007/s00415-010-5653-x

Krupp, L. B., & Macallister, W. S. (2005). Treatment of pediatric multiple sclerosis. *Current Treatment Options in Neurology, 7*(3), 191–199.

Kuo, H. (2009). Common conditions: Related resources and evidence. In E. B. Crepeau, E. S. Cohn, & B. A. B. Schell (Eds.), *Willard & Spackman's occupational therapy* (11 ed., pp. 977–981). Philadelphia, PA: Lippincott Williams & Wilkins.

Kwong, J. C., Vasa, P. P., Campitelli, M. A., Hawken, S., Wilson, K., Rosella, L. C., . . . Deeks, S. L. (2013). Risk of Guillain-Barre syndrome after seasonal influenza vaccination and influenza health-care encounters: A self-controlled study. *Lancet Infectious Diseases, 13*(9), 769–776. doi:10.1016/s1473-3099(13)70104-x

Marder, K., Logroscino, G., Alfaro, B., Mejia, H., Halim, A., Louis, E., . . . Mayeux, R. (1998). Environmental risk factors for Parkinson's disease in an urban multiethnic community. *Neurology, 50*(1), 279–281.

Multiple Sclerosis Trust. (2013). *Prevalence and incidence of multiple sclerosis.* Retrieved from http://www.mstrust.org.uk/atoz/prevalence_incidence.jsp

National Institute on Aging. (2014). *2013–2014 Alzheimer's disease: Insight and challenge.* Bethesda, MD: DHHS. Retrieved from http://www.nia.nih.gov/alzheimers/publication/2013-2014-alzheimers-disease-progress-report/

National Institute of Neurological Disorders and Stroke. (2013). *Amyotrophic lateral sclerosis.* Bethesda, MD: DHHS. Retrieved from http://www.ninds.nih.gov/disorders/amyotrophiclateralsclerosis/ALS.htm

National Institute of Neurological Disorders and Stroke. (2014a). *Deep brain stimulation for Parkinson's disease fact sheet.* Bethesda, MD: DHHS. Retrieved from http://www.ninds.nih.gov/disordersdeep_brain_stimulation/detail_deep_brain_stimulation.htm

National Institute of Neurological Disorders and Stroke. (2014b). *Parkinson's disease: Hope through research.* Bethesda, MD: DHHS. Retrieved from http://www.ninds.nih.gov/disorders/parkinsons_disease/detail_parkinsons_disease.htm

National Multiple Sclerosis Society. (2015). *About MS.* Retrieved from http://www.nationalmssociety.org/What-is-MS/Who-Gets-MS

Neudert, C., Wasner, M., & Borasio, G. D. (2004). Individual quality of life is not correlated with health-related quality of life or physical function in patients with amyotrophic lateral sclerosis. *Journal of Palliative Medicine, 7*(4), 551–557. doi:10.1089/1096621041838443

Noseworthy, J. H., Lucchinetti, C., Rodriguez, M., & Weinshenker, B. G. (2000). Multiple sclerosis. *New England Journal of Medicine, 343*(13), 938–952. doi:10.1056/NEJM200009283431307

Polman, C. H., Reingold, S. C., Banwell, B., Clanet, M., Cohen, J. A., Filippi, M., . . . Wolinsky, J. S. (2011). Diagnostic criteria for multiple sclerosis: 2010 revisions to the McDonald criteria. *Annals of Neurology, 69*(2), 292–302. doi:10.1002/ana.22366

Ramachandran, T. S. (2012). *Acute inflammatory demyelinating polyradiculoneuropathy workup.* Retrieved from http://emedicine.medscape.com/article/1169959-workup#a0723

Robberecht, W., & Brown, R. H. (1996). Etiology and pathogenesis of ALS: Biochemical, genetic, and other theories. In J. M. Belsh & P. L. Schiffman (Eds.), *ALS diagnosis and management for the clinician.* Armonk, NY: Futura.

Rodriguez-Oroz, M. C., Obeso, J. A., Lang, A. E., Houeto, J. L., Pollak, P., Rehncrona, S., . . . Van Blercom, N. (2005). Bilateral deep brain stimulation in Parkinson's disease: A multicentre study with 4 years follow-up. *Brain, 128*(Pt 10), 2240–2249. doi:10.1093/brain/awh571

Schultz-Krohn, W., Foti, D., & Glogoski, C. (2013). *Degenerative diseases of the central nervous system* (7th ed.). St. Louis, MO: Elsevier.

Takahashi, K., & Huang, P. (2009). Parkinson's disease. In H. S. Willard, E. B. Crepeau, E. S. Cohn, & B. A. B. Schell (Eds.), *Willard & Spackman's occupational therapy* (11th ed., pp. 976–980). Baltimore, MD: Wolters Kluwer Health/Lippincott Williams & Wilkins.

Trapp, B. D., & Nave, K. A. (2008). Multiple sclerosis: An immune or neurodegenerative disorder? *Annual Review of Neuroscience, 31,* 247–269. doi:10.1146/annurev.neuro.30.051606.094313

Trapp, B. D., Peterson, J., Ransohoff, R. M., Rudick, R., Mörk, S., & Bö, L. (1998). Axonal transection in the lesions of multiple sclerosis. *New England Journal of Medicine, 338*(5), 278–285. doi:10.1056/NEJM199801293380502

van Doorn, P. A., Ruts, L., & Jacobs, B. C. (2008). Clinical features, pathogenesis, and treatment of Guillain-Barre syndrome. *Lancet Neurology, 7*(10), 939–950. doi:10.1016/s1474-4422(08)70215-1

Occupational Functioning: Physical Disabilities (Musculoskeletal and Orthopedics) Days 10–14

Orthopedic Conditions of the Shoulder

Darren Gustitus, Jeffrey Placzek, and Fredrick D. Pociask

Learning Objectives

- Describe standardized assessments designed to assess functional limitations of the upper extremity.
- Describe the components of a shoulder assessment and apply these findings to a treatment plan.
- Describe key pathology, etiology, and epidemiology for proximal humeral fractures, clavicle fractures, acromioclavicular separation, shoulder dislocation, rotator cuff tendinosis and tears, labral tears, adhesive capsulitis, and shoulder arthritis.
- Compare and contrast clinical presentation for the shoulder conditions listed above.
- Describe diagnostic tests for the shoulder conditions listed above.
- Describe medical and surgical procedures for the shoulder conditions listed above.
- List medical/surgical precautions and contraindications for the shoulder conditions listed above.
- Describe physical agent modalities and manual techniques used for pain management.
- Describe the treatment interventions of manual techniques, range of motion, and strengthening.
- Describe techniques utilized to address activities of daily living (ADLs) limitations.
- Describe conservative and postsurgical therapeutic interventions for diagnoses listed above.

Key Terms

- *Arthroscopy*: Examination, diagnosis, and/or treatment of a joint using an endoscope that is inserted through a small incision in the skin.
- *Avascular necrosis*: Death of bone tissue secondary to a lack of blood supply.
- *Computed tomography (CT)*: CT is a noninvasive imaging technology that utilizes a rotating x-ray emitter to generate detailed cross-sectional computer images of body tissues.
- *Concentric contraction*: A contraction in which the muscle is actively shortening.
- *Eccentric contraction*: A contraction in which the muscle is actively lengthening.
- *Hypermobility*: Movement greater than normal.
- *Idiopathic*: Any disease or disease process for which the cause is unknown.
- *Isokinetic contraction*: A contraction in which movement occurs at a constant speed.
- *Isometric contraction*: A contraction in which the muscle length and joint angle do not change.
- *Isotonic contraction*: A contraction in which the length of the muscle changes; may be either concentric or eccentric.
- *Magnetic resonance imaging (MRI)*: MRI is a noninvasive imaging technology that utilizes a magnetic field and radio waves to create detailed computer images of body tissues.

Introduction

The shoulder is a complicated structure comprised of dynamic movements occurring between the scapula, rib cage, clavicle, sternum, and humerus. Any disruption within this system may result in a significant loss of function secondary to pain, loss of motion, weakness, and/or instability. Treatment of these conditions requires a thorough understanding of this system, communication with the physician, and the ability to apply appropriate treatment strategies to alleviate the client's symptoms and return them to an acceptable level of function.

Standardized Assessments

Orthopedic conditions of the shoulder follow similar screening, assessment, and evaluation procedures to the rest of the body. The following provides an outline of commonly used screening and assessments.

- *The Disabilities of the Arm, Shoulder, and Hand (DASH)*: The DASH is a 30-question assessment that addresses both the client's level of disability and symptoms as related to their upper extremity pathology/disability (Beaton et al., 2001).
- *American Shoulder and Elbow Surgeons (ASES) Shoulder Score*: Utilizes both a client-derived subjective assessment and physician-derived objective assessment. The subjective assessment addresses both pain and function. The ASES is often used to assess clients with shoulder instability, rotator cuff disease, and glenohumeral arthritis (Kocher et al., 2005).
- *Shoulder Disability Questionnaire (SDQ)*: Developed to primarily assess the change over time in pain-related disability as related to shoulder pathology. The items within the questionnaire were chosen to detect clinically relevant changes as related to shoulder pathology (de Winter, van der Heijden, Scholten, van der Windt, & Bouter, 2007).
- *Shoulder Pain and Disability Index (SPADI)*: Designed for use in an outpatient setting, this assessment attempts to measure current shoulder pain and disability (Breckenridge & McAuley, 2011).
- *Quantitative Test of Upper Extremity Function*: Assesses the ability to perform general arm and hand activities of daily living (ADLs). It utilizes simple materials to perform daily tasks: gripping using various grasp patterns, fine prehension, pronation, supination, arm elevation, external rotation, and writing skills (Kasch & Walsh, 2013).

Shoulder Assessment Components

History

A thorough assessment is necessary to identify the client's disorder, condition or injury, and impact on function. The history should minimally include the client's age, hand dominance, occupation, mechanism of injury, medical and surgical treatment received thus far, and further surgery or conservative interventions that may be planned.

Inspection

In terms of inspection, it is important to observe for symmetry, abnormal cervical and thoracic curvatures, muscle atrophy evident in the periscapular muscles, altered scapular position(s), skin integrity/wound status, and guarded and antalgic positioning (Kasch & Walsh, 2013).

Palpation

Palpation of the following structures is necessary in order to formulate an appropriate treatment plan. This includes, but is not limited to, palpation of the greater and lesser tuberosities, sternoclavicular joint, acromioclavicular (AC) joint, long head of the biceps/bicipital groove, the periscapular muscles, and the cervical spine.

Range of Motion (ROM) Assessment

ROM measurements include both active range of motion (AROM) and passive range of motion (PROM). To assess for AROM, it is optimal to observe shoulder motion during ADLs or while performing a functional ROM assessment. ROM assessment helps determine the need for assistive devices, and to document progress. The therapist should also note the client's fluidity of movement and pain occurring with movement. Assessment of PROM provides information about the joint capsule, associated ligaments, muscle extensibility, and end-feel (Brun, 2012).

Soft-Tissue Assessment

Limitations can happen in joint play (i.e., accessory motion) secondary to trauma, immobilization, or disuse. Limitations or pain with performance may be indicative of potential tightness in the joint capsule, soft-tissue restrictions, muscle guarding, ligamentous tightness, or adherence (Kasch & Walsh, 2013).

Strength/Manual Muscle Testing

Assessment of a muscle provides objective data on the client's ability to resist movement. Manual muscle testing scores the strength of shoulder muscles based on the amount of resistance perceived by the therapist via manual resistance, or by means of a handheld force dynameter. Muscle weakness with shoulder injuries typically occurs as a result of the injury, as well as from disuse (i.e., inactivity) and immobilization. Muscle strength is evaluated in order to:

1. Establish a baseline and assess progress.
2. Facilitate diagnosis in some neuromuscular conditions.
3. Determine effects of weakness on functional performance.
4. Assess the need for compensatory techniques or assistive devices.
5. Identify muscle imbalances (Poole, 2009).

Activities of Daily Living

Utilization of function using an aforementioned standardized assessment, including DASH, ASES, SDQ, SPADI, and the Quantitative Test of Upper Extremity Function, can provide insight into the client's ADLs. In addition, a formal interview with the client, as well as observed performance of functional tasks that may be limited by the client's pathology (e.g., placing items overhead, hair care, tucking in a shirt, and donning a belt), should be included in the assessment.

Upper Quarter Neurologic Screen

This screen is performed by a therapist with training in performance. Improper assessment of this region can result in aggravation of the client's condition (Kasch & Walsh, 2013). Screening includes a postural assessment and AROM of the cervical and thoracic spine. **Table 14-1** describes "key" regions of sensory loss (i.e., dermatomal changes), weakness (i.e., myotomal changes), and potential diminished or absent reflexes, as they relate to cervical spine nerve root irritation (i.e., radiculopathy).

Interventions

Although each shoulder condition will include specific interventions, the following outline provides a guide of commonly used interventions for orthopedic conditions of the shoulder and shoulder complex.

Pain Management Techniques

Various pain management techniques can be incorporated into treatment of orthopedic shoulder conditions. These typically include the following:

1. *Transcutaneous electrical nerve stimulation (TENS)*: Used to stimulate the afferent A fibers. High frequency to stimulate release of morphine-like neural hormones. Low frequency to stimulate encephalin release.
2. *Elastic therapeutic taping*: Provides support to weakened muscles, decreases swelling by stimulating the lymphatic system, and decreases pain by increasing the somatosensory system.
3. *Moist heat packs*: Used prior to AROM, PROM, joint mobilizations, and soft-tissue mobilizations to reduce pain and muscle spasms, and increase extensibility of collagen.

Table 14-1 Nerve Root (NR) and Key Neurological Findings

NR	Dermatome	Myotome	Reflex
C4	Supraclavicular region	None (diaphragm)	
C5	Lateral shoulder and upper arm	Biceps brachii, supraspinatus, and infraspinatus	Biceps brachii (C5 and **C6**)
C6	Lateral lower arm and forearm, and the first two digits	Brachioradialis and wrist extensors	Biceps brachii (C5 and **C6**) Brachioradialis (C5, **C6**, and C7)
C7	Dorsal forearm and the third digit Medial and lateral aspects of the second and fourth digits, respectively, with some variation	Triceps long head, wrist flexors, finger extensors, and abductor pollicis brevis	Triceps brachii (C6, **C7**, and C8)
C8	Medial forearm and the fourth and fifth digits	Flexor digitorum, adductor pollicis, and abductor digiti minimi	
T1	Medial distal arm and medial proximal forearm	Interossei	

Notes: Neurological distributions will vary slightly between individuals as a function of normal variation. Bolded reflex NR levels reflect primary innervation; primary innervation for the biceps brachii reflex varies between references.

Data from Adler, C. (2013). Spinal Cord Injury. In L. W. Pedretti, H. M. Pendleton, & W. Schultz-Krohn (Eds.), Pedretti's occupational therapy: practice skills for physical dysfunction (7th ed., pp. 954–982). St. Louis, Mo.: Elsevier.

4. *Deep heat ultrasound*: Used to decrease soft-tissue tightness and to treat subacute (i.e., in some instances) and chronic inflammation.
5. *Cold packs*: Used to help manage acute inflammation and edema.
6. *Iontophoresis*: Used to decrease pain and to help manage acute inflammation (Poole, 2009).

Manual Techniques

Manual techniques are used in cooperation with thermal modalities, electrical stimulation, dynamic splinting, and A/PROM for the treatment of joint stiffness. Grades I and II joint mobilizations are helpful for pain relief and preparation for A/PROM. Occupational therapy practitioners not trained in performance in manual techniques, including joint mobilization, should not attempt performing these techniques (Donatelli, Ruivo, Thurner, & Ibrahim, 2014).

Range of Motion

Table 14-2 provides a description of the type of ROM and corresponding definitions, resistance, and precautions.

Strengthening

The following provides an outline and examples of various types of muscle contractions and their definitions:

- *Isometric without resistance*: Contraction of muscle for five seconds. Used when motion is prohibited.
- *Isotonic resistance*: Isotonic contractions against resistance provided by dumbbells, TheraBand, springs, and weights changes the length of the muscle (i.e., concentric shortens, eccentric lengthens).
- *Isometric resistance*: Isometric contraction against an immovable surface.

- *Isokinetic exercise*: Exercise using a machine that controls the speed of the contraction within a specified ROM.

Physical Agent Modalities

Physical agent modalities are preparatory treatment techniques used to prepare a client for engagement into functional tasks, which may include the following:

- Moist and dry heat
- Cold packs and ice massage
- Ultrasound
- Electrotherapy

Activities of Daily Living

Functional engagement in ADLs is the ultimate goal of occupational therapy. When orthopedic shoulder pathologies are involved, this may include training in the following:

- Utilization of adaptive devices.
- Utilization of adaptive/compensatory techniques for temporary use.
- Instruction of precautions related to diagnosis and/or surgical procedure.
- Instruction in energy conservation and work simplification techniques.

Shoulder Complex Pathology

Proximal Humeral Fractures

Description: Proximal humeral fractures result from a fall on an outstretched arm or from a direct fall on the shoulder itself and account for approximately 4–5% of

Table 14-2 ROM Types		
Type	**Definition**	**Precautions**
PROM	Passive range of motion that is typically used on joints that are inactive.	Inflammation and limited sensation for pain
Isotonic AAROM	Active contraction through available ROM, followed by assistance from an external source through additional ROM	Increasing ROM should be gradual with attention to pain and weakness
Isotonic AROM	Movement through available ROM that is typically fully controlled and completed by the client.	Poor muscles move in gravity-eliminated plane. Fair muscles move against gravity

Data from Poole, J. (2009). Musculoskeletal factors. In H. S. Willard, E. B. Crepeau, E. S. Cohn, & B. A. B. Schell (Eds.), Willard & Spackman's occupational therapy (11th ed., pp. 658–680). Philadelphia: Wolters Kluwer Health/Lippincott Williams & Wilkins.

all fractures (Bell, 2013; Bell & Cadet, 2014). Proximal humeral fractures occur most commonly in the elderly, older than age 65 (e.g., secondary due to low energy trauma), but can occur in younger adults (e.g., higher energy trauma) (Bell, 2013). Fractures of the proximal humerus often result in long-term ROM deficits; however, most deficits are well tolerated if acceptable overall function is obtained (Bell, 2013; Bell & Cadet, 2014). Neer's classification system recognizes four parts to the proximal humerus including the head, lesser tuberosity, greater tuberosity, and proximal shaft. Fragments are counted when displaced greater than 1 centimeter or angulated 45°; fracture fragments are displaced by the deforming forces acting on them by shoulder musculature. Complications include axillary and suprascapular nerve injury, and avascular necrosis can result from four part fractures disrupting the blood flow to the humeral head (Bell, 2013; Carofino & Leopold, 2013).

Clinical presentation: The affected extremity will exhibit evidence of trauma, such as ecchymosis and swelling. Neurovascular injury may be present, particularly with high energy trauma (Bell & Cadet, 2014).

Common diagnostic tests: X-rays including true anteroposterior (AP), outlet, and axillary views are typically sufficient to evaluate proximal humeral fractures. A computed tomography (CT) scan is indicated for severely comminuted and displaced fractures; magnetic resonance imaging (MRI) may be useful in determining the integrity of the rotator cuff when deciding between open reduction internal fixation (ORIF) and arthroplasty (Bell, 2013).

Common medical and surgical procedures: The majority of proximal humeral fractures are minimally displaced and may be treated with a sling for three to four weeks and then with a progressive therapy program. Most clients can expect 130° of elevation with minor weakness and functional rotation. Displaced fractures can be treated with locked proximal humeral plates, intermedullary nails for displaced neck fractures, or shoulder arthroplasty. Reverse shoulder arthroplasty may be useful in the elderly with a severe fracture, or concurrent arthritis or rotator cuff tear (Bell, 2013; Carofino & Leopold, 2013).

Precautions and contraindications: Early aggressive PROM or AROM may further displace fracture or tuberosities.

Interventions

The primary goals of conservative treatment include pain relief, increased ROM, and increased strength, while allowing for the approximation and healing of the bony fragments. Clinically, treatment protocols are based on the classification of the fracture and surgical procedure performed. Conservative treatments for proximal humeral fractures are described below.

- *Immobilization*: Immobilization typically includes use of a sling for up to eight weeks (Maher, 2014).
- *Manual techniques*: Manual techniques include PROM and passive stretching. However, there is disagreement in the orthopedic profession with regard to the safety of performing PROM with fractures. It is extremely important that the occupational therapy practitioners be aware of the physician's views on this topic. Similarly, passive stretching is contraindicated during the early phases of treatment, but may be utilized upon fracture healing to achieve end-range motions (Maher, 2014).
- *Therapeutic exercise*: Exercise includes progression from PROM to active-assistive range of motion (AAROM) in a scapular plane and external rotation within an arc of motion dictated by the physician's treatment protocols. Further progression includes AROM and light self-care as indicated with discontinuation of the sling at eight weeks and strengthening beginning at eight weeks (Maher, 2014).
- *Home exercise program (HEP)*: Home exercise programming may include pendulum exercises for management of pain and stiffness, and active use of noninvolved joints above and below the site of injury. Progression of home exercise begins with PROM, which progresses to AAROM, and AROM within a controlled arc of motion dictated by the physician's treatment protocols, and progressive strengthening as tolerated with an emphasis placed on glenohumeral and scapular stabilization (Maher, 2014).
- *Physical agent modalities*: Use of modalities may include cold packs, hot packs, ultrasound as appropriate, and electrical stimulation (e.g., TENS) for symptom management.

Clavicle Fractures

Description: Clavicle fractures typically result from a direct fall on the shoulder or direct blow to the shoulder itself. Clavicle fractures are typically from higher energy injuries to the lateral shoulder itself. Clavicle fractures are described by the location, such as proximal third, middle third, or distal third, with the middle third fractures accounting for approximately 80% of clavicular fractures (Bell & Cadet, 2014; Dunwoody & McKee, 2013). The annual reported incidents of clavicular fractures is approximately 29 per 100,000 population or approximately 2.6–4% of all fractures, with fractures occurring more commonly in males younger than 20 years of age (Dunwoody & McKee, 2013; Sajadi, 2014a).

Clinical presentation: Clavicle fractures present with swelling and ecchymosis about the clavicle. Significant displacement may result in tenting of the skin and shoulder ptosis (Sajadi, 2014a).

Common diagnostic tests: Two view clavicle x-rays are usually sufficient to evaluate clavicle fractures. A CT scan may be needed to evaluate comminuted or far medial or lateral intraarticular fractures (Dunwoody & McKee, 2013; Sajadi, 2014a).

Common medical and surgical procedures: Most minimally displaced or angulated fractures do not require surgery and can be treated in a sling or figure eight brace (Sajadi, 2014b). Fractures that are comminuted, completely displaced, or shortened greater than 2 centimeters can be repaired with plate and screw fixation or an intramedullary screw (Bell & Cadet, 2014; Dunwoody & McKee, 2013).

Precautions and contraindications: Aggressive early motion is contraindicated as glenohumeral stiffness rarely occurs after clavicle fractures.

Interventions

Nonoperative management of clavicle fractures is uncommon. Operative management of clavicle fractures is more likely due to a secondary instance of malunion. Clients with malunion are more likely to have increased pain and weakness, with decreased ROM typically in abduction (Edwards, Whittle, & Wood, 2000). Therapy is also more likely in instances of brachial plexus irritation or the development of thoracic outlet syndrome secondary to the clavicle fracture (Oh, Kim, Lee, Shin, & Gong, 2011). Typically, most medial and lateral clavicle fractures can be treated nonsurgically with satisfactory outcomes (van der Meijden, Gaskill, & Millett, 2012). Clients involved in athletics are typically allowed to return to noncontact sports at six weeks postinjury. Those clients returning to contact sports typically return 8–12 weeks postinjury (Pujalte & Housner, 2008).

AC Separation

Description: AC separations occur after a fall on the tip of the shoulder with the arm in an adducted position or a direct blow to the superior aspect of the shoulder. The AC joint is most frequently injured in physically active individuals, such as athletes competing in contact sports (Ahmad & Levine, 2014; Klepps, 2013). AC separations result in the disruption of the AC ligaments and coracoclavicular (CC) ligaments with subsequent elevation of the clavicle in relation to the acromion (Klepps, 2013).

Clinical presentation: Clinical presentation typically includes pain in the anterosuperior shoulder and directly over the AC joint, as well as pain with horizontal adduction, and with combined shoulder extension and internal rotation. Pain may also be reproduced with an active compression test and with anterior–posterior stresses applied to the clavicle (Ahmad & Levine, 2014). Clinical presentation, diagnostic tests, and treatment for AC separation are further described in **Table 14-3**.

Table 14-3 Clinical Presentation, Diagnostic Tests, and Treatment of AC Separation

Type	AC Ligaments	CC Ligaments	Radiographs	Treatment
Type I	Sprained	Intact	Normal	Rest/therapy
Type II	Torn	Sprained	Normal or slight elevation	Rest/therapy
Type III	Torn	Torn	Elevated 25–100%	Conservative or surgical
Type IV	Torn	Torn	Posterior/superior displacement of the clavicle	Surgical
Type V	Torn	Torn	Clavicle elevated 100–300%	Surgical
Type VI	Torn	Torn	Clavicle displaced inferior to the coracoid	Surgical

Modified from Klepps, S. (2013). Classification and Treatment of Acromioclavicular Separations In G. P. Nicholson (Ed.), Orthopaedic Knowledge Update: Shoulder and Elbow 4 (4 ed., pp. 467–475). Rosemont, IL: American Academy of Orthopaedic Surgeons.

Common diagnostic tests: Pain is typically elicited with horizontal crossed arm adduction and with O'Brien's testing (Cleland, Koppenhaver, & Netter, 2011). Special radiographs include Zanca view (i.e., AC Joint AP view with 15° of superior angulation) or weighted stress views where a 10-pound weight is suspended around the wrists and bilateral AP views are obtained (Carofino & Leopold, 2013).

Common medical and surgical procedures: Surgical procedures include any number of procedures which attempt to reduce the clavicle (e.g., pins, screws, and sutures). Most procedures utilize a tendon graft, suture, or Dacron® tape around or through the coracoid which is then secured over the top of the clavicle, recreating the trapezoid and conoid ligaments (Klepps, 2013).

Precautions and contraindications: Avoid early aggressive motion to help prevent severe hypermobility at the AC joint.

Interventions

There are three types of interventions that include variations of home programs, modalities, manual techniques, exercise, and ADLs.

- *Type 1*: Consists of a mild sprain of the AC ligament with no tearing of the ligamentous structures at the AC or CC joints. Treatment includes an ice pack for the first 24–48 hours, a sling for 7–10 days, gentle ROM, and pendulum exercises on days 2–3 and gentle AROM; manual techniques are not indicated. In terms of ADLs, it is important for individuals to avoid heavy ADLs until ROM is painless and the client has no point tenderness at the AC joint (Manske, 2011).

- *Type 2*: Consists of a complete tear of the AC ligament with a sprain to the CC ligament. Treatment includes an ice pack for 1–2 days, a sling for 1–2 weeks, and gentle ROM on day 7; manual techniques are not indicated. ADLs may include use of the client's arm for light ADLs beginning on day 7, and potential use in heavy lifting, pushing, pulling, and contact sports at week 6 (Manske, 2011).

- *Type 3*: A complete tearing of the CC and AC ligaments, with an inferiorly displaced shoulder. Treatment is indicated for operative treatment in active and laboring clients. The home program includes an ice pack for 1–2 days and sling use. Manual techniques can ensue with gentle PROM on day 7 and exercise with functional ROM on day 7, as well as full ROM at 2–3 weeks (Manske, 2011).

Postsurgical treatment is indicated for AC joint stabilization. Interventions typically include AAROM for flexion, external rotation, and internal rotation, pendulums, capsular stretching, pulleys into flexion (i.e., although it is important to restrict horizontal adduction and abduction), and progression to an appropriate home program as indicated in **Table 14-4**. Physical agent modalities

Table 14-4 Exercises for Postsurgical AC Joint Stabilization	
Time Line	**Exercises**
Weeks 1–2	• AAROM for flexion, external rotation, and internal rotation • Isometric strengthening for external rotation, internal rotation, abduction, extension, biceps, and triceps. Resisted shoulder flexion is not performed • Isotonic strengthening for external rotation and internal rotation
Week 3	• Isotonic strengthening for abduction, extension, internal rotation, external rotation, biceps, and triceps • Scapular strengthening • PNF patterns
Week 6	• Add light strengthening into flexion at week 6 • Upper extremity endurance training at week 6
Weeks 8–16	• Continue strengthening • Add resistance to PNF patterns • Scapular strengthening • Rhythmic stabilization • Plyometrics to upper extremity

PNF, Proprioceptive neuromuscular facilitation.
Data from Manske, R. C. (2011). Shoulder Injuries. In S. B. Brotzman & K. E. Wilk (Eds.), Clinical Orthopaedic Rehabilitation: An Evidence-Based Approach (3rd ed., pp. 82–210). Philadelphia: Mosby.

include heat, ice, electrical stimulation, and ultrasound. Manual techniques can begin during the first week with capsular stretching. Ultimately, the goal of treatment is to progress to full functional recovery by 16 weeks postsurgery.

Shoulder Dislocation

Description: Most shoulder dislocations occur in an anterior inferior direction due to anteriorly directed trauma to a shoulder in an abducted and externally rotated position. Posterior dislocations may occur after grand mal seizure due to the strong pull of the internal rotators or after a fall on an adducted, internally rotated arm (Van Thiel, Heard, Romeo, & Provencher, 2013). Dislocation of the shoulder requires and results in tears of the joint capsule and glenoid labrum. The incidence of shoulder dislocation reported for the United States in 2010 was approximately 24 per 100,000 population, with greater prevalence in males, and in individuals between the age of 15 and 29, and 70 years of age and older (Van Thiel et al., 2013).

Clinical presentation: The arm is usually held across the body in internal rotation with varying degrees of abduction depending on the direction of the dislocation, with complaints of severe acute pain (Van Thiel et al., 2013).

Common diagnostic tests: X-rays in three views—true AP, axillary, and scapular lateral—are sufficient to diagnose an acute dislocation. CT scan or MRI may be used to evaluate Hill–Sachs lesions (i.e., compression fracture of the posterior lateral humeral head) or rotator cuff tears and labral tears. A Bankart lesion is a tear of the anterior inferior labrum off the glenoid rim (Van Thiel et al., 2013).

Common medical and surgical procedures: Acute reduction is undertaken in the emergency room after radiographs are taken. Immobilization up to six weeks may be required to reduce the risk of redislocation in young adults. Immediate gentle motion is indicated in older adults to prevent adhesive capsulitis. Arthroscopic repair of the glenoid labrum is indicated in cases of recurrent dislocation. Tuberosity fractures may require ORIF if displaced greater than 3–5 millimeters. Rotator cuff tears may require repair if large and symptomatic (Van Thiel et al., 2013).

Precautions and contraindications: Rotator cuff tears, axillary nerve injuries, and fractures may accompany a shoulder dislocation. Rotator cuff tears are more common in client's over 40 years of age (Van Thiel et al., 2013).

Interventions

- *HEP*: Home programs for shoulder dislocations vary given the age of the client. Sling immobilization is indicated for 6 weeks with less than 20-year olds, for 2–3 weeks for 20–30-year olds, for 10–14 days for greater than 30-year olds, and for 3–5 days for greater than 40-year olds (Manske, 2011).
- *Physical agent modalities*: Include moist heat, ice packs, ultrasound, and high volt stimulation.
- *Manual techniques*: Include PROM per age appropriate immobilization protocol as described above, and avoidance of provocative positions that may cause instability (i.e., abduction with external rotation or extension). At weeks 3–4, the goal of ROM is 140° of flexion and 40° of external rotation with the arm at the side. At weeks 4–8, the goal is 160° of flexion and 40° of external rotation with the arm at 30°–45° of abduction, and at weeks 8–12, the goal is end range and posterior capsular stretching (Manske, 2011).
- *Exercise*: Exercises for nonoperative anterior shoulder instability are outlined in **Table 14-5**.
- *ADLs*: At 12–16 weeks, clients typically prepare to return to normal functioning and sports activities (Manske, 2011).

Rotator Cuff Tendinosis and Tears

Description: Rotator cuff tendons degenerate with age resulting in progressive degeneration and often tearing of the tendon from the tuberosity. Most cuff tears are degenerative in nature, although some are traumatic in origin (Ilkhani-Pour, Dunkman, & Soslowsky, 2013). The rotator cuff has a relative avascular zone that degenerates with normal aging. Rotator cuff pathology may be accelerated by extrinsic factors such as compression from acromial osteophytes, and intrinsic factors such as vascularity, metabolic factors (e.g., diabetes), and genetic factors (Sugaya, 2013). Rotator cuff tears are typically classified as partial thickness or full thickness. Full-thickness tears are described based on size, small <1 centimeter, medium 1–3 centimeters, large 3–5 centimeters, and massive >5 centimeters (Cofield, 1982). Cadaver and MRI studies have reported a prevalence of

Table 14-5 Exercise Protocol for Nonoperative Anterior Shoulder Instability

Timeline	Exercises
Week 3	• PROM/AAROM/AROM within 140° of flexion, and 40° of external rotation with the arm at the side • Closed chain isometric strengthening of internal rotation, external rotation, and flexion • Closed chain isometric scapular stabilization strengthening
Weeks 4–8	• PROM/AAROM/AROM within 160° of flexion, and 40° of external rotation with the arm in 30°–45° of abduction • Strengthening of rotator cuff and scapular stabilizers • Closed chain progressing to open chain; to strengthen external rotation, internal rotation, abduction, and flexion
Weeks 8–12	• Posterior capsule stretching • Continued strengthening
Weeks 12–16	• Functional strengthening

Data from Manske, R. C. (2011). Shoulder Injuries. In S. B. Brotzman & K. E. Wilk (Eds.), Clinical Orthopaedic Rehabilitation: An Evidence-Based Approach (3rd ed., pp. 82–210). Philadelphia: Mosby.

full-thickness rotator cuff tears between approximately 13 and 32%, and a prevalence of 20% in asymptomatic individuals as determined by MRI (Lo, 2013). The prevalence of full-thickness rotator cuff tears in individuals 50 years of age and older is approximately 50%, with the prevalence of massive rotator cuff tears ranging from 10 to 40% (Hampton, Delaney, & Higgins, 2013; Krishnan, Rudolph, & Garofalo, 2013).

Clinical presentation: Pain is typically felt in the anterior lateral shoulder and down the upper arm. Tendinopathy results in pain, limited ROM, impingement signs, and night pain limiting rest. Further tearing can result in worsening the above complaints and significant weakness and disability (Edwards & Galatz, 2014; Sugaya, 2013).

Common diagnostic tests: Strength testing of the rotator cuff along with impingement signs is highly predictive of rotator cuff tears. MRI and ultrasound are highly sensitive for diagnosing rotator cuff tears (Edwards & Galatz, 2014; Sugaya, 2013).

Common medical and surgical procedures: Most rotator cuff tendinopathies will resolve with time, exercise, modalities, and the use of cortisone injections when necessary. Arthroscopic or open repair of the rotator cuff is considered with symptomatic tears that are unresponsive to conservative treatment (Jobin & Yamaguchi, 2013). Better strength outcomes are achieved with complete healing of the rotator cuff. Proximal migration of the humeral head, fatty infiltration of the rotator cuff, diabetes, smoking, and age >65 are negative prognostic surgical

factors (Angeline & Dines, 2013; Edwards & Galatz, 2014; Sugaya, 2013).

Precautions and contraindications: Exercises for the rotator cuff should not produce impingement-like pain. Mobility in the postoperative period needs to be limited per the surgeon's instructions to allow adequate healing time for the rotator cuff (i.e., typically up to six weeks). Strengthening is delayed until 12 weeks postoperatively (Manske, 2011).

Interventions

Rotator cuff tears require essential training, communication for client education, and activity modification.

- *Home program*: Sleeping postures, such as an avoidance of sleeping with the arm above the head or sleeping in an adducted and internally rotated position is important to communicate with the client, as well as awareness that therapy and their home program should be pain free. Equally, painful and aggravating movements or ADLs should be avoided. Home exercises should correlate with treatment provided, with an emphasis placed on pain management, PROM, and strengthening per the client's tolerance (Maher, 2014).
- *Physical agent modalities*: Include moist heat (e.g., to stimulate blood flow and decrease pain and stiffness), electrical stimulation, and cold packs (Itoi, 2013).
- *Manual techniques*: Include PROM to maintain or increase ROM of the shoulder.

- *Therapeutic exercise*: Includes AROM once there is decreased pain, and isometric and isotonic strengthening exercises for increased rotator cuff and scapular stabilization (Itoi, 2013).

Postsurgical interventions: Client education and activity modification on sleeping postures, awareness that therapy and ADLs should be pain free, and training in one-handed ADL techniques can be performed if necessary (Conti et al., 2009). Therapy for large to massive-sized tears requires a slower progression of treatment, frequent communication with the surgeon, and lower expectations for functional outcomes.

The size of the tear and orders from the physician will dictate exercise selection and timeline. For small to medium-sized tears, the postoperative home program typically includes the following:

- Pendulum exercises for the management of pain and stiffness.
- Passive shoulder elevation while lying in supine.
- Passive shoulder internal and external rotation using a dowel rod with the shoulder in slight abduction while lying in supine.
- Overhead pulleys can be used if the surgeon has requested their use; however, excessive exercises in flexion may irritate the repair.
- Progression of HEP in accordance with treatment for AAROM, AROM, and strengthening (Conti et al., 2009).

It is also important for the clients to wear a shoulder immobilizer with an abduction pillow between exercises. Modalities typically include moist heat and ultrasound. Manual techniques usually involve pain-free PROM within established limits of the surgeon's protocol. Progression to stretching to achieve end-range motion of the shoulder is indicated by the physician. Exercises typically include the following:

- AAROM with a progression of AROM occurs per physician's orders. Care should be taken not to perform activities that cause any aggravation to the repair.
  - ROM should begin with gravity-eliminated techniques and progress to exercise against gravity.
- Strengthening of the rotator cuff and scapular stabilizers can occur as indicated by the referring physician.
- Progress to functional strengthening as appropriate.

- Progress to sport-specific strengthening as appropriate (Conti et al., 2009).

ADLs: Light ADLs can be initiated at six to eight weeks and progress as tolerated. Light ADLs above the shoulder level can be performed as tolerated in therapy. A full return to ADL performance can typically occur between 4 and 6 months postoperative (Harwin, Birns, Mbabuike, Porter, & Galano, 2014).

Labral Tears

Description: Tears of the glenoid labrum may occur from overuse (e.g., repetitive overhead athletics), trauma (e.g., fall on an outstretched arm), or degenerative conditions (Chang, Mohana-Borges, Borso, & Chung, 2008). Tears are described as anterior, posterior, circumferential, or superior (Andrews & Shore, 2013; Mazzocca et al., 2011). Superior labral tears or SLAP tears (i.e., superior labrum, anterior to posterior) are subdivided into four types—Type I: degenerative fraying, Type II: avulsion of superior labrum and biceps, Type III: bucket handle tear with biceps intact, and Type IV: bucket handle tear with extension into the biceps (Andrews & Shore, 2013). Current data suggest a substantial increase in both the number of arthroscopic SLAP repairs performed annually, and the age of the client undergoing arthroscopic SLAP repairs (Onyekwelu, Khatib, Zuckerman, Rokito, & Kwon, 2012).

Clinical presentation: Clients typically present with complaints of pain, especially with overhead activities, decreased shoulder strength, endurance, and ROM, as well as mechanical symptoms, which may include clicking, locking, and signs and symptoms of instability (Manske, 2011; Manske & Prohaska, 2010).

Common diagnostic tests: Physical examination tests such as load and shift, apprehension, O'Brien's Test, and SLAP test may be present; generally having higher specificity than sensitivity (Cleland et al., 2011). MRI and arthroscopy are typically used to diagnose labral tears with increased sensitivity noted with the concurrent use of intraarticular gadolinium (Andrews & Shore, 2013).

Common medical and surgical procedures: Clients with ongoing pain despite shoulder stabilization strength training often do well with arthroscopic repair of the glenoid labrum and concurrent capsulorrhaphy if needed (Andrews & Shore, 2013).

Precautions and contraindications: Joint mobilization in the direction of the labral repair should not be done in the acute postoperative period.

Interventions

General guidelines for treating a Type 2 SLAP include the following interventions.

- *Home program*: Sling use is typically recommended for four to six weeks. PROM within restrictions (i.e., avoid extension, and end-range external and internal rotation), elbow and hand ROM, and submaximal isometrics for shoulder musculature are recommended. No shoulder extension or active/resisted elbow flexion with shoulder flexion for six weeks. Progress to end-range stretching/PROM at seven to nine weeks, along with gentle isotonic strengthening to rotator cuff and scapular musculature. Manual techniques and exercises should be completed through weeks 7–20. Progression with a HEP should be completed in accordance with indications for therapy (Manske, 2011).

- *Manual techniques*: PROM is initiated postsurgery to increase flexion, external rotation, and internal rotation at weeks 0–2. Increase PROM for external rotation in the scapular plane to 10°–15° and internal rotation in the scapular plane to 45°. PROM should move toward flexion to 90°, abduction to 75°–85°, external rotation to 25°–30°, and internal rotation to 55°–60°. At weeks 5–6, flexion to 145°, external rotation to 45°–50° in 45° abduction, and internal rotation to 55°–60° in 45° abduction. Weeks 7–9 typically include flexion to 180°, external rotation to 90° in 90° abduction, and internal rotation to 70°–75° in 90° abduction (Manske, 2011).

- *Therapeutic exercise*: May include submaximal isometrics for shoulder musculature at weeks 0–2 and AROM at the elbow and hand. AAROM and AROM within pain-free range, scapular training exercises are indicated. At weeks 6–12, gentle isotonic strengthening for internal and external rotation with progression to scaption, abduction, retraction, and protraction. Strengthening and ROM exercises (e.g., PNF, endurance training and plyometrics) are progressed as tolerated (Manske, 2011).

- *ADLs*: Include functional training to allow return to activities and/or sports by weeks 12–14, restricted light sports at weeks 14–16, and unrestricted sport activities 6–9 months postsurgery (Manske, 2011).

Adhesive Capsulitis

Description: Adhesive capsulitis, also known as "frozen shoulder," is characterized by a painful, gradual loss of active and passive glenohumeral ROM in multiple planes, decreased glenohumeral joint space, capsular thickening, and corresponding loss of function (Manske, 2011; Neviaser & Neviaser, 2011). The underlying etiology and pathophysiology of adhesive capsulitis is poorly understood and the diagnosis may be complicated by the number of factors (i.e., intrinsic and extrinsic to the shoulder) that may contribute to shoulder pain and stiffness (Manske, 2011; Neviaser & Hannafin, 2010). Additionally, adhesive capsulitis may be described as primary adhesive capsulitis (i.e., occurs in the presence of a primary disease process such as rotator cuff disease) or as idiopathic adhesive capsulitis (i.e., occurs in the absence of identified or directly causal factors) (Scott & Green, 2013). Adhesive capsulitis is characterized by progressive capsular inflammation with fibrosis, adhesions, and contracture of the glenohumeral joint capsule and potential obliteration of the axillary folds (Hsu, Anakwenze, Warrender, & Abboud, 2011; Neviaser & Neviaser, 2011). Incidence of adhesive capsulitis is typically reported as 2–5% of the general population; however, this figure has been scrutinized (Hsu et al., 2011; Scott & Green, 2013). Approximately 60–80% of individuals with adhesive capsulitis are female, onset frequently occurs between the ages of 40 and 60, approximately 20–30% of those affected will develop the condition in the contralateral shoulder, and occurrence in the nondominant upper extremity may be slightly more common (Neviaser & Hannafin, 2010; Scott & Green, 2013). Risk factors for the development of adhesive capsulitis have been associated with diabetes mellitus, thyroid dysfunction, hyperlipidemia, cardiovascular disease, Dupuytren's contractures, autoimmune disease, treatment of breast cancer, and minor trauma (Hsu et al., 2011; Lo et al., 2014; Neviaser & Neviaser, 2011).

Clinical presentation: Adhesive capsulitis is typically described as progressing through a series of stages or phases as characterized by arthroscopic and histologic findings, as well as client-reported symptoms and clinical findings. The four stages of clinical symptoms of adhesive capsulitis as described by Neviaser and Hannafin (2010) are as follows: (1) pain referred to the deltoid insertion and pain at night; (2) severe night pain and

Table 14-6 Adhesive Capsulitis: Common Diagnostic Tests and Possible Findings

Test	Possible Findings
Arthrogram	Arthrography may reveal joint volume to be reduced by at least 50% (e.g., the volume may be 5–10 ml, as compared to normal volumes of 28–35 ml).
Plain film radiograph	Useful for ruling out other pathologies but not helpful for diagnosing adhesive capsulitis.
MRI and MRI arthrogram	Thickening of the cortical humeral ligament, thickening of the capsule, thickening and fibrotic changes in the axillary recess, and identification of other shoulder pathologies.

MRI, magnetic resonance imaging.

Modified from Neviaser and Neviaser (2011); Scott and Green (2013).

Table 14-7 Adhesive Capsulitis: Common Medical and Surgical Procedures

Procedure	Description
Arthroscopic capsular release	Sharp or thermal incision of joint capsule adjacent to glenoid.
Translational MUA	Joint glides are performed inferiorly, anteriorly in abduction and adduction, and posteriorly to tear adhesions.
Long lever MUA	Long lever arm (i.e., angular) stretching of joint capsule.
Distension arthrography	Injection of a large volume of local anesthetic and steroid intraarticularly to distend the joint capsule.
Steroid injection	Intraarticular injection of steroids; presents with inconsistent pain relief and improved outcome measures.

MUA, manipulation under anesthesia.

Data from: Neviaser and Hannafin (2010); Scott and Green (2013).

stiffness; (3) profound stiffness and pain occurring only at the end ROM; and (4) profound stiffness with minimal pain. Common diagnostic tests and possible findings are described in **Table 14-6** and common medical and surgical procedures are described in **Table 14-7**.

Precautions and contraindications: Aggressive-painful stretching and joint mobilizations are typically poorly tolerated and may exacerbate underlying synovial pathology (Manske, 2011).

Interventions

The goals of treatment with adhesive capsulitis are to achieve a permanent increase in ROM with decreased complaints of pain. This is achieved through progressive joint mobilizations, stretching, and ROM procedures to increase length of restricted tissues, such as joint capsule, extracapsular ligaments, and tendons of the rotator cuff (Griggs, Ahn, & Green, 2000).

- *HEPs*: Includes ROM and stretching in four directions—passive forward elevation/flexion, passive external rotation, passive internal rotation, and passive horizontal adduction. Pendulum exercises may be used early to address ROM, pain, and stiffness.

- *Physical agent modalities*: Include pain management modalities prior to treatment to decrease pain and stiffness (e.g., heat, electrical stimulation, and ultrasound).

- *Manual techniques*: Include joint mobilizations per the client's tolerance to increase humeral glide within the glenoid fossa. Occupational therapy practitioners should be competent in performing these techniques. Overaggressive treatment may cause symptoms to worsen.

- *Therapeutic exercise*: Includes therapeutic exercise based on the client's tolerance, as overaggressive treatment may cause symptoms to worsen. Glenohumeral and scapular stabilization strengthening can be initiated per tolerance. Isometric exercises can be utilized first, followed by progression to isotonic strengthening.

Postsurgical treatment following manipulation under anesthesia (MUA) includes a HEP that begins the day of surgery to maintain manipulation gains in flexion, internal rotation, external rotation, and horizontal adduction. Initiation of strengthening exercises for the rotator cuff and scapular stabilizers can be introduced as tolerated (Griggs et al., 2000).

- *Physical agent modalities*: Include cryotherapy to help manage pain and edema during the initial inflammatory phase of treatment or following manipulation. Additionally, electrical stimulation can be utilized for pain management (e.g., TENS). As inflammation and pain subside, moist heat and ultrasound may be used prior to treatment (Griggs et al., 2000).
- *Manual techniques*: Grade 1 and 2 mobilizations can be used to decrease pain and stiffness in preparation for ROM. Stretching into end-range motions can be used to maximize shoulder ROM. Joint mobilization techniques, stretching, and AAROM can be used to maintain ROM gains achieved during MUA per the client tolerance.
- *Therapeutic exercise*: Includes AAROM/AROM exercises to maximize forward elevation, external rotation, internal rotation, and horizontal abduction, and strengthening exercises initiated and progressed based on the client's tolerance. Strengthening includes isometric exercises to increase strength of the glenohumeral and scapular stabilizers with a progression to isotonics, and a return to functional activities per the client's tolerance (Griggs et al., 2000).

Shoulder Arthritis

Description: Glenohumeral osteoarthritis is the most common degenerative condition affecting the shoulder joint (Jobin & Bigliani, 2014). The prevalence of osteoarthritis increases with age, particularly after the sixth decade, and affects women more frequently than men (Jobin & Bigliani, 2014). Primary osteoarthritis has no apparent cause while secondary osteoarthritis is due to previous trauma. Joint space narrowing and osteophyte formation are key features of glenohumeral arthritis. Shoulder arthritis can also be caused by inflammatory disorders such as rheumatoid arthritis, gout, pseudogout, or avascular necrosis. Degenerative osteoarthritis typically causes posterior glenoid erosion while rheumatoid arthritis typically causes global joint erosion (Jobin & Bigliani, 2014; Millett, Gobezie, & Boykin, 2008). End-stage osteoarthritis and associated degenerative conditions are common indications for surgery; shoulder replacement surgery is the third most common joint replacement surgery following knee and hip arthroplasty (Jacobs & King, 2009; Norris & Iannotti, 2002).

Clinical presentation: Clients typically present with diffuse pain which is present at rest and worsens with increased activity, as well as loss of active and passive glenohumeral ROM, joint effusion, painful crepitus, palpable grinding with mechanical stresses placed on the glenohumeral joint, and associated loss of function (Millett et al., 2008). Common medical and surgical procedures for glenohumeral arthritis are described in **Table 14-8**.

Common diagnostic tests: Radiographs reveal joint space narrowing, spurring of the humeral neck, sclerosis, and cystic changes. CT may be helpful in evaluating glenoid wear and MRI is helpful in evaluating the rotator cuff if joint arthroplasty is being considered (Denard & Walch, 2013; Jobin & Bigliani, 2014).

Precautions and contraindications: Care needs to be taken to protect the subscapularis during early rehab as this is incised and repaired during the surgical procedure (Jobin & Bigliani, 2014). Rupture of the subscapularis after total shoulder arthroplasty (TSA) results in weakness and instability (Sacevich, Athwal, & Lapner, 2015).

Interventions

Treatment of shoulder arthritis includes client education on joint protection and energy conservation techniques (i.e., as outlined below), adaptive equipment to assist with reaching tasks, and heat modalities to decrease pain and stiffness.

Table 14-8 Common Medical and Surgical Procedures

Procedure	Description
Steroid injection	Temporizing relief from intraarticular injections.
TSA	Utilizes a cobalt chrome or titanium head on polyethylene glenoid; offers consistent pain relief, elevation to approximately 130°–140° and complication rates are low.
Reverse TSA	Used when rotator cuff is deficient. The glenoid is changed to a glenosphere, and the head is removed and replaced with a concave humeral component. Lengthens and improves function of deltoid, offers good pain relief, but complication rates are higher than with a standard TSA.

Data from: Cheung, Safran, and Costouros (2013); Farshad and Gerber (2010); Jobin and Bigliani (2014).

- *Joint protection*: Respecting pain, utilization of proper body mechanics, avoidance of prolonged postures, and prolonged repetitive postures, especially those spent in an aggravating position, using the strongest joint/muscle possible, a healthy combination of balance rest and stress, and never starting an activity that cannot be stopped, are the key points included in client education on joint protection techniques (Poole, 2009).
- *Energy conservation techniques*: Common energy conservation techniques include teaching clients to plan ahead, paying attention to their pace, prioritizing necessary tasks, incorporating work simplification techniques, as well as maintaining good posture (Poole, 2009).

Postsurgical management of TSA: Postsurgical management of TSA includes the following interventions:

- *HEP*: Includes early pendulum exercises, as well as PROM for shoulder elevation while lying in supine. The noninvolved upper extremity should perform the motion of the involved side. Passive external rotation using a dowel rod while lying in supine is appropriate; however, note that depending on the surgical approach used, the integrity of the subscapularis muscle may be disrupted. Performance of external rotation PROM must be accomplished in accordance with the physician's direction, in order to avoid potential disruption of the tendon. Progression to AAROM, AROM, and strengthening is in accordance with clinical treatment and pain should not be present with exercises.
- *Physical agent modalities*: Include cold packs following surgery for symptom management during the inflammatory phase of healing, and hot packs initiated when decreased acute inflammation allows. Hot packs and ultrasound can be used to decrease pain and stiffness prior to treatment (Maher, 2014).
- *Manual techniques*: Include passive shoulder elevation when lying in supine with the noninvolved hand to assist, and passive to active-assistive external rotation using a dowel rod while lying in supine. Note that depending on the surgical approach used, the integrity of the subscapularis muscle may be disrupted. Performance of external rotation PROM must be accomplished in accordance with the physician's direction in order to avoid potential disruption of

the tendon. It is commonly appropriate to initiate passive internal rotation, extension, and horizontal adduction at six weeks postsurgery (Maher, 2014).
- *Therapeutic exercise*: Therapy starts within two days after surgery, exercises should be pain free, and no weight bearing is allowed for six months postsurgery. Progression to isometric strengthening is followed by progression to isotonic strengthening for internal and external rotation. There may be delayed strengthening for internal rotation if the subscapularis was released and repaired during surgery. Treatment can typically progress to include isotonic exercises and ADLs between 8 and 12 weeks of treatment, including rotation and elevation of the shoulder (Maher, 2014).
- *ADLs*: The client can perform nonresistive activities while maintaining the shoulder at the side. The client is allowed to perform light elevated activities at 8–12 weeks as tolerated (Maher, 2014).

Referrals and Discharge Considerations

Throughout the course of occupational therapy, the client is reassessed and progressed to increase ROM, strength, endurance, speed, confidence, and functional use of their involved upper extremity. The physician, therapist, and caregiver ultimately work together with the client for a full return to meaningful activities and full participation in their vocational and avocational roles. Once the client has met his or her goals in therapy, or reached a plateau, the therapist ensures the client's competence in completing a HEP to maintain or further promote their autonomy.

Management and Standards of Practice

In any setting it is important for occupational therapy practitioners to participate in professional development and continuing education. This not only ensures continued certification, but also helps therapists to maintain and enhance knowledge of musculoskeletal disorders and injuries. Maintaining open communication with physicians and staff involved with client care is also necessary in this area of practice. Many issues that arise in orthopedic practice can be addressed if communication between the occupational therapist and physician is open and clear. It is also crucial here, and in any other area of practice, to maintain clear and concise medical records of all treatment provided, as well as treatment planned.

Chapter 14 Self-Study Activities (Answers Are Provided at the End of the Chapter)

1. The following are all examples of a physical agent modalities, except:
   A. Electrical stimulation
   B. Splinting
   C. Ultrasound
   D. Iontophoresis
   E. Moist heat

2. When treating a proximal humerus fracture, early in care it is important to perform aggressive PROM to avoid the development of a frozen shoulder. True or false? Please explain why the answer is true or false.

3. Prepare a thorough HEP for an individual with a nondisplaced proximal humerus fracture during the first weeks of treatment. Please address symptom management, exercise, and client education.

4. Mr. Johnson is referred to you for therapy with a diagnosis of shoulder pain. He presents with a reported negative shoulder MRI, tests negative with performance of all provocative shoulder tests (e.g., Empty Can, O'Brien's, Hawkins–Kennedy, and Neer's), and no pain with elevation and external rotation. He does report lateral shoulder pain and has weakness with deltoid manual muscle testing. What is a possible secondary diagnosis? Be specific to anatomical location.

5. Match the following cervical NRs to their associated key myotome and dermatome distributions.

Term	Key Myotome and Dermatome
A. C5	1. Tip of middle finger, dorsal forearm, triceps long head, wrist flexors, finger extensors, and abductor pollicis brevis.
B. C6	2. Tip of little finger, ulnar side of forearm, flexor digitorum, adductor pollicis, and abductor digiti minimi.
C. C7	3. Proximal lateral shoulder sensation, biceps brachii, supraspinatus, and infraspinatus.
D. C8	4. Medial distal arm, medial forearm, and interossei.
E. T1	5. Tip of thumb, radial side of forearm, brachioradialis, and wrist extensors.

6. Most rotator cuff injuries require surgery secondary to a tendon's inability to spontaneously repair? True or false? Please explain why the answer is true or false.

7. Please describe the recommended sleeping positions for an individual with shoulder pathology such as rotator cuff irritation.

8. Place the following options in order of the progression of care for client's recovering from rotator cuff surgery.
   A. AROM
   B. AAROM
   C. PROM
   D. Functional strengthening
   E. Sport-specific strengthening
   F. Rotator cuff and scapular stabilization strengthening

9. A client presents with anterolateral shoulder pain especially at night, and pain and weakness with active external rotation and abduction. The client has a negative O'Brien's, positive Neer's, and a positive empty can test. What is the most likely diagnosis?
   A. Proximal humerus fracture
   B. AC joint pathology
   C. Labrum tear
   D. Rotator cuff pathology
   E. Adhesive capsulitis

10. The client is a 50-year-old female with diabetes and a 3-month history of shoulder pain and stiffness. She does not remember injuring the shoulder. Her pain is most severe at night. AROM measurements are most limited with elevation at 60° and functional internal rotation to the gluteal muscles. She has no pain with resistance to internal rotation or external rotation in neutral. Her passive measurements are not significantly higher than her AROM measurements. What is her likely diagnosis? Why?

_____

_____

_____

_____

_____

11. Aggressive stretching is essential with the treatment of an individual with adhesive capsulitis in order to eliminate adhesions within the glenohumeral joint capsule. True or false? Please explain your answer.

_____

_____

_____

_____

_____

_____

_____

12. Name three common indications/diagnoses that may choose to have a TSA.
    A.
    B. _____
    C. _____

13. PROM into external rotation is sometimes contraindicated early in the treatment of a TSA only if the surgeon had to disrupt the continuity of the _____ tendon(s) during the prosthetic implantation.
    A. Anterior deltoid
    B. Long head of the biceps
    C. Subscapularis
    D. Supraspinatus
    E. C and D
    F. B and C

14. Common diagnostic tests indicative of AC joint irritation include:
    A. Empty Can Test
    B. Hawkins–Kennedy Test
    C. O'Brien's Test
    D. Horizontal abduction
    E. Horizontal adduction
    F. A and C
    G. C and E
    H. C and D

15. Shoulder dislocations are most common in what direction?
    A. Anterior
    B. Posterior
    C. Lateral
    D. Medial

16. Shoulder anatomy self-study activity

    Please list the origin, insertion, action, and innervation for muscles identified below using a format of your choosing (e.g., blank sheet of paper or a computer-generated table). Please use the anatomy textbook recommended by your occupational therapy program to check your answers as needed; minor differences between anatomy references should be expected.

    While the inclusion of an anatomy recall question (i.e., origin, insertion, action, and innervation question) on the board examination is highly unlikely, you may be required to apply knowledge of anatomy. For example, given an affected muscle or muscle group, determine the most appropriate functional task for a given assessment or intervention.

    • Biceps brachii
    • Deltoid—anterior
    • Deltoid—middle
    • Deltoid—posterior
    • Infraspinatus
    • Latissimus dorsi
    • Levator scapulae
    • Pectoralis major—clavicular
    • Pectoralis major—sternal
    • Pectoralis minor
    • Rhomboids major
    • Rhomboids minor
    • Serratus anterior
    • Subscapularis
    • Supraspinatus
    • Teres major
    • Teres minor
    • Trapezius—lower
    • Trapezius—middle
    • Trapezius—upper
    • Triceps brachii

Chapter 14 Self-Study Answers

1. B. Splinting
2. False, early aggressive PROM or AROM may further displace fractures or tuberosities.
3. During the early phases of proximal humerus healing, it is important for the client to be instructed in symptom management techniques, including moist heat and/or cold packs. Pendulum exercises are typically also performed for symptom management. Gentle PROM of the shoulder into flexion within an arc of motion dictated by the physician is indicated via table stretch, manual performance supine, or chair stretch. Caution should be taken and cleared by the physician with performance

of PROM into rotation secondary to possible involvement of the greater and or lesser tuberosities (i.e., insertions of the rotator cuff), PROM into internal rotation and/or external rotation may displace fracture fragments. Early AROM of the shoulder could also potentially further displace the fracture fragments and is not appropriate.

4. C5 NR pathology. The client's MRI of the shoulder did not indicate any pathology, and diagnostic testing of the shoulder was negative for pathology. However, the client has pain at the shoulder and lateral arm, as well as weakness of his deltoids. This could potentially be C5 NR pathology.

5. **A.** C7
   B. C8
   C. C5
   D. T1
   E. C6

6. False, most tendinopathies will resolve with time, exercise, modalities, and the use of cortisone injections when necessary.

7. Proper sleeping positions for individuals with rotator cuff pathology include sleeping postures, such as an avoidance of sleeping with the arm above the head or sleeping in an adducted and internally rotated position, which is important to communicate with the client. Sleeping supine or on the noninvolved shoulder is recommended. When sleeping on the noninvolved side, the client should use a bolster to support the involved upper extremity and prevent internal rotation and adduction of the shoulder.

8. C, B, A, F, D, E (PROM, AAROM, AROM, RC and scapular strengthening, functional strengthening, and sport-specific strengthening).

9. D, rotator cuff pathology: pain in the shoulder at night, with weakness in abduction and external rotation, and positive diagnostic testing for RC pathology are all indicators that the client's rotator cuff is likely involved.

10. The client most likely has adhesive capsulitis of the idiopathic sort. This condition is characterized by night pain, painful limitations in PROM and AROM, and the absence of pain with resistance applied to the RC muscles.

11. False. Aggressive-painful stretching and joint mobilizations are typically poorly tolerated and may exacerbate underlying synovial pathology.

12. TSAs are used to treat end-stage arthritic changes at the glenohumeral joint. These changes can be caused by primary osteoarthritis, secondary osteoarthritis, rheumatoid arthritis, gout, pseudogout, or avascular necrosis.

13. C, subscapularis.

14. G, horizontal crossed arm adduction and O'Brien's testing. Pain may also be produced with an active compression test and with anterior–posterior stresses applied to the clavicle.

15. A, anterior. Most shoulder dislocations occur in an anterior inferior direction due to anteriorly directed trauma to a shoulder in an abducted and externally rotated position. Posterior dislocations may occur after grand mal seizures due to the strong pull of the internal rotators or after a fall on an adducted, and internally rotated arm.

16. Please use the anatomy textbook recommended by your occupational therapy program to check your answers.

References

Adler, C. (2013). Spinal cord injury. In L. W. Pedretti, H. M. Pendleton, & W. Schultz-Krohn (Eds.), *Pedretti's occupational therapy: Practice skills for physical dysfunction* (7th ed., pp. 954–982). St. Louis, MO: Elsevier.

Ahmad, C. S., & Levine, W. N. (2014). Shoulder and elbow disorders in the athlete. In L. K. Cannada (Ed.), *Orthopaedic knowledge update 11* (11th ed., pp. 373–386). Rosemont, IL: American Academy of Orthopaedic Surgeons.

Andrews, J. R., & Shore, B. (2013). Superior labrum anterior and to posterior lesions. In G. P. Nicholson (Ed.), *Orthopaedic knowledge update: Shoulder and elbow 4* (4th ed., pp. 307–319). Rosemont, IL: American Academy of Orthopaedic Surgeons.

Angeline, M. E., & Dines, J. S. (2013). Factors affecting the outcome of rotator cuff surgery. In G. P. Nicholson (Ed.), *Orthopaedic knowledge update: Shoulder and elbow 4* (4th ed., pp. 217–228). Rosemont, IL: American Academy of Orthopaedic Surgeons.

Beaton, D. E., Katz, J. N., Fossel, A. H., Wright, J. G., Tarasuk, V., & Bombardier, C. (2001). Measuring the whole or the parts? Validity, reliability, and responsiveness of the Disabilities of the Arm, Shoulder and Hand outcome measure in different regions of the upper extremity. *Journal of Hand Therapy, 14*(2), 128–146. Retrieved from http://www.ncbi.nlm.nih.gov/pubmed/11382253

Bell, J. E. (2013). Proximal humeral fractures. In G. P. Nicholson (Ed.), *Orthopaedic knowledge update: Shoulder and elbow 4* (4th ed., pp. 409–418). Rosemont, IL: American Academy of Orthopaedic Surgeons.

Bell, J. E., & Cadet, E. R. (2014). Shoulder trauma: Bone. In L. K. Cannada (Ed.), *Orthopaedic knowledge update 11* (11th ed., pp. 319–337). Rosemont, IL: American Academy of Orthopaedic Surgeons.

Breckenridge, J. D., & McAuley, J. H. (2011). Shoulder Pain and Disability Index (SPADI). *Journal of Physiotherapy, 57*(3), 197. doi:10.1016/S1836-9553(11)70045-5

Brun, S. (2012). Shoulder injuries—Management in general practice. *Australian Family Physician, 41*(4), 188–194.

Carofino, B. C., & Leopold, S. S. (2013). Classifications in brief: The Neer classification for proximal humerus fractures. *Clinical Orthopaedics and Related Research, 471*(1), 39–43. doi:10.1007/s11999-012-2454-9

Chang, D., Mohana-Borges, A., Borso, M., & Chung, C. B. (2008). SLAP lesions: Anatomy, clinical presentation, MR imaging diagnosis and characterization. *European Journal of Radiology, 68*(1), 72–87. doi:10.1016/j.ejrad.2008.02.026

Cheung, E. V., Safran, M., & Costouros, J. (2013). Arthroscopic treatment of the arthritic shoulder. In G. P. Nicholson (Ed.), *Orthopaedic knowledge update: Shoulder and elbow 4* (4th ed., pp. 321–329). Rosemont, IL: American Academy of Orthopaedic Surgeons.

Cleland, J., Koppenhaver, S., & Netter, F. H. (2011). *Netter's orthopaedic clinical examination: An evidence-based approach* (2nd ed.). Philadelphia, PA: Saunders/Elsevier.

Cofield, R. H. (1982). Cofield classification of rotator cuff tears. *Surgery, Gynecology & Obstetrics, 154*(5), 667–672.

Conti, M., Garofalo, R., Delle Rose, G., Massazza, G., Vinci, E., Randelli, M., & Castagna, A. (2009). Post-operative rehabilitation after surgical repair of the rotator cuff. *La Chirurgia degli Organi di Movimento, 93*(Suppl. 1), S55–S63. doi:10.1007/s12306-009-0003-9

Denard, P. J., & Walch, G. (2013). Current concepts in the surgical management of primary glenohumeral arthritis with a biconcave glenoid. *Journal of Shoulder and Elbow Surgery, 22*(11), 1589–1598. doi:10.1016/j.jse.2013.06.017

de Winter, A. F., van der Heijden, G. J., Scholten, R. J., van der Windt, D. A., & Bouter, L. M. (2007). The Shoulder Disability Questionnaire differentiated well between high and low disability levels in patients in primary care, in a cross-sectional study. *Journal of Clinical Epidemiology, 60*(11), 1156–1163. doi:10.1016/j.jclinepi.2007.01.017

Donatelli, R., Ruivo, R. M., Thurner, M., & Ibrahim, M. I. (2014). New concepts in restoring shoulder elevation in a stiff and painful shoulder patient. *Physical Therapy in Sport, 15*(1), 3–14. doi:10.1016/j.ptsp.2013.11.001

Dunwoody, J. M., & McKee, M. D. (2013). Clavicular fractures. In G. P. Nicholson (Ed.), *Orthopaedic knowledge update: Shoulder and elbow 4* (4th ed., pp. 447–454). Rosemont, IL: American Academy of Orthopaedic Surgeons.

Edwards, S., & Galatz, L. M. (2014). Shoulder instability and rotator cuff disease. In L. K. Cannada (Ed.), *Orthopaedic knowledge update 11* (11th ed., pp. 357–371). Rosemont, IL: American Academy of Orthopaedic Surgeons.

Edwards, S. G., Whittle, A. P., & Wood, G. W., II. (2000). Nonoperative treatment of ipsilateral fractures of the scapula and clavicle. *The Journal of Bone and Joint Surgery, American Volume, 82*(6), 774–780. Retrieved from http://www.ncbi.nlm.nih.gov/pubmed/10859096

Farshad, M., & Gerber, C. (2010). Reverse total shoulder arthroplasty—From the most to the least common complication. *International Orthopaedics, 34*(8), 1075–1082. doi:10.1007/s00264-010-1125-2

Griggs, S. M., Ahn, A., & Green, A. (2000). Idiopathic adhesive capsulitis. A prospective functional outcome study of nonoperative treatment. *The Journal of Bone and Joint Surgery, American Volume, 82-A*(10), 1398–1407. Retrieved from http://www.ncbi.nlm.nih.gov/pubmed/11057467

Hampton, D. M., Delaney, R. A., & Higgins, L. D. (2013). Massive rotator cuff tears. In G. P. Nicholson (Ed.), *Orthopaedic knowledge update: Shoulder and elbow 4* (4th ed., pp. 197–208). Rosemont, IL: American Academy of Orthopaedic Surgeons.

Harwin, S. F., Birns, M. E., Mbabuike, J. J., Porter, D. A., & Galano, G. J. (2014). Arthroscopic tenodesis of the long head of the biceps. *Orthopedics, 37*(11), 743–747. doi:10.3928/01477447-20141023-03

Hsu, J. E., Anakwenze, O. A., Warrender, W. J., & Abboud, J. A. (2011). Current review of adhesive capsulitis. *Journal of Shoulder and Elbow Surgery, 20*(3), 502–514. doi:10.1016/j.jse.2010.08.023

Ilkhani-Pour, S., Dunkman, A. A., & Soslowsky, L. J. (2013). Basic science of rotator cuff tendons and healing. In G. P. Nicholson (Ed.), *Orthopaedic knowledge update: Shoulder and elbow 4* (4th ed., pp. 13–29). Rosemont, IL: American Academy of Orthopaedic Surgeons.

Itoi, E. (2013). Rotator cuff tear: Physical examination and conservative treatment. *Journal of Orthopaedic Science, 18*(2), 197–204. doi:10.1007/s00776-012-0345-2

Jacobs, J. J., & King, T. (2009). US bone and joint decade prepares for the future. *Arthritis & Rheumatology, 61*(11), 1470–1471. doi:10.1002/art.24974

Jobin, C. M., & Bigliani, L. U. (2014). Shoulder reconstruction. In L. K. Cannada (Ed.), *Orthopaedic knowledge update 11* (11th ed., pp. 339–355). Rosemont, IL: American Academy of Orthopaedic Surgeons.

Jobin, C. M., & Yamaguchi, K. (2013). Arthroscopic repair of rotator cuff tears. In G. P. Nicholson (Ed.), *Orthopaedic knowledge update: Shoulder and elbow 4* (4th ed., pp. 247–263). Rosemont, IL: American Academy of Orthopaedic Surgeons.

Kasch, M. C., & Walsh, M. (2013). Hand and upper extremity injuries. In H. M. Pendleton & W. Schultz-Krohn (Eds.), *Pedretti's occupational therapy: Practice skills for physical dysfunction* (7th ed., pp. 1037–1073). St. Louis, MO: Elsevier.

Klepps, S. (2013). Classification and treatment of acromioclavicular separations. In G. P. Nicholson (Ed.), *Orthopaedic knowledge update: Shoulder and elbow 4* (4th ed., pp. 467–475). Rosemont, IL: American Academy of Orthopaedic Surgeons.

Kocher, M. S., Horan, M. P., Briggs, K. K., Richardson, T. R., O'Holleran, J., & Hawkins, R. J. (2005). Reliability, validity, and responsiveness of the American Shoulder and Elbow Surgeons subjective shoulder scale in patients with shoulder instability, rotator cuff disease, and glenohumeral arthritis. *The Journal of Bone and Joint Surgery, American Volume, 87*(9), 2006–2011. doi:10.2106/JBJS.C.01624

Krishnan, S. G., Rudolph, G. H., & Garofalo, R. (2013). Surgical treatment of full-thickness rotator cuff tears. In G. P. Nicholson (Ed.), *Orthopaedic knowledge update: Shoulder and elbow 4* (4th ed., pp. 187–195). Rosemont, IL: American Academy of Orthopaedic Surgeons.

Lo, I. K. Y. (2013). Partial-thickness rotator cuff tears. In G. P. Nicholson (Ed.), *Orthopaedic knowledge update: Shoulder and elbow 4* (4th ed., pp. 177–185). Rosemont, IL: American Academy of Orthopaedic Surgeons.

Lo, S. F., Chu, S. W., Muo, C. H., Meng, N. H., Chou, L. W., Huang, W. C., . . . Sung, F. C. (2014). Diabetes mellitus and accompanying hyperlipidemia are independent risk factors for adhesive capsulitis: A nationwide population-based cohort study (Version 2). *Rheumatology International, 34*(1), 67–74. doi:10.1007/s00296-013-2847-4

Maher, C. M. (2014). Orthopaedic conditions. In M. V. Radomski & C. A. T. Latham (Eds.), *Occupational therapy for physical dysfunction* (7th ed., pp. 1103–1128). Philadelphia, PA: Wolters Kluwer Health/Lippincott Williams & Wilkins.

Manske, R. C. (2011). Shoulder injuries. In S. B. Brotzman & K. E. Wilk (Eds.), *Clinical orthopaedic rehabilitation: An evidence-based approach* (3rd ed., pp. 82–210). Philadelphia, PA: Mosby.

Manske, R., & Prohaska, D. (2010). Superior Labrum Anterior to Posterior (SLAP) rehabilitation in the overhead athlete. *Physical Therapy in Sport, 11*(4), 110–121. doi:10.1016/j.ptsp.2010.06.004

Mazzocca, A. D., Cote, M. P., Solovyova, O., Rizvi, S. H. H., Mostofi, A., & Arciero, R. A. (2011). Traumatic shoulder instability involving anterior, inferior, and posterior labral injury: A prospective clinical evaluation of arthroscopic repair of 270° labral tears. *The American Journal of Sports Medicine, 39*(8), 1687–1696. doi:10.1177/0363546511405449

Millett, P. J., Gobezie, R., & Boykin, R. E. (2008). Shoulder osteoarthritis: Diagnosis and management. *American Family Physician, 78*(5), 605–611. Retrieved from http://www.ncbi.nlm.nih.gov/pubmed/18788237

Neviaser, A. S., & Hannafin, J. A. (2010). Adhesive capsulitis: A review of current treatment. *The American Journal of Sports Medicine, 38*(11), 2346–2356. doi:10.1177/0363546509348048

Neviaser, A. S., & Neviaser, R. J. (2011). Adhesive capsulitis of the shoulder. *Journal of the American Academy of Orthopaedic Surgeons, 19*(9), 536–542. Retrieved from http://www.ncbi.nlm.nih.gov/pubmed/21885699

Norris, T. R., & Iannotti, J. P. (2002). Functional outcome after shoulder arthroplasty for primary osteoarthritis: A multicenter study. *Journal of Shoulder and Elbow Surgery, 11*(2), 130–135. Retrieved from http://www.ncbi.nlm.nih.gov/pubmed/11988723

Onyekwelu, I., Khatib, O., Zuckerman, J. D., Rokito, A. S., & Kwon, Y. W. (2012). The rising incidence of arthroscopic Superior Labrum Anterior and Posterior (SLAP) repairs. *Journal of Shoulder and Elbow Surgery, 21*(6), 728–731. doi:10.1016/j.jse.2012.02.001

Oh, J. H., Kim, S. H., Lee, J. H., Shin, S. H., & Gong, H. S. (2011). Treatment of distal clavicle fracture: A systematic review of treatment modalities in 425 fractures. *Archives of Orthopaedic and Trauma Surgery, 131*(4), 525–533.

Poole, J. (2009). Musculoskeletal factors. In H. S. Willard, E. B. Crepeau, E. S. Cohn, & B. A. B. Schell (Eds.), *Willard & Spackman's occupational therapy* (11th ed., pp. 658–680). Philadelphia, PA: Wolters Kluwer Health/Lippincott Williams & Wilkins.

Pujalte, G. G., & Housner, J. A. (2008). Management of clavicle fractures. *Current Sports Medicine Reports, 7*(5), 275–280. doi:10.1249/JSR.0b013e3181873046

Sacevich, N., Athwal, G. S., & Lapner, P. (2015). Subscapularis management in total shoulder arthroplasty. *The Journal of Hand Surgery, 40*(5), 1009–1011. doi:10.1016/j.jhsa.2015.01.032

Sajadi, K. R. (2014a). Clavicle fractures: Epidemiology, clinical evaluation, imaging, and classification. In J. D. Zuckerman (Ed.), *Disorders of the shoulder: Trauma* (3rd ed., pp. 99–107). Philadelphia, PA: Lippincott Williams & Wilkins/Wolters Kluwer Health.

Sajadi, K. R. (2014b). Non-operative management of clavicle fractures: Indications, techniques, and outcomes.

In J. D. Zuckerman (Ed.), *Disorders of the shoulder: Trauma* (3rd ed., pp. 108–117). Philadelphia, PA: Lippincott Williams & Wilkins/Wolters Kluwer Health.

Scott, D., & Green, A. (2013). Frozen shoulder. In G. P. Nicholson (Ed.), *Orthopaedic knowledge update: Shoulder and elbow 4* (4th ed., pp. 613–621). Rosemont, IL: American Academy of Orthopaedic Surgeons.

Sugaya, H. (2013). Anatomy, pathogenesis, natural history, and nonsurgical treatment of rotator cuff disorders. In G. P. Nicholson (Ed.), *Orthopaedic knowledge update: Shoulder and elbow 4* (4th ed., pp. 165–176). Rosemont, IL: American Academy of Orthopaedic Surgeons.

van der Meijden, O. A., Gaskill, T. R., & Millett, P. J. (2012). Treatment of clavicle fractures: Current concepts review. *Journal of Shoulder and Elbow Surgery, 21*(3), 423–429. doi:10.1016/j.jse.2011.08.053

Van Thiel, G. S., Heard, W., Romeo, A. A., & Provencher, M. T. (2013). Acute and chronic shoulder dislocations. In G. P. Nicholson (Ed.), *Orthopaedic knowledge update: Shoulder and elbow 4* (4th ed., pp. 77–91). Rosemont, IL: American Academy of Orthopaedic Surgeons.

Orthopedic Conditions of the Elbow and Forearm

Jennifer Siegert, Kurt Krueger, Jeffrey Placzek, and Fredrick D. Pociask

Learning Objectives

- Describe key pathology, etiology, and epidemiology for distal humeral, olecranon and radial head fractures, elbow dislocations, epicondylitis, biceps tendinosis and ruptures, and elbow arthritis.
- Compare and contrast clinical presentation for the orthopedic conditions of the elbow and forearm listed above.
- Describe diagnostic tests for the elbow and forearm disorders listed above.
- Describe medical and surgical procedures for the orthopedic conditions of the elbow and forearm listed above.
- List medical and surgical precautions, and contraindications for the orthopedic conditions of the elbow and forearm listed above.
- Describe physical agent modalities typically used for the management of elbow and forearm disorders.
- Describe the treatment interventions of manual techniques, range of motion, and strengthening used for the management of elbow and forearm disorders.
- Describe techniques utilized to address elbow and forearm activity of daily living limitations.
- Describe conservative and postsurgical therapeutic interventions for the orthopedic conditions of the elbow and forearm listed above.

Key Terms

- *Arthroplasty*: The surgical replacement or reconstruction of a joint.
- *Arthroscopy*: Examination, diagnosis, and/or treatments of a joint using an endoscope that is inserted through a small incision in the skin.

- *Computed tomography (CT)*: CT is a noninvasive imaging technology that utilizes a rotating x-ray emitter to generate detailed cross-sectional computer images of body tissues.
- *Concentric contraction*: A contraction in which the muscle is actively shortening.
- *Eccentric contraction*: A contraction in which the muscle is actively lengthening.
- *Fibrosis*: The development of fibrous connective tissue as a result of injury, disease, or abnormal healing.
- *Isometric contraction*: A contraction in which the muscle length and joint angle do not change.
- *Isotonic contraction*: A contraction in which the length of the muscle changes; may be either concentric or eccentric.
- *Magnetic resonance imaging (MRI)*: MRI is a noninvasive imaging technology that utilizes a magnetic field and radio waves to create detailed computer images of body tissues.
- *Orthoses*: External orthopedic devices used to prevent, control, or correct deformities or to improve function.

Common Fractures and Disorders of Bones and Joints

Distal Humeral Fractures

Description: Fractures of the distal humerus in an older adult typically result from a direct fall on the elbow or a fall on an outstretched hand (Kuhnel, Athwal, & King, 2014; Ring, 2013). Distal humeral fractures occurring in younger adults are typically caused by high-energy trauma, such as a sport- or industrial-related injury (Kuhnel et al., 2014). Distal humeral fractures in adults have an incidence of 5.7 per 100,000 person-years and occur with an increasing incidence in women beginning in the sixth decade (Kuhnel et al., 2014). Distal humeral fractures are most common in children between the ages of 5 and 9 with supracondylar fractures accounting for 65–75% of all pediatric elbow fractures (Kim, Szabo, & Marder, 2012; Lord & Sarraf, 2011).

Fractures may be described as supracondylar, epicondylar, transcondylar, or intercondylar; several different classification schemes are used to comprehensively classify distal humeral fractures (Kuhnel et al., 2014). The Orthopaedic Trauma Association classification scheme for distal humeral fractures subdivides fractures into three types (i.e., extraarticular, partial articular, and complete articular fractures); the three types are further divided into subtypes to designate increasing degrees of comminution or to further describe the location of the fracture (Nauth, McKee, Ristevski, Hall, & Schemitsch, 2011).

Clinical presentation: Clients frequently present with a flaccid deformed elbow and extreme pain exacerbated by motion.

Common diagnostic tests: X-rays are sufficient for the diagnosis of the fracture. Computed tomography (CT) scans are often useful for surgical planning (Kuhnel et al., 2014).

Common medical and surgical procedures: Open reduction and internal fixation (ORIF) with parallel plating is often utilized to stabilize the fracture and to allow for early or immediate range of motion (ROM) (Kuhnel et al., 2014; Ring, 2013).

Precautions and contraindications: A thorough pre- ~~and postoperative physical and occupational~~ examination ~~...~~ th et al., ~~...~~ ken as ~~...~~ aggressive ~~...~~ hetero-

limitations. Whether a practitioner chooses to use a top-down, bottom-up, or a combination of these assessments, the outcome should be goal setting that addresses the client's limitations as they relate to his or her life roles (Brown & Chien, 2010; Maher, 2014). Some of the more common assessments are as follows:

- The Patient-Rated Elbow Evaluation (PREE) is a 20-item, self-report form consisting of 15 questions regarding function and 5 questions pertaining to pain (MacDermid & Michlovitz, 2006).
- The Disabilities of the Arm, Shoulder, and Hand (DASH) is a 30-item, client-rated questionnaire that was designed to measure functional disabilities of the upper extremity (UE), as well as symptoms, social and work function, sleep, and confidence in using the arm (Beaton et al., 2001).
- Michigan Hand Outcome Questionnaire (MHQ) consists of 37 hand-specific questions about UE status (Schwartz, 2010).
- Client history including the client's age, hand dominance, occupational and avocational responsibilities, prior UE injuries, comorbidities, family issues, psychological issues, broader social issues, and economic issues (Kasch & Walsch, 2013; Vaughn, 2014).
- Mechanism and date of injury, structures involved, type and extent of medical and surgical intervention, concomitant injuries, stability of fixation, limitation in ROM due to joint instability, and future treatment planned (Bano & Kahlon, 2006).
- Physical assessment may include the following:
  - Pain (e.g., location, type, quality, and intensity).
  - Ability to participate in life roles.
  - Color, temperature, and signs of compromised circulation or compartment syndrome.
  - Edema (e.g., circumferential measurements).
  - Sensory and motor function.
  - Skin integrity and wound assessment.
    - Wound or surgical incision observation and inspection (e.g., location, size, integrity of closure, exposure of pins or hardware, and signs of infection).
    - Scar observation and inspection (e.g., location, size, adherence, hypertrophy, blanching with motion, pliability, and sensitivity).
  - Soft tissue assessment.
  - Active/passive ROM (A/PROM) of adjacent/ uninvolved joints (e.g., shoulder, wrist, and hand).

Handwritten notes (overlaid):

Supracondylar Fracture:
Injury to hummerus or upper arm bone @ its narrowest point, just above the elbow.
* most common in children

Epicondyle Fracture:
avulsion "tearing away" injury of attachment of the common flexors for the forearm.
extra-articular / elbow dislocation

Trans/intracondylar Fracture:
T or Y shape displacement b/w the condyles + humerus.

- Active ROM (AROM) of elbow and forearm in the stable arc of motion.
- Functional movements of the UE.
- Manual muscle testing (MMT) is deferred until fracture is stable (Bano & Kahlon, 2006).

Interventions

The primary objective of occupational therapy intervention is to assist the client in restoring independence in life roles by maximizing the function of the affected arm. Specific occupational therapy interventions in orthopedic rehabilitation of the elbow will vary according to the type of injury sustained, stage of recovery, and surgical intervention (Maher, 2014).

Client education: The involvement of the client in rehabilitation cannot be underestimated; therefore, it is very important for the client to understand his or her role in the process. Client and family education consists of fracture precautions, orthotic management, edema management, wound and scar management, activity of daily living (ADL) training, adapted equipment, and a thorough home exercise program (HEP).

Compensatory methods: Compensatory methods teach the client adaptive techniques to maintain independence during recovery. Teaching functional one-handed use through strategies and devices, as well as techniques for using stronger, uninvolved muscles to compensate for immobilized joints and activity and/or environmental modifications are all examples of compensatory methods to address occupational performance (Maher, 2014).

Preparatory methods: Preparatory methods may include the following skilled interventions and procedures to optimize functional use of the arm:

- *Orthoses*: Orthoses provide distinctive functions at varied stages of healing including protection and support to healing structures while maintaining stability and preventing further injury, decreasing pain by providing support, and assist with improving ROM and function during the later stages of healing (Davila, 2011). The specific type of orthosis used with a distal humerus fracture will depend on the extent of injury, surgical procedure, elbow stability, and the surgeon's preference (Davila, 2011). A long arm orthosis with the elbow positioned at 90° of flexion or a hinged splint are two of the commonly used orthoses with the acute distal humerus fractures. Immobilization is generally less than two weeks to avoid elbow stiffness.

A hinged splint will allow controlled elbow flexion and extension while providing protection from varus and valgus stresses if protection is desired for a greater period of time (Beredjiklian, 2011). If the progression of elbow range is slower than desired and the fracture site is stable, a serial static orthosis, a night extension orthosis, or a static progressive orthosis may be incorporated at four to eight weeks to improve end ROM.

- *Manual techniques*: The experienced occupational therapist (OT) and occupational therapy assistant uses various skilled manual techniques to decrease pain and swelling, assist with wound and scar management, increase musculotendinous length, joint play and ROM, and ultimately improve the functional use of the affected UE. Soft tissue mobilization beginning the first week and controlled stretching at four to six weeks assists with decreasing muscle tension and increasing ROM and musculotendinous length. Edema management techniques initiated in the first few days after surgery may include compression wraps, elevation, massage, and/or manual edema mobilization (MEM). Joint mobilizations include grade I/II oscillations to decrease pain and edema around four weeks, and grade III/IV to increase ROM but caution must be used to not mobilize at this level until after bony stability is achieved. Discuss bony stability with the surgeon prior to initiating PROM, stretching, or joint mobilization techniques. The occupational therapy practitioner must also avoid ulnohumeral mobilizations until the fracture site is stable.

- *Therapeutic exercise*: Therapeutic exercise includes a variety of techniques implemented at appropriate stages of healing. Some of these procedures and techniques include:
  - A/AAROM of uninvolved joints (e.g., digits, wrist, and shoulder) initiated immediately.
  - Elbow ROM and forearm rotation within stable arc of motion initiated within the first week postoperatively, but not later than two weeks after.
  - Isolated biceps and triceps contractions (i.e., adhere to precautions with surgical repair of respective musculature).
  - Avoidance of shoulder substitution patterns during elbow ROM.
  - Gentle PROM to lengthen tissue; however, take care to avoid exacerbating an inflammatory

response or increasing pain, and avoid forceful PROM.

- o Strengthening according to a stable arc of motion and stage of healing, progressing from submaximal isometric muscle contraction to isotonic exercise with low resistance and then to progressive resistance exercises (PREs) at 8–12 weeks (Beredjiklian, 2011; Davila, 2011).
- *Therapeutic activity*: No lifting or weight-bearing activities should be implemented during the inflammatory phase. Encourage participation in light ADLs as soon as bone healing allows, maintain fine motor control, and increase proximal strength and endurance with a gradual increase in functional ADLs (Kasch & Walsch, 2013).
- *Physical agent modalities*: Moist hot packs and fluidotherapy may be used to increase blood flow, decrease pain, decrease muscle tightness, decrease joint stiffness, and increase tissue extensibility in preparing the soft tissue for functional movement and activity (Davila, 2011). Ultrasound may be used for selective heating of deeper muscles and the joint capsule. Neuromuscular electrical stimulation, high voltage galvanic stimulation (HVGS) and transcutaneous electrical nerve stimulation (TENS) may assist with decreasing muscle spasms, pain, edema, and increasing circulation if indicated (Cameron, 2013). Cryotherapy may be used if acute inflammation, swelling, and pain are present.

Rehabilitation following a fracture is often divided into three physiological phases of treatment, thus allowing progressive stress to the tissues to promote motion and improve function without causing tissue damage or compromised healing.

- *Inflammatory phase*: The focus during the inflammatory phase is to decrease pain and edema, promote healing, protect healing structures, provide and maintain stability, and maintain ROM.
- *Reparative phase*: This phase focuses on decreasing edema, increasing ROM, function, and participation in light ADLs.
- *Remodeling phase*: The goal in this phase is to increase ROM, strength, endurance, and independence in functional activities (Davila, 2011; Maher, 2014).

Olecranon Fractures

Description: Olecranon fractures typically occur from a direct fall on the elbow from a standing height (e.g., a fall on an outstretched hand) or indirectly secondary to the forceful contraction of the triceps against resistance, and may result in a loss of extension strength secondary to loss of triceps insertional stability (Kuhnel et al., 2014; Wiegand, Bernstein, & Ahn, 2012). Olecranon fractures in the elderly are typically associated with low-energy trauma and olecranon fractures in young individuals typically result from high-energy trauma (Kuhnel et al., 2014). Olecranon fractures account for approximately 10% of all elbow fractures, with open fractures accounting for roughly 6% of all olecranon fractures (Kuhnel et al., 2014). Fractures of the olecranon are intra-articular and can result in loss of motion and significant loss of strength if nonunited or malunited (Kuhnel et al., 2014).

Clinical presentation: Fractures of the olecranon may result in ecchymosis of the posterior elbow and loss of extension strength secondary to involvement of the triceps insertion.

Common diagnostic tests: X-rays are usually sufficient in the diagnosis and surgical planning for ORIF (Kuhnel et al., 2014).

Common medical and surgical procedures: Nondisplaced fractures can be treated in a cast for three weeks in extension followed by slow progressive ROM. Transverse fractures can be treated with a tension band wire technique, and displaced and comminuted fractures are treated with plate and screw fixation (Kuhnel et al., 2014; Wiegand et al., 2012).

Precautions and contraindications: Care should be taken to avoid resisted triceps activity until full healing of the fracture has occurred.

Screening and Assessments

Appropriate top-down to bottom-up screening and assessments include:

- The PREE (MacDermid & Michlovitz, 2006).
- The DASH (Beaton et al., 2001).
- The MHQ (Schwartz, 2010).
- Client history including: Client's age, hand dominance, occupational and avocational responsibilities, prior UE injuries, comorbidities, family issues, psychological issues, broader social issues, and economic issues (Kasch & Walsch, 2013; Vaughn, 2014).

- Mechanism and date of injury, structures involved, type and extent of medical and surgical intervention, concomitant injuries, stability of fixation, limitation in ROM due to joint instability, and future treatment planned (Bano & Kahlon, 2006).
- Physical assessment may include the following:
  - Pain (e.g., location, type, quality, and intensity).
  - Ability to participate in life roles.
  - Color, temperature, and signs of compromised circulation or compartment syndrome.
  - Edema (e.g., circumferential measurements).
  - Sensory and motor function.
  - Skin integrity and wound assessment.
  - Wound or surgical incision observation and inspection (e.g., location, size, integrity of closure, exposure of pins or hardware, and signs of infection).
  - Scar observation and inspection (e.g., location, size, adherence, hypertrophy, blanching with motion, pliability, and sensitivity).
  - ROM should include the following:
    - A/PROM of adjacent/uninvolved joints (e.g., shoulder, wrist, and hand).
    - AROM of elbow and forearm in the stable arc of motion.
    - Functional movements of the UE.

Interventions

Client education: The participation of the client in the elbow rehabilitation process is crucial. Client and family education consists of fracture precautions, orthotic management, edema management, wound and scar management, ADL training, adapted equipment, and a thorough HEP.

Compensatory methods: Compensatory methods teach the client adaptive techniques to maintain independence during recovery. These methods include strategies and devices for completing tasks with functional one-handed use, as well as techniques for using stronger and uninvolved muscle groups to compensate for immobilized joints. Modifications of activities or environments are appropriate in order to enhance activity performance. Teaching the client with an elbow fracture how to don a button down shirt with the affected arm first is an example of an activity modification.

Preparatory methods: Preparatory methods may include the following skilled interventions and procedures to optimize functional use of the arm:

- *Orthoses*: Nonoperative treatment of the nondisplaced olecranon fracture includes placing the elbow in a long arm orthoses at 45°–90° for one to three weeks. This may be followed by a hinged brace with flexion blocked at 90°. Postoperatively, the client wears an Orthoplast® long arm orthosis with the elbow at 45°–70° and the forearm in neutral for two to four weeks. The orthosis is removed multiple times a day for exercise and wound care during the inflammatory phase, and light functional activity during the reparative phase. A static progressive or serial static orthosis may be used to improve rotation or flexion/extension once there is bony stability at the fracture site and there is no longer concern of reinjury to the triceps (Davila, 2011; Placzek, 2006).
- *Manual techniques*: The occupational therapy practitioner may incorporate edema management, compression garments or wraps, elevation, MEM, wound and scar management, and sensory reeducation including desensitization, stretching, massage, soft tissue mobilization, and joint mobilization.
- *Therapeutic exercise*: During therapy, the aim is to minimize muscle weakness and joint stiffness while maintaining fracture reduction and joint stability in order to maximize the client's functional performance (Davila, 2011).
  - A/AAROM of uninvolved joints (e.g., digits, wrist, and shoulder) initiated immediately. However, avoid shoulder flexion beyond 90° if the triceps has been repaired.
  - Elbow and forearm A/AAROM within a stable arc of motion. Flexion performed while the client is supine with elbow vertical allowing gravity to assist motion. Extension performed with the client in a seated position, and forearm rotation performed in a seated position with the elbow at 90°.
  - With a triceps repair, avoid active extension and limit A/PROM elbow flexion to 90° during the early phases of healing and increase 10° per week.
  - Isolate triceps contractions at three to four weeks posttriceps repair.
  - Add PREs at six to eight weeks (Beredjiklian, 2011; Davila, 2011).
- *Physical agent modalities*: Moist hot packs may be used to increase blood flow, decrease pain, decrease muscle tightness, decrease joint stiffness, and increase tissue extensibility in preparing the

soft tissue for functional movement and activity if indicated. Ice and neuromuscular electrical stimulation (e.g., HVGS and TENS) may be used for pain management, and ultrasound may be used for selective heating of deeper muscles and the joint capsule if indicated (Cameron, 2013).

Radial Head Fractures

Description: Radial head fractures often occur from a fall on the outstretched hand where the radial head is compressed against the capitellum (Kuhnel et al., 2014; Yoon & King, 2013). Radial head fractures are the most common elbow fracture with a reported incidence of 5.5 to 10,000 per year. Radial head fractures occur most frequently in older women (e.g., a fragility fracture secondary to osteoporosis), as well as in younger individuals, predominately men, secondary to high-energy trauma (Kuhnel et al., 2014; Yoon & King, 2013).

Fractures may occur along the neck of the radius or extend through the head into the radiocapitellar joint space (Kuhnel et al., 2014; Yoon & King, 2013). Nondisplaced or minimally displaced fractures do not typically present with associated injuries. However, a high prevalence of associated fractures or ligamentous injuries is associated with displaced, unstable, or comminuted radial head fractures (Lapner & King, 2013; Yoon & King, 2013). **Table 15-1** describes the different types of radial head fractures and related surgical management.

Clinical presentation: Radial head fractures present with pain and hemarthrosis. Limited rotational movement, a bony block, ligamentous, and/or neurovascular injury may also be present, particularly with a displaced radial head fracture, or radial head fracture with concurrent elbow fracture or dislocation (Yoon & King, 2013).

Common diagnostic tests: X-rays are usually sufficient to diagnose radial head fractures and magnetic resonance imaging (MRI) or a CT scan may be indicated if a block in motion is identified during physical examination (Yoon & King, 2013).

Common medical and surgical procedures: Most radial head fractures are treated by sling protection and early ROM. Displaced fractures can be treated with ORIF and severely comminuted fractures are best treated with excision or radial head replacement (Ruchelsman, Christoforou, & Jupiter, 2013; Yoon & King, 2013).

Precautions and contraindications: Active-assistive ROM needs to be done immediately to avoid long-term ROM loss (Lapner & King, 2013). Care needs to be taken during ORIF to avoid hardware placement in the articular portion of the proximal radial ulnar joint (Yoon & King, 2013).

Screening and Assessments

Appropriate top-down to bottom-up screening and assessments include:

- The PREE (MacDermid & Michlovitz, 2006).
- The DASH (Beaton et al., 2001).
- The MHQ (Schwartz, 2010).
- Client history including: client's age, hand dominance, occupational and avocational responsibilities, prior UE injuries, comorbidities, family issues, psychological issues, broader social issues, and economic issues (Kasch & Walsch, 2013; Vaughn, 2014).
- Mechanism and date of injury, structures involved, type and extent of medical and surgical intervention, concomitant injuries, stability of fixation, limitation in ROM due to joint instability, and future treatment planned (Bano & Kahlon, 2006).
- Physical assessment may include the following:
  - Pain (e.g., location, type, quality, and intensity).
  - Ability to participate in life roles.

Table 15-1 Classification and Surgical Management of Radial Head Fractures

Fracture	Description	Management
Type I	Undisplaced	Short-term splint and ROM
Type II	Marginal fracture greater than 25% with displacement	Splint if minimally displaced or ORIF if displaced greater than 3 mm or angled greater than 30°
Type III	Comminuted	Excision vs. prosthetic replacement
Type IV	Associated with dislocation or fracture	Reduce, repair ligaments, and fracture, ORIF or excise radial head

Data from Kuhnel, Athwal, & King, 2014; Yoon & King, 2013.

- Color, temperature, and signs of compromised circulation or compartment syndrome.
- Edema (e.g., circumferential measurements).
- Sensory and motor function.
- Skin integrity and wound assessment:
  - Wound or surgical incision observation and inspection (e.g., location, size, integrity of closure, exposure of pins or hardware, and signs of infection).
  - Scar observation and inspection (e.g., location, size, adherence, hypertrophy, blanching with motion, pliability, and sensitivity).
- Soft tissue assessment.
- A/PROM of adjacent/uninvolved joints (e.g., shoulder, wrist, and hand).
- AROM of elbow and forearm in the stable arc of motion.
- Functional movements of the UE.

Interventions

Education: Client and family education consists of fracture precautions, orthotic management, edema management, wound and scar management, ADL training, adapted equipment, and a ROM HEP.

Compensatory methods: Include strategies and devices for completing tasks with functional one-handed use and techniques for using stronger and uninvolved muscle groups to compensate for immobilized joints. Modification of activity or environments can enhance activity performance.

Preparatory methods: Preparatory methods may include the following skilled interventions and procedures to optimize functional use of the arm:

- *Orthoses*: The specific type of orthosis used with radial head fractures will depend on the type of fracture sustained. Type I and minimally displaced type II fractures are typically immobilized in a sling for one week (Bano & Kahlon, 2006; Beredjiklian, 2011). Type II fractures require ORIF and type III fractures are immobilized in a long arm orthoses or cast at 90° of elbow flexion and restricted forearm rotation for up to three weeks (Bano & Kahlon, 2006). The forearm position is dependent on ligament involvement. If the medial collateral ligament (MCL) is involved, splint the forearm in supination and if the lateral collateral ligament (LCL) is involved, splint the forearm in pronation to protect against varus/valgus stresses, and if both the MCL

and LCL are involved, position the forearm in neutral (Bano & Kahlon, 2006; Davila, 2011; King, 2011). The hinged elbow splint can allow controlled movement while protecting against valgus and varus stresses (i.e., blocks set for acceptable range and motion during exercise and locked between exercises), and can be worn for three to six weeks (Bano & Kahlon, 2006; Davila, 2011). Static progressive or serial static night extension orthoses may be necessary for complex radial head fractures at the four- to six-week mark if the desired ROM has not been achieved (Adams & Steinmann, 2011; Bano & Kahlon, 2006).

- *Manual techniques*: Similar to other elbow injuries, manual techniques may include edema management, wound and scar management, sensory reeducation, stretching, massage, and soft tissue and joint mobilization. Joint mobilizations must be used cautiously with type II and III fractures, ulnohumeral joint mobilizations are avoided until bony stability is achieved, and radiocapitellar joint mobilizations are contraindicated with radial head excision or arthroplasty (Bano & Kahlon, 2006).

- *Therapeutic exercise*: Prolonged immobilization of the elbow following injury significantly increases risks of adhesions and joint stiffness (Bano & Kahlon, 2006); therefore, ROM exercises are encouraged as early as possible and may include:
  - A/AAROM of uninvolved joints (e.g., digits, wrist, and shoulder).
  - Elbow ROM within a stable arc of motion; with elbow extension is typically initiated within the first week, and no later than 10 days.
  - Forearm rotation is generally performed in sitting with the elbow at 90° to protect the collateral ligament integrity; valgus and varus stresses must be avoided.
  - Gentle PROM and stretching may begin at four to six weeks for a simple and stable fracture; however, according to King (2011), this may be delayed until six to eight weeks for more complex fractures.
  - The therapist will progress strengthening according to the stable arc of motion and stage of healing. Submaximal wrist isometrics may be introduced at two weeks, followed by submaximal isometrics at the elbow and forearm at three to four weeks. Strengthening is then progressed to PREs to the

elbow, wrist, and forearm at 4–6 weeks; however, this may be delayed to 8–12 weeks if the fracture and ligaments are healed (Bano & Kahlon, 2006; King, 2011).

- *Physical agent modalities*: Moist hot packs and fluidotherapy may be used to increase blood flow, decrease pain, decrease muscle tightness, decrease joint stiffness, and increase tissue extensibility in preparation of the soft tissue for functional movement and activity. Ice and neuromuscular electrical stimulation (e.g., HVGS and TENS) may be used for pain management, and ultrasound may be used for selective heating of deeper muscles and the joint capsule if indicated (Cameron, 2013).

Elbow Dislocations

Description: Elbow dislocations can occur from a rotatory, hyperextension, or varus/valgus force exerted through an outstretched hand and is typically described by the position of the ulna and radius in relation to the distal humerus (Kuhnel et al., 2014; O'Driscoll, Morrey, Korinek, & An, 1992). Dislocations typically occur beginning with tearing of the radial collateral ligaments, progressing across the anterior and posterior capsule and finally rupturing the MCL (O'Driscoll et al., 1992).

Elbow dislocations comprise approximately 11–28% of all injuries of the elbow joint and is one of the most common dislocations in children (Manske, 2011a). Stoneback et al. (2012) reported the incidence of elbow dislocations in the U.S. population at 5.21 per 100,000 person-years with the highest incidence occurring between the ages of 10 and 19, with males at the highest risk.

Clinical presentation: Posterior lateral dislocations are the most common and present with the deformity of a slightly flexed elbow held against the body (Manske, 2011a). Simple dislocations involve soft tissue injury only, whereas complex dislocations are also associated with fractures (O'Driscoll et al., 1992).

Common diagnostic tests: X-ray is sufficient to diagnose elbow dislocations and their reduction. A CT scan may be indicated to evaluate concurrent fractures of the coronoid or radial head, and to develop a treatment plan (Kuhnel et al., 2014).

Common medical and surgical procedures: Most elbow dislocations are treated with gentle ROM and brief immobilization, as immobilization beyond three weeks may result in ongoing elbow stiffness. Early end of range

extension should be avoided in cases with instability beyond 30° (Geissler & Craft, 2010; Manske, 2011a). Cases of instability that continue even with the elbow flexed to 40° may require reconstruction of the collateral ligaments. Triad injuries that involve the radial head and coronoid should undergo ORIF or replacement of the radial head, ORIF of the coronoid, and repair of the radial collateral ligament (Geissler & Craft, 2010; Kuhnel et al., 2014). Even with simple dislocations, loss of approximately 6°–15° of extension along with slight decreases in strength is common (Lin et al., 2012; Manske, 2011a).

Precautions and contraindications: Nonsteroidal anti-inflammatory drugs should be given to help prevent heterotopic ossification. Aggressive early stretching should also be avoided to decrease hypertrophic ossification and prevent ongoing instability (Geissler & Craft, 2010; Manske, 2011a).

Screening and Assessments

Appropriate top-down to bottom-up screening and assessments include:

- The PREE (MacDermid & Michlovitz, 2006).
- The DASH (Beaton et al., 2001).
- The MHQ (Schwartz, 2010).
- Client history including: client's age, hand dominance, occupational and avocational responsibilities, prior UE injuries, comorbidities, family issues, psychological issues, broader social issues, and economic issues.
- Mechanism and date of injury, structures involved, type and extent of medical and surgical intervention, concomitant injuries, stability of fixation, and limitation in ROM due to joint instability (Bano & Kahlon, 2006).
- Physical assessment may include the following:
  - Pain (e.g., location, type, quality, and intensity).
  - Ability to participate in life roles.
  - Color, temperature, and signs of compromised circulation or compartment syndrome.
  - Edema (e.g., circumferential measurements).
  - Sensory and motor function.
  - Soft tissue assessment.
  - A/PROM of adjacent/uninvolved joints (e.g., shoulder, wrist, and hand).
  - AROM of elbow and forearm in the stable arc of motion.
  - Functional movements of the UE.

Interventions

Client education: Client and family education should include fracture precautions (i.e., if applicable), orthotic management, edema management, wound and scar management, ADL training, adapted equipment, and a ROM HEP.

Compensatory methods: Occupational therapy includes strategies and devices for completing tasks with functional one-handed use, as well as techniques for using stronger and uninvolved muscle groups to compensate for immobilized joints. Modification of activity or environments may be necessary to enhance occupational performance.

Preparatory methods: Preparatory methods may include the following skilled interventions and procedures to optimize functional use of the arm:

- *Orthoses*: The client with an elbow dislocation is placed in a long arm orthosis or cast with the forearm in neutral and the elbow at 90° of elbow flexion (i.e., at 20°–30° more flexion than the position of instability) or a hinged elbow brace with blocks to limit ROM for the first four to six weeks (Adams & Steinmann, 2011). For a simple dislocation, the splint will remain on for a maximum of two weeks. For a complex elbow dislocation (i.e., one associated with other ligament or bony injuries), the splint should remain on for four to eight weeks; however, the splint must be removed for exercise and wound care (Davila, 2011). According to Beredjiklian (2011), immobilization longer than three weeks yields poor results in nine-tenths of clients.
- *Manual techniques*: The manual techniques may include edema management, stretching, massage, soft tissue mobilization, and joint mobilization as appropriate.
- *Therapeutic exercise*: Exercise consists of the following ROM and strengthening components:
  - ROM for a simple dislocation can progress from as early as a few days postinjury with minimal restrictions regarding range.
  - ROM for a complex dislocation will vary according to concomitant injuries sustained. The surgeon will determine the stable arc of motion (i.e., generally limiting extension by 30° for two to three weeks and then gradually increasing this range by 10° per week).
  - For the complex dislocation with associated fracture or ligament injuries, care must be taken to protect the LCL and MCL during rotation. The therapist will ensure forearm rotation with the elbow flexed to 90°.
- A progressive strengthening program will be initiated according to a stable arc of motion and stage of healing and then progress to full return to activity by three to six months.
- *Physical agent modalities*: Moist hot packs may be used to increase blood flow, decrease pain, decrease muscle tightness, decrease joint stiffness, and increase tissue extensibility in preparation of the soft tissue for functional movement and activity. Ice and neuromuscular electrical stimulation (e.g., HVGS and TENS) may be used for pain and edema management if indicated. Ultrasound may be used for selective heating of deeper muscles and the joint capsule (Cameron, 2013).

Throughout therapy, the client is reassessed and progressed to increase ROM, strength, endurance, speed, confidence, and functional use of their involved arm. The goal of therapy is to return the client to their prior level of function with vocational and avocational activities. Once the client has met his or her goals in therapy or reached a plateau, the therapist ensures the client's competence in completing a HEP to maintain or further progress their independence.

Elbow Arthritis

Description: Arthritis may be degenerative, inflammatory, or posttraumatic. Progressive osteoarthritis (OA) results in articular cartilage degeneration, subchondral bone sclerosis, osteophyte formation, joint effusion, joint instability, stiffness, and radiographic joint space narrowing, as well as limited mobility and pain with ADLs (Shen & Chen, 2014; Stern, Elfar, & Shuler, 2010). OA is the most common form of arthritis affecting approximately 15% of the overall population, 50% of individuals aged 65 years and older, and 85% of individuals 75 years and older (Hunter, 2009; Shen & Chen, 2014). In contrast, symptomatic OA of the elbow joint is relatively uncommon and affects less than 2% of the general population (Armstrong & Murthi, 2014).

Rheumatoid arthritis (RA), the most common form of inflammatory arthritis, affects approximately 1% of the population and is most common in middle-aged women. RA results in swelling, stiffness, nodules, and joint and bone destruction that may lead to instability (Armstrong & Murthi, 2014; Stern et al., 2010).

Posttraumatic degeneration may occur after elbow fracture or dislocation. Presentation of posttraumatic elbow arthritis is typically delayed following an elbow fracture and may take months or years to progress (Stern et al., 2010).

Clinical presentation: Degenerative forms of arthritis typically present with pain during active functional activities, decreased ROM, and mild effusion and tenderness at the joint line (Armstrong & Murthi, 2014; Stern et al., 2010). RA presents with large effusions, synovitis, and elbow instability; pain and loss of ROM are the initial symptoms that typically develop as a result of synovitis (Armstrong & Murthi, 2014; Stern et al., 2010).

Common diagnostic tests: X-rays are sufficient for the diagnosis of OA; CT scan may be useful if planning osteocapsular arthroplasty. RA factor (i.e., positive in approximately 80% of clients with RA), also described as seropositive if present, is the classic marker for active rheumatoid disease (Stern et al., 2010).

Common medical and surgical procedures: Conservative care includes therapy and steroid injections. Operative interventions include arthroscopy or open osteocapsular arthroplasties or total elbow replacement. Clients with RA do better with total joint replacement than osteoarthritic or posttraumatic clients. Older clients are more satisfied than younger clients after joint replacement (Armstrong & Murthi, 2014; Hurt & Savoie, 2013; Stern et al., 2010).

Precautions and contraindications: Motion should not be forced if limited by osteophytes.

Screening and Assessments

Appropriate top-down to bottom-up screening and assessments include:

- The PREE (MacDermid & Michlovitz, 2006).
- The DASH (Beaton et al., 2001).
- Client history including: client's age, hand dominance, occupational and avocational, responsibilities, prior UE injuries, duration of contracture, and comorbidities.
- Physical assessment may include the following:
  - Pain (e.g., location, type, quality, and intensity).
  - Edema.
  - Neurovascular function.
  - Skin integrity and wound assessment (i.e., postarthroplasty).
    - Wound or surgical incision observation and inspection (e.g., location, size, integrity of closure, and signs of joint infection or pin tract infection).
    - Scar observation and inspection (e.g., location, size, adherence, hypertrophy, blanching with motion, pliability, and sensitivity).
  - A/PROM of adjacent/uninvolved joints (e.g., shoulder, wrist, and hand).
  - ROM, mobility, and stability of elbow and forearm.
  - Muscle/tendon length.
  - Joint play and end feel.
  - Intrinsic versus extrinsic versus mixed contracture.
  - Functional movement and limitations: elbow restriction limits ability to position hand in space to complete ADLs.
  - Ability to participate in life roles.

Interventions

Compensatory methods: Adaptive equipment such as a reacher, long-handled tools, sock aide, buttonhook, and zipper pulls to increase function of the involved arm. Strategies and devices for completing tasks with functional one-handed use, as well as modification of activities or environments to enhance activity performance with significant postural and spatial adaptation are useful in treatment. Joint protection and energy conservation include avoiding prolonged immobilization, rest, and avoidance of activities that cause pain.

Preparatory methods: Preparatory methods may include the following skilled interventions and procedures to optimize functional use of the arm:

- Treatment includes client and family education consisting of precautions, orthotic management, edema management, wound and scar management (i.e., postsurgical), ADL training, and a ROM HEP. Splinting can include continuous passive motion and compressive wraps or elbow pads.
- *Manual techniques*: Interventions include stretching (e.g., contract–relax techniques), massage, and soft tissue mobilization.
- *Therapeutic exercise*: Includes A/AA/PROM for elbow flexion and extension, supination and pronation, and a progressive strengthening program.
- *Physical agent modalities*: Moist hot packs may be used to increase blood flow, decrease pain, decrease muscle tightness, decrease joint stiffness, and

increase tissue extensibility in preparation of the soft tissue for functional movement and activity if indicated. Neuromuscular electrical stimulation (e.g., HVGS and EMG biofeedback) may be used if indicated. Ultrasound may be used for selective heating of deeper muscles and the joint capsule (Cameron, 2013).

When treating a client with elbow arthritis, the primary goal is to increase ROM and function without increasing pain. The accepted arc of elbow flexion and extension for completing most functional ADLs is 30°–130° of motion (Altman, 2011).

Disorders of Muscles and Tendons

Lateral Epicondylitis

Description: Lateral epicondylitis, also known as "tennis elbow," is chronic tendon degeneration that is more accurately classified as angiofibroblastic tendinosis (i.e., secondary to a lack of signs of inflammation) or histologically as angiofibroblastic hyperplasia (Budoff, 2010; Hurt & Savoie, 2013). Angiofibroblastic hyperplasia is characterized by the presence of dense populations of hypertrophic fibroblasts, vascular hyperplasia, disorganized collagen, fibrosis, and the absence of acute inflammatory cells (Budoff, 2010). The extensor carpi radialis brevis is the most frequently involved tendon; however, the extensor digitorum communis, extensor radialis longus, and extensor carpi ulnaris may also be involved (Ahmad & Levine, 2014). Lateral epicondylitis is widely thought to originate from repetitive overuse or microtrauma which results in microtears and progressive degeneration secondary to continued faulty healing and progressive tendinosis (Binaghi, 2015). Avascular zones within the tendon may compromise the normal healing process (Bales, Placzek, Malone, Vaupel, & Arnoczky, 2007).

Lateral epicondylitis is one of the most common UE musculoskeletal disorders with an estimated prevalence of 1–3% of adults, particularly during the fourth and fifth decades of life, with men and women affected equally (Descatha, Dale, Silverstein, Roquelaure, & Rempel, 2015; Faro & Wolf, 2007; Tosti, Jennings, & Sewards, 2013). Additionally, while fewer than 10% of clients with lateral epicondylitis are tennis players, it is reported that approximately 50% of tennis players will experience some form of lateral elbow pain in their lifetimes (Tosti et al., 2013). In the general population, individuals with lateral epicondylitis frequently participate in work or recreational activities that require repetitive and vigorous use of the wrist and forearm (Cooper & Martin, 2007). Common medical and surgical interventions for lateral epicondylitis are described in **Table 15-2**.

Table 15-2 Common Medical and Surgical Intervention for Epicondylitis

Procedure	Description
Corticosteroid injections	Corticosteroid injections provide predictable short-term symptom relief, typically lasting less than 6 weeks, with high recurrence rates. Additionally, there is little to no evidence supporting long-term benefits. Conversely, corticosteroid injections may contribute to tendon degeneration, fatty atrophy, and skin depigmentation.
Autologous whole blood or platelet-rich plasma injections	Small amounts of platelet-rich plasma or autologous whole blood is injected into the tendon itself. There is limited and mixed evidence supporting these therapies, as well as clinically meaningful outcomes, with platelet-rich plasma typically reported as providing more favorable results as compared to autologous whole blood.
ESWT	ESWT applied to the tendon origin presents with varied and mixed findings reported in the literature, with no difference as compared to placebo reported in many studies.
Percutaneous debridement	Percutaneous debridement has a success on the order of 80% with risk of damage to the radial collateral ligament present, and limited evidence supporting the procedure.
Open debridement	Open debridement encompasses the excision of mucoid tissue followed by direct repair (i.e., tendon to tendon or tendon to bone), with success rates reported as high as 85%.

ESWT, extracorporeal shockwave therapy.

Data from (Ahmad & Levine, 2014; Budoff, 2010; Calfee, Patel, DaSilva, & Akelman, 2008; Childress & Beutler, 2013; Cincere & Nirschl, 2013; Foster, Voss, Hatch, & Frimodig, 2015; Speed, 2014; Thanasas, Papadimitriou, Charalambidis, Paraskevopoulos, & Papanikolaou, 2011; Wang, 2012).

Clinical presentation: Clinical presentation frequently includes lateral elbow pain with pain that may radiate down the forearm, as well as pain reported with maximum passive wrist flexion, gripping, resisted long finger extension, resisted wrist extension while the elbow is fully extended, and decreased grip strength (Ahmad & Levine, 2014; Budoff, 2010; Faro & Wolf, 2007). However, maximal tenderness seen over the origin of the extensor carpi radialis brevis, within 1–2 centimeters of the lateral epicondyle, is typically a hallmark symptom (Budoff, 2010). Differential diagnosis includes cervical radiculopathy, proximal neurovascular entrapment, and radial tunnel syndrome, arthritis or articular calcifications (Cooper, 2014a, 2014b).

Common diagnostic tests: Radiographs are typically unremarkable but calcium deposits may be occasionally observed in the proximal aspects of the tendon (Budoff, 2010). MRI may show increased signal and evidence of degeneration at the tendon origin (Ahmad & Levine, 2014).

Precautions and contraindications: Surgical interventions require great care to avoid injury to the radial collateral ligament.

Screening and Assessments

Common clinical examination procedures for lateral epicondylitis and possible findings are described in **Table 15-3**. Appropriate top-down to bottom-up screening and assessments include:

- The PREE (MacDermid & Michlovitz, 2006).
- The DASH (Beaton et al., 2001).

- Client history including: client's age, hand dominance, occupational and avocational responsibilities, prior UE injuries, comorbidities, family issues, psychological issues, broader social issues, and economic issues.
- Mechanism and date of injury, structures involved, type and extent of medical and surgical intervention, concomitant injuries, stability of fixation, and limitations in ROM due to joint instability (Bano & Kahlon, 2006).
- Physical assessment may include the following:
  - Pain (e.g., location, type, quality, and intensity).
  - Ability to participate in life roles.
  - Color, temperature, and signs of compromised circulation or compartment syndrome.
  - Edema (e.g., circumferential measurements).
  - Sensory and motor function.
  - Soft tissue assessment.
  - A/PROM of adjacent/uninvolved joints (e.g., shoulder, wrist, and hand).
  - AROM of elbow and forearm in the stable arc of motion.
  - Functional movements of the UE.
  - MMT including the proximal scapular muscle strength (Cooper & Martin, 2007).

Interventions

Treatment for lateral epicondylitis includes adaptive equipment such as built-up handles, and splinting the wrist at 0°–30° of extension with a counterforce strap used during activity. However, precautions must be

Table 15-3 Common Clinical Examination Procedures and Possible Findings

Test	Description	Possible Findings
Mills Tennis Elbow Test	With the client's shoulder in neutral, the examiner palpates the tender area near the lateral epicondyle, then pronates the forearm and flexes the wrist while moving the elbow from flexion to extension.	Pain in the lateral epicondyle is a positive test result for lateral epicondylitis.
Cozen's Test	The client's elbow is stabilized by the thumb of the examiner at the lateral epicondyle. With the elbow pronated, the client makes a fist and then extends and radially deviates the wrist, while the examiner resists the wrist motion.	Severe and sudden pain in the lateral epicondyle is a positive test for lateral epicondylitis.
Middle finger or Maudsley's Test	With the client's wrist positioned in neutral, the examiner resists extension of the middle finger distal to the proximal intraphalangeal joint.	Pain with resisted finger extension is a positive test for radial tunnel syndrome.
Tapping or Tinel's Test	The examiner taps over the radial nerve in a proximal to distal direction.	If paresthesia is reported, the test is positive for radial tunnel syndrome.

Data from Magee, D. J. (2014). Orthopedic physical assessment (6th edition. ed.). St. Louis, Missouri: Elsevier.

taken, as an overly tight epicondylitis strap may lead to radial tunnel syndrome. Strengthening should focus on proximal conditioning and scapular strengthening, isometric strengthening, and the gradual addition of eccentric exercise as pain improves (Cooper, 2014b; Cooper & Martin, 2007).

Medial Epicondylitis

Description: Medial epicondylitis, also known as "golfer's elbow," is characterized by point tenderness at the medial epicondyle at the common flexor and pronator origin. Symptoms are typically attributable to repetitive wrist flexion or forearm pronation activities (e.g., golf, racquetball sports, football, and weight lifting) and occupations such as carpentry and plumbing (Ahmad & Levine, 2014; Cooper & Martin, 2007). The pronator teres and flexor carpi radialis are the muscles most often involved; however, the flexor carpi ulnaris and the flexor digitorum superficialis may also be involved (Cooper & Martin, 2007).

Clinical presentation: Symptoms typically include complaints of medial elbow pain exacerbated by wrist flexion or forearm pronation activities and tenderness at the tendon origin on the medial condyle.

Common medical and surgical procedures: Interventions are analogous to those used in the management of lateral epicondylitis; see Table 15-2 for common medical and surgical interventions for medial epicondylitis.

Common diagnostic tests: Radiographs are typically negative but calcium deposits may be occasionally observed in the tendon. MRI may show increased signal and evidence of degeneration at the tendon origin (Ahmad & Levine, 2014).

Precautions and contraindications: Care needs to be taken with surgical procedures or injections to avoid inadvertent injury to the MCL and ulnar nerve.

Screening and Assessments

Appropriate top-down to bottom-up screening and assessments include:

- The PREE (MacDermid & Michlovitz, 2006).
- The DASH (Beaton et al., 2001).
- Client history including: client's age, hand dominance, occupational and avocational responsibilities, prior UE injuries, comorbidities, family issues, psychological issues, broader social issues, and economic issues.

- Mechanism and date of injury, structures involved, type and extent of medical and surgical intervention, concomitant injuries, stability of fixation, and limitation in ROM due to joint instability (Bano & Kahlon, 2006).
- Physical assessment may include the following:
  - Pain (e.g., location, type, quality, and intensity).
  - Ability to participate in life roles.
  - Color, temperature, and signs of compromised circulation or compartment syndrome.
  - Edema (e.g., circumferential measurements).
  - Sensory and motor function.
  - Soft tissue assessment.
  - A/PROM of adjacent/uninvolved joints (e.g., shoulder, wrist, and hand).
  - AROM of elbow and forearm in the stable arc of motion.
  - Functional movements of the UE.

Interventions

Treatment for medial epicondylitis includes adaptive equipment such as built-up handles, and splinting with the wrist in neutral including a counterforce strap when in use. However, precautions must be taken, as an overly tight epicondylitis strap may lead to radial tunnel syndrome. Exercises should include proximal conditioning and scapular strengthening, as well as isometric strengthening and gradual eccentric exercise as pain improves (Cooper & Martin, 2007).

Biceps Ruptures

Description: Distal biceps ruptures typically occur after a rapid and unexpected eccentric extension force while the elbow is positioned in midflexion (Cincere & Nirschl, 2013). Most distal biceps ruptures present as an acute avulsion from the radial tuberosity; however, ruptures at the musculotendinous junction and within the tendon have also been reported (Cincere & Nirschl, 2013; Manske, 2011b). Possible predisposing factors for distal biceps rupture include tendinosis (i.e., chronic degenerative changes within the tendon) and impingement (Ahmad & Levine, 2014). Additionally, distal biceps tendon ruptures have been found to be associated with smoking and elevated body mass index (Kelly, Perkinson, Ablove, & Tueting, 2015). Distal biceps tendon tears typically occur in the dominant extremity of physically active men aged 40–60 years with a national estimated incidence of 2.55 per 100,000 patient-years (Cincere & Nirschl, 2013; Kelly et al., 2015).

Clinical presentation: Clients will typically describe a popping sensation and pain localized to the anterior elbow at the level of the radial tuberosity with consequent swelling and ecchymosis (Ahmad & Levine, 2014; Manske, 2011b). Physical examination typically reveals a deformity of the biceps (i.e., proximal retraction of the muscle belly with a change in contour) and weakness; particularly with the elbow positioned at 90° of flexion with full supination of the forearm (Ahmad & Levine, 2014).

Common diagnostic tests: Pain and weakness are noted with resisted supination more so than elbow flexion, which is more severe if a portion of the tendon is still attached. Clinical examination is usually sufficient for diagnosis and MRI is helpful in the case of partial thickness tears, as well as for the evaluation of tear severity (Cincere & Nirschl, 2013).

Common medical and surgical procedures: Nonoperative treatment can be considered for less active individuals, particularly in their nondominant arm. Clients will have approximately 30% deficit in elbow flexion strength, 40% deficit in supination strength, and an 86% decrease in supination endurance (Manske, 2011b). The brachialis and brachioradialis substitute well for elbow flexion but the isolated supinator does not have the strength to substitute well for the loss of biceps supination strength and endurance. Repair can be done through a one incision or two incision technique. A two incision technique repairs the biceps to its anatomic origin more precisely than a one incision technique. Fixation may be through bone tunnels, anchors, interference screws, buttons, or a combination of these. Good results are typical with ROM and strength of 90% or better when compared with the contralateral side (Cincere & Nirschl, 2013).

The client with a surgical repair of a biceps rupture may opt for outpatient therapy or receive an exercise program to complete the exercises at home. After surgical repair of a biceps rupture, one can generally expect full elbow flexion and extension to return in two to three weeks, and full or near to full rotation to return in approximately one month (Adams & Steinmann, 2011). Two to three months postsurgery, the client can expect to return to premorbid activities per the surgeon's recommendation. If the client is not a surgical candidate, or elects to not have surgery, the expected outcome is approximately 30–40% loss of strength with flexion and supination (Adams & Steinmann, 2011; Blackmore, 2011).

Precautions and contraindications: Rehabilitation of partial tears may take many months to complete. Surgical complications include neurovascular injury, particularly to the superficial radial nerve, lateral antebrachial cutaneous nerve, or posterior interosseous nerve. Heterotopic ossification can occur as radioulnar synostosis (Ahmad & Levine, 2014; Cincere & Nirschl, 2013).

Screening and Assessments

Appropriate top-down to bottom-up screening and assessments include:

- The PREE (MacDermid & Michlovitz, 2006).
- The DASH (Beaton et al., 2001).
- Client history including: client's age, hand dominance, occupational and avocational responsibilities, prior UE injuries, comorbidities, and tobacco use.
- Mechanism and date of injury, type and extent of medical and surgical intervention.
- Physical assessment may include the following:
  - Pain (e.g., location, type, quality, and intensity).
  - Ability to participate in life roles.
  - Edema (e.g., circumferential measurements).
  - Sensory and motor function.
  - Skin integrity and wound assessment (i.e., if surgery performed).
    - Wound or surgical incision observation and inspection (e.g., location, size, integrity of closure, and signs of infection).
    - Scar observation and inspection (e.g., location, size, adherence, hypertrophy, blanching with motion, pliability, and sensitivity).
  - A/PROM of adjacent/uninvolved joints (e.g., shoulder, wrist, and hand).
  - AROM of elbow and forearm per surgeon.
  - Functional movements of the UE.

Interventions

Compensatory methods: Treatment includes strategies and devices for completing tasks with functional one-handed use and techniques for using stronger and uninvolved muscle groups to compensate for immobilized joints.

Preparatory methods: Preparatory methods may include the following skilled interventions and procedures to optimize functional use of the arm:

- *Orthoses*: The client with a biceps rupture will be placed in a long arm orthosis or cast, with the elbow at 90° of flexion and the forearm in neutral or pronation for two days to two weeks depending on the surgeon and surgical technique (Blackmore, 2011). Alternative management includes a hinge brace locked at 90° of flexion for the first week and then adjusted to block at 30°–45° of flexion and allowing full flexion at two to three weeks. At this point of healing, the physician may elect to allow increased extension by 10° per week until full extension is achieved. Education regarding splints/orthoses should include the purpose of the splint, wearing schedule, the donning/doffing process, and skin care precautions.

- *Manual techniques*: Edema management includes compression garments or wraps, elevation, and MEM. Other manual techniques include gentle stretching, massage, and soft tissue mobilization.
- *Therapeutic exercise*:
  - AROM to the shoulder, wrist, and digits; especially if stiffness or swelling is a concern.
  - Active extension against gravity with gradual lengthening of the biceps musculotendinous unit.
  - PROM for elbow flexion or gravity-assisted elbow flexion in the supine position, which help to decrease guarding.
  - PROM supination and pronation with the elbow at 90°.
  - A progressive strengthening program may be initiated pending approval from the referring surgeon.
- *Physical agent modalities*: Moist hot packs may be used to increase blood flow, decrease pain, decrease muscle tightness, decrease joint stiffness, and increase tissue extensibility in preparing the soft tissue for functional movement and activity if indicated. Ice packs may be used for pain and edema management, and electrical stimulation may be used for pain management, neuromuscular reeducation, and muscle strengthening. Ultrasound may be used to selectively heat deeper muscles and joint structures if indicated (Cameron, 2013).

Referrals and Discharge Considerations

Throughout the course of occupational therapy, the client is reassessed and progressed to increase ROM, strength, endurance, speed, confidence, and functional use of their involved UE. The physician, therapist, and caregiver ultimately work together with the client for a full return to meaningful activities and full participation in their vocational and avocational roles. Once the client has met his or her goals in therapy, or reached a plateau, the therapist ensures the client's competence in completing a HEP to maintain or further promote their autonomy.

Management and Standards of Practice

In any setting, it is important for occupational therapy practitioners to participate in professional development and continuing education. This not only ensures continued certification, but also helps therapists to maintain and enhance knowledge of musculoskeletal disorders and injuries. Maintaining open communication with physicians and staff involved with client care is also necessary in this area of practice. Many issues that arise in orthopedic practice can be addressed if communication between the OT and physician is open and clear. It is also crucial to maintain clear and concise medical records of all treatment provided, as well as treatment planned.

Chapter 15 Self-Study Activities (Answers Are Provided at the End of the Chapter)

Match the UE orthopedic test with the correct finding:

	Test Name	Answer	Possible Findings
1.	Mills Tennis Elbow Test	B	A. Pain with resisted finger extension.
2.	Cozen's Test	C	B. Pain in the lateral epicondyle is considered a positive test.
3.	Maudsley's Test	A	C. Severe and sudden pain in the lateral epicondyle.
4.	Tinel's Test	D	D. Tapping over nerve distribution results in tingling.

5. A patient reports pain along the lateral epicondyle region of the humerus and weakness secondary to pain. Which of the following tests MOST likely produced these findings?
   A. Tinel's sign
   B. Cozen's Test
   C. Golfer's Elbow Test
   D. Finkelstein's Test
   E. Phalen's Test

6. A patient reports pain along the medial aspect of the elbow. Which of the following tests MOST likely produced these findings?
   A. Tinel's sign
   B. Cozen's Test
   C. Golfer's Elbow Test
   D. Finkelstein's Test
   E. Phalen's Test

Match the UE orthopedic assessment with the correct description:

	Assessment	Answer	Description
7.	The Patient-Rated Elbow Evaluation (PREE)		A. A 37-item self-administered questionnaire on general hand functioning.
8.	The Disabilities of the Arm, Shoulder, and Hand (DASH)		B. A 20-item questionnaire to measure pain and disability of ADLs specific to the elbow.
9.	Michigan Hand Outcome Questionnaire (MHQ)		C. A 30-item self-report on physical functioning of the UE.

Match the following physical agent modality (PAM) with the correct definition:

	PAM	Answer	Definition
10.	Cold		A. Effects of this modality include vasoconstriction.
11.	Paraffin		B. This modality is useful for larger joints, requires approximately six towel layers, and is applied for 15–20 min.
12.	Ultrasound		C. Heating occurs through convection and the modality is useful for hypersensitive injuries.
13.	Fluidotherapy		D. Heating occurs through conduction and the modality is frequently used before stretching.
14.	Moist heat		E. High frequency acoustic energy is used to enhance tissue healing, reduce pain, and restore mobility.

15. Elbow and forearm anatomy self-study activity

Please list the origin, insertion, action, and innervation for muscles identified below using a format of your choosing (e.g., blank sheet of paper or a computer-generated table). Please use the anatomy textbook recommended by your occupational therapy program to check your answers as needed; minor differences between anatomy references should be expected.

While the inclusion of an anatomy recall question (i.e., origin, insertion, action, and innervation question) on the board examination is highly unlikely, you may be required to apply knowledge of anatomy. For example, given an affected muscle or muscle group, determine the most appropriate functional task for a given assessment or intervention.

- Anconeus
- Biceps brachii short head
- Brachialis
- Brachioradialis
- Coracobrachialis
- Extensor carpi radialis brevis
- Extensor carpi radialis longus
- Extensor carpi ulnaris
- Flexor carpi radialis
- Flexor carpi ulnaris
- Pronator teres
- Supinator
- Triceps brachii

Chapter 15 Self-Study Answers

1. B
2. C
3. A
4. D
5. B
6. C
7. B
8. C
9. A
10. A
11. D
12. E
13. C
14. B
15. Please use the anatomy textbook recommended by your occupational therapy program to check your answers.

References

Adams, J., & Steinmann, S. (2011). Distal biceps rupture. In S. W. Wolfe, R. N. Hotchkiss, & D. P. Green (Eds.), *Green's operative hand surgery* (6th ed., pp. 931–944). Philadelphia, PA: Elsevier.

Ahmad, C. S., & Levine, W. N. (2014). Shoulder and elbow disorders in the athlete. In L. K. Cannada (Ed.), *Orthopaedic knowledge update 11* (11th ed., pp. 373–386). Rosemont, IL: American Academy of Orthopaedic Surgeons.

Altman, E. (2011). Therapist's management of the stiff elbow. In T. M. Skirven, L. Osterman, J. Fedorczyk, & P. C. Amadio (Eds.), *Rehabilitation of the hand and upper extremity* (6th ed., pp. 1075–1088). Philadelphia, PA: Elsevier/Mosby.

Armstrong, A. D., & Murthi, A. (2014). Elbow instability and reconstruction. In L. K. Cannada (Ed.), *Orthopaedic knowledge update 11* (11th ed., pp. 407–417). Rosemont, IL: American Academy of Orthopaedic Surgeons.

Bales, C. P., Placzek, J. D., Malone, K. J., Vaupel, Z., & Arnoczky, S. P. (2007). Microvascular supply of the lateral epicondyle and common extensor origin. *Journal of Shoulder and Elbow Surgery, 16*(4), 497–501. doi:10.1016/j.jse.2006.08.006

Bano, K. Y., & Kahlon, R. S. (2006). Radial head fractures—Advanced techniques in surgical management and rehabilitation. *Journal of Hand Therapy, 19*(2), 114–135. doi:10.1197/j.jht.2006.02.011

Beaton, D. E., Katz, J. N., Fossel, A. H., Wright, J. G., Tarasuk, V., & Bombardier, C. (2001). Measuring the whole or the parts? Validity, reliability, and responsiveness of the Disabilities of the Arm, Shoulder and Hand outcome measure in different regions of the upper extremity. *Journal of Hand Therapy, 14*(2), 128–146. Retrieved from http://www.ncbi.nlm.nih.gov/pubmed/11382253

Beredjiklian, P. (2011). Management of fractures and dislocations of the elbow. In T. M. Skirven, L. Osterman, J. Fedorczyk, & P. C. Amadio (Eds.), *Rehabilitation of the hand and upper extremity* (6th ed., pp. 1049–1060). Philadelphia, PA: Elsevier/Mosby.

Binaghi, D. (2015). MR imaging of the elbow. *Magnetic Resonance Imaging Clinics of North America, 23*(3), 427–440. doi:10.1016/j.mric.2015.04.005

Blackmore, S. (2011). Therapy following distal biceps and triceps ruptures. In T. M. Skirven, L. Osterman, J. Fedorczyk, & P. C. Amadio (Eds.), *Rehabilitation of the hand and upper extremity* (6th ed., pp. 1122–1133). Philadelphia, PA: Elsevier/Mosby.

Brown, T., & Chien, C.-W. (2010). Top-down or bottom-up occupational therapy assessment: Which way do we go? *The British Journal of Occupational Therapy, 73*(3), 95. doi:10.4276/030802210x12682330090334

Budoff, J. E. (2010). Tendinopathies of the hand, wrist and elbow. In T. E. Trumble, G. M. Rayan, M. E. Baratz, & J. E. Budoff (Eds.), *Principles of hand surgery and therapy* (2nd ed., pp. 327–351). Philadelphia, PA: Saunders.

Calfee, R. P., Patel, A., DaSilva, M. F., & Akelman, E. (2008). Management of lateral epicondylitis: Current concepts. *Journal of the American Academy of Orthopaedic Surgeons, 16*(1), 19–29. Retrieved from http://www.ncbi.nlm.nih.gov/pubmed/18180389

Cameron, M. H. (2013). *Physical agents in rehabilitation: From research to practice* (4th ed.). St. Louis, MO: Elsevier/Saunders.

Childress, M. A., & Beutler, A. (2013). Management of chronic tendon injuries. *American Family Physician, 87*(7), 486–490. Retrieved from http://www.ncbi.nlm.nih.gov/pubmed/23547590

Cincere, B., & Nirschl, R. P. (2013). Tendon injuries and conditions of the elbow: Biceps, triceps, lateral and medial epicondylitis. In G. P. Nicholson (Ed.), *Orthopaedic knowledge update: Shoulder and elbow 4* (4th ed., pp. 479–493). Rosemont, IL: American Academy of Orthopaedic Surgeons.

Cooper, C. (2014a). Elbow, wrist, and hand tendinopathies. In C. Cooper (Ed.), *Fundamentals of hand therapy: Clinical reasoning and treatment guidelines for common diagnoses of the upper extremity* (2nd ed., pp. 383–393). St. Louis, MO: Elsevier/Mosby.

Cooper, C. (2014b). Hand impairments. In M. V. Radomski & C. A. T. Latham (Eds.), *Occupational therapy for physical dysfunction* (7th ed., pp. 1129–1167). Philadelphia, PA: Wolters Kluwer Health/Lippincott Williams & Wilkins.

Cooper, C., & Martin, H. A. (2007). Common forms of tendinitis/tendinosis. In C. Cooper (Ed.), *Fundamentals of hand therapy: Clinical reasoning and treatment guidelines for common diagnoses of the upper extremity* (pp. 286–300). St. Louis, MO: Elsevier/Mosby.

Davila, S. (2011). Therapist's management of fractures and dislocations of the elbow. In T. M. Skirven, L. Osterman, J. Fedorczyk, & P. C. Amadio (Eds.), *Rehabilitation of the hand and upper extremity* (6th ed., pp. 1061–1074). Philadelphia, PA: Elsevier/Mosby.

Descatha, A., Dale, A. M., Silverstein, B. A., Roquelaure, Y., & Rempel, D. (2015). Lateral epicondylitis: New evidence for work relatedness. *Joint Bone Spine, 82*(1), 5–7. doi:10.1016/j.jbspin.2014.10.013

Faro, F., & Wolf, J. M. (2007). Lateral epicondylitis: Review and current concepts. *The Journal of Hand Surgery, 32*(8), 1271–1279. doi:10.1016/j.jhsa.2007.07.019

Foster, Z. J., Voss, T. T., Hatch, J., & Frimodig, A. (2015). Corticosteroid injections for common musculoskeletal conditions. *American Family Physician, 92*(8), 694–699. Retrieved from http://www.ncbi.nlm.nih.gov/pubmed/26554409

Geissler, W. B., & Craft, J. A. (2010). Elbow arthroscopically and instability. In T. E. Trumble, G. M. Rayan, M. E. Baratz, & J. E. Budoff (Eds.), *Principles of hand surgery and therapy* (2nd ed., pp. 543–554). Philadelphia, PA: Saunders.

Hunter, D. J. (2009). Insights from imaging on the epidemiology and pathophysiology of osteoarthritis. *Radiologic Clinics of North America, 47*(4), 539–551. doi:10.1016/j.rcl.2009.03.004

Hurt, J. A., & Savoie, F. H. (2013). Advanced elbow arthroscopy. In G. P. Nicholson (Ed.), *Orthopaedic knowledge update: Shoulder and elbow 4* (4th ed., pp. 561–571). Rosemont, IL: American Academy of Orthopaedic Surgeons.

Kasch, M., & Walsch, M. (2013). Hand and upper extremity injuries. In L. W. Pedretti, H. M. Pendleton, & W. Schultz-Krohn (Eds.), *Pedretti's occupational therapy: Practice skills for physical dysfunction* (7th ed., pp. 1037–1071). St. Louis, MO: Elsevier.

Kelly, M. P., Perkinson, S. G., Ablove, R. H., & Tueting, J. L. (2015). Distal biceps tendon ruptures: An epidemiological analysis using a large population database. *American Journal of Sports Medicine, 43*(8), 2012–2017. doi:10.1177/0363546515587738

Kim, S. H., Szabo, R. M., & Marder, R. A. (2012). Epidemiology of humerus fractures in the United States: Nationwide emergency department sample, 2008. *Arthritis Care & Research, 64*(3), 407–414. doi:10.1002/acr.21563

King, G. (2011). Fractures of the head of the radius. In S. W. Wolfe, R. N. Hotchkiss, & D. P. Green (Eds.), *Green's operative hand surgery* (6th ed., pp. 783–819). Philadelphia, PA: Elsevier.

Kuhnel, S. P., Athwal, G. S., & King, G. J. W. (2014). Elbow and forearm trauma. In L. K. Cannada (Ed.), *Orthopaedic knowledge update 11* (11th ed., pp. 387–406). Rosemont, IL: American Academy of Orthopaedic Surgeons.

Lapner, M., & King, G. J. W. (2013). Radial head fractures. *The Journal of Bone & Joint Surgery, 95*(12), 1136–1143. Retrieved from http://jbjs.org/jbjsam/95/12/1136.full.pdf

Lin, K.-Y., Shen, P.-H., Lee, C.-H., Pan, R.-Y., Lin, L.-C., & Shen, H.-C. (2012). Functional outcomes of surgical reconstruction for posterolateral rotatory instability of the elbow. *Injury, 43*(10), 1657–1661. doi:10.1016/j.injury.2012.04.023

Lord, B., & Sarraf, K. M. (2011). Paediatric supracondylar fractures of the humerus: Acute assessment and management. *British Journal of Hospital Medicine (London), 72*(1), M8–M11. Retrieved from http://www.ncbi.nlm.nih.gov/pubmed/21240129

MacDermid, J. C., & Michlovitz, S. L. (2006). Examination of the elbow: Linking diagnosis, prognosis, and outcomes as a framework for maximizing therapy interventions. *Journal of Hand Therapy, 19*(2), 82–97. doi:10.1197/j.jht.2006.02.018

Magee, D. J. (2014). *Orthopedic physical assessment* (6th ed.). St. Louis, MO: Elsevier.

Maher, C. M. (2014). Orthopaedic conditions. In M. V. Radomski & C. A. T. Latham (Eds.), *Occupational therapy for physical dysfunction* (7th ed., pp. 1103–1128). Philadelphia, PA: Wolters Kluwer Health/Lippincott Williams & Wilkins.

Manske, R. C. (2011a). Elbow injuries. In S. B. Brotzman & K. E. Wilk (Eds.), *Clinical orthopaedic rehabilitation: An evidence-based approach* (3rd ed., pp. 82–210). Philadelphia, PA: Mosby.

Manske, R. C. (2011b). Shoulder injuries. In S. B. Brotzman & K. E. Wilk (Eds.), *Clinical orthopaedic rehabilitation: An evidence-based approach* (3rd ed., pp. 82–210). Philadelphia, PA: Mosby.

Nauth, A., McKee, M. D., Ristevski, B., Hall, J., & Schemitsch, E. H. (2011). Distal humeral fractures in adults. *The Journal of Bone & Joint Surgery, 93*(7), 686–700. doi:10.2106/jbjs.j.00845

O'Driscoll, S. W., Morrey, B. F., Korinek, S., & An, K.-N. (1992). Elbow subluxation and dislocation: A spectrum of instability. *Clinical Orthopaedics and Related Research, 280*, 186–197.

Placzek, J. D. (2006). Elbow fractures and dislocations. In J. D. Placzek & D. Boyce (Eds.), *Orthopaedic physical therapy secrets* (2nd ed.). Philadelphia, PA: Elsevier.

Ring, D. (2013). Fractures of the distal humerus. In G. P. Nicholson (Ed.), *Orthopaedic knowledge update: Shoulder and elbow 4* (4th ed., pp. 543–552). Rosemont, IL: American Academy of Orthopaedic Surgeons.

Ruchelsman, D. E., Christoforou, D., & Jupiter, J. B. (2013). Fractures of the radial head and neck. *The Journal of Bone & Joint Surgery, 95*(5), 469–478. doi:10.2106/jbjs.j.01989

Schwartz, D. A. (2010). Responsiveness of the Michigan Hand Outcomes Questionnaire and the Disabilities of the Arm, Shoulder and Hand questionnaire in patients with hand injury. *Journal of Hand Therapy, 23*(4), 428. doi:10.1016/j.jht.2010.06.004

Shen, J., & Chen, D. (2014). Recent progress in osteoarthritis research. *Journal of the American Academy of Orthopaedic Surgeons, 22*(7), 467–468. doi:10.5435/JAAOS-22-07-467

Speed, C. (2014). A systematic review of shockwave therapies in soft tissue conditions: Focusing on the evidence. *British Journal of Sports Medicine, 48*(21), 1538–1542. doi:10.1136/bjsports-2012-091961

Stern, P., Elfar, J. C., & Shuler, M. S. (2010). Arthritis. In T. E. Trumble, G. M. Rayan, M. E. Baratz, & J. E. Budoff (Eds.), *Principles of hand surgery and therapy* (2nd ed., pp. 352–384). Philadelphia, PA: Saunders.

Stoneback, J. W., Owens, B. D., Sykes, J., Athwal, G. S., Pointer, L., & Wolf, J. M. (2012). Incidence of elbow dislocations in the United States population. *The Journal of Bone & Joint Surgery, 94*(3), 240–245. doi:10.2106/jbjs.j.01663

Thanasas, C., Papadimitriou, G., Charalambidis, C., Paraskevopoulos, I., & Papanikolaou, A. (2011). Platelet-rich plasma versus autologous whole blood for the treatment of chronic lateral elbow epicondylitis: A randomized controlled clinical trial. *American Journal of Sports Medicine, 39*(10), 2130–2134. doi:10.1177/0363546511417113

Tosti, R., Jennings, J., & Sewards, J. M. (2013). Lateral epicondylitis of the elbow. *The American Journal of Medicine, 126*(4), 357.e351–357.e356. doi:10.1016/j.amjmed.2012.09.018

Vaughn, P. (2014). Appendix I common conditions, resources, and evidence: Substance abuse disorders. In B. A. B. Schell, G. Gillen, & M. E. Scaffa (Eds.), *Willard & Spackman's occupational therapy* (12th ed., pp. 1161–1163). Philadelphia, PA: Wolters Kluwer Health/Lippincott Williams & Wilkins.

Wang, C. J. (2012). Extracorporeal shockwave therapy in musculoskeletal disorders. *Journal of Orthopaedic Surgery and Research, 7*, 11. doi:10.1186/1749-799X-7-11

Wiegand, L., Bernstein, J., & Ahn, J. (2012). Fractures in brief: Olecranon fractures. *Clinical Orthopaedics and Related Research, 470*(12), 3637–3641. doi:10.1007/s11999-012-2393-5

Yoon, A., & King, G. J. W. (2013). Radial head and neck fractures. In G. P. Nicholson (Ed.), *Orthopaedic knowledge update: Shoulder and elbow 4* (4th ed., pp. 531–541). Rosemont, IL: American Academy of Orthopaedic Surgeons.

Orthopedic Conditions of the Wrist and Hand

Marie Eve Pepin, Kurt Krueger, and Jeffrey Placzek

Learning Objectives

- Describe key pathology, etiology, and epidemiology for wrist/hand fractures, thumb arthritis, finger tendon pathologies, and mononeuropathies of the forearm and hand.
- Compare and contrast clinical presentation for the orthopedic conditions of the wrist and hand listed above.
- Describe diagnostic tests for the wrist/hand disorders listed above.
- Describe medical and surgical procedures for orthopedic conditions of the wrist and hand listed above.
- List medical/surgical precautions and contraindications for orthopedic conditions of the wrist and hand listed above.
- List what should be included in an occupational therapy (OT) examination of the pathologies covered in this chapter.
- Describe the OT intervention for the wrist and hand pathologies described in this chapter.

Key Terms

- *Angulation*: When the alignment of the bone is affected and the distal fragment points in a different direction.
- *Arthroscopy*: Examination, diagnosis, and/or treatment of a joint using an endoscope that is inserted through a small incision in the skin.
- *Capsulodesis*: Correction of joint instability by cutting, tightening, and re-attaching the capsule with sutures.
- *Computed tomography (CT)*: Noninvasive imaging technology that utilizes a rotating x-ray emitter to generate detailed cross-sectional computer images of body tissues.

- *Extensor lag*: An inability to actively extend a joint to its passive ability.
- *Fibrosis*: The development of fibrous connective tissue as a result of injury, disease, or abnormal healing.
- *Magnetic resonance imaging (MRI)*: Noninvasive imaging technology that utilizes a magnetic field and radio waves to create detailed computer images of body tissues.
- *Neurolysis*: Application of certain agents to a nerve in order to cause a temporary degeneration of the nerve's fibers to interrupt the transmission of pain signals.
- *Tenodesis*: Stabilizing a joint by anchoring the tendons that move that joint.
- *Tenodesis grasp*: Due to development of tension in the finger flexor tendons and muscles, extension of the wrist will make the fingers flex slightly while wrist flexion will cause a release or extension of the fingers.
- *Tenosynovitis*: Inflammation of the tendon sheath.
- *Ulnocarpal impaction syndrome*: Degenerative wrist condition caused by the ulnar head impacting upon the triangular fibrocartilage complex.
- *Wallerian degeneration*: Process of degeneration of the axon distal to a site of transection.

Common Fractures and Disorders of Bones and Joints

Distal Radius Fracture

Description: Distal radius fractures are among the most common fractures, accounting for 25% of all fractures in children and up to 18% of all fractures in the elderly

(Nellans, Kowalski, & Chung, 2012). Due to a variety of factors, incidence seems to be on the rise (Nellans et al., 2012). The two most common types of distal radius fractures are Colles' and Smith's fractures (Moscony, 2007; Moscony & Shank, 2014). Colles' fracture is a fracture of the distal radius with dorsal displacement of the distal fragment while Smith's fracture is a fracture of the distal radius with palmar displacement of the distal fragment (Moscony & Shank, 2014). Colles' and Smith's fractures occur most commonly in postmenopausal women with osteoporotic bone and typically occur as a result of a fall on an outstretched hand (Moscony, 2007; Moscony & Shank, 2014). Children and adolescents are also at high risk, as up to 25% of all fractures in this population occur at the distal radius (Nellans et al., 2012).

Clinical presentation: Wrist deformity, pain, limited range of motion (ROM), swelling, and ecchymosis are common. The Colles' fracture deformity is often referred to as a dinner fork deformity due to the shape of the forearm after the displacement of the distal segment.

Common diagnostic tests: X-rays are usually sufficient to diagnose wrist fractures. Computerized axial tomography (i.e., CAT) or CT scans are occasionally used for preoperative planning.

Common medical and surgical procedures: The American Academy of Orthopaedic Surgeons (2008) (AAOS) recommends surgery for distal radius fractures when there is postreduction shortening >3 millimeters, dorsal angulation > 10°, or intraarticular displacement >2 millimeters (Yoon & Grewal, 2012). In cases of extra-articular fractures, there is inconclusive evidence as to which method, closed reduction with casting or external fixation, leads to the best outcomes (Yoon & Grewal, 2012).

Precautions and contraindications: Aggressive therapy should be avoided. Redness over the joint or temperature elevation may indicate the treatment is causing an inflammatory response and should be modified (Cooper, 2014c). Arthrosis commonly develops in clients who have joint incongruity (91%) and is seen radiographically in all clients with an intraarticular incongruity of 2 millimeters or more (Yoon & Grewal, 2012).

Screening and Assessments

Similar to other orthopedic conditions of the upper extremity, there are various top-down and bottom-up approaches to examination. **Tables 16-1** through **16-3** provide a list of appropriate screening and assessments

Table 16-1 Screening and Assessments for Distal Radius Fracture (Immobilization Phase)

Screening and Assessments	Description
Observation	Incision and pins if present, skin color, edema, autonomic signs which could indicate CRPS, and cast fitting
ROM	Assessment of the noninvolved joints (e.g., shoulder, elbow, forearm, and digit ROM) if not casted. Gentle passive ROM and PROM of the involved elbow only with physician approval
Sensory	Moving or static two-point discrimination or monofilament testing
Circulation	Skin color, pulses, and capillary refill
Edema	Circumferential measurements
ADL assessment	DASH

Data from Cooper, 2014c; Kasch and Walsh, 2013.

Table 16-2 Screening and Assessments for Distal Radius Fracture (Mobilization Phase)

Screening and Assessments	Description
Observation	Skin redness and warmth may indicate inflammation (e.g., from doing too much too soon)
ROM	Assessment of wrist AROM and PROM with physician approval. Reassessment of shoulder, elbow, forearm, and hand
Sensory	Moving or static two-point discrimination or monofilament testing
Edema	Circumferential measurements
ADL assessment	DASH and PRWE
Assess scar adhesions and sensitivity	Determine if the underlying tissues are adherent and limiting normal tendon-gliding

Data from Cooper, 2014c; Kasch and Walsh, 2013.

during the immobilization, mobilization, and strengthening phases of rehabilitation, respectively.

Interventions

The main objective of the OT intervention after a wrist and/or hand injury is to restore function and independence in life roles. Before discussing interventions, it

Table 16-3 Screening and Assessments for Distal Radius Fracture (Strengthening Phase)

Screening and Assessments	Description
Grip and pinch testing	Dynamometer and pinch gauge. Isolate actions of the specific muscle (e.g., intrinsics from extensor digitorum)
MMT	Testing of the shoulder, elbow, and wrist

Data from Cooper, 2014c; Kasch and Walsh, 2013.

is important to note that interventions must be carefully matched to the stage of injury and recovery (e.g., whether the client is in the immobilization or mobilization phase).

Interventions for the immobilization phase:

- Education regarding pin site care for clients with percutaneous pinning or external fixation, precautions related to the cast, monitoring for adverse reactions (e.g., cast too tight and complex regional pain syndrome [CRPS]), home exercise program, and discontinuation of a sling (Cooper, 2014c; Kasch & Walsh, 2013).
- Edema management during the immobilization phase of rehabilitation is critical and techniques may include active ROM (AROM) in a nondependent position, elevation, retrograde massage, and compression (Moscony, 2007; Moscony & Shank, 2014).
- AROM to adjoining joints, which may begin as early as possible, and may include shoulder ROM (e.g., flexion, extension, abduction, internal and external rotation) and elbow ROM (e.g., flexion and extension). Reduction in the use of the sling may be advised when appropriate.
- Instruction in finger ROM, and tendon-gliding exercises.
- Activity instruction and modification to help maintain independence with activities of daily living (ADLs) (Cooper, 2014c; Kasch & Walsh, 2013).

Interventions for the mobilization phase:

- A custom-fabricated volar wrist orthosis may be used to protect the injured joint, limit motion, decrease pain, and help the client avoid resting

the wrist in a flexed posture. The client should be instructed to wean off the splint per physician orders (Cooper, 2014c; Moscony, 2007; Moscony & Shank, 2014).

- Edema management is continued through the mobilization phase of rehabilitation in conjunction with ROM and pain management techniques (Cooper, 2014c; Moscony, 2007; Moscony & Shank, 2014).
- Adherent scars and fibrosis should be addressed with active tendon-gliding techniques, scar massage, pressure garments, gel sheeting, and thermal agents (i.e., modalities), which may aid in improving scar mobility (Kasch & Walsh, 2013). If applicable, a desensitization program may be implemented to address scar sensitivity.
- AROM exercises for shoulder, elbow, forearm, and digits are continued until normalized ROM is achieved. For example:
  o Retrain the extensor carpi radialis longus (ECRL) by having the client extend the wrist while making a gentle fist with the fingers, and retrain the extensor carpi radialis brevis (ECRB) by having the client hold the fingers gently in extension while performing wrist flexion.
  o Instruct the client in tendon glides for the flexor digitorum superficialis (FDS) and hook fist exercises to encourage extensor digitorum communis (EDC) gliding and promote interphalangeal (IP) flexion. The hook fist position will also stretch the intrinsic hand muscles.
- Grasp-and-release activities that reinforce tenodesis grasp (Cooper, 2014c; Kasch & Walsh, 2013).
- Dexterity activities such as cat's cradle, pickup sticks, folding, and buttoning (Cooper, 2014c; Kasch & Walsh, 2013).

Intervention considerations:

- Treatment planning will be dependent on the severity of the wrist injury and the surrounding tissues; the OT practitioner will adjust interventions to address individual client factors and needs.
- The therapist must strictly follow physician's recommendations as the AAOS recommends with moderate strength not to start early wrist ROM in clients post stable wrist fixation (Yoon & Grewal, 2012).
- Aggressive therapy should be avoided. Redness over the joint or temperature elevation may indicate the

treatment is causing an inflammatory response and should be modified (Cooper, 2014c).

- Client goals will also need to address individual client factors such as occupation and interest, overall health, previous functional level, hand dominance, cognition, and finances (Moscony, 2007; Moscony & Shank, 2014).

Scaphoid Fracture

Description: The scaphoid is the most commonly fractured carpal bone and scaphoid fractures make up to 80% of all carpal bone fractures (American Academy of Orthopaedic Surgeons, 2011). Scaphoid fractures occur from a fall on an outstretched hand especially with the wrist in extension or radial deviation (Cheung, Tang, & Fung, 2014; Gupta, Rijal, & Jawed, 2013). Fractures of the scaphoid may occur at the distal end, the wrist, or the proximal pole (Cheung et al., 2014). The main blood supply to the scaphoid enters distally and works in a retrograde fashion to supply the proximal pole (American Academy of Orthopaedic Surgeons, 2011). Therefore, blood supply disruption due to a fracture increases the risks of complications such as delayed healing or avascular necrosis (Cheung et al., 2014; Gupta et al., 2013). **Table 16-4** lists the classification of scaphoid fractures.

Clinical presentation: Clients with a scaphoid fracture typically present with pain upon pinching tasks, pain with forearm pronation, limited wrist flexion and radial deviation ROM, and reduced grip strength (Cheung et al., 2014). Positive examination techniques include tenderness to palpation of the scaphoid (e.g., in the anatomical snuff box) and a positive scaphoid compression test (Cheung et al., 2014).

Common diagnostic tests: Plain film radiographs can identify 70–90% of all scaphoid fractures (Cheung et al., 2014). If radial wrist pain persists, repeat radiographs,

MRI, bone scintigraphy, or a CT scan should be undertaken to diagnose a scaphoid fracture (Cheung et al., 2014; Steinmann & Adams, 2006).

Common medical and surgical procedures: Due to good blood supply, distal pole fractures usually heal well and are immobilized with a short arm thumb spica cast for four to six weeks. Undisplaced, stable wrist fracture requires longer immobilization (8–12 weeks) (Cheung et al., 2014). A new trend favors internal fixation for clients who are active and for whom the prolonged immobilization would be impractical (Cheung et al., 2014). Nonunion fractures may require internal fixation and bone grafting (Cheung et al., 2014).

Precautions and contraindications: A client with radial-sided wrist pain that persists or is reproduced upon palpation of the scaphoid should be immobilized and sent for repeat radiographs or other testing. Missed radial fractures (i.e., approximately 12% of scaphoid fractures) can lead to complications such as nonunion and osteonecrosis (Cheung et al., 2014). Osteonecrosis is frequent, occurring in 13–50% of all scaphoid fractures (Steinmann & Adams, 2006).

Screening and Assessments

Screening and assessments are similar throughout the various orthopedic conditions of the upper extremity with slight variations. Below is a list of top-down approaches that address the symptoms, as well as the impact of the symptoms on the person's roles, contexts, and environment, followed by bottom-up approaches that are symptom specific:

- Client history including the client's age, hand dominance, occupational and avocational responsibilities, prior injuries, comorbidities, family issues, psychological issues, broader social issues, and economic issues.
- Mechanism and date of injury, structures involved, type and extent of medical and surgical intervention, concomitant injuries, and future treatment planned.
- Client-reported symptoms.
- Physical assessment includes the following:
  - Baseline physical evaluation to assess limitations not related to the injury.
  - Observations of pain or fear with rest and movement.
  - Color, temperature, and signs of compromised circulation or compartment syndrome.

Table 16-4 Classification of Scaphoid Fractures	
Fracture	**Description**
Type A	Stable acute fractures (i.e., distal pole or partial wrist fractures)
Type B	Unstable acute fractures (i.e., proximal pole or complicated fractures of the wrist and distal pole)
Type C	Delayed union after cast immobilization
Type D	Established nonunions

Data from Cheung, Tang, & Fung, 2014.

- Edema (e.g., circumferential and volumetric).
- Sensory and motor function.
- Coordination.
- Skin integrity and wound assessment.
  - *Wound or surgical incision*: Note location, size, integrity of closure, exposure of pins or hardware, and signs of infection.
  - *Scar*: Note location, size, adherence, hypertrophy, blanching with motion, pliability, and sensitivity.
- A/PROM of adjacent and uninvolved joints.
- AROM of involved joint if approved by the physician.
- Manual muscle testing (MMT) can be performed once there is evidence of bone healing.
- *Diagnostic special tests*: Scaphoid compression test (i.e., scaphoid pain upon compression of the first metacarpal into the scaphoid).
- *Palpation*: Scaphoid, especially in the snuffbox.
- Cognitive assessment.
- Ability to participate in life roles.
- Assessment of basic and instrumental ADLs (e.g., disabilities of the arm, shoulder, and hand [DASH] and Patient-Rated Wrist Evaluation [PRWE]).
- Functional mobility (Lawson & Murphy, 2013).

Interventions

Treatment of scaphoid fractures follow similar rehabilitation guidelines as distal radius fractures (Cooper, 2014c; Kasch & Walsh, 2013). Treatment must be in accordance with physician guidelines and knowledge about fracture stability and healing times (Cooper, 2014c; Kasch & Walsh, 2013). Interventions post immobilization should target the particular deficits found in the examination. Common interventions include pain and edema management, desensitization, ROM of the wrist, thumb and adjoining joints, motor and coordination retraining, progressive strengthening, tendongliding exercises, and ADL retraining. In some scaphoid fractures, immobilization may be prolonged (i.e., up to 12 weeks), and secondary deficits and contractures may be significant.

Metacarpal Fracture

Description: Metacarpal fractures are relatively common hand fractures and account for 18–44% of all hand fractures (Kollitz, Hammert, Vedder, & Huang, 2014). The most common metacarpal fracture is one of the neck of the fifth metacarpal (Kollitz et al., 2014). Fifth metacarpal fractures are often referred to as a Boxer's fracture because it occurs most frequently when the ulnar aspect of a closed fist strikes against an object (Brotzman & Manske, 2011). Fractures to other metacarpals occur primarily from a direct blow to the dorsum of the hand (Cotterell & Richard, 2015). The majority of metacarpal fractures are isolated injuries, simple, closed, and stable (Kollitz et al., 2014). Metacarpal bones have good blood supply and usually heal well in six weeks or less (Brotzman & Manske, 2011; Kollitz et al., 2014).

Clinical presentation: Common findings with metacarpal fractures include pain while making a fist or while moving the fingers, decreased grip strength, pain to palpation of the metacarpal bone, and possible swelling (Brotzman & Manske, 2011). At times, deformity of the metacarpal bone may be palpated on the dorsum of the hand (Brotzman & Manske, 2011; Kollitz et al., 2014).

Common diagnostic tests: Common diagnostic tests include plain film radiographs.

Common medical and surgical procedures: Nonsurgical treatment is usually recommended for nondisplaced fractures or those with small angulations, and surgery is usually warranted when multiple fractures are present, with oblique or open fractures or with large angulations (American Academy of Orthopaedic Surgeons, 2011; Brotzman & Manske, 2011). See **Table 16-5** for nonoperative treatment of metacarpal fractures of digits II through IV.

Precautions and contraindications: Prevent loss of metacarpophalangeal (MCP) flexion after a fracture and maintain tendon excursion of EDC due to the tendency to develop adhesions and joint stiffness (Brotzman & Manske, 2011). Rotation or bone angulation in excess of 30° may result in long-term grip weakness (Kollitz et al., 2014). A displaced metacarpal fracture should not be reduced until radiographic examination has been performed (Cotterell & Richard, 2015).

Screening and Assessments

Screening and assessments are similar throughout the various orthopedic conditions of the upper extremity with slight variations. Below is a list of top-down approaches that address the symptoms, as well as the impact of the symptoms on the person's roles, contexts, and

Table 16-5 Nonoperative Treatment Recommendations for Simple Closed, Isolated Metacarpal Fractures of Digits II Through IV

Fracture Type	Recommended Treatment	Comments
Fifth metacarpal neck or shaft	No reduction needed; Buddy tape with immediate mobilization or splint/cast immobilization for 4 weeks (level of evidence: III)*	Fingers may be splinted in neutral or flexion (level of evidence: I).*
Index, middle, and ring finger metacarpal shaft fractures	Palmar wrist splint with immediate mobilization or splint/cast immobilization for 4 weeks (level of evidence: III)*	Initial extensor lag may be seen with palmar wrist splint, which will likely resolve

*Levels of evidence refer to research hierarchy where level I studies are the most rigorous (e.g., random control trials) and levels IV through VII have less rigor (e.g., case studies and opinion papers).
Data from Kollitz et al., 2014.

environment, followed by bottom-up approaches that are symptom specific:

- Client history including the client's age, hand dominance, occupational and avocational responsibilities, prior injuries, comorbidities, family issues, psychological issues, broader social issues, and economic issues.
- Mechanism and date of injury, structures involved, type and extent of medical and surgical intervention, concomitant injuries, and future treatment planned.
- Client-reported symptoms.
- Physical assessment includes the following:
  o Baseline physical evaluation to assess limitations not related to the injury.
  o Observations of pain or fear with rest and movement.
  o Color, temperature, and signs of compromised circulation or compartment syndrome.
  o Edema (e.g., circumferential and volumetric).
  o Sensory and motor function.
  o Coordination.
  o Skin integrity and wound assessment.
    ▪ *Wound or surgical incision*: Note location, size, integrity of closure, exposure of pins or hardware, and signs of infection.
    ▪ *Scar*: Note location, size, adherence, hypertrophy, blanching with motion, pliability, and sensitivity.
  o A/PROM of adjacent/uninvolved joints.
  o AROM
    ▪ Finger extension ROM should be performed to check for an extensor lag and rule out an

associated extensor tendon injury (Brotzman & Manske, 2011).
  o MMT can be performed once there is evidence of bone healing.
  o Cognitive assessment.
  o Ability to participate in life roles.
  o Assessment of basic and instrumental ADLs (e.g., DASH and PRWE).
  o Functional mobility (Lawson & Murphy, 2013).

Interventions

Similar to other fractures, interventions post immobilization should target the particular deficits found in the examination. Treatment must be in accordance with physician guidelines and knowledge about fracture stability and healing times (Cooper, 2014c; Kasch & Walsh, 2013). Common interventions include pain and edema management, desensitization, ROM of the wrist, fingers and adjoining joints, motor and coordination retraining, progressive strengthening, tendon-gliding exercises, and ADL retraining. If allowed by the physician, early ROM and edema reduction are a high priority to decrease the risks of contractures and atrophy (Cooper, 2014c; Kasch & Walsh, 2013).

Phalangeal Fractures

Description: Fractures of a proximal, middle, or distal phalanx of the hand are usually the result of a direct blow, fall, or crush injury (Cotterell & Richard, 2015). Phalangeal fractures are generally more unstable than metacarpal fractures (Brotzman & Manske, 2011). Because of lumbrical, interossei, and central slip attachment of the FDS, proximal phalanx fractures often lead to a volar angulation deformity. In contrast, fractures of the middle phalanges have unpredictable deformities while fractures of the distal phalanges are usually nondisplaced (Cotterell & Richard, 2015). Fractures are most prevalent over the distal phalanges (Hile & Hile, 2015).

Clinical presentation: Common findings with phalangeal fractures include pain while making a fist or moving the fingers, decreased grip strength, pain to palpation of the involved phalanx, and possible swelling.

Common diagnostic tests: Plain film radiographs are usually the prime mode of examination. In rare instances, a CT or an MRI scan is ordered to supplement radiographs (Pope, Bloem, Beltran, Morrison, & Wilson, 2014).

Common medical and surgical procedures: Immobilization is the most common treatment method but it depends on the type and the extent of the fracture. Generally, immobilization beyond three weeks is not recommended. Slings are not recommended for hand injuries (Cotterell & Richard, 2015).

Precautions and contraindications: Reduction of a deformed finger should not be attempted before a radiographic evaluation is performed (Cotterell & Richard, 2015). During immobilization, clients are advised to continue to perform ROM of uninvolved fingers and wrist to prevent contractures (Cotterell & Richard, 2015). Complete bony union and resolution of symptoms may take several months (McKinnis, 2014).

Screening and Assessments

Screening and assessments are similar throughout the various orthopedic conditions of the upper extremity with slight variations. Below is a list of top-down approaches that address the symptoms, as well as the impact of the symptoms on the person's roles, contexts, and environment, followed by bottom-up approaches that are symptom specific:

- Client history including the client's age, hand dominance, occupational and avocational responsibilities, prior injuries, comorbidities, family issues, psychological issues, broader social issues, and economic issues.
- Mechanism and date of injury, structures involved, type and extent of medical and surgical intervention, concomitant injuries, and future treatment planned.

- Physical assessment includes the following:
  - Baseline physical evaluation to assess limitations not related to the injury.
  - Observations of pain or fear with rest and movement.
  - Observation of extensor lag, which would indicate an extensor tendon injury.
  - Color, temperature, and signs of compromised circulation or compartment syndrome.
  - Edema (e.g., circumferential and volumetric).
  - Sensory and motor function.
  - Coordination.
  - Skin integrity and wound assessment.
    - *Wound or surgical incision*: Note location, size, integrity of closure, exposure of pins or hardware, and signs of infection.
    - *Scar*: Note location, size, adherence, hypertrophy, blanching with motion, pliability, and sensitivity.
  - A/PROM of adjacent and uninvolved joints.
  - *AROM*: Be observant for lack of active distal IP (DIP) extension in situations when full passive DIP extension is seen as this could indicate an extensor tendon injury.
  - MMT can be performed once there is evidence of bone healing.
  - Cognitive assessment.
  - Ability to participate in life roles.
  - Assessment of basic and instrumental ADLs (e.g., DASH and PRWE).
  - Functional mobility (Lawson & Murphy, 2013).

Interventions

Similar to other fractures, interventions post immobilization should target the particular deficits found in the examination. Treatment must be in accordance with physician guidelines and knowledge about fracture stability and healing times (Cooper, 2014c; Kasch & Walsh, 2013). Common interventions include pain and edema management, desensitization, ROM of the wrist, fingers, and adjoining joints, motor and coordination retraining, progressive strengthening, tendon-gliding exercises, and ADL retraining. When the middle phalanx is involved, isolated FDS exercises are recommended. In both proximal and distal phalangeal fractures, ROM is essential to prevent finger contractures (Cooper, 2014c; Kasch & Walsh, 2013).

CMC Arthritis of the Thumb

Description: Arthritis of the carpometacarpal (CMC) joint of the thumb is also known as trapeziometacarpal joint arthritis or basal joint arthritis. It is the second most common location of arthritis of the hand, after the DIP joints (American Academy of Orthopaedic Surgeons, 2011). The prevalence of basal thumb arthritis increases with age and is seen predominantly in postmenopausal women. The female to male ratio is 6:1. The most common etiology is a deficiency of the anterior oblique ligament causing instability of the CMC joint (American Academy of Orthopaedic Surgeons, 2011).

Clinical presentation: Clients frequently report pain with daily activities that require forceful pinching and gripping (American Academy of Orthopaedic Surgeons, 2011). As the disorder progresses, clients may also report weakness and constant pain at the base of the thumb and over the thenar eminence (Dias, Chandrasenan, Rajaratnam, & Burke, 2007). Pain may also be reproduced with palpation of the CMC joint of the thumb (Wyrick & Marik, 2010).

Common diagnostic tests: Typically, plain film radiographs are the main diagnostic test used to diagnose and stage the disease (American Academy of Orthopaedic Surgeons, 2011).

Common medical and surgical procedures: **Table 16-6** provides a list of common medical and surgical procedures for CMC arthritis of the thumb.

Precautions and contraindications: Aggressive stretching of the CMC joint should be avoided after CMC arthroplasty (Cooper, 2014b, 2014c).

Screening and Assessments

Screening and assessments are similar throughout the various orthopedic conditions of the upper extremity with slight variations. Below is a list of top-down approaches that address the symptoms, as well as the impact of the symptoms on the person's roles, contexts, and environment, followed by bottom-up approaches that are symptom specific:

- Client history including the client's age, hand dominance, occupational and avocational responsibilities, prior injuries, comorbidities, family issues, psychological issues, broader social issues, and economic issues.
- Type of symptoms, onset of symptoms, activities that aggravate or alleviate symptoms, type and

Table 16-6 Common Medical and Surgical Procedures for CMC Arthritis of the Thumb

Procedure	Description
Cortisone injections	Good temporary relief but little long-term benefit. Increases risks of tendon degeneration, fatty atrophy, and skin blanching
Custom splinting	A short thumb spica splint can be fabricated from low temperature thermoplastics. The purpose of the splint is to stabilize the CMC joint by placing the thumb in gentle palmar abduction. In the presence of MCP joint hyperextension, the splint should also include the MCP, which should be placed in slight flexion (Cooper, 2014c)
Prefabricated splints	Neoprene splints with additional strapping may be used to stabilize the CMC joint (Cooper, 2014c)
Surgical procedures	CMC interposition arthroplasty and/or CMC fusion

Data from Beasley, 2014; Biese, 2007; Cooper, 2014b

extent of medical intervention, concomitant injuries, and future treatment planned.

- Physical assessment includes the following:
  - Baseline physical evaluation to assess limitations not related to the thumb.
  - Observations of pain or fear with rest and movement.
  - Color, temperature, and signs of inflammation.
  - Edema (e.g., circumferential and volumetric) if needed.
  - Sensory and motor function.
  - Coordination.
  - Skin integrity.
  - A/PROM of adjacent and uninvolved joints.
  - AROM.
  - *MMT*: Pinch strength.
  - *Special tests*: Ligament stress test at the thumb to determine if instability is present.
  - *Palpation*: CMC joint.
  - Cognitive assessment.
  - Ability to participate in life roles.
  - Assessment of basic and instrumental ADLs (e.g., DASH and PRWE).
  - Functional mobility (Lawson & Murphy, 2013).

Interventions

The purpose of OT intervention for CMC arthritis is threefold:

- Symptom reduction through education and joint protection techniques.
- Splinting and provision of assistive devices to assist with ADLs.
- Education to avoid repetitive or forceful gripping and pinching activities. A hand-based thumb spica orthosis can help support the joint and relieve symptoms (Cooper, 2014c; Kasch & Walsh, 2013).

Disorders of Muscles and Tendons

Flexor Tendon Injuries

Description: Flexor tendon injuries can result from (1) lacerations to the palm from sharp objects (e.g., knifes or glass), (2) crush injuries (e.g., often in contact sports), or (3) fractures (American Academy of Orthopaedic Surgeons, 2011; Griffin, Hindocha, Jordan, Saleh, & Khan, 2012). The injury is classified depending on the location or anatomical zone of the hand where the injury occurred. The zones of injury are described in **Table 16-7**.

Clinical presentation: A client with a flexor tendon injury may report pain and difficulty or inability to bend the fingers (Griffin et al., 2012). On observation, a wound or swelling may be noticed and tendon bowstringing may be visualized if the A2 and A4 pulleys are also disrupted (American Academy of Orthopaedic Surgeons, 2011; Griffin et al., 2012). Clients with laceration of both the FDS and the flexor digitorum profundus (FDP) will present with an extended finger position at rest (Lutsky, Giang, & Matzon, 2015). On examination, the client will have decreased active finger flexion ROM and decreased finger flexion strength.

Common diagnostic tests: Diagnosis of flexor tendon injuries is done with a clinical exam. Depending on the tendon involved and the extent of injury, the contractile ability of FDS and FDP may be diminished or lost. Isolated FDS activity can be evaluated by holding the other digits in full extension while asking the client to flex the involved digit. FDP activity can be evaluated by isolating active or resisted flexion at the DIP joint (Lutsky et al., 2015). The tenodesis grasp with passive wrist flexion and extension is often lost. A thorough neurological examination should be performed to rule out nerve injuries (Griffin et al., 2012). Plain film radiographs are routinely performed to rule out foreign bodies or concomitant fractures (Griffin et al., 2012; Lutsky et al., 2015).

Table 16-7 Mechanism of Injury and Treatment for Each Zone of Flexor Tendon Injury

Zone of Injury	Mechanism of Injury	Treatment
Zone I: FDP is avulsed from the distal phalanx or transected distal to A4 pulley	Eccentric contraction of FDP during forced hyperextension of the DIP joint	FDP only is repaired and is sutured to the distal phalanx
Zone II: (Clavert et al., 2009) Between A1 and A4 pulleys. Both FDS and FDP can be involved		Repair of FDS and FDP with at least four-strand core stitch which would ideally be performed within 7–14 days of injury. Complicated to repair. Highest chance of developing adhesions and failed repair
Zone III: Between the A1 pulley and the distal margin of the transverse carpal ligament		Less evidence regarding repair techniques. Typically less difficult to treat compared to extensor tendon injuries
Zone IV: Under the transverse carpal ligament		Less evidence regarding repair techniques. Typically less difficult to treat compared to extensor tendon injuries
Zone V: Proximal to the transverse carpal ligament		Difficult to repair as the tendons are in close proximity to the carpal tunnel

Data from Lutsky et al., 2015

Common medical and surgical procedures: Flexor tendon injuries do not heal by themselves so surgery is almost always indicated (Griffin et al., 2012). See Table 16-7 for a list of common medical and surgical procedures for flexor tendon injuries.

Precautions and contraindications: Tendon re-rupture requires urgent surgical repair. Rupture of tendons can occur from swelling, misuse, or overly aggressive AROM or stretching. Adhesions are a common complication, and as many as 20% of clients will develop adhesions that require surgical intervention. AROM has shown to prevent adhesion but may also increase the rate of ruptures (Griffin et al., 2012).

Screening and Assessments

Screening and assessments are similar throughout the various orthopedic conditions of the upper extremity with slight variations. Below is a list of top-down approaches that address the symptoms, as well as the impact of the symptoms on the person's roles, contexts, and environment, followed by bottom-up approaches that are symptom specific:

Screening and Assessments: Early Phase

These examination techniques would be appropriate in the intermediate phase post extension tendon repair (i.e., approximately four to six weeks).

- Client history including the client's age, hand dominance, occupational and avocational responsibilities, prior injuries, comorbidities, family issues, psychological issues, broader social issues, and economic issues.
- Mechanism and date of injury, structures involved, type and extent of medical and surgical intervention, concomitant injuries, and current symptoms.
- Client-reported symptoms.
- Physical assessment includes the following:
  - Baseline physical evaluation to assess limitations not related to the surgery.
  - Observations of pain or fear with rest and movement. Observation of bowstringing, swelling, and normal hand resting position.
  - Color, temperature, and signs of compromised circulation or infection.
  - Edema (e.g., circumferential and volumetric).
  - Sensory (e.g., monofilament and two-point discrimination).

- Skin integrity and wound assessment.
  - *Wound or surgical incision*: Note location, size, integrity of closure, exposure of pins or hardware, and signs of infection.
  - *Scar*: Note location, size, adherence, hypertrophy, blanching with motion, pliability, and sensitivity.
- A/PROM of adjacent and uninvolved joints.
- AROM and tenodesis grasp, with physician approval.
- Cognitive assessment.
- Ability to participate in life roles.
- Assessment of basic and instrumental ADLs (e.g., DASH and PRWE).
- Functional mobility (Lawson & Murphy, 2013).

Screening and Assessments: Late Phase (Approximately Six to Eight Weeks)

Grip and pinch strength, PROM, and coordination should be assessed when allowed by particular protocol, often by weeks 6–8. Assessment of heavy lifting and sports activities is usually delayed until 12 weeks postsurgery.

Interventions

General principles of rehabilitation: Rehabilitation of flexor tendon injuries requires close communication with the referring physician. Treatment will depend on the zone involved and the procedure used, but protected motion protocols are typically used (Brotzman & Manske, 2011). In a systemic review, passive protocols had a statistically lower risk of tendon rupture but a higher risk of ROM deficits as compared to active protocols (Lutsky et al., 2015). Many surgical technique components may or may not improve the repair. Which technique is best remains controversial and depends on the injury type and the surgeon's skills. A number 6–8 strand repair technique offers the stability to stand up to immediate active motion. Locking loop-type sutures, epitendinous sutures, higher suture caliber, and core sutures placed dorsally seem to increase the strength of the repair (Griffin et al., 2012). Nonsteroidal anti-inflammatory drugs (NSAIDs), such as ibuprofen, may help decrease tendon adhesions during the healing phase but its effect on tendon healing is still uncertain (Tan et al., 2010). Improved tendon healing may occur in healthy individuals, who are younger, nonsmokers, and motivated (Brotzman & Manske, 2011). Clients who scar excessively, who have injuries in zone II or IV, and who have a more severe or crush-type injury may have poorer outcomes (Brotzman & Manske, 2011).

Protocols: Refer to **Table 16-8** for commonly used rehab protocols following flexor tendon repair (Kasch & Walsh, 2013).

Intervention protocols for flexor tendon injuries— subacute phase: Usually starts when the client is allowed and able to perform active finger flexion—typically around four to six weeks (Cooper, 2014a).

Early active mobilization protocols: These protocols involve carefully controlled active flexion and extension of the involved digits (Kasch & Walsh, 2013). This is possible due to the advancement in surgical techniques. Early active mobilization requires a repair technique capable of withstanding higher forces generated by early mobilization, usually initiated between two and four days. The client must be compliant and able to understand the exercise protocol. The therapist should also be experienced in tendon rehabilitation and able to communicate closely with the physician.

Splinting: Continue with splinting between exercises. The splint can be adjusted to position the wrist in neutral (Klein, 2007, 2014). Clients with protective splints are discharged between six and eight weeks depending on physician preference. If proximal interphalangeal (PIP) joint flexion contractures are present but smaller than 25°, PROM exercises and splinting can be effective; if the flexion contracture is greater than 25°, static splinting would be most effective (Kasch & Walsh, 2013).

Exercises: Wrist ROM exercises, as well as tendon glides including hook fist, straight fist, and composite fist. After three to four days, compare active flexion to passive flexion. If passive flexion is 50° greater than active flexion, add blocking exercises to promote individual gliding of the FDP and FDS tendons (Klein, 2007, 2014). If no improvement is noted after one week, light resistive gripping can be added. Resistance may only be added at this stage if patency of the tendons can be confirmed. Adding resistance too early can result in tendon ruptures.

Table 16-8 Intervention Protocols for Flexor Tendon Injuries (Acute Phase)

Protocol	Splint	Exercise	Notes
Immobilization	Cast or custom dorsal blocking splint. The wrist is placed in 30° of flexion; positioning the MCPs in flexion and the IPs in extension (3–4 weeks)	No exercise is performed to the digits. Perform ROM to elbow and shoulder	This protocol is reserved for very young children or noncompliant clients
Early passive flexion Kleinert protocol	Dorsal blocking splint. The MCP joints are placed in 60° of flexion and the wrist is placed in 30° of flexion; the splint should allow for full IP extension. Rubber band traction is applied to the fingertip and runs through a palmar pulley to ensure flexion at both IP joints. This splint is worn at all times for 3 weeks	Active extension of the digits to the limits of the splint. The rubber bands flex the fingers	This exercise promotes tendon healing by improving blood flow and tendon nutrition while minimizing tendon adhesions
Controlled passive motion Duran and Houser protocol	Dorsal blocking splint. The MCP joints positioned in 60° of flexion and the wrist positioned in 30° of flexion; the splint should allow for full IP extension. Between exercise sessions, the digits are strapped in extension (4½ weeks). At 4½ weeks, rubber band traction is attached to a wristband. Active extension and passive flexion are performed until discharged by the physician	Begin passive flexion and extension exercises on the third postoperative day: 1. The MCP and PIP are flexed, and the DIP is extended 2. The MCP and DIP are flexed, and the PIP is extended	This exercise is designed to allow 3–5 mm of tendon excursion to prevent tendon adhesions

Data from Kasch and Walsh, 2013.

Extensor Tendon Injuries

Description: Extensor tendon injuries can result from lacerations to the dorsum of the hand, crush injuries, or fractures. The anatomical zone of the hand where the laceration took place classifies these injuries. Zones I, III, V, and VII are over the DIP, PIP, MCP, and wrist joints, respectively. Zones II, IV, and VI are in between zones I, III, V, and VII and are over the respective phalanges and metacarpals. Zone VIII is proximal to the extensor retinaculum and zone IX is at the proximal musculotendinous junction (Cooper, 2014c). A common mechanism of injury includes forced flexion of the finger, often from the impact of a ball (Brotzman & Manske, 2011).

Clinical presentation: Depending on the extensor tendon injury zone, clinical presentations vary. Clients often have a wound laceration, have pain over the involved finger, report lack of ability to move the finger, and may demonstrate a loss of normal hand resting position (Matzon & Bozentka, 2010). A client with a zone I injury will have a typical mallet deformity while a client with zone III may develop a boutonniere deformity (Matzon & Bozentka, 2010). A client with a mallet deformity will present with a flexed DIP that can be extended passively but not actively. A boutonniere deformity will present as a flexion of the PIP and hyperextension of the DIP.

Common diagnostic tests: Diagnosis of extensor tendon laceration is usually made after a physical examination. Testing of the central slip is performed by flexing the PIP joint to 90° (i.e., to keep the central band taut and the lateral bands loose) followed by PIP extension with a counterforce applied to the middle phalanx. Active PIP extension with a floppy DIP indicates an intact central slip. An absence of active PIP extension with a taut and slightly extended DIP indicates injury of the central slip.

Common medical and surgical procedures: Refer to **Table 16-9** for medical interventions of extensor tendon injuries in each zone.

Precautions and contraindications: Clients need to be compliant with the extension splinting regimen because if the finger is allowed to flex once, the immobilization period needs to be re-initiated (Brotzman & Manske, 2011). Fingers are prone to contractures so mobilize uninvolved joints and involved joints when safe and allowed by physician.

Screening and Assessments

Screening and assessments are similar throughout the various orthopedic conditions of the upper extremity with slight variations. Below is a list of top-down approaches that address the symptoms, as well as the impact of the symptoms on the person's roles, contexts, and environments, followed by bottom-up approaches that are symptom specific.

Intermediate phase: These examination techniques would be appropriate in the intermediate phase post extensor tendon repair:

- Client history including the client's age, hand dominance, occupational and avocational responsibilities, prior injuries, comorbidities, family issues, psychological issues, broader social issues, and economic issues.
- Mechanism and date of injury, structures involved, type and extent of medical and surgical intervention, concomitant injuries, and current symptoms.
- Client-related symptoms.
- Physical assessment includes the following:
  - Baseline physical evaluation to assess limitations not related to the surgery.
  - Observations of pain or fear with rest and movement, resting hand position, and deformities.
  - Color, temperature, and signs of compromised circulation or infection.
  - Edema (e.g., circumferential and volumetric).
  - Sensory (e.g., monofilament and two-point discrimination).
  - Skin integrity/wound assessment.
    - *Wound or surgical incision*: Note location, size, integrity of closure, exposure of pins or hardware, and signs of infection.
    - *Scar*: Note location, size, adherence, hypertrophy, blanching with motion, pliability, and sensitivity.
  - A/PROM of adjacent and uninvolved joints.
  - AROM with physician approval.
  - Cognitive assessment.
  - Ability to participate in life roles.
  - Assessment of basic and instrumental ADLs (e.g., DASH and PRWE).
  - Functional mobility (Lawson & Murphy, 2013).

Late phase: Grip and pinch strength, PROM, and coordination should be assessed when allowed by the physician's protocol. Assessment of heavy lifting and sports activities are usually delayed until the final stage of rehabilitation.

Table 16-9 Zone-Specific Intervention and Presentation of Extensor Tendon Injuries

Zones	Presentation	Intervention
Zone I: Mallet injury	Injury over the DIP. Lack of active DIP extension. Presents with a Mallet deformity	Continuous splinting × 6 weeks followed by 3–6 weeks of night and sport splinting. Criteria for surgery are controversial but open injuries, instability at the DIP, inability to comply with splinting regimen, or large fracture fragments are indications
Zone II	Injury over the middle phalanx; most often from laceration	Continuous splinting for 1–2 weeks if the tear is partial with normal active finger extension, and without extensor lag. Complete tears should be treated surgically
Zone III	Injury over the PIP with disruption of the central slip, and typically entails a subtle presentation. Clients present with swelling over the PIP, mild PIP extensor lag, and weak resisted extension at the PIP. The Elson test may be positive. Attenuation of the central slip tendon may only occur weeks after initial injury and/or a boutonniere deformity may develop	Closed injuries are treated with continuous extension splinting of the PIP × 6 weeks if full passive PIP extension and DIP flexion can be achieved, followed by an additional 6 weeks of night splinting. Perform DIP ROM while maintaining PIP extension throughout the course of treatment. Surgery is performed for open injuries, displaced avulsion fractures, PIP instability, and failed nonsurgical treatment
Zone IV	Injury, occurring most often from laceration (i.e., often partial) over the proximal phalanx. Extension weakness may be very subtle	Nonsurgical treatment with splinting and early ROM is indicated when there is no loss of extension AROM. Tendon repair is indicated when loss of extension AROM is present
Zone V	Injury occurs at MCP joint, which is the most common location of extensor tendon injury. The injury frequently occurs from a clenched fist hitting someone else's teeth (i.e., fight bite). In this instance, a risk of infection from mouth bacteria is high. Nonfight bites typically occur from blunt trauma. Lack of finger extension and noticeable ulnar subluxation of the tendons are common following injury	Fight bite injuries are treated with surgical debridement, intravenous antibiotics, and splinting. Acute nonfight bite injuries are treated with extension splinting of the MCP for 6 weeks
Zone VI	Injury of the metacarpals and typically have favorable outcomes. Diagnosis may be challenging as extensor indicis and extensor digiti minimi may be able to assist MCP extension (i.e., watch for compensations when testing for extension weakness at MCP)	Surgical treatment with core suture is advised
Zone VII	The injury involves the extensor retinaculum	Surgical treatment with core suture is advised. A partial or full release of the extensor retinaculum is necessary to visualize the tendon for repair
Zones VIII and IX	The location of injury is in the forearm	Challenging repair due to difficulty in finding tissue for sutures and repair

Data from Brotzman and Manske 2011; Matzon and Bozentka, 2010.

Interventions

General principles in rehabilitation: Rehabilitation of extensor tendon injuries requires close communication with the referring physician. Treatment of extensor tendon injuries is dependent on the zone where the laceration took place and the surgical intervention technique used (Cooper, 2014c; Kasch & Walsh, 2013). Recently, early ROM protocols have gained favor but research shows that static splinting is equivalent to early ROM protocols for distal and uncomplicated injuries (Brotzman & Manske, 2011). In general, extensor tendon injuries affected in distal zones in children younger than 5 and with a complete laceration have a poorer prognosis post repair (Brotzman & Manske, 2011).

Table 16-10 highlights splinting and exercise recommendations based on the zone of injury (Cooper, 2014c; Kasch & Walsh, 2013).

Intersection Syndrome

Description: Intersection syndrome is an uncommon disorder. It is described as a cluster of symptoms at the crossing point between an extensor compartment and a muscle or tendon (Brotzman & Manske, 2011; Zhari, Edderai, Boumdine, Amil, & En-Nouali, 2015). It can be further divided into proximal (PIS) and distal intersection syndrome (DIS). PIS is an inflammation at the intersection of the first dorsal compartment tendons abductor pollicis longus (AbPL) and extensor pollicis brevis (EPB), with the second compartment tendons (i.e., ECRB and ECRL) approximately 4 centimeters proximal to the Lister's tubercle. DIS is an inflammation at the intersection of the (extensor pollicis longus) EPL tendon (i.e., third compartment) with ECRL and ECRB tendons (Zhari et al., 2015). Pathophysiology is unclear but the two most common theories are (1) inflammation from crossing of a muscle with a tendon sheath and (2) stenosis within a compartment (Brotzman & Manske, 2011). Controversy also exists as to whether this causes a tenosynovitis or a pure tendinitis (Sutliff, 2009). Intersection syndrome is usually caused by repetitive wrist flexion and extension, or less commonly from a direct trauma (Zhari et al., 2015). It is most common in skiers and from occupational exposure to spraying, cementing, threshing, planting, and hammering activities (Sutliff, 2009).

Clinical presentation: Intersection syndrome presents as pain upon wrist flexion and extension, swelling, and crepitus over the dorsal radial aspect of the forearm. A specific tender area to palpation is 4–8 centimeters proximal to the radial styloid process (Sutliff, 2009; Zhari et al., 2015). This is an important distinguishing feature from De Quervain's tenosynovitis which causes pain closer to the radial styloid process.

Common diagnostic tests: The diagnosis is usually made clinically but may be augmented with an ultrasound and/or MRI (Zhari et al., 2015).

Common medical and surgical procedures: Clients are treated conservatively and symptoms usually resolve within two to three weeks for 60% of clients. Conservative treatment may include rest, therapy, NSAIDs, and splinting (Sutliff, 2009). Corticosteroid injections may be given if conservative care is unsuccessful (Sutliff, 2009), while surgical tenosynovectomy and/or fasciotomy of AbPL may be indicated for those recalcitrant cases (Zhari et al., 2015).

Precautions and contraindications: Avoid repetitive wrist flexion and extension during early rehabilitation as the condition may be easily exacerbated.

Table 16-10 Extensor Tendon Injury Zone Clinical Presentation, Splinting, and Exercise Protocol

Zone of Injury	Splinting	Exercise
I and II	DIP extension splinting for 6–8 weeks. Nighttime extension splinting may be used to prevent an extensor lag during the mobilization phase	Maintain ROM of the MCP and PIP joints during the immobilization period. Add active flexion while monitoring for extensor lag at the DIP joint following splint removal
III and IV	*Nonoperative:* The PIP is splinted in full extension for 6 weeks. Prevent PIP hyperextension using a static splint that allows PIP flexion (e.g., a figure eight splint). Splints should be used during activity to improve functional prehensile patterns *Operative:* Follow physician guidelines	*Nonoperative:* DIP active and passive flexion *Operative:* Follow physician guidelines
V, VI, and VII	*Evans protocol:* Wrist 45° of extension, MCPs and IPs 0° with dynamic traction and a palmar block to limit flexion of the MCPs to 30°. The flexion block is removed at 3 weeks, and the splint can be removed at 6 weeks. Flexion splinting can begin at 8 weeks if flexion deficits are present	*1–3 weeks:* Active MCP flexion up to the block *3 weeks:* The volar block is removed and active flexion is permitted in the splint *6 weeks:* Active finger extension and wrist flexion are permitted, as well as mild strengthening

Data from Cooper, 2014c; Kasch and Walsh, 2013; Klein, 2014; Moscony, 2014.

Screening and Assessments

Screening and assessments are similar throughout the various orthopedic conditions of the upper extremity with slight variations. Below is a list of top-down approaches that address the symptoms, as well as the impact of the symptoms on the person's roles, contexts, and environment, followed by bottom-up approaches that are symptom specific:

- Client history including the client's age, hand dominance, occupational and avocational responsibilities, prior injuries, comorbidities, family issues, psychological issues, broader social issues, and economic issues.
- Type of symptoms, onset of symptoms, activities that aggravate or alleviate symptoms, type and extent of medical intervention, concomitant injuries, and future treatment planned.
- Physical assessment includes the following:
  - Baseline physical evaluation to assess limitations not related to the wrist/hand.
  - Observations of pain or fear with rest and movement.
  - Color, temperature, and signs of inflammation.
  - Edema (e.g., circumferential and volumetric).
  - Sensory and motor function.
  - Coordination.
  - Skin integrity.
  - A/PROM of adjacent and uninvolved joints.
  - AROM at the wrist and all digits: Listen for crepitus with wrist ROM.
  - MMT.
  - Palpation with attention to the point of pain, 4–8 centimeters distal to the radial styloid process.
  - Cognitive assessment.
  - Ability to participate in life roles.
  - Assessment of basic and instrumental ADLs (e.g., DASH and PRWE).
  - Functional mobility (Lawson & Murphy, 2013).

Interventions

Interventions should target the particular deficits found in the examination. Common interventions include modalities to decrease pain and inflammation, ROM of the wrist, hand, and adjoining joints, motor and coordination retraining, progressive strengthening, tendon-gliding exercises, and ADL retraining. Generally, clients should be educated to avoid painful resisted wrist extension activities, as well as forceful gripping (Cooper, 2014c; Kasch & Walsh, 2013).

Manual workers should be instructed on how to limit high occupational forces through optimizing body and arm position, avoid prolonged arm vibrations, and limit high repetitions of wrist motions and on the use of lighter weight tools (Sutliff, 2009). Alpine skiers should avoid deep pole planting and pole dragging and should decrease their pole length by 2 inches (Sutliff, 2009). If a splint is needed, a forearm-based thumb spica with a mobile IP joint (Cooper, 2014c) or a splint supporting the wrist in 15° of extension can be used (Sutliff, 2009).

De Quervain's Tenosynovitis

Description: De Quervain's disease is a tenosynovitis that affects the tendons within the first dorsal compartment, the AbPL, and the EPB (Cooper, 2014a; Cooper & Martin, 2007). Women are four times more likely than men to have De Quervain's disease. Risks increase in those who are pregnant or are mothers of young children. This condition is common with activities involving repeated ulnar and radial deviation, such as with hammering, cross country skiing, or lifting a child or pet (Adams & Habbu, 2015).

Clinical presentation: Clients typically report pain over the radial styloid process with thumb extension or abduction that can radiate proximally or distally (Cooper, 2014a; Cooper & Martin, 2007). Examination shows swelling and/or tenderness of the tendons of the first compartment over the radial wrist (Darowish & Sharma, 2014). Finkelstein's test, which is an ulnar deviation of the wrist while the client grasps the thumb in the palm, is typically positive (Adams & Habbu, 2015; Magee, 2014).

Common diagnostic tests: The diagnosis of De Quervain's tenosynovitis is made through a physical examination. Plain film radiographs are usually negative but may be used to rule out bone pathology, CMC arthritis, or calcification (Adams & Habbu, 2015).

Common medical and surgical procedures: De Quervain's disease is treated with oral anti-inflammatories, corticosteroid injections, thumb spica splinting, therapy, and/or surgical release of the tendon sheath. Splinting alone is successful in about 14–18% of clients (Adams & Habbu, 2015) while a corticosteroid injection in the first dorsal compartment is curative in 60–100% of cases (Adams & Habbu, 2015). The benefit of adding therapy and/or splinting has not been demonstrated (Adams & Habbu, 2015).

Precautions and contraindications: Avoid repetitive resisted thumb extension or abduction, as well as resisted wrist radial deviation and extension in the acute phase.

Screening and Assessments

Screening and assessments are similar throughout the various orthopedic conditions of the upper extremity with slight variations. Below is a list of top-down approaches that address the symptoms, as well as the impact of the symptoms on the person's roles, contexts, and environments, followed by bottom-up approaches that are symptom specific:

- Client history including the client's age, hand dominance, occupational and avocational responsibilities, prior injuries, comorbidities, family issues, psychological issues, broader social issues, and economic issues.
- Type of symptoms, onset of symptoms, activities that aggravate or alleviate symptoms, type and extent of medical intervention, concomitant injuries, and future treatment planned.
- Physical assessment includes the following:
  - Baseline physical evaluation to assess limitations not related to the thumb.
  - Observations of pain or fear with rest and movement.
  - Color, temperature, and signs of inflammation.
  - Edema (e.g., circumferential and volumetric).
  - Sensory and motor function.
  - Coordination.
  - Skin integrity.
  - A/PROM of adjacent and uninvolved joints.
  - *AROM*: Wrist and thumb.
  - *MMT*: Focus on the wrist and the thumb.
  - *Special tests*: Finkelstein's test.
  - *Palpation*: Especially AbPL and EPB close to the radial styloid process.
  - Cognitive assessment.
  - Ability to participate in life roles.
  - Assessment of basic and instrumental ADLs (e.g., DASH and PRWE).
  - Functional mobility (Lawson & Murphy, 2013).

Interventions

Interventions should target the particular deficits found in the examination. Common interventions include modalities to decrease pain and inflammation, ROM of the wrist, thumb, and adjoining joints, motor and coordination retraining, progressive strengthening, tendon-gliding exercises, and ADL retraining. Clients should be educated to avoid prolonged thumb hyperabduction when using the computer space bar and to avoid wrist ulnar or radial deviation while performing pinching tasks (Cooper, 2014c; Kasch & Walsh, 2013). A forearm-based thumb spica-type splint can be used while carefully monitoring for irritation of the first dorsal compartment on the radial edge of the splint (Cooper, 2014c; Kasch & Walsh, 2013).

Trigger Finger (Stenosing Tenosynovitis)

Description: Trigger finger is also known as a stenosing tenosynovitis. Trigger finger occurs when the A1 pulley becomes thick and constricts the FDS and FDP tendons making it difficult for the tendons to glide freely (Cooper, 2014a; Cooper & Martin, 2007). The disease naturally progresses from painless clicking upon ROM, to painful triggering, and ultimately to a flexed, locked digit (Giugale & Fowler, 2015). Women develop a trigger finger more often than men. The ring finger and thumb are most often involved followed by the index and fourth and fifth digits. Associated diagnoses include diabetes, rheumatoid arthritis (RA), gout, carpal tunnel syndrome (CTS), and Dupuytren's contracture.

Clinical presentation: Subjectively, the client may report stiffness, lack of finger ROM, and catching during either finger flexion or extension. Examiners may find tenderness and/or a palpable nodule over the A1 pulley and lack of ROM of the involved finger (Cooper, 2014c).

Common diagnostic tests: The diagnosis is usually made with a clinical examination and imaging is usually unnecessary (Giugale & Fowler, 2015). The most helpful clinical test is to ask the client to make a full fist and subsequently extend the fingers fully while noticing and asking for catching (Brotzman & Manske, 2011).

Common medical and surgical procedures: **Table 16-11** provides a list of common medical and surgical procedures for trigger finger.

Precautions and contraindications: Repetitive finger flexion exercises in the acute phase may further increase inflammation and symptoms (Giugale & Fowler, 2015).

Table 16-11 Medical and Surgical Procedures for Trigger Finger

Injections	Cortisone injections will eliminate symptoms in approximately 70% of cases
Splinting	The MCP joints of the affected digits should be splinted in neutral to prevent composite flexion. The client is instructed in hook fisting and hold fisting
Adaptive ADL techniques	Built-up handles, padded gloves, and pacing strategies are helpful
Surgical release	Surgical release of the A1 pulley may be required if symptoms do not improve with conservative treatment

Data from Cooper, 2014a; Cooper and Martin, 2007.

Screening and Assessments

Screening and assessments are similar throughout the various orthopedic conditions of the upper extremity with slight variations. Below is a list of top-down approaches that address the symptoms, as well as the impact of the symptoms on the person's roles, contexts, and environment, followed by bottom-up approaches that are symptom specific. Occupation-based guidelines for screenings and assessments of trigger finger are limited (Langer, Luria, Maeir, & Erez, 2014).

- Client history includes the client's age, hand dominance, occupational and avocational responsibilities, prior injuries, comorbidities, family issues, psychological issues, broader social issues, and economic issues.
- Type of symptoms, onset of symptoms, activities that aggravate or alleviate symptoms, type and extent of medical intervention, concomitant injuries, and future treatment planned.
- Physical assessment includes the following:
  - Baseline physical evaluation and interview to assess limitations not related to the hand.
  - Observations of pain or fear with rest and movement.
  - Color, temperature, and signs of inflammation.
  - Edema (e.g., circumferential and volumetric).
  - Sensory and motor function.
  - Coordination.
  - Skin integrity.
  - A/PROM of adjacent/uninvolved joints.
  - *AROM*: Ask the client to make a full fist and subsequently extend the fingers fully while noticing and asking for catching or locking.
  - MMT.
  - *Palpation*: Tenderness and/or thickening of the A1 pulley.
  - Cognitive assessment.
  - Ability to participate in life roles.
  - Assessment of basic and instrumental ADLs (e.g., DASH and PRWE).
  - Functional mobility (Lawson & Murphy, 2013).

The standard assessments most commonly used by OT practitioners in one study included grip strength, pinch strength, ROM, pain assessment, sensation testing with monofilaments, two-point discrimination, and the Purdue Pegboard Test (Langer et al., 2014).

Interventions

The most common interventions used by OT practitioners for trigger finger includes orthoses (e.g., MCP joint blocking splints), physical agent modalities (e.g., ultrasound), exercise and activity, and environment modification (Langer et al., 2014). Finger ROM and tendon-gliding exercises are often recommended. Adaptive equipment such as place-and-hold fisting and padded gloves may be helpful. Clients should be educated on how to avoid triggering the finger and the use of pacing strategies (Cooper, 2014c; Kasch & Walsh, 2013).

Disorders of Ligaments and Soft Tissues

Scapholunate Ligament Sprain

Description: A scapholunate sprain is a tensile injury to the ligaments stabilizing the scaphoid to the lunate. The scapholunate interosseous ligament (SLIL) is an intraarticular ligament bathed in synovial fluid, which decreases its ability to heal (Pappou, Basel, & Deal, 2013). SLIL injuries are the most common cause of traumatic wrist instability (American Academy of Orthopaedic Surgeons, 2011). If left untreated, they can lead to wrist arthritis and carpal bone collapse (American Academy of Orthopaedic Surgeons, 2011).

Clinical presentation: Clients typically report wrist pain and weakness upon loading, as well as painful clicks and snapping sounds with wrist movements. Swelling may be apparent over the scapholunate joint area (American Academy of Orthopaedic Surgeons, 2011).

Common diagnostic tests: Plain film radiographs are usually sufficient for scapholunate injuries in stages IV, V, and VI while the best imaging techniques for diagnosing stages I through III remains controversial (see **Table 16-12** for a description of stages). Magnetic resonance angiogram (MRA) seems superior to MRI while multidetector CT arthrogram seems better than MRA for partial ligament tears (Pappou et al., 2013). See Table 16-12 for diagnostic tests specific to each stage of scapholunate injury.

Common medical and surgical procedures: Immobilization or arthroscopic debridement is usually prescribed for partial tears while full tears usually require a ligament reconstruction (American Academy of Orthopaedic Surgeons, 2011). See Table 16-12 for procedures associated with each stage of scapholunate injury.

Precautions and contraindications: Wrist loading should be limited at the end range of wrist flexion or extension.

Screening and Assessments

Screening and assessments are similar throughout the various orthopedic conditions of the upper extremity with slight variations. Below is a list of top-down approaches that address the symptoms, as well as the impact of the symptoms on the person's roles, contexts, and environment, followed by bottom-up approaches that are symptom specific:

- Client history including the client's age, hand dominance, occupational and avocational responsibilities, prior injuries, comorbidities, family issues, psychological issues, broader social issues, and economic issues.
- Mechanism and date of injury, structures involved, type and extent of medical and surgical intervention, concomitant injuries, and future treatment planned.
- Physical assessment includes the following:
  o Baseline physical evaluation and interview to assess limitations not related to the injury.
  o Observations of pain and fear with rest and movement.
  o Color, temperature, and signs of compromised circulation or inflammation.
  o Edema: Special attention to the scapholunate area.
  o Sensory and motor function.
  o Coordination.

Table 16-12 Stages of Scapholunate Injury with Associated Diagnostic Tests and Surgical Procedures

Stages	Diagnostic Test	Surgical Procedures
Stage 1: Partial scapholunate ligament injury	MRI, MRA, plain arthrography and MDCTA, arthroscopy, and direct surgical observation	Arthroscopic debridement without reconstruction or repair
Stage 2: Complete disruption with repairable ligament	Dynamic radiographs, cineradiography, MRI, MRA, plain arthrography, MDCTA, arthroscopy, and direct surgical observation	Direct ligament repair with or without supplementary capsulodesis
Stage 3: Complete disruption with irreparable ligament but normal alignment	Dynamic radiographs, cineradiography, MRI, MRA, plain arthrography, MDCTA, arthroscopy, and direct surgical observation	Reconstruction of the scapholunate ligament only
Stage 4: Complete disruption with irreparable ligament and reducible rotary subluxation of the scaphoid	Plain film radiographs	Ligament reconstruction with many different techniques of arthrodesis, capsulodesis, and tenodesis
Stage 5: Complete disruption with irreducible malalignment and intact cartilage	Plain film radiographs and intraoperative diagnosis	Salvage procedure with aggressive soft tissue release and mobilization of the scar and adhesions
Stage 6: Chronic SLIL disruption with cartilage loss—SLAC	Plain film radiographs	Neurectomies, proximal row carpectomy, and partial or total wrist fusion

MDCTA, multidetector CT arthrogram; SLAC, scapholunate advanced collapse.
Data from Pappou, Basel, & Deal, 2013.

- Skin integrity and wound assessment.
  - *Wound or surgical incision if present*: Note location, size, integrity of closure, exposure of pins or hardware, and signs of infection.
  - *Scar*: Note location, size, adherence, hypertrophy, blanching with motion, pliability, and sensitivity.
- A/PROM of adjacent and uninvolved joints.
- *AROM*: Listen for clicking or snapping sounds with wrist ROM.
- MMT can be performed in the subacute phase of healing.
- Cognitive assessment.
- Ability to participate in life roles.
- Assessment of basic and instrumental ADLs (e.g., DASH and PRWE).
- Functional mobility (Lawson & Murphy, 2013).

Interventions

The main objective of the OT intervention after a wrist/hand injury is to restore function and independence in life roles. Intervention of scapholunate ligament sprain will vary depending on the severity or stage of the sprain, stage of healing, medical intervention, and client-specific factors. Nonetheless, it should focus on restoring the objective deficits seen during the examination and geared toward a return to function. The therapist must be careful to avoid axial loading of the wrist, especially in end range wrist positions.

Lunotriquetral Ligament Sprain and Instability

Description: A lunotriquetral ligament (LTL) injury occurs rarely in isolation (American Academy of Orthopaedic Surgeons, 2011). A fall on a pronated forearm with an extended and radially deviated or fully flexed wrist is the prime mechanism of injury for an isolated LTL sprain. This mechanism is often the result of a backward fall on an outstretched hand (American Academy of Orthopaedic Surgeons, 2011). The injury is classified as either acute or chronic (i.e., >3 months), traumatic or degenerative, with or without carpal collapse, and as an isolated or part of a perilunate instability (van de Grift & Ritt, 2016).

Clinical presentation: Signs and symptoms vary depending on the injury classification but generally acute injuries will cause ulnar wrist pain, swelling, limited grip

strength, and decreased ROM. The clients with more chronic injuries report instability, crepitus, and/or clicking with ulnar deviation (van de Grift & Ritt, 2016). Wrist deformity and severe wrist dysfunctions may be seen with carpal collapse and perilunate instability (van de Grift & Ritt, 2016).

Common diagnostic tests: Plain film radiographs, MRI, arthrography, and cineradiography have different purposes and goals in the evaluation of LTL injuries but arthroscopy is the gold standard for the examination of LTL tears (American Academy of Orthopaedic Surgeons, 2011; van de Grift & Ritt, 2016). Specials tests can be performed to aid in diagnosis and commonly include the lunotriquetral ballottement (Reagan's) test and the lunotriquetral shear test.

Common medical and surgical procedures: Immobilization if the tear is stable, with a corticosteroid injection or arthroscopic debridement if symptoms persist. Surgery, such as direct ligament repair, is usually necessary for unstable tears (American Academy of Orthopaedic Surgeons, 2011). Ligament reconstruction using tendon grafts, limited intercarpal fusions, and ulnar shortening may be performed in recalcitrant cases (Nicoson & Moran, 2015).

Precautions and contraindications: Avoid putting the wrist in a position that replicates the initial injury or reproduces instability symptoms.

Screening and Assessments

Screening and assessments are similar throughout the various orthopedic conditions of the upper extremity with slight variations. Below is a list of top-down approaches that address the symptoms, as well as the impact of the symptoms on the person's roles, contexts, and environment, followed by bottom-up approaches that are symptom specific:

- Client history including the client's age, hand dominance, occupational and avocational responsibilities, prior injuries, comorbidities, family issues, psychological issues, broader social issues, and economic issues.
- Mechanism and date of injury, structures involved, type and extent of medical and surgical intervention, concomitant injuries, and future treatment planned.
- Physical assessment includes the following:
  - Baseline physical evaluation and interview to assess limitations not related to the injury.

- Observations of pain or fear at rest and with movement, while looking for wrist deformities.
- Color, temperature, and signs of compromised circulation or inflammation.
- Edema (e.g., circumferential and volumetric).
- Sensory and motor function.
- Coordination.
- Skin integrity and wound assessment.
  - *Wound or surgical incision if present*: Note location, size, integrity of closure, exposure of pins or hardware, and signs of infection.
  - *Scar*: Note location, size, adherence, hypertrophy, blanching with motion, pliability, and sensitivity.
- A/PROM of adjacent/uninvolved joints.
- *AROM*: Notice clicking upon wrist movements.
- MMT can be performed in the subacute phase of healing.
- *Special tests*: Lunotriquetral ballottement (i.e., Reagan's) test and lunotriquetral shear test (see **Table 16-13**).
- Cognitive assessment.
- Ability to participate in life roles.
- Assessment of basic and instrumental ADLs (e.g., DASH and PRWE).
- Functional mobility (Lawson & Murphy, 2013).

Interventions

The main objective of OT intervention is to restore function and independence of life roles affected by disorders of the arm and wrist. Intervention for LTL sprains vary depending on the severity or stage of the sprain, stage of

Table 16-13 Special Tests for Lunotriquetral Ligament Sprain and Instability

Special Test	Description	Positive Test
Lunotriquetral ballottement test	The therapist stabilizes the triquetrum and moves the lunate in a palmar and dorsal direction	Pain, laxity, or crepitus indicates a positive test for LTL instability
Lunotriquetral shear test	The therapist stabilizes the lunate and shears the triquetrum palmarly and dorsally	Pain, laxity, and crepitus suggests possible lunotriquetral interosseous ligament injury

Data from Magee, 2014.

healing, medical intervention, and client-specific factors. Nonetheless, it should focus on restoring the objective deficits seen during the examination and geared toward a return to function. Initially, the OT practitioner can work in positions away from instability and symptoms and progress toward these positions in later stages of healing.

PIP/DIP Joint Ligament Injuries

Description: PIP is the most commonly injured joint in sports (Prucz & Friedrich, 2015). There is a continuum of injuries to the starting of PIP and DIP with a simple volar plate or collateral sprain to a complete joint dislocation. Volar plate sprains occur with finger hyperextension and are common in ball-handling sports (Prucz & Friedrich, 2015). Collateral ligament sprains occur with varus or valgus stresses. Dorsal dislocations occur when there is injury to the volar plate, both collateral ligaments, and the dorsal joint capsule (Prucz & Friedrich, 2015). These dislocations occur from an impact to a finger that causes axial loading and forced hyperextension (Prucz & Friedrich, 2015). Volar dislocations are rare, but when they occur, they can damage the extensor tendon central slip (Prucz & Friedrich, 2015). Finally, a dislocation can also cause a fracture of one of the phalanges.

Clinical presentation: Clients with volar sprains may have excessive and painful hyperextension of the fingers and tenderness to palpation of the volar plate. Collateral ligament injuries present with excessive movement on varus or valgus testing and pain upon palpation of the ligaments. Dislocations present with deformity, pain, and decreased ROM.

Common diagnostic tests: MRI and MRA are the imaging modalities of choice for collateral ligament injuries (Prucz & Friedrich, 2015). Radiographs are helpful to rule out avulsion fractures, to help in the treatment decision making post-dislocation, and to ensure success of closed reduction post-dislocation (Freiberg, 2007).

Common medical and surgical procedures: Immobilization for up to three weeks, protected motion, traction, closed reduction, open reduction, and internal fixation are procedures that can be used depending on the location and the extent of injury. Dorsal dislocations without fractures are usually manually reduced and then immobilized with a dorsal blocking splint in 30° of flexion followed by Buddy taping and early mobilization. A volar dislocation usually requires six weeks of immobilization in full extension once reduced (Prucz & Friedrich, 2015). Collateral ligaments are treated conservatively and do not require surgery. In most PIP injuries, open reduction and internal fixation should be avoided due to the high risk of associated contractures (Freiberg, 2007).

Precautions and contraindications: Safe, early ROM and frequent mobility monitoring may reduce the high risk of contractures.

Screening and Assessments

Screening and assessments are similar throughout the various orthopedic conditions of the upper extremity with slight variations. Below is a list of top-down approaches that address the symptoms, as well as the impact of the symptoms on the person's roles, contexts, and environment, followed by bottom-up approaches that are symptom specific:

- Client history including the client's age, hand dominance, occupational and avocational responsibilities, prior injuries, comorbidities, family issues, psychological issues, broader social issues, and economic issues.
- Mechanism and date of injury, structures involved, type and extent of medical and surgical intervention, concomitant injuries, and future treatment planned.
- Physical assessment includes the following:
  - Baseline physical evaluation to assess limitations not related to the injury.
  - Observations of pain or fear at rest and with movement.
  - Observation for finger deformities.
  - Color, temperature, and signs of compromised circulation or inflammation.
  - Edema (e.g., circumferential and volumetric).
  - Sensory and motor function.
  - Coordination.
  - Skin integrity and wound assessment.
    - *Wound or surgical incision if present*: Note location, size, integrity of closure, exposure of pins or hardware, and signs of infection.
    - *Scar*: Note location, size, adherence, hypertrophy, blanching with motion, pliability, and sensitivity.
  - A/PROM of adjacent and uninvolved joints.
  - AROM.
  - MMT can be performed in the subacute phase of healing.
  - *Special tests*: Varus or valgus stress tests at the fingers.
  - Cognitive assessment.
  - Ability to participate in life roles.
  - Assessment of basic and instrumental ADLs (e.g., DASH and PRWE).
  - Functional mobility (Lawson & Murphy, 2013).

Interventions

The main objective of OT intervention is to restore function and independence of life roles affected by disorders of the arm and wrist. Intervention of PIP/DIP joint ligament injuries will vary depending on the severity of the sprain, stage of healing, medical intervention, and client-specific factors. Nonetheless, it should focus on restoring the objective deficits seen during the examination and geared toward a return to function. The focus should be placed on early ROM (i.e., as soon as permissible per physician approval) secondary to the high risk of finger contractures with this condition.

Gamekeeper's Thumb (Skier's Thumb)

Description: Gamekeeper's thumb is an injury to the ulnar collateral ligament (UCL) of the thumb. It is common in sports activities and manual labor occupations and is most often the result of an MCP joint hyperabduction or hyperextension movement or fall on an outstretched hand (Avery, Caggiano, & Matullo, 2015). The term came initially from the gamekeepers in Scotland who got this injury from sacrificing rabbits (Gagliardi & Agarwal, 2012). The term "skier's thumb" is used due to the frequency of this injury in skiers. It occurs when the skier falls while his ski pole is planted, causing a radial stress to the thumb and injury to the UCL. The UCL most often tears within its distal portion; however, rupture can occur proximally or within the substance of the ligament (Avery et al., 2015). A Stener lesion occurs when the torn end of the ligament becomes displaced and is trapped superficial to the adductor aponeurosis (Gagliardi & Agarwal, 2012). With a Stener lesion, the ligament is unable to heal back unto the proximal phalanx and surgical repair is usually required.

Clinical presentation: Swelling and ecchymosis are noted over the MCP joint and clients often report weakness and pain with pinching activities. Pain is elicited upon palpation of the UCL and a palpable mass on the ulnar aspect of the joint is present with a Stener lesion (Avery et al., 2015).

Common diagnostic tests: Clinical examination is usually sufficient for the diagnosis of an UCL injury and a ligament stress test is the most important component of the clinical examination (Avery et al., 2015). Complete tears will demonstrate laxity of the UCL when stressed in both an extended and flexed position. In acute injuries and in clients that are guarded, performing the test after local anesthesia improves the accuracy of the test (Avery et al., 2015). Plain film radiographs are usually ordered to rule out a subluxation, fracture, or bony avulsion of the UCL (Avery et al., 2015). Stress radiographs are often useful to evaluate the extent of joint laxity when the clinical examination is inconclusive (Avery et al., 2015). Ultrasound or MRI may be ordered when there is an uncertain clinical picture (Avery et al., 2015).

Common medical and surgical procedures: Grade I and II sprains are commonly treated nonoperatively while grade III sprains (i.e., complete ruptures) are often treated surgically. Conservative treatment includes MCP immobilization and mobility of the IP joint. Immobilization is typically maintained for four weeks although it can be as short as 10 days with small grade I sprains and as much as six weeks for more severe sprains. As far as surgical techniques are concerned, both repair and reconstruction have shown similar outcomes for grade III sprains. Despite the frequency, of surgical repairs of grade III sprains, conservative treatment and immobilization have shown to produce good outcomes (Avery et al., 2015).

Precautions and contraindications: Precise repair of the ligament insertion is critical to maximize ROM, as slight deviations from the normal insertion can significantly decrease MCP motion.

Screening and Assessments

Screening and assessments are similar throughout the various orthopedic conditions of the upper extremity with slight variations. Below is a list of top-down approaches that address the symptoms, as well as the impact of the symptoms on the person's roles, contexts, and environment, followed by bottom-up approaches that are symptom specific:

- Client history including the client's age, hand dominance, occupational and avocational responsibilities, prior injuries, comorbidities, family issues, psychological issues, broader social issues, and economic issues.

- Mechanism and date of injury, structures involved, type and extent of medical and surgical intervention, concomitant injuries, and future treatment planned.
- Physical assessment includes the following:
  - Baseline physical evaluation and interview to assess limitations not related to the injury.
  - Observations of pain or fear at rest and with movement.
  - Color, temperature, and signs of compromised circulation or inflammation.
  - Edema.
  - Sensory and motor function.
  - Coordination.
  - Skin integrity and wound assessment.
    - *Wound or surgical incision if present*: Note location, size, integrity of closure, exposure of pins or hardware, and signs of infection.
    - *Scar*: Note location, size, adherence, hypertrophy, blanching with motion, pliability, and sensitivity.
  - A/PROM of adjacent and uninvolved joints.
  - AROM.
  - MMT can be performed in the subacute phase of healing.
  - *Special tests*: UCL stress test.
  - *Palpation*: Palpate the UCL for the presence of a mass and for symptom reproduction.
  - Cognitive assessment.
  - Ability to participate in life roles.
  - Assessment of basic and instrumental ADLs (e.g., DASH and PRWE).
  - Functional mobility (Lawson & Murphy, 2013).

Interventions

The main objective of OT intervention is to restore function and independence of life roles affected by disorders of the arm and wrist. Intervention of Gamekeeper's thumb will vary depending on the severity of the sprain, stage of healing, medical intervention, and client-specific factors. Nonetheless, it should focus on restoring the objective deficits seen during the examination and geared toward a return to function. If the client is casted, interventions may begin with thumb AROM exercises with emphasis placed on IP motion once the cast is removed. Improvement in MCP flexion may remain limited in older clients (Cooper, 2014c). Following physician approval, resistive pinch exercises can begin with lateral pinch; tip-to-tip pinch may be delayed until 12 weeks because of the stress placed on the UCL (Cooper, 2014c). A hand-based thumb spica splint may be useful to protect the healing ligament (Cooper, 2014c).

Triangular Fibrocartilaginous Complex Tears

Description: The triangular fibrocartilaginous complex (TFCC) is composed of an articular disk, dorsal and volar radioulnar ligaments, a meniscus, UCL, and the sheath of the extensor carpi ulnaris (ECU) (American Academy of Orthopaedic Surgeons, 2011). The TFCC transmits load from the ulna to the proximal carpal row, significantly contributing to the stability of the distal radioulnar (DRU) joint and less strongly to ulnocarpal joint stability. Due to its stabilizing role, an injury to the TFCC will threaten DRU joint stability. Tear of the TFCC occurs most commonly from landing on an extended and ulnarly deviated hand or a fully pronated or supinated forearm (Sachar, 2008). The injuries are classified by the mechanism of injury including traumatic (type I) and degenerative (type II) with subclasses depending on location and amount of disruption (American Academy of Orthopaedic Surgeons, 2011; Roenbeck & Imbriglia, 2011; Sachar, 2008). Similar to the meniscus at the knee, the central portion of the TFCC has poor vascularity, making central tears difficult to heal (Brotzman & Manske, 2011).

Clinical presentation: Clients will report pain on the ulnar side of the wrist reproduced with end range wrist extension, ulnar deviation and/or axial loading (Sachar, 2008), clicking, and crepitus with forearm pronation, and gripping or ulnar deviation of the wrist (Brotzman & Manske, 2011). On examination, palpation of the TFCC of the wrist may reproduce symptoms. Provocative tests may be performed to reproduce symptoms and assist in diagnosis.

Common diagnostic tests: Radiographs, CT, MRI, MRI arthrograms, and arthroscopy aid in the diagnosis of TFCC injuries (American Academy of Orthopaedic Surgeons, 2011; Sachar, 2008). Arthroscopy may be the most accurate method to detect defects in the TFCC.

Common medical and surgical procedures: Common interventions include conservative treatment, surgical debridement, and arthroscopic repair (American Academy of Orthopaedic Surgeons, 2011). See **Table 16-14** for the types of TFCC injuries and associated treatment.

Precautions and contraindications: Axial loading and shear forces through the wrist should be avoided.

Screening and Assessments

Screening and assessments are similar throughout the various orthopedic conditions of the upper extremity with slight variations. Below is a list of top-down approaches that address the symptoms, as well as the impact of the symptoms on the person's roles, contexts, and environment, followed by bottom-up approaches that are symptom specific:

- Client history including the client's age, hand dominance, occupational and avocational

Table 16-14 Types of TFCC Injuries with Associated Treatment

Type of Injury	Description	Treatment
1A	Isolated central disk perforation	*Starts with conservative treatment*: Activity modification, immobilization, NSAIDs, corticosteroid if symptoms persist, and arthroscopic debridement for recalcitrant cases
1B	Peripheral ulnar-sided tear of TFCC—in the vascular zone (i.e., with or without an ulnar styloid fracture)	Open or arthroscopic repair followed by 4–6 weeks of immobilization in supination
1C	Distal TFCC disruption (i.e., disruption from distal ulnocarpal ligaments)	Not described
1D	Radial TFCC disruption (i.e., with or without a sigmoid notch fracture)	Some advocate repair while others recommend arthroscopic debridement with early ROM
II	Degenerative	Nonoperative for at least 3 months before surgery is recommended. Extraarticular ulnar shortening is sometimes necessary

Data from Brotzman and Manske 2011; Sachar, 2008.

responsibilities, prior injuries, comorbidities, family issues, psychological issues, broader social issues, and economic issues.

- Mechanism and date of injury, structures involved, type and extent of medical and surgical intervention, concomitant injuries, and future treatment planned.
- Physical assessment includes the following:
  o Baseline physical evaluation and interview to assess limitations not related to the injury.
  o Observations of pain or fear at rest and with movement.
  o Color, temperature, and signs of compromised circulation or inflammation.
  o Edema (e.g., circumferential and volumetric).
  o Sensory and motor function.
  o Coordination.
  o Skin integrity and wound assessment.
    ▪ *Wound or surgical incision if present*: Note location, size, integrity of closure, exposure of pins or hardware, and signs of infection.
    ▪ *Scar*: Note location, size, adherence, hypertrophy, blanching with motion, pliability, and sensitivity.
  o A/PROM of adjacent and uninvolved joints.
  o *AROM*: Notice clicking upon wrist movements.
  o *MMT*: Can be performed in the subacute phase of healing.
  o *Special tests*: See special tests in **Table 16-15**.
  o *Palpation*: TFCC.
  o Cognitive assessment.
  o Ability to participate in life roles.

  o Assessment of basic and instrumental ADLs (e.g., DASH and PRWE).
  o Functional mobility (Lawson & Murphy, 2013).

Interventions

The main objective of OT intervention is to restore function and independence of life roles affected by disorders of the arm and wrist. Intervention of TFCC injuries will vary depending on the severity or type of injury, stage of healing, medical intervention, and client-specific factors. Nonetheless, it should focus on restoring the objective deficits seen during the examination and geared toward a return to function. The therapist must be careful as to not create excessive loading or shear forces through the wrist during the interventions.

Upper Extremity Mononeuropathies and Lacerations

Nerve injuries can occur as a result from lacerations, crush injuries, or from other traumatic injuries such as fractures. Nerve injuries can be classified into three categories (Depukat et al., 2014; Kasch & Walsh, 2013).

1. *Neurapraxia*: Injury to the nerve without Wallerian degeneration. Usually due to mechanical compression and once compression is removed, full recovery can occur in a few weeks.

Table 16-15 TFCC Special Tests

Special Test	Description	Positive Test
TFCC load test (Sharpey's)	Ulnar deviation of the wrist with axial load, while shearing the wrist palmarly and dorsally	Pain, crepitus, and clicking in the area of the TFCC
Ulnar fovea sign test	Palpation of the fovea (i.e., the depression between the ulnar styloid process and pisiform and just next to the flexor carpi ulnaris tendon)	Pain or tenderness reproduced with palpation
Ulnar styloid triquetral impaction provocation test	The wrist is fully extended and the forearm is pronated. The forearm is then supinated while maintaining wrist extension	Pain over the ulnar styloid process is positive for ulnocarpal impaction syndrome
Ulnomeniscotriquetral dorsal glide test	One hand stabilizes the ulna and the contralateral hand is used to apply a dorsal glide to the pisiform–triquetrum complex	Excessive movement and/or pain

Data from Magee, 2014.

2. *Axonotmesis*: Injury to the nerve results in distal degeneration. Axonal conduction altered but Schwann coating is normal. Nerve recovery may be complete but depends on the location and timing of the injury.

3. *Neurotmesis*: A complete laceration of nerve fibers with interruption of axonal conduction and damage to Schwann coating. Surgical intervention is required and full recovery rarely occurs.

Nerve injuries warrant specific test and measures to establish neurological status and document recovery. Some tests and measures that can be applied to a variety of nerve problems include (Kasch & Walsh, 2013) the following:

1. *Tests for motor function*: Testing motor ability and strength of muscles innervated by a certain nerve and distal to the lesion.

2. *Sensory mapping*: Requires finding the location where skin goes from having normal to abnormal sensation, documenting, and repeating the process every month during the nerve regeneration process.

3. *Nerve compression (Tinel's sign)*: Involves tapping on the nerve gently starting distally and moving proximally. The most proximal point where symptoms are reproduced indicates the possible location of entrapment. This test is also used after surgery to evaluate the extent of sensory axon healing. Axonal regeneration may occur at a rate of 1 millimeter per day in the postoperative period.

4. *Nerve tension*: Tensioning the involved nerve through upper limb tension tests may reproduce nerve symptoms.

5. *Vibration*: Vibratory sensation with a 30- or 256-Hz tuning fork. Return of vibratory sensation may indicate a return of nerve function, which may provide a guide to start a sensory re-education program.

6. *Touch pressure*: Tests the clients' ability to perceive touch-pressure changes (e.g., with light or heavy pressure, or with moving or constant pressure). With early nerve injuries, sensation testing with Semmes–Weinstein monofilaments may be the most accurate for assessing pressure thresholds.

7. *Two-point discrimination*: Moving or stationary pressures are applied with two adjacent points, randomly alternating with one-point touch. The therapist finds the minimal distance at which the client can distinguish between the two-point and one-point stimuli.

8. *Modified Moberg pickup test*: Tests for tactile gnosis which is the ability to recognize common objects using touch only.

Median Nerve

Median nerve injuries include the following three types of syndromes:
- Pronator teres syndrome (PTS)
- Anterior interosseous syndrome (AIS)
- CTS

Pronator Teres Syndrome

Description: PTS is a rare proximal median nerve entrapment causing symptoms of vague anterior forearm pain and paresthesia (Rodner, Tinsley, & O'Malley, 2013). It is named because of the possible compression of the median nerve between the two heads of the pronator teres but it may also be compressed in the proximal arch of FDS, at the ligament of Struthers, by the bicipital aponeurosis or accessory head of the flexor pollicis longus (FPL) (Rodner et al., 2013). It is most common in women in their fifth decade of life (American Academy of Orthopaedic Surgeons, 2011). It develops in clients who do repetitive forearm activities or have a hypertrophic forearm (American Academy of Orthopaedic Surgeons, 2011).

Clinical presentation: PTS mainly causes sensory changes in the median nerve cutaneous distribution of the hand. As opposed to CTS, the sensory changes affect the palmar cutaneous branch and may cause sensory changes in the radial palm and medial aspect of the thenar eminence. There may be pain with resisted pronation, with resisted elbow flexion with the forearm supinated, or with contraction of FDS (American Academy of Orthopaedic Surgeons, 2011). Lengthening of pronator teres with elbow extension and forearm supination may also provoke symptoms.

Common diagnostic tests: Electrodiagnostic tests may be done in addition to a physical examination but are not reliable for making a diagnosis of PTS (American Academy of Orthopaedic Surgeons, 2011; Rodner et al., 2013). A positive PTS test is the most common sign of PTS but resisted pronation and resisted FDS may also provoke symptoms (Rodner et al., 2013).

Common medical and surgical procedures: Treatment of PTS includes activity modification, NSAIDs, splinting, and surgery if conservative care fails. It is estimated that up to 50% of clients with PTS will require surgery (American Academy of Orthopaedic Surgeons, 2011). When surgery is indicated, a complete decompression of the median nerve throughout its course in the proximal forearm is usually recommended. After surgery, early ROM is encouraged and return to normal activities is expected after six to eight weeks (Rodner et al., 2013).

Precautions and contraindications: Repetitive contractions or lengthening of the pronator teres may aggravate symptoms.

Screening and Assessments

Screening and assessments are similar throughout the various orthopedic conditions of the upper extremity with slight variations. Below is a list of top-down approaches that address the symptoms, as well as the impact of the symptoms on the person's roles, contexts, and environment, followed by bottom-up approaches that are symptom specific:

- Client history including the client's age, hand dominance, occupational and avocational responsibilities, prior injuries, comorbidities, family issues, psychological issues, broader social issues, and economic issues.
- Mechanism and date of injury, structures involved, type and extent of medical and surgical intervention, concomitant injuries, and future treatment planned.
- *Symptoms*: Pain, paresthesias, numbness, weakness, stiffness, and/or lack of coordination.
- Physical assessment includes the following:
  - Baseline physical evaluation to assess limitations not related to the injury.
  - Observations of pain or fear at rest and with movement, while looking for atrophy.
  - Color, temperature, and signs of compromised circulation or inflammation.
  - Edema.
  - *Sensory and motor function*: Being a sensory neuropathy, sensation testing will be especially important. Testing with monofilament or two-point discrimination is indicated.
  - Coordination.
  - Skin integrity/wound assessment.
  - A/PROM of adjacent and uninvolved joints. A posture and cervical screen is most likely warranted.
  - *AROM*: Elbow extension and forearm supination may provoke symptoms.
  - *MMT*: Resisted pronation, resisted elbow flexion with the forearm supinated, or resisted FDS may reproduce symptoms. Muscles innervated by medial nerve should be strong.
  - *Special tests*: Test for PTS (**Table 16-16**).
  - *Palpation*: Pain and tenderness is typically noted over the proximal anterior aspect of the forearm.
  - Cognitive assessment.
  - Ability to participate in life roles.
  - Assessment of basic and instrumental ADLs (e.g., DASH and PRWE).
  - Functional mobility (Lawson & Murphy, 2013).

Interventions

The main objective of OT intervention is to restore function and independence of life roles affected by disorders of the arm and wrist. Intervention of PTS will vary depending on the cause of nerve compression, stage of healing, medical intervention, and client-specific factors. Nonetheless, it should focus on relieving nerve symptoms, restoring the objective deficits seen during the examination, and restoring function. Repetitive contractions or lengthening of the pronator teres should be avoided initially as to not aggravate symptoms. Splinting may be used as part of the treatment, in a position of 90°–100° of elbow flexion with the forearm in neutral. If the nerve entrapment is suspected to be under the FDS arch, the splint should be made with the wrist in a neutral position (Moscony, 2007).

Anterior Interosseous Syndrome

Description: AIS is a rare proximal nerve entrapment causing vague forearm pain and weakness in muscles innervated by the anterior interosseous branch of the median nerve (Rodner et al., 2013). The pathophysiology and etiology is uncertain but the most often proposed theories include an idiopathic neuritis or a nerve

Table 16-16 Special Tests for PTS		
Special Test	**Description**	**Positive Test**
Test for PTS	The client sits with the elbow flexed to 90° and the therapist resists pronation as the elbow is extended	Tingling and paresthesia in the medial nerve distribution

Data from Magee, 2014.

insult as part of a brachial plexus neuralgia (Rodner et al., 2013).

Clinical presentation: Similar to PTS, it causes vague ventral forearm pain but unlike PTS, it causes motor rather than sensory dysfunctions (Rodner et al., 2013). Muscle weakness primarily affects the FPL and pronator quadratus but the FDP to the second and third digits may also be affected. Clients may have a positive "OK" sign.

Common diagnostic tests: Physical examination and electrodiagnostic studies are useful, although imaging may not be helpful for the diagnosis and management of AIS (Rodner et al., 2013). MRI is usually not helpful other than to diagnose a brachial plexus neuralgia and/or to identify a rare mass causing compression (Chi & Harness, 2010).

Common medical and surgical procedures: Due to a lack of evidence, controversy exists in regard to management of AIN, compounded by the fact that many clients recover spontaneously. Conservative treatment is usually the first and best option (Rodner et al., 2013). Surgical decompression is advised when a mass is visualized or if symptoms persist >1 year.

Precautions and contraindications: Activities that aggravate nerve symptoms should be avoided.

Screening and Assessments

Screening and assessments are similar throughout the various orthopedic conditions of the upper extremity with slight variations. Below is a list of top-down approaches that address the symptoms, as well as the impact of the symptoms on the person's roles, contexts, and environment, followed by bottom-up approaches that are symptom specific:

- Client history including the client's age, hand dominance, occupational and avocational responsibilities, prior injuries, comorbidities, family issues, psychological issues, broader social issues, and economic issues.
- Mechanism and date of injury, structures involved, type and extent of medical and surgical intervention, concomitant injuries, and future treatment planned.
- *Symptoms*: Pain, paresthesias, numbness, weakness, stiffness, and/or lack of coordination.
- Physical assessment includes the following:
  - Baseline physical evaluation to assess limitations not related to the injury.
  - Observations of pain or fear at rest and with movement, while looking for atrophy.
  - Color, temperature, and signs of compromised circulation or inflammation.
  - Edema.
  - Sensory and motor function: Sensory testing should be normal.
  - Coordination.
  - Skin integrity and wound assessment.
  - A/PROM of adjacent and uninvolved joints (e.g., posture and cervical screen warranted).
  - AROM.
  - *MMT*: Resisted FPL, pronator quadratus, and FDP to second and third digits may show weakness.
  - *Special tests*: Positive OK sign (see **Table 16-17**).
  - Palpation.
  - Cognitive assessment.
  - Ability to participate in life roles.
  - Assessment of basic and instrumental ADLs (e.g., DASH and PRWE).
  - Functional mobility (Lawson & Murphy, 2013).

Interventions

The main objective of OT intervention is to restore function and independence of life roles affected by disorders of the arm and wrist. Intervention for AIS will vary depending on the cause of nerve compression, stage of healing, medical intervention, and client-specific factors. Nonetheless, it should focus on relieving nerve symptoms, restoring the objective deficits seen during the examination, and restoring function. Tchoryk (2000) advises treatment of the whole upper extremity: stretching/relaxation of tight muscles, mobilization of stiff joints, strengthening weak muscles, and re-educating in correct movement patterns to improve the whole kinetic chain. If splinting is advised, a static DIP blocking splint is usually used (Moscony, 2007).

Table 16-17 Special Tests for AIS

Special Test	Description	Positive Test
OK sign	The client is asked to make a tip-to-tip pinch with the index finger and thumb	The client demonstrates a pulp-to-pulp pinch (i.e., DIP extended rather than flexed). Indicates weakness/paralysis of the flexors of the second digit and thumb

Data from Magee, 2014.

Carpal Tunnel Syndrome

Description: CTS is a constellation of hand symptoms associated with a median entrapment in the carpal tunnel. The carpal tunnel is located in the ventral wrist and is bounded by the scaphoid tubercle and trapezium medially, the hook of hamate and pisiform laterally, transverse carpal ligament superiorly, and the carpal bones inferiorly. CTS is the most prevalent peripheral neuropathy (Brotzman & Manske, 2011) affecting up to 5% of the U.S. population (Keith et al., 2010). It is most common in clients older than 40 and is twice as frequent in women as in men (Brotzman & Manske, 2011). Any structures causing physical narrowing of the canal or causing median nerve ischemia may be at the origin of CTS. Occupations requiring repetitive wrist and finger movements, as well as fluid overload such as with hemodialysis, pregnancy, or oral contraceptive intake increase the risks of CTS. Other risk factors include the following: diabetes, obesity, strong family history, hypothyroidism, autoimmune diseases, rheumatologic diseases, arthritis, renal diseases, infectious diseases, and substance abuse (American Academy of Orthopaedic Surgeons, 2008).

Clinical presentation: Characteristic symptoms include pain, numbness, and tingling in the medial nerve distribution distal to the wrist. Pain and paresthesia symptoms are often worse at night, aggravated by daily activities and sometimes relieved by hand shaking (Brotzman & Manske, 2011). In contrast to PTS, the palmar cutaneous branch is usually unaffected, so that part of the radial palm and medial aspect of the thenar eminence is spared (Magee, 2014). Muscle weakness can be found in the flexor pollicis brevis, abductor pollicis brevis, opponens pollicis, and lateral two lumbricals. Several provocative special tests may aid in diagnosis (see **Table 16-18**).

Common diagnostic tests: Electrodiagnostic studies may be appropriate in the presence of thenar atrophy or persistent symptoms and should be performed with clinical presentation suggesting CTS and when surgical management is considered (Brotzman & Manske, 2011).

Common medical and surgical procedures: The American Academy of Orthopaedic Surgeons recommends conservative treatment for most clients with CTS. AAOS recommends surgery when there is evidence of median nerve denervation or if symptoms persist beyond seven weeks. Conservative interventions advised by the AAOS are local steroid injections and splinting, but oral corticosteroids and ultrasound may also be helpful. Strong evidence supports surgical release of the flexor retinaculum when indicated (American Academy of Orthopaedic Surgeons, 2008).

Precautions and contraindications: Prolonged wrist flexion or extension positions should be avoided. Repetitive finger contractions or poor work ergonomics may also aggravate symptoms.

Screening and Assessments

Screening and assessments are similar throughout the various orthopedic conditions of the upper extremity with slight variations. Below is a list of top-down

Table 16-18 CTS Special Tests		
Special Test	**Method**	**Positive Result**
Phalen's (wrist flexion) test	The client holds the dorsum of the hands together then flexes the shoulders maximally for one minute (i.e., to create maximal wrist flexion)	Tingling and/or paresthesia in the median nerve distribution
Reverse Phalen's (prayer) test	The client brings the palms together and brings the hands toward the wrists to create wrist extension	Tingling or paresthesia in the median nerve distribution
Two-point discrimination	In the median nerve sensory distribution, apply pressure with two adjacent points, randomly alternating with one-point touch. Find the minimal distance at which the client can distinguish between the two-point and one-point stimuli	Greater than 6 mm indicates sensory loss (i.e., which is common with CTS)
Tinel's sign	Tap with the index finger over the carpal tunnel and the median nerve	Tingling or paresthesia in the median nerve distribution

Data from Cooper, 2014c; Magee, 2014.

approaches that address the symptoms, as well as the impact of the symptoms on the person's roles, contexts, and environment, followed by bottom-up approaches that are symptom specific:

- Client history including the client's age, hand dominance, occupational and avocational responsibilities, prior injuries, comorbidities, family issues, psychological issues, broader social issues, and economic issues.
- Mechanism and date of injury, structures involved, type and extent of medical and surgical intervention, concomitant injuries, and future treatment planned.
- *Symptoms*: Pain, paresthesias, numbness, weakness, stiffness, and/or lack of coordination.
- Physical assessment includes the following:
  - Baseline physical evaluation and interview to assess limitations not related to the injury.
  - Observations of pain or fear at rest and with movement, while looking for atrophy.
  - Color, temperature, and signs of compromised circulation or inflammation.
  - Edema.
  - Sensory and motor function (e.g., monofilament and two-point discrimination).
  - Coordination.
  - Skin integrity and wound assessment.
  - A/PROM of adjacent and uninvolved joints. A posture and cervical screen is most likely warranted.
  - AROM.
  - *MMT*: Muscle testing of flexor pollicis brevis, abductor pollicis brevis, opponens pollicis, and the lateral two lumbricals may show weakness. Assessing grip and pinch strength is also useful.
  - *Special tests*: See special tests (Table 16-18).
  - *Palpation*: Palpate for possible atrophy of thenar eminence.
  - Cognitive assessment.
  - Ability to participate in life roles.
  - Assessment of basic and instrumental ADLs (e.g., DASH and PRWE).
  - Functional mobility (Lawson & Murphy, 2013).

Interventions

The main objective of OT intervention is to restore function and independence of life roles affected by disorders of the arm and wrist. Intervention of CTS will vary depending on the cause of nerve compression, stage of healing, medical intervention, and client-specific factors. Nonetheless, it should focus on relieving nerve symptoms, restoring the objective deficits seen during the examination and restoring function. It is also important to respect pain and avoid activities that aggravate nerve symptoms. Worsening neurological deficits warrant a referral back to the physician. The following are guidelines for conservative treatment of CTS (Cooper, 2014c):

1. Provision of adaptive equipment such as built-up handles, jar openers, and buttonhooks.
2. Night or occupational splinting with the wrist in a neutral or slightly extended position (Beasley, 2014).
3. Median nerve-gliding exercises.
4. Flexor tendon-gliding exercises.
5. Aerobic exercises and proximal conditioning.
6. Ergonomic modification.
7. Client education.
   - Avoid extremes of forearm rotation and wrist motion.
   - Avoid sustained or forceful grip.
   - Padded gloves and steering wheel or built-up handles may also be beneficial (Cooper, 2014c).
8. Compensatory strategies for sensory and motor loss with focus on injury prevention.
9. Postural training.

If the client had surgery, treatment can often begin as soon as 24–48 hours after surgery but may be delayed by several weeks. The therapist is advised to follow the surgeon's rehabilitation protocol. The following provides an outline for treatment of CTS postoperatively (Cooper, 2014c):

1. ROM exercises.
2. Mobilization including tendon-gliding and median nerve-gliding exercises.
3. Wound and scar care. After suture removal, the use of silicone gel or Micropore tape may improve scar cosmesis.
4. Pain and edema management.
5. Desensitization.
6. Strengthening may be delayed until the third week postsurgery or later depending on the physician. Start with gentle strengthening and encourage participation in light ADLs until the client can progress to advanced strengthening at five to six weeks (Moscony, 2014).

Radial Nerve

Radial nerve injuries include the following two types of syndromes:

- Radial tunnel syndrome (RTS)
- Posterior interosseous syndrome (PIS)

Radial Tunnel Syndrome

Description: This syndrome is caused by a compression of the radial nerve in the radial tunnel, which extends from the lateral epicondyle to the supinator muscle (Clavert et al., 2009). The arcade of Frohse is the most common but not exclusive compression site of the radial nerve in the radial tunnel (Clavert et al., 2009). The arcade of Frohse is a fibrous arch formed by the superficial head of the supinator muscle (Clavert et al., 2009). The syndrome is most prevalent in the dominant arm of women between the ages of 30 and 50 (Moradi, Ebrahimzadeh, & Jupiter, 2015).

Clinical presentation: RTS causes lateral elbow and forearm pain that is aggravated by repeated forearm pronation and supination (Clavert et al., 2009) and is often worse at night (Moradi et al., 2015). It is often mistaken as lateral epicondylitis (American Academy of Orthopaedic Surgeons, 2011) but RTS causes a point tenderness over the radial nerve, 5 centimeters distal to the lateral epicondyle rather than directly over it (Moradi et al., 2015). Symptoms may be provoked by a radial nerve tension test (Magee, 2014) or components of the radial nerve tension test (e.g., wrist flexion, elbow extension, and forearm pronation). The superficial radial nerve is a purely sensory nerve so insults to it do not usually cause motor deficits (American Academy of Orthopaedic Surgeons, 2011; Bevelaqua, Hayter, Feinberg, & Rodeo, 2012); this is an important distinguishing feature between RTS and PIS (American Academy of Orthopaedic Surgeons, 2011; Moradi et al., 2015).

Common diagnostic tests: A good clinical examination is most important in making a diagnosis as electrodiagnostic studies and other imaging techniques are usually negative (American Academy of Orthopaedic Surgeons, 2011; Moradi et al., 2015).

Common medical and surgical procedures: Nonsurgical treatment is indicated in most cases (American Academy of Orthopaedic Surgeons, 2011). Rest, NSAIDs, injections, and therapy may be prescribed but often bring only temporary relief (Moradi et al., 2015). A radial nerve block may help alleviate or resolve symptoms (Moradi et al., 2015). If three months of these conservative interventions fail, surgical decompression is recommended (Moradi et al., 2015).

Precautions and contraindications: Avoid stretches, positioning, and repetitive movements that overly stretch or compress the radial nerve (e.g., repetitive pronation and/or supination activities, and prolonged elbow extension, forearm pronation, and wrist flexion) (Moradi et al., 2015).

Screening and Assessments

Screening and assessments are similar throughout the various orthopedic conditions of the upper extremity with slight variations. Below is a list of top-down approaches that address the symptoms, as well as the impact of the symptoms on the person's roles, contexts, and environment, followed by bottom-up approaches that are symptom specific:

- Client history including the client's age, hand dominance, occupational and avocational responsibilities, prior injuries, comorbidities, family issues, psychological issues, broader social issues, and economic issues.
- Mechanism and date of injury, structures involved, type and extent of medical and surgical intervention, concomitant injuries, and future treatment planned.
- Symptoms: Pain, paresthesias, numbness, weakness, stiffness, and/or lack of coordination.
- Physical assessment includes the following:
  - Baseline physical evaluation and interview to assess limitations not related to the injury.
  - Observations of pain or fear at rest and with movement, while looking for atrophy.
  - Color, temperature, and signs of compromised circulation or inflammation.
  - Edema.
  - *Sensory function*: This is mainly a sensory nerve, so examination of sensation is very important. Consider two-point discrimination and/or monofilament test.
  - Coordination.
  - Skin integrity and wound assessment.
  - A/PROM of adjacent/uninvolved joints. A posture and cervical screen is most likely warranted.

o *AROM/PROM*: Passive or active wrist flexion, elbow extension, and forearm pronation may provoke symptoms.

o *MMT*: No motor deficits expected but important in the differential diagnosis.

o *Special tests*: *Radial nerve tension test (ULNT3)*: Shoulder girdle depression, glenohumeral abduction, elbow extension, forearm pronation, wrist flexion, and ulnar deviation.

o *Palpation*: Palpation over the radial nerve, approximately 5 centimeters distal to the lateral epicondyle.

o Cognitive assessment.

o Ability to participate in life roles.

o Assessment of basic and instrumental ADLs (e.g., DASH and PRWE).

o Functional mobility (Lawson & Murphy, 2013).

Interventions

The main objective of OT intervention is to restore function and independence of life roles affected by disorders of the arm and wrist. RTS treatment will vary depending on the cause of nerve compression, stage of healing, medical intervention, and client-specific factors. Nonetheless, it should focus on relieving nerve symptoms, restoring the objective deficits seen during the examination, and restoring function. The OT practitioner must initially avoid stretches, positioning, and repetitive movements that excessively stretch or compress the radial nerve. Repetitive pronation/supination activities and prolonged positions with elbow extension, forearm pronation, and wrist flexion should therefore be avoided (Moradi et al., 2015).

Posterior Interosseous Syndrome

Description: PIS is an entrapment of the deep branch of the radial nerve outside of the radial tunnel (Bevelaqua et al., 2012). As a primary motor nerve, posterior interosseous nerve (PIN) compression often leads to weakness in finger and thumb extension without sensory loss (American Academy of Orthopaedic Surgeons, 2011; Bevelaqua et al., 2012). It is a rare form of entrapment, accounting for less than 0.7% of all upper extremity neuropathies (Bevelaqua et al., 2012). PIN syndrome is usually caused by trauma or space occupying a lesion, but may also be idiopathic in presentation (American Academy of Orthopaedic Surgeons, 2011; Bevelaqua et al., 2012).

Clinical presentation: Clients may present with weakness of finger and thumb extension at the MCP joint and weakness of thumb abduction due to a weak abductor pollicis longus. Extension of the IP, as well as strength of the lumbricals and interossei is usually preserved. The wrist may radially deviate due to unopposed contraction of the ECRL (i.e., if ECU is affected) as ECRL and ECRB are usually spared (Bevelaqua et al., 2012). Typically, no sensory loss is observed (American Academy of Orthopaedic Surgeons, 2011; Bevelaqua et al., 2012).

Common diagnostic tests: A diagnosis is usually made with a physical examination with or without electrodiagnostic studies. An MRI can be ordered if a mass is suspected as the cause of compression (American Academy of Orthopaedic Surgeons, 2011).

Common medical and surgical procedures: Conservative treatment is usually initiated. Nerve decompression or tendon transfer is recommended with either a lack of improvement or disease progression (American Academy of Orthopaedic Surgeons, 2011).

Precautions and contraindications: More extensive and progressing nerve involvement is possible if not treated in a timely manner (Cooper, 2014c).

Screening and Assessments

Screening and assessments are similar throughout the various orthopedic conditions of the upper extremity with slight variations. Below is a list of top-down approaches that address the symptoms, as well as the impact of the symptoms on the person's roles, contexts, and environment, followed by bottom-up approaches that are symptom specific:

- Client history including the client's age, hand dominance, occupational and avocational responsibilities, prior injuries, comorbidities, family issues, psychological issues, broader social issues, and economic issues.
- Mechanism and date of injury, structures involved, type and extent of medical and surgical intervention, concomitant injuries, and future treatment planned.
- *Symptoms*: Pain, paresthesias, numbness, weakness, stiffness, and/or lack of coordination.
- Physical assessment includes the following:
  o Baseline physical evaluation and interview to assess limitations not related to the injury.
  o Observations of pain or fear at rest and with movement, while looking for atrophy.

- Color, temperature, and signs of compromised circulation or inflammation.
- Edema.
- Sensory and motor function.
- Coordination.
- Skin integrity and wound assessment.
- A/PROM of adjacent/uninvolved joints. A posture and cervical screen is most likely warranted.
- *AROM*: Watch for radial deviation of the wrist during wrist extension.
- *MMT*: Weakness expected with MCP extension of the fingers, and especially thumb ADB.
- *Special tests*: *Radial nerve tension test (ULNT3)*: Shoulder girdle depression, GH ABD 110, elbow extension, forearm pronation, wrist flexion, and ulnar deviation.
- *Palpation*: Palpate for tenderness in the supinator muscle 4–5 centimeters distal to the lateral epicondyle.
- Cognitive assessment.
- Ability to participate in life roles.
- Assessment of basic and instrumental ADLs (e.g., DASH and PRWE).
- Functional mobility (Lawson & Murphy, 2013).

Interventions

The main objective of OT intervention is to restore function and independence of life roles affected by disorders of the arm and wrist. PIS treatment will vary depending on the cause of nerve compression, stage of healing, medical intervention, and client-specific factors. Nonetheless, it should focus on relieving nerve symptoms, maintaining PROM, restoring the objective deficits and function, and preventing deformity through orthotic prescription (Cooper, 2014c). If needed, a splint that positions the wrist, MCPs, and thumb in extension may prevent excessive stretching of the extensors during the acute phase and maintain an optimal position for functional tasks. A dynamic splint is also commonly used (Kasch & Walsh, 2013).

Ulnar Nerve

Ulnar nerve injuries were the most frequent acute nerve injury resulting in hospital admission, as compared to medial, radial, and brachial plexus injuries, between 1993 and 2006 (Woo, Bakri, & Moran, 2015). Injuries are most frequent in working males aged 18–45 years old (Woo et al., 2015). To improve outcomes of traumatic ulnar nerve injuries, early repair is paramount and incomplete recovery resulting in functional loss is common (Woo et al., 2015). Chronic ulnar nerve injuries include the following three types of syndromes:

- Cubital tunnel syndrome
- Bowler's thumb
- Guyon's canal syndrome

Cubital Tunnel Syndrome

Description: Compression of the ulnar nerve in the cubital tunnel is the second most common peripheral neuropathy after CTS (American Academy of Orthopaedic Surgeons, 2011). The ulnar nerve is compressed in a tunnel formed by the medial epicondyle of the humerus, the olecranon process of the ulna, and the Osbourne ligament joining the humeral and ulnar heads of the flexor carpi ulnaris (Palmer & Hughes, 2010).

Clinical presentation: Symptoms include paresthesia or numbness in the fourth and fifth digits, clumsiness with fine motor skills, and occasionally pain over the medial aspect of the elbow (American Academy of Orthopaedic Surgeons, 2011; Palmer & Hughes, 2010). Some special tests such as the Tinel's sign over the cubital tunnel, the upper limb tension test, and the elbow flexion test may be positive (Magee, 2014). More severe compressions will cause weakness in muscles innervated by the ulnar nerve distal to the lesion (e.g., hypothenar muscles, palmar and dorsal interossei, the third and fourth lumbricals, and adductor pollicis). Severe or long-standing denervation of the hand intrinsics causes a claw or intrinsic-minus deformity, which is a hyperextension of the proximal phalanx with flexion of the middle and distal phalanges of the fourth and fifth digits (American Academy of Orthopaedic Surgeons, 2011; Palmer & Hughes, 2010). A positive Froment's paper sign may be present and may indicate paralysis of the adductor pollicis (Magee, 2014).

Common diagnostic tests: Electromyography (EMG) and nerve conduction studies can supplement the physical examination for the purpose of making a diagnosis (American Academy of Orthopaedic Surgeons, 2011). Radiographs may be taken to rule out impingement of the ulnar nerve from osteophytes (Palmer & Hughes, 2010).

Common medical and surgical procedures: Usually nonsurgical management is the first option. It includes night splinting and rehabilitation, which may include nerve mobilizations, and education to avoid end range elbow flexion and pressure on the ulnar nerve (Palmer & Hughes, 2010). When signs and symptoms persist or progress, surgical procedures such as decompression, medial epicondylectomy, or anterior transposition may be indicated (American Academy of Orthopaedic Surgeons, 2011).

Precautions and contraindications: Clients should avoid leaning on the medial elbow and flexing the elbow for a prolonged period of time.

Screening and Assessments

Screening and assessments are similar throughout the various orthopedic conditions of the upper extremity with slight variations. Below is a list of top-down approaches that address the symptoms, as well as the impact of the symptoms on the person's roles, contexts, and environments, followed by bottom-up approaches that are symptom specific:

- Client history including the client's age, hand dominance, occupational and avocational responsibilities, prior injuries, comorbidities, family issues, psychological issues, broader social issues, and economic issues.
- Mechanism and date of injury, structures involved, type and extent of medical and surgical intervention, concomitant injuries, and future treatment planned.
- *Symptoms*: Pain, paresthesias, numbness, weakness, stiffness, and/or lack of coordination.
- Physical assessment includes the following:
  - Baseline physical evaluation and interview to assess limitations not related to the injury.
  - Observations of pain or fear at rest and with movement, while looking for atrophy. Also observe for a claw hand or intrinsic-minus deformity.
  - Color, temperature, and signs of compromised circulation or inflammation.
  - Edema.
  - Sensory and motor function.
  - Coordination.
  - Skin integrity and wound assessment.
  - A/PROM of adjacent/uninvolved joints. A posture and cervical screen is most likely warranted.
  - *AROM*: Elbow flexion might reproduce symptoms.

- *MMT*: With focus on hypothenar muscles, palmar and dorsal interossei, the third and fourth lumbricals, and the adductor pollicis. Grip and pinch strength should also be assessed.
- *Special tests*: See **Table 16-19**.
- Palpation.
- Cognitive assessment.
- Ability to participate in life roles.
- Assessment of basic and instrumental ADLs (e.g., DASH and PRWE).
- Functional mobility (Lawson & Murphy, 2013).

Interventions

The main objective of OT intervention is to restore function and independence of life roles affected by disorders of the arm and wrist. Cubital tunnel syndrome treatment will vary depending on the cause of nerve compression, stage of healing, medical intervention, and client-specific factors. Nonetheless, it should focus on relieving nerve symptoms, restoring the objective deficits and function, and preventing deformity through orthotic prescription.

Table 16-19 Common Diagnostic Tests for Cubital Tunnel Syndrome

Test	Possible Findings
Tinel's sign at the elbow	Pain and numbness in the ulnar nerve distribution
Elbow flexion test	Pain and numbness in the ulnar nerve distribution
Upper limb tension test	Symptoms are reproduced with tensioning of the ulnar nerve with shoulder girdle depression, shoulder abduction and external rotation, elbow flexion, and wrist extension
Wartenberg sign	The small finger is held in an abducted position when the hand is placed on a table, without being able to be adducted. Indicates weakness of interosseous muscles
Monofilament testing	Lack of sensation may be found with the filament test. Reliable and sensitive test for early detection of nerve compression (Kasch & Walsh, 2013)
Froment's paper sign	The client is unable to hold the paper with a key pinch and thumb IP flexion is seen. Indicates paralysis of the adductor pollicis often from ulnar nerve injury (Magee, 2014)

Data from Cooper, 2014c; Magee, 2014.

Below is a list of common interventions for conservative and postoperative management:

Conservative Treatment

1. Fabricate a long arm gutter splint positioning the elbow in 45°–60° of flexion with the wrist and forearm in a neutral position; recommended for use at night to prevent prolonged elbow flexion.
2. If clawing is present, provide a hand-based splint to block hyperextension of the MCP joints and allow MCP and IP flexion and extension to neutral.
3. Provide an elbow pad to limit pressure on the nerve when the elbow is resting on a hard surface. This pad can also be used at night, with the pad turned around on the volar surface of the elbow to limit elbow flexion at night (i.e., if a custom splint is not available).
4. Instruct the client in activity modification such as avoiding sustained elbow flexion, repetitive elbow flexion, and extension activity, or positioning the elbow on a hard surface.
5. Ulnar nerve glides (Moscony, 2014).

Postsurgical Treatment

Protective phase (day 1 to 3 weeks):

1. *Splinting*: Long arm gutter placing the elbow in 70°–90° of flexion with the wrist and forearm in neutral. Provide an anticlaw splint if clawing is present.
2. AROM of uninvolved joints.
3. AROM of the elbow will begin one to two weeks postoperatively depending on the surgical procedure performed. The goal is to achieve functional AROM while limiting pain (Moscony, 2014).
4. Scar management can begin following suture removal.
5. Edema control techniques.
6. Desensitization techniques when hypersensitivity is present.
7. Pain management techniques (Moscony, 2014).

Strengthening phase (weeks 5–7):

1. *Splinting*: Continue with anticlaw splint if muscle imbalances remain. Padding of the elbow may also continue if hypersensitivity remains.
2. Assess grip and pinch strength, and address deficits found.
3. Assess muscle strength in the ulnar nerve distribution using MMT; address deficits.
4. Isolated strengthening should begin with isometric exercises.

5. A work rehab program may be needed to address back to work issues including conditioning and work activity modifications (Moscony, 2014).

Bowler's Thumb

Description: Bowler's thumb is an acute or chronic neuropathy involving the ulnar digital nerve of the thumb. It gets its name because it affects tenpin bowlers who keep their thumb in the bowling ball for an extended time when attempting to create a spin on the ball (Halsey, Therattil, Viviano, Fleegler, & Lee, 2015). This syndrome may happen in other populations such as dressmakers (i.e., from overuse of scissors), jewelers, and massage therapists, but in all cases, nerve compression, traction, or irritation of the ulnar digital nerve causes the symptoms and a neuroma may also develop (Halsey et al., 2015; Waldman, 2012).

Clinical presentation: Subjectively, the client may report pain and tenderness in the second web space, numbness, or paresthesia along the medial aspect of the thumb and difficulty using scissors (Halsey et al., 2015; Waldman, 2012). On examination, a small mass or thickening along the ulnar digital nerve may be palpable; diminished two-point discrimination over the involved skin area or positive Tinel's or nerve compression sign may be found (Halsey et al., 2015; Swanson, Macias, & Smith, 2009; Waldman, 2012).

Common diagnostic tests: EMG and nerve conduction studies can supplement the physical examination but may or may not be positive. MRI can help in furthering the examination of a neuroma (Halsey et al., 2015) and plain film radiographs may help in ruling out spurs or cysts as a cause of nerve compression (Waldman, 2012).

Common medical and surgical procedures: A period of conservative treatment is usually initiated which includes rest, activity modification, and splinting. If conservative treatment fails, various surgical techniques can be performed: neurolysis, neuroma resection with or without nerve grafting, and nerve transposition (Halsey et al., 2015). Very little evidence exists comparing the outcomes of these various interventions.

Precautions and contraindications: Continued bowling should be avoided if symptoms persist.

Screening and Assessments

Screening and assessments are similar throughout the various orthopedic conditions of the upper extremity with slight variations. Below is a list of top-down approaches that address the symptoms, as well as the impact of the symptoms on the person's roles, contexts, and environment, followed by bottom-up approaches that are symptom specific:

- Client history including the client's age, hand dominance, occupational and avocational responsibilities, prior injuries, comorbidities, family issues, psychological issues, broader social issues, and economic issues.
- Mechanism and date of injury, structures involved, type and extent of medical and surgical intervention, concomitant injuries, and future treatment planned.
- *Symptoms*: Pain, paresthesias, numbness, weakness, stiffness, and/or lack of coordination.
- Physical assessment includes the following:
  - Baseline physical evaluation to assess limitations not related to the injury.
  - Observations of pain or fear at rest and with movement, while looking for atrophy.
  - Color, temperature, and signs of compromised circulation or inflammation.
  - Edema.
  - *Sensory and motor function*: Consider two-point discrimination testing or monofilament.
  - Coordination.
  - Skin integrity and wound assessment.
  - A/PROM of adjacent/uninvolved joints. A posture and cervical screen is most likely warranted.
  - AROM.
  - MMT.
  - *Special tests*: Positive Tinel's sign over the ulnar digital nerve.
  - *Palpation*: Over ulnar digital nerve and first web space.
  - Cognitive assessment.
  - Ability to participate in life roles.
  - Assessment of basic and instrumental ADLs (e.g., DASH and PRWE). Assess ability to use scissors.
  - Functional mobility (Lawson & Murphy, 2013).

Interventions

The main objective of OT intervention is to restore function and independence of life roles affected by disorders of the arm and wrist. Treatment of Bowler's thumb will vary depending on the cause of nerve compression, stage of healing, medical intervention, and client-specific

factors. Nonetheless, it should focus on relieving nerve symptoms, restoring the objective deficits and function, and preventing deformity through orthotic prescription. Modification of offending movements is of paramount importance. Clients that have stopped bowling tend to have marked improvement of their symptoms. For those who decide not to stop bowling, a thumb neoprene sleeve or splinting can be recommended, as well as changing the weight, size, or type of bowling ball, training parameters, or throwing technique (Halsey et al., 2015).

Guyon's Canal Syndrome

Description: Uncommonly, the ulnar nerve gets compressed in the Guyon's canal, a canal bounded by the pisiform and pisohamate ligament, the hook of the hamate, and the superficial palmar carpal ligament. It is most often due to an acute injury, repetitive trauma, or a space occupying lesion such as a ganglia (American Academy of Orthopaedic Surgeons). Less commonly, metabolic diseases, diseases of neighboring blood vessels, degenerative joint disease of the wrist, or idiopathic causes are at fault (Depukat et al., 2014). The syndrome can be subdivided into three categories, depending on what nerve branch is involved (Depukat et al., 2014). **Table 16-20** describes the types of ulnar nerve injuries in the Guyon's canal.

Clinical presentation: Presentation may vary depending on the type of injury (see Table 16-20): Sensory or motor deficits (or both) are possible, depending on the exact location of compression (American Academy of Orthopaedic Surgeons, 2011; Depukat et al., 2014). The client may present with complaints of ulnar-sided palm pain, grip weakness, and/or numbness/tingling in the medial hand (Chen & Tsai, 2014). On examination, the client may present with sensory and/or motor changes in the skin or muscles innervated by the ulnar nerve distal to the lesion. The Guyon's canal is distal to the branching off of the dorsal ulnar cutaneous nerve so the dorsal aspect of the hand is usually spared from sensory deficits (Chen & Tsai, 2014). Similar to many peripheral neuropathies, a positive Tinel's sign may be present.

Common diagnostic tests: EMG and nerve conduction studies can supplement the physical examination for the purpose of making a diagnosis. Occasionally, plain film radiographs or MRI are ordered to supplement the examination findings especially if a mass is suspected to cause the symptoms (Depukat et al., 2014). Allen's test or palpation of ulnar and radial pulses can help in ruling

Table 16-20 Types of Ulnar Nerve Injuries in Guyon's Canal and Common Presentations

Type	Description	Presentation
Type I	The ulnar nerve is affected at the very beginning of Guyon's canal or within Guyon's canal but before the bifurcation of the superficial and deep branches	Cutaneous (i.e., sensory) distribution of the ulnar nerve (i.e., medial half of the fourth digit, fifth digit, and the ulnar aspect of palm, while sparing the dorsum of the hand) and/or motor deficits (i.e., abductor digiti minimi, flexor digiti minimi, opponens digiti minimi, dorsal interossei, palmar interossei, lumbricals #3 and 4, and adductor pollicis). Froment's sign and claw hand deformity are both possible
Type II	Compression of the deep branch of the ulnar nerve	Causes motor deficits only (i.e., similar to those of type I) unless the compression occurs distal to branching to the hypothenar muscles, in which case sparing of the hypothenar muscles will typically occur. Froment's sign and claw hand deformity are both possible
Type III	Compression affecting the superficial branch of the ulnar nerve. Occurs most commonly due to an abnormal muscle or a thrombosis within the ulnar artery	Sensory deficits over the superficial branch of the ulnar nerve (i.e., palmar aspect of the fifth digit and medial half of the fourth digit while sparing most of the palm and the dorsum of the hand). Affects motor fibers to palmaris brevis, which rarely causes functional deficits

Data from Chen and Tsai, 2014; Depukat et al., 2014; Clavert et al., 2009.

out a vascular cause of symptoms or nerve irritation (Chen & Tsai, 2014).

Common medical and surgical procedures: Conservative treatment may include education to avoid putting pressure on the ulnar side of the hand, immobilization, protective braces, NSAIDs, activity modification, and discontinuation of provocative activities. Surgical release is indicated when there is a physical compressive insult, when symptoms progress or persist, or with major motor deficits (Chen & Tsai, 2014). Surgical treatment includes exploration, removal of lesions, decompression of the ulnar tunnel, and pisohamate hiatus (Chen & Tsai, 2014).

Precautions and contraindications: Clients should avoid leaning on the ulnar side of the hand. Acute sensory loss post-fracture or surgical interventions require immediate referral for possible and timely surgical exploration/decompression (Chen & Tsai, 2014).

Screening and Assessments

Screening and assessments are similar throughout the various orthopedic conditions of the upper extremity with slight variations. Below is a list of top-down approaches that address the symptoms, as well as the impact of the symptoms on the person's roles, contexts, and environment, followed by bottom-up approaches that are symptom specific:

- Client history including the client's age, hand dominance, occupational and avocational responsibilities, prior injuries, comorbidities, family issues, psychological issues, broader social issues, and economic issues.
- Mechanism and date of injury, structures involved, type and extent of medical and surgical intervention, concomitant injuries, and future treatment planned.
- *Symptoms*: Pain, paresthesias, numbness, weakness, stiffness, and/or lack of coordination.
- Physical assessment includes the following:
  - Baseline physical evaluation to assess limitations not related to the injury.
  - Observations of pain or fear at rest and with movement, while looking for atrophy. Also observe for possible clawing of the hand.
  - Color, temperature, and signs of compromised circulation or inflammation.
  - Edema.
  - Sensory and motor function: Consider two-point discrimination testing or monofilament testing.
  - Coordination.
  - Skin integrity and wound assessment.
  - A/PROM of adjacent/uninvolved joints. A postural assessment and cervical screen is most likely warranted.
  - AROM.
  - *MMT*: Flexor digiti minimi, opponens digiti minimi, dorsal interossei, palmar interossei,

lumbricals #3 and 4, adductor pollicis, and abductor digiti minimi.
  - *Special tests*: Tinel's sign over Guyon's canal, Froment's sign, and tests to rule out circulatory causes for symptoms (e.g., palpation of pulses and Allen's test).
  - *Palpation*: Tender over Guyon's canal.
  - Cognitive assessment.
  - Ability to participate in life roles.
  - Assessment of basic and instrumental ADLs (e.g., DASH and PRWE).
  - Functional mobility (Lawson & Murphy, 2013).

Interventions

The main objective of OT intervention is to restore function and independence of life roles affected by disorders of the arm and wrist. Treatment of Guyon's canal syndrome will vary depending on the cause of nerve compression, stage of healing, medical intervention, and client-specific factors. Nonetheless, it should focus on relieving nerve symptoms, restoring the objective deficits and function, and preventing deformity through orthotic prescription. When paralysis of hand intrinsics is present, a dynamic ulnar nerve splint that blocks MCP hyperextension while allowing MCP flexion and extension to neutral is recommended (Kasch & Walsh, 2013). Client education can focus on avoiding pressure on the ulnar side of the hand, modifying provoking activities, and using protective bracing as needed (Chen & Tsai, 2014).

Complex Regional Pain Syndrome

Description: CRPS (i.e., current terminology) may also be referred to as reflex sympathetic dystrophy, reflex neurovascular dystrophy, or causalgia (i.e., to name a few). Clients with CRPS display pain and dysfunction out of proportion to those normally expected (Kasch & Walsh, 2013).

Clinical presentation: The signs and symptoms of CRPS are pain, swelling, blotchy, or shiny skin. Coolness of the extremity, excessive sweating, or dryness may also be present. Hypersensitivity to light touch is common. CRPS can be divided into three types.

Type I follows a noxious event that does not include injuries to nerves. Pain does not follow distribution of a single peripheral nerve. Pain is spontaneous and is disproportionate to the noxious event; *type II* develops after a nerve injury. Pain is spontaneous and is disproportionate to the noxious event; and *type III* includes clients that do not fall into category I or II (Cooper, 2014c; Kasch & Walsh, 2013). There are three stages to CRPS. **Table 16-21** outlines these three stages along with their clinical presentation.

Common medical and surgical management: CRPS is treated conservatively and treatment is most effective in stage I (Kasch & Walsh, 2013).

Precautions and contraindications: No PROM should be performed until pain and edema start to decrease (Kasch & Walsh, 2013).

Screening and Assessments

Screening and assessments are similar throughout the various orthopedic conditions of the upper extremity with slight variations. Below is a list of top-down approaches that address the symptoms, as well as the impact of the symptoms on the person's roles, contexts, and environment, followed by bottom-up approaches that are symptom specific:

- Client history including the client's age, hand dominance, occupational and avocational responsibilities, prior injuries, comorbidities, family issues, psychological issues, broader social issues, and economic issues.
- Mechanism and date of injury, structures involved, type and extent of medical and surgical intervention, concomitant injuries, and future treatment planned.

Table 16-21 Stages of CRPS	
Stage	**Description**
Stage I (traumatic stage)	May last 3 months. The client displays pain, pitting edema, and discoloration
Stage II (dystrophic stage)	May last an additional 6–9 months. The client displays pain, brawny edema, stiffness, redness, heat, and bony demineralization. The hand frequently has a glossy appearance. Pain intensity usually peaks in stage II
Stage III (atrophic stage)	May last several years or indefinitely. Pain may decrease. Hard edema may be present but is nonresponsive. Thickening around the joints may lead to contractures. The hand may be pale, dry, and cool

Data from Kasch and Walsh, 2013.

- *Symptoms*: Pain, paresthesias, numbness, weakness, stiffness, and/or lack of coordination.
- Physical assessment includes the following:
  - Baseline physical evaluation to assess limitations not related to the injury.
  - Observations of pain or fear at rest and with movement, while looking for atrophy, as well as skin appearance.
  - Color, temperature, and signs of compromised circulation or inflammation.
  - Edema: Document volumetric measurements.
  - *Sensory and motor function*: Consider two-point discrimination or monofilament test.
  - *Sympathetic function*: Sudomotor (e.g., sweating), vasomotor (e.g., temperature discrimination, and skin color), pilomotor (e.g., gooseflesh response), and trophic changes (e.g., skin texture, nail, and hair growth) (Kasch & Walsh, 2013).
  - Coordination.
  - Skin integrity and wound assessment.
  - A/PROM of adjacent and uninvolved joints.
  - AROM.
  - MMT.
  - *Palpation*: Palpatory findings may include generalized and point tenderness, allodynia (i.e., pain with gentle touch or contact), edema, temperature changes (e.g., regionally or right/left), increased moisture (i.e., sweating) or dry skin, muscle and joint tenderness, and/or muscle spasms.
  - Cognitive assessment.
  - Ability to participate in life roles.
  - Assessment of basic and instrumental ADLs (e.g., DASH and PRWE).
  - Functional mobility (Lawson & Murphy, 2013).

Interventions

The main objective of OT intervention is to restore function and independence of life roles affected by disorders of the arm and wrist. CRPS treatment will vary depending on the type and stage of the disorder, medical intervention, and client-specific factors. Nonetheless, conservative treatment of CRPS is geared at decreasing sympathetic stimulation, pain, and hypersensitivity. It is most effective in stage I (Kasch & Walsh, 2013). Below

is a list of common interventions for CRPS (Kasch & Walsh, 2013):

1. Edema control techniques:
   a. Elevation and manual edema mobilization.
   b. Contrast baths.
   c. High-volt direct current in water.
2. Stress-loading program.
3. Desensitization techniques (e.g., gentle handling of the hand, acupressure, and desensitization with various textures).
4. Physical agent modalities:
   a. Transcutaneous electrical nerve stimulation should be used for intervention periods not to exceed 20 minutes at a time.
   b. Surface EMG-biofeedback training may help decrease muscle spasms and improve blood flow.
   c. Fluidotherapy at low heat or warm moist heat.
5. AROM for the entire extremity. Avoid painful positions and painful PROM. Consider gravity-eliminated exercises (e.g., table top in a horizontal plane or in water) if well tolerated and shoulder ROM exercises early in the disease.
6. Functional activities that involve the whole upper quadrant.

This concludes the section of the chapter on wrist and hand pathologies; general intervention guidelines for wrist and hand pathologies are covered below.

Evidence-Based Practice

Evidence for OT interventions for work-related injuries and conditions of the forearm, wrist, and hand are described in **Table 16-22**.

Referrals and Discharge Considerations

Clients are ready for discharge when they are reporting a return to functional use of their upper extremity and are independent with a home exercise program. Referrals for additional therapies and services are discussed with the team and provided prior to discharge.

Table 16-22 Evidence of OT Interventions for Work-Related Injuries

Intervention	Evidence
Silicone gel sheeting	Reduces hypertrophic scarring and improves scar elasticity
Scar massage	Reduces pain and itching from scars
Splinting	Effective for CMC arthritis and CTS regardless of style
Early mobilization (<21 days after injury)	Effective at decreasing pain, swelling, and facilitating a return to work after acute hand injuries or fractures
Low-level laser therapy	May decrease pain and increase function in clients with RA and CTS
Cryotherapy	Combining ice with exercise may be effective for decreasing pain after sprains or surgery
Low-level heat wraps	Decreases pain and improves function in CTS, OA, and strain or sprain
Contrast baths	No significant effects
Exercises	Decreases pain and increases strength and function for hand OA and RA
Ultrasound	Effective for CTS
ADL simulations	Better improvement as compared to traditional exercises
Sensory re-education	Superficial tactile techniques show limited evidence for effectiveness
Ergonomic modifications	Limited evidence showing effectiveness at reducing symptoms due to repetitive activities (e.g., such as using a keyboard)

OA, osteoarthritis.
Data from Amini, 2011.

Management and Standards of Practice

Occupational therapy assistants (OTAs) can be valuable team members when treating upper extremities. OTAs can deliver OT services under the supervision of an occupational therapist. The amount of supervision required can depend on the medical complexity of the client and the skill level of the OTA. State regulations and facility rules can also dictate levels of supervision required. Following the evaluation and establishment of the treatment plan, OTAs may provide daily treatment, splinting, and client education activities.

Chapter 16 Self-Study Activities (Answers Are Provided at the End of the Chapter)

Match the following special test with the appropriate positive finding:

1. OK sign	E	A. Tingling and paresthesia in the median nerve distribution
2. Tinel's sign—wrist	A	B. Pain with ulnar deviation of the wrist while the client grasps the thumb in the palm
3. Phalen's test	A	C. Pain, laxity, or crepitus for LTL instability
4. Sharpey's	D	D. Pain, crepitus, and clicking in the TFCC
5. Test for PTS	A	E. Unable to bring tip-to-tip pinch of thumb and second finger
6. Reagan's test	C	
7. Finkelstein's test	B	

Match the correct splint with the appropriate diagnosis:

8. Figure eight splint	A. De Quervain's tenosynovitis
9. Dorsal blocking splint with the wrist positioned in 30° of flexion, the MCPs flexed, and the IPs extended	B. Index, middle, and ring finger metacarpal shaft fractures
	C. Fifth metacarpal neck or shaft fracture
10. Dorsal blocking splint with the wrist positioned in 30° of flexion, the MCPs positioned in 60° of flexion, and the IPs positioned in full extension, with rubber bands through the fingertip and palmar pulley	D. Flexor tendon injury—Immobilization phase
	E. Flexor tendon injury—Early passive flexion Kleinert protocol
	F. Flexor tendon injury—Duran and Houser protocol

11. Palmer wrist splint		**G.** Extensor tendon injury zones I and II	
12. Buddy tape		**H.** Extensor tendon injury zones III and IV	
13. MCP joint blocking splints		**I.** Extensor tendon injury zones V, VI, and VII	
14. DIP extension splinting		**J.** Intersection syndrome	
15. Thumb spica		**K.** Trigger finger	
16. Forearm-based thumb spica with mobile IP joint			
17. Evan's protocol with the wrist positioned in 45° of extension, and the MCPs and IPs positioned in neutral (i.e., 0°)			
18. Dorsal blocking splint with the wrist positioned in 30° flexed, the MCPs positioned in 60° of flexion, with full IP extension and the digits strapped in extension with rubber bands attached to the wristband			

19. Which of the following conservative treatment methods should be used for cubital tunnel syndrome?

   A. Fabricate a long arm gutter splint positioning the elbow in 45°–60° of flexion, wrist and forearm in a neutral position, and recommend wearing at night to prevent prolonged elbow flexion.

   B. If clawing is present, provide a hand-based splint to block hyperextension of the MCP joints and allow MCP and PIP flexion.

   C. A static or dynamic splint that provides wrist extension, MCP extension, and thumb extension. The purpose of the splint is to prevent overstretching of the extensor muscles and promote functional use of the hand during the healing phase.

   D. Both A and B.

20. A client with PIN syndrome will likely display a loss of finger extension strength.

   A. True

   B. False

21. A client with basal joint arthritis can be splinted with a custom or prefabricated hand-based thumb spica as long as the _____ joint is supported by the splint.

22. A boutonniere deformity is a common deformity in a zone III extensor tendon injury. Which of the following provides the most accurate clinical presentation of a boutonniere deformity (i.e., zone III extensor tendon injury)?

   A. The finger presents with the PIP in flexion and the DIP in extension.

   B. The finger presents with a hyperextension of the PIP joint and DIP flexion.

   C. The finger presents with MCP hyperextension and PIP and DIP flexion.

23. When treating a zone II flexor tendon injury with a Kleinert protocol on postop day 3, the therapist should fabricate a splint then instruct the client in which of the following exercises? (There is more than one correct answer.)

   A. No exercise is performed to the digits.

   B. Perform ROM to the elbow and the shoulder.

   C. Active extension of the digits to the limits of the splint and rubber bands to flex the fingers.

   D. Passive flexion and extension exercises.

   E. MP and PIP flexed; the DIP is extended.

   F. MP and DIP flexed; the PIP is extended.

24. Anatomy self-study activity

   Please list the origin, insertion, action, and innervation for muscles identified below using a format of your choice (e.g., blank sheet of paper and a computer-generated table). Please use the anatomy textbook recommended by your OT program to check your answers as needed; minor differences between anatomy references should be expected.

   While the inclusion of an anatomy recall question (i.e., origin, insertion, action, and innervation question) on the board exam is highly unlikely, you will be required to apply knowledge of anatomy. For example, given an affected muscle or muscle group, determine the most appropriate functional task for a given assessment or intervention.

   • Abductor pollicis brevis
   • Abductor pollicis longus

- Extensor digiti minimi
- Extensor digitorum
- Extensor indices
- Extensor pollicis brevis
- Extensor pollicis longus
- Flexor digiti minimi brevis
- Flexor digitorum profundus
- Flexor digitorum superficialis
- Flexor pollicis brevis
- Flexor pollicis longus
- Interossei
- Lumbricals
- Opponens digiti minimi
- Opponens pollicis
- Palmaris longus
- Palmer interosseous

Chapter 16 Self-Study Answers

1. E
2. A
3. A
4. D
5. A
6. C
7. B
8. H
9. D
10. E
11. B
12. C
13. K
14. G
15. A
16. J
17. I
18. F
19. D. Both A. and B.
    A and B are correct due to the following:
    A. Fabricate a long arm gutter splint positioning the elbow in 45°–60° of flexion and with the wrist and forearm in a neutral position; to wear at night to prevent prolonged elbow flexion (Moscony, 2014).
    B. If clawing is present, provide a hand-based splint to block hyperextension of the MCP joints and allow MCP and IP flexion (Moscony, 2014).
    C. This was not a correct answer. A static or dynamic splint that provides wrist extension,

MCP extension, and thumb extension. The purpose of the splint is to prevent over-stretching of the extensors and promote functional use of the hand during the healing phase. This splint is used to treat a radial nerve injury (Kasch & Walsh, 2013).

20. A. True
    There is commonly a loss of finger extension strength (Kasch & Walsh, 2013).
21. CMC joint. The purpose of the splint is to stabilize the CMC joint by placing the thumb in gentle palmar abduction (Beasley, 2014).
22. A. The finger with a boutonniere deformity presents with the PIP in flexion and the DIP in extension (Kasch & Walsh, 2013).
23. B. Perform ROM to elbow and shoulder.
    C. Active extension of the digits to the limits of the splint and rubber bands to flex the fingers (Kasch & Walsh, 2013).
24. Please use the anatomy textbook recommended by your occupational therapy program to check your answers.

References

Adams, J. E., & Habbu, R. (2015). Tendinopathies of the hand and wrist. *Journal of the American Academy of Orthopaedic Surgeons, 23*(12), 741–750. doi:10.5435/JAAOS-D-14-00216

American Academy of Orthopaedic Surgeons. (2008). *Clinical practice guideline on the treatment of carpal tunnel syndrome*. Retrieved from http://www.aaos.org/search/?srchtext=Clinical+practice+guideline+on+the+treatment+of+carpal+tunnel+syndrome

American Academy of Orthopaedic Surgeons. (2011). *Orthopaedic knowledge update 10*. Rosemont, IL: American Academy of Orthopaedic Surgeons.

Amini, D. (2011). Occupational therapy interventions for work-related injuries and conditions of the forearm, wrist, and hand: A systematic review. *American Journal of Occupational Therapy, 65*(1), 29–36. Retrieved from http://www.ncbi.nlm.nih.gov/pubmed/21309369

Avery, D. M., Caggiano, N. M., & Matullo, K. S. (2015). Ulnar collateral ligament injuries of the thumb: A comprehensive review. *Orthopedic Clinics of North America, 46*(2), 281–292. doi:10.1016/j.ocl.2014.11.007

Beasley, J. (2014). Arthritis. In C. Cooper (Ed.), *Fundamentals of hand therapy: Clinical reasoning and treatment guidelines for common diagnoses of the upper extremity* (2nd ed., pp. 457–478). St. Louis, MO: Elsevier/Mosby.

Bevelaqua, A. C., Hayter, C. L., Feinberg, J. H., & Rodeo, S. A. (2012). Posterior interosseous neuropathy: Electrodiagnostic evaluation. *HSS Journal, 8*(2), 184–189. doi:10.1007/s11420-011-9238-8

Biese, J. (2007). Arthritis. In C. Cooper (Ed.), *Fundamentals of hand therapy: Clinical reasoning and treatment guidelines for common diagnoses of the upper extremity* (pp. 348–375). St. Louis, MO: Mosby/Elsevier.

Brotzman, S. B., & Manske, R. C. (2011). *Clinical orthopaedic rehabilitation: An evidence-based approach* (3rd ed.). Philadelphia, PA: Mosby.

Chen, S. H., & Tsai, T. M. (2014). Ulnar tunnel syndrome. *Journal of Hand Surgery American Volume, 39*(3), 571–579. doi:10.1016/j.jhsa.2013.08.102

Cheung, J. P., Tang, C. Y., & Fung, B. K. (2014). Current management of acute scaphoid fractures: A review. *Hong Kong Medical Journal, 20*(1), 52–58. doi:10.12809/hkmj134146

Chi, Y., & Harness, N. G. (2010). Anterior interosseous nerve syndrome. *Journal of Hand Surgery American Volume, 35*(12), 2078–2080. doi:10.1016/j.jhsa.2010 .08.018

Clavert, P., Lutz, J. C., Adam, P., Wolfram-Gabel, R., Liverneaux, P., & Kahn, J. L. (2009). Frohse's arcade is not the exclusive compression site of the radial nerve in its tunnel. *Orthopaedics & Traumatology · Surgery & Research, 95*(2), 114–118. doi:10.1016/j. otsr.2008.11.001

Cooper, C. (2014a). Elbow, wrist, and hand tendinopathies. In C. Cooper (Ed.), *Fundamentals of hand therapy: Clinical reasoning and treatment guidelines for common diagnoses of the upper extremity* (2nd ed., pp. 383–393). St. Louis, MO: Elsevier/Mosby.

Cooper, C. (2014b). *Fundamentals of hand therapy: Clinical reasoning and treatment guidelines for common diagnoses of the upper extremity* (2nd ed.). St. Louis, MO: Elsevier/Mosby.

Cooper, C. (2014c). Hand impairments. In M. V. Radomski & C. A. T. Latham (Eds.), *Occupational therapy for physical dysfunction* (7th ed., pp. 1129–1167). Philadelphia, PA: Wolters Kluwer Health/Lippincott Williams & Wilkins.

Cooper, C., & Martin, H. A. (2007). Common forms of tendinitis/tendinosis. In C. Cooper (Ed.), *Fundamentals of hand therapy: Clinical reasoning and treatment guidelines for common diagnoses of the upper extremity* (pp. 286–300). St. Louis, MO: Mosby/Elsevier.

Cotterell, I. H., & Richard, M. J. (2015). Metacarpal and phalangeal fractures in athletes. *Clinical Journal of Sport Medicine, 34*(1), 69–98. doi:10.1016/j.csm .2014.09.009

Darowish, M., & Sharma, J. (2014). Evaluation and treatment of chronic hand conditions. *Medical Clinics of North America, 98*(4), 801–815, xii. doi:10.1016/j. mcna.2014.03.006

Depukat, P., Mizia, E., Zwinczewska, H., Bonczar, T., Mazur, M., Dzikowska, M., . . . Matuszyk, A. (2014). Topography of ulnar nerve and its variations with special respect to carpal region. *Folia Medica Cracoviensia, 54*(4), 45–58. Retrieved from http://www.ncbi.nlm .nih.gov/pubmed /25891242

Dias, R., Chandrasenan, J., Rajaratnam, V., & Burke, F. D. (2007). Basal thumb arthritis. *Postgraduate Medical Journal, 83*(975), 40–43. doi:10.1136/pgmj .2006.046300

Freiberg, A. (2007). Management of proximal interphalangeal joint injuries. *Canadian Journal of Plastic Surgery, 15*(4), 199–203. Retrieved from http://www.ncbi.nlm .nih.gov/pubmed/19554177

Gagliardi, J. A., & Agarwal, A. (2012). Gamekeeper's thumb (Skier's thumb). *Applied Radiology, 41*, 7–8.

Giugale, J. M., & Fowler, J. R. (2015). Trigger finger: Adult and pediatric treatment strategies. *Orthopedic Clinics of North America, 46*(4), 561–569. doi:10.1016/j. ocl.2015.06.014

Griffin, M., Hindocha, S., Jordan, D., Saleh, M., & Khan, W. (2012). An overview of the management of flexor tendon injuries. *Open Orthopedic Journal, 6*, 28–35. doi:10.2174/1874325001206010028

Gupta, V., Rijal, L., & Jawed, A. (2013). Managing scaphoid fractures. How we do it? *Journal of Clinical Orthopaedics and Trauma, 4*(1), 3–10. doi:10.1016/j.jcot .2013.01.009

Halsey, J. N., Therattil, P. J., Viviano, S. L., Fleegler, E. J., & Lee, E. S. (2015). Bowler's thumb: Case report and review of the literature. *Eplasty, 15*, e47. Retrieved from http://www.ncbi.nlm.nih.gov/pubmed/26528379

Hile, D., & Hile, L. (2015). The emergent evaluation and treatment of hand injuries. *Emergency Medicine Clinics of North America, 33*(2), 397–408. doi:10.1016/j. emc.2014.12.009

Kasch, M. C., & Walsh, M. (2013). Hand and upper extremity injuries. In H. M. Pendleton & W. Schultz-Krohn (Eds.), *Pedretti's occupational therapy: Practice skills for physical dysfunction* (7th ed., pp. 1037–1073). St. Louis, MO: Elsevier.

Keith, M. W., Masear, V., Chung, K. C., Amadio, P. C., Andary, M., Barth, R. W., . . . McGowan, R. (2010). American Academy of Orthopaedic Surgeons: Clinical practice guideline on the treatment of carpal tunnel syndrome. *Journal of Bone and Joint Surgery, 92*(1), 218–219. doi:10.2106/JBJS.I.00642

Klein, L. J. (2007). Tendon injury. In C. Cooper (Ed.), *Fundamentals of hand therapy: Clinical reasoning and treatment guidelines for common diagnoses of the upper extremity* (pp. 320–347). St. Louis, MO: Mosby/Elsevier.

Klein, L. J. (2014). Flexor tendon injury. In C. Cooper (Ed.), *Fundamentals of hand therapy: Clinical reasoning and treatment guidelines for common diagnoses of the upper extremity* (2nd ed., pp. 412–425). St. Louis, MO: Elsevier/Mosby.

Kollitz, K. M., Hammert, W. C., Vedder, N. B., & Huang, J. I. (2014). Metacarpal fractures: Treatment and complications. *Hand (New York), 9*(1), 16–23. doi:10.1007/s11552-013-9562-1

Langer, D., Luria, S., Maeir, A., & Erez, A. (2014). Occupation-based assessments and treatments of trigger finger: A survey of occupational therapists from Israel and the United States. *Occupational Therapy International, 21*(4), 143–155. doi:10.1002/oti.1372

Lawson, S., & Murphy, L. F. (2013). Hip fractures and lower extremity joint replacement. In L. W. Pedretti, H. M. Pendleton, & W. Schultz-Krohn (Eds.), *Pedretti's occupational therapy: Practice skills for physical dysfunction* (7th ed., pp. 1074–1090). St. Louis, MO: Elsevier.

Lutsky, K. F., Giang, E. L., & Matzon, J. L. (2015). Flexor tendon injury, repair and rehabilitation. *Orthopedic Clinics of North America, 46*(1), 67–76. doi:10.1016/j.ocl.2014.09.004

Magee, D. J. (2014). *Magee orthopedic physical assessment* (6th ed.). St. Louis, MO: Saunders.

Matzon, J. L., & Bozentka, D. J. (2010). Extensor tendon injuries. *Journal of Hand Surgery, 35*(5), 854–861. doi:10.1016/j.jhsa.2010.03.002

McKinnis, L. N. (2014). *Fundamentals of musculoskeletal imaging* (4th ed.). Philadelphia, PA: F.A. Davis Company.

Moradi, A., Ebrahimzadeh, M. H., & Jupiter, J. B. (2015). Radial tunnel syndrome, diagnostic and treatment dilemma. *Archives of Bone and Joint Surgery, 3*(3), 156–162. Retrieved from http://www.ncbi.nlm.nih.gov/pubmed/26213698

Moscony, A. M. B. (2007). Common wrist and hand fractures. In C. Cooper (Ed.), *Fundamentals of hand therapy: Clinical reasoning and treatment guidelines for common diagnoses of the upper extremity* (pp. 251–285). St. Louis, MO: Mosby/Elsevier.

Moscony, A. M. B. (2014). Peripheral nerve problems. In C. Cooper (Ed.), *Fundamentals of hand therapy: Clinical reasoning and treatment guidelines for common diagnoses of the upper extremity* (2nd ed., pp. 272–311). St. Louis, MO: Elsevier/Mosby.

Moscony, A. M. B., & Shank, T. M. (2014). Wrist fractures. In C. Cooper (Ed.), *Fundamentals of hand therapy: Clinical reasoning and treatment guidelines for common diagnoses of the upper extremity* (2nd ed., pp. 312–335). St. Louis, MO: Elsevier/Mosby.

Nellans, K. W., Kowalski, E., & Chung, K. C. (2012). The epidemiology of distal radius fractures. *Hand Clinics, 28*(2), 113–125. doi:10.1016/j.hcl.2012.02.001

Nicoson, M. C., & Moran, S. L. (2015). Diagnosis and treatment of acute lunotriquetral ligament injuries. *Hand Clinics, 31*(3), 467–476. doi:10.1016/j.hcl.2015.04.005

Palmer, B. A., & Hughes, T. B. (2010). Cubital tunnel syndrome. *Journal of Hand Surgery American Volume, 35*(1), 153–163. doi:10.1016/j.jhsa.2009.11.004

Pappou, I. P., Basel, J., & Deal, D. N. (2013). Scapholunate ligament injuries: A review of current concepts. *Hand, 8*(2), 146–156. doi:10.1007/s11552-013-9499-4

Pope, T., Bloem, H. L., Beltran, J., Morrison, W. B., & Wilson, D. J. (2014). *Musculoskeletal imaging* (2nd ed.). Philadelphia, PA: United Elsevier—Health Sciences Division.

Prucz, R. B., & Friedrich, J. B. (2015). Finger joint injuries. *Clinics in Sports Medicine, 34*(1), 99–116. doi:10.1016/j.csm.2014.09.002

Rodner, C. M., Tinsley, B. A., & O'Malley, M. P. (2013). Pronator syndrome and anterior interosseous nerve syndrome. *Journal of the American Academy of Orthopaedic Surgeons, 21*(5), 268–275. doi:10.5435/JAAOS-21-05-268

Roenbeck, K., & Imbriglia, J. E. (2011). Peripheral triangular fibrocartilage complex tears. *Journal of Hand Surgery American Volume, 36*(10), 1687–1690. doi:10.1016/j.jhsa.2011.05.007

Sachar, K. (2008). Ulnar-sided wrist pain: Evaluation and treatment of triangular fibrocartilage complex tears, ulnocarpal impaction syndrome, and lunotriquetral ligament tears. *Journal of Hand Surgery American Volume, 33*(9), 1669–1679. doi:10.1016/j.jhsa.2008.08.026

Steinmann, S. P., & Adams, J. E. (2006). Scaphoid fractures and nonunions: Diagnosis and treatment. *Journal of*

Orthopaedic Science, 11(4), 424–431. doi:10.1007/s00776-006-1025-x

Sutliff, L. S. (2009). Intersection syndrome. *Clinical Reviews, 19*(4), 12–14.

Swanson, S., Macias, L. H., & Smith, A. A. (2009). Treatment of Bowler's neuroma with digital nerve translocation. *Hand (New York, NY), 4*(3), 323–326. doi:10.1007/s11552-009-9170-2

Tan, V., Nourbakhsh, A., Capo, J., Cottrell, J. A., Meyenhofer, M., & O'Connor, J. P. (2010). Effects of nonsteroidal anti-inflammatory drugs on flexor tendon adhesion. *Journal of Hand Surgery American Volume, 35*(6), 941–947.

Tchoryk, J. (2000). Median and anterior interosseous nerve entrapment syndromes versus carpal tunnel syndrome: A study of two cases. *Journal of the Canadian Chiropractic Association, 44*(2), 103–112.

van de Grift, T. C., & Ritt, M. J. (2016). Management of lunotriquetral instability: A review of the literature. *Journal of Hand Surgery European Volume, 41*(1), 72–85. doi:10.1177/1753193415595167

Waldman, S. D. (2012). *Atlas of pain management injection techniques* (3rd ed.). Philadelphia, PA: Saunders.

Woo, A., Bakri, K., & Moran, S. L. (2015). Management of ulnar nerve injuries. *Journal of Hand Surgery American Volume, 40*(1), 173–181. doi:10.1016/j.jhsa.2014.04.038

Wyrick, T. O., & Marik, T. L. (2010). Arthritis. In R. R. Bindra & T. L. Brininger (Eds.), *Advanced concepts of hand pathologyans surgery: Application to hand therapy practice* (pp. 279–323). Rosemont, IL: American Society for Surgery of the Hand.

Yoon, A., & Grewal, R. (2012). Management of distal radius fractures from the North American perspective. *Hand Clinics, 28*(2), 135–144. doi:10.1016/j.hcl.2012.02.002

Zhari, B., Edderai, M., Boumdine, H., Amil, T., & En-Nouali, H. (2015). Dual intersection syndrome of the forearm: A case report. *Pan African Medical Journal, 21*, 325. doi:10.11604/pamj.2015.21.325.4105

Orthopedic Conditions of the Lower Extremity

Darren Gustitus, Jeffrey Placzek, and Fredrick D. Pociask

Learning Objectives

- Describe key pathology, etiology, and epidemiology for hip fractures, hip and knee arthritis, and hip and knee arthroplasty.
- Compare and contrast clinical presentations for the orthopedic conditions of the lower extremity listed above.
- Describe diagnostic tests for the lower extremity disorders listed above.
- Describe medical and surgical procedures for the orthopedic conditions of the lower extremity listed above.
- List medical/surgical precautions and contraindications for the orthopedic conditions of the lower extremity listed above.
- List weight-bearing restrictions for hip fracture and total hip arthroplasty (THA).
- List movement restrictions for hip fracture and THA.
- Describe adapted techniques for activities of daily living following hip fracture surgery, THA, and total knee arthroplasty (TKA).
- Describe typical symptom management techniques for knee and hip arthritis.
- Describe the concepts of energy conservation, work simplification, and joint protection.

Key Terms

- *Arthroplasty*: The surgical replacement or reconstruction of a joint.
- *Intramedullary fixation*: A metal rod or nail that is placed into the medullary cavity of a bone; typically used in the management of fractures.
- *Magnetic resonance imaging (MRI)*: MRI is a noninvasive imaging technology that utilizes a magnetic field and radio waves to create detailed computer images of body tissues.
- *Movement restrictions*: Restrictions of movement implemented by the physician indicating positions that need to be avoided during treatment to avoid damage to the THA.
- *Neoplasm*: An abnormal growth in tissue that is typically uncontrolled and progressive; may be benign or malignant.
- *Weight-bearing restrictions*: Restrictions implemented by the physician indicating the amount of weight the involved lower extremity is allowed to bear.

Hip Fractures

Description: More than 340,000 hip fractures occur yearly in the United States, with the majority of fractures occurring in individuals older than 65 years (Stoneback & Ziran, 2014). More than 95% of hip fractures are accounted for by falls, but they may also be caused by motor vehicle accidents or pathologic fractures due to neoplasms or infection (Scherger & Mak, 2010). Hip fractures may be divided into different categories including femoral neck (FN) fractures, intertrochanteric (IT) fractures, and subtrochanteric (ST) fractures with various grading systems within each category (Fpoa, 2014). Common risk factors for hip fracture include advancing age, osteoporosis, smoking, and falls (Stoneback & Ziran, 2014).

Clinical presentation: Clients often present in severe pain with the hip held flexed and internally rotated in the case of FN and IT fractures, and often externally rotated with ST fractures. The leg may appear shorter than the unaffected limb with a complete break (Scherger & Mak, 2010).

Common diagnostic tests: X-rays are usually sufficient to diagnose and categorize hip fractures. magnetic resonance imaging can be useful to detect nondisplaced fractures (Scherger & Mak, 2010).

Common medical and surgical procedures: Clients should typically be hospitalized, started on heparin, and undergo surgical fixation as soon as possible (Mak, Cameron, & March, 2010). Nonoperative treatment is only considered in clients who are too ill to undergo the operation or were nonambulatory prior to the fracture (Scherger & Mak, 2010). Ten to thirty percent of clients will die within the first year after a hip fracture (Scherger & Mak, 2010). Other complications include decubitus ulcers, nonunion, infection, deep vein thrombosis (DVT), heterotopic ossification, and hardware failure (Fpoa, 2014). Surgical management of hip fractures is further described in **Table 17-1**.

Precautions and contraindications: Weight-bearing restrictions should be followed as strictly as possible to facilitate tissue healing and to help reduce hardware-related complications. Displaced FN fractures carry the risk of compromising the blood supply leading to avascular necrosis and flattening of the femoral head (Scherger & Mak, 2010).

Screening and Assessments

Screening and assessments are similar throughout the various orthopedic conditions of the lower extremity with some variation. There are various top-down and bottom-up approaches to evaluation in orthopedics. Below is a list of top-down approaches that not only address the symptoms but also address the impact of the symptoms on the person's roles, contexts, and environments, followed by bottom-up approaches that are symptom specific. They are as follows:

- Client history including the client's age, hand dominance, occupational and avocational responsibilities, prior injuries, comorbidities, family issues, psychological issues, broader social issues, and economic issues (Lawson & Murphy, 2013).
- Mechanism and date of injury, structures involved, type and extent of medical and surgical intervention, concomitant injuries, and future treatment planned (Lawson & Murphy, 2013).

Physical assessments include the following:

- Baseline physical evaluation/interview to assess limitations not related to the surgery.
- Pain (e.g., location, type, quality, intensity).
- Color, temperature, and signs of compromised circulation or compartment syndrome.
- Edema (e.g., circumferential measurements).
- Sensory and motor function.
- Coordination.
- Skin integrity and wound assessment.
  - *Wound or surgical incision*: Note location, size, integrity of closure, exposure of pins or hardware, and signs of infection.
  - *Scar*: Note location, size, and adherence, hypertrophy, blanching with motion, pliability, and sensitivity.
- Active/passive range of motion (A/PROM) of adjacent/uninvolved joints.
- Cognitive assessment.
- Ability to participate in life roles.
- The occupational therapist (OT) will also need to have an understanding of the site, type, and cause of fracture, as well as the phases of healing (Lawson & Murphy, 2013).

Interventions

Occupational therapy treatment is similar throughout the various orthopedic conditions of the lower extremity with some variation. Occupational therapy treatment includes compensatory, preparatory, and remedial approaches. Compensatory approaches attempt to teach adaptive strategies or incorporate adaptive equipment in order to achieve functional outcomes, whereas preparatory activities seek to prepare individuals for

Table 17-1 Surgical Management of Hip Fractures

Fracture	Surgery
FN fractures	Reduction and cannulated screw fixation or hemiarthroplasty in low-demand clients. THA can be considered if the hip has severe preexisting arthritis.
IT fractures	Dynamic hip screw or intramedullary fixation.
ST fractures	Intramedullary fixation or fixed angle plating.

Modified from Fpoa, 2014

occupational engagement and remediation seeks to improve performance. It's important to understand the following weight-bearing restrictions:

1. *Nonweight-bearing*: No weight-bearing on the affected lower extremity. The client utilizes a walker or crutches for ambulation.
2. *Toe-touch weight-bearing*: The affected toe can be used for balance; 85–90% of weight is placed on the uninvolved lower extremity. The client utilizes a walker or crutches for ambulation.
3. *Partial weight-bearing*: Thirty to fifty percent of weight on the involved lower extremity. The client utilizes a walker or crutches for ambulation.
4. *Weight-bearing at tolerated*: Weight-bearing on the involved lower extremity with minimal pain. The client utilizes a cane for ambulation.
5. *Full weight-bearing*: Seventy-five to one hundred percent weight-bearing is allowed. A cane is utilized as necessary for ambulation (Lawson & Murphy, 2013; Maher, 2014).

Awareness of movement restrictions following hip surgery must be clearly communicated with the client. See specific restrictions outlined in the hip arthroplasty section of this chapter.

Mobility and weight-bearing restrictions are based on multiple factors, including severity and location of fracture, surgical approach, fixation integrity, prosthesis integrity, bone integrity, client's weight, and cognitive status (Maher, 2014). The role of the OT practitioner is to instruct clients in activity of daily living (ADL) performance while following modifications and precautions or restrictions of care. For example, modified techniques may include instructions on rising from a regular-height seat or similar transfer while maintaining hip precautions (Maher, 2014). Most restrictions are discontinued between 8 and 12 weeks postop (Maher, 2014). Additionally, treatment progression is based on fracture healing and the client's tolerance for care. The client should also be instructed in adapted techniques for activities related to following all hip precautions. Typical problems and adaptations are described in **Table 17-2**.

Hip Arthritis

Description: Hip arthritis has been reported as the most common cause of disability among adults in the United States, as well as a leading cause of hospitalization

Table 17-2 Typical Problems and Adaptations

Problem	Adaptation
Bathe feet	Long-handled sponge
Get in and out of tub	Nonskid bathmat, grab bar, and tub bench
Don and doff shoes	Extended-handled shoehorn (i.e., medial side for posterior surgical approach and lateral for anterior approach) and elastic laces
Don and doff socks	Sock aide
Don pants	Reacher or dressing stick
Transfer to and from the toilet, tub, and bed	Raised toilet seat, increased height of chair and bed
Sit in and rise from chair	Wedge cushion with thick end of the wedge at the back of the chair
Open and close cabinets	Relocate frequently used items to eliminate the need to bend, and implement use of a reacher

Modified from Maher, 2014

(Sassoon & Haidukewych, 2014). Hip arthritis may be degenerative (i.e., noninflammatory), inflammatory, or posttraumatic in origin. The most common joint disease is osteoarthritis (OA), a noninflammatory arthritis, which affects 60% of men and 70% of women over age 65 (Goodman, 2009). Joint space narrowing, occurrence of osteophyte formation, and cystic changes in subchondral bone are common features of degenerative arthritis (Wold, Unni, Sim, Sundaram, & Adler, 2008). Severe joint destruction is seen with inflammatory arthritis, which includes rheumatoid arthritis, systemic lupus erythematous, gout, and spondyloarthropathies (Mortazavu & Parvizi, 2011). Hypermobility, obesity, abnormal biomechanics or alignment, and a history of high-impact activity can predispose an individual to OA, while inflammatory arthritis tends to carry a genetic risk (Goodman, 2009; Mortazavu & Parvizi, 2011).

Clinical presentation: Clients typically present with antalgic gait and pain in the groin and buttocks; knee pain referred via a branch of the obturator nerve may also be present (Sassoon & Haidukewych, 2014). Physical examination typically reveals pain with end of range hip flexion and rotation, and limited ROM is common. Additional findings typically include activity-related pain (e.g., walking long distances), pain that is worse at night, stiffness and crepitus, and difficulty with specific ADLs (e.g., donning and doffing socks and footwear and getting in and out of an automobile) (Mortazavu & Parvizi, 2011; Sassoon & Haidukewych, 2014).

Common diagnostic tests: Weight-bearing anteroposterior x-rays as well as lateral views may reveal hip arthritis. The radiographic classification scheme of OA by Tönnis describes three grades of OA, with grade 0 describing no signs of OA, grade 1 describing increased sclerosis of the head of the femur and acetabulum, grade 2 describing small cyst formation, moderate joint space narrowing, and moderate loss of head sphericity, and grade 3 describing large cyst formation, significant joint space narrowing, severe femoral head deformity, and signs of necrosis (Sassoon & Haidukewych, 2014). However, it is important to note that the extent of radiographic changes is poorly correlated with clinical symptoms (Mortazavu & Parvizi, 2011; Sassoon & Haidukewych, 2014).

Common medical and surgical procedures: Nonsurgical approaches typically include nonsteroidal anti-inflammatory drug (NSAID) therapy and cortisone injections for the management of mild to moderate degenerative arthritis and disease-modifying antirheumatic drugs for inflammatory arthritis (Mortazavu & Parvizi, 2011). total hip arthroplasty (THA) is the most commonly used surgical approach for severe arthritic changes and ongoing pain (Mortazavu & Parvizi, 2011). Currently, there is no evidence for cartilage regeneration procedures (Mortazavu & Parvizi, 2011).

Precautions and contraindications: Clients should be educated on the benefits of therapeutic exercise in the treatment of OA but care should be taken to maintain the safety of the older individual during exercise interventions (Goodman, 2009). Postsurgically, the client will likely need to follow specific precautions depending on the surgical procedure performed.

Screening and Assessments

Screening and assessments are similar throughout the various orthopedic conditions of the lower extremity with some variation. There are various top-down and bottom-up approaches to evaluation in orthopedics. Below is a list of top-down approaches that not only address the symptoms but also address the impact of the symptoms on the person's roles, contexts, and environments, followed by bottom-up approaches that are symptom specific. They are as follows:

- Client history including the client's age, hand dominance, occupational and avocational responsibilities, prior injuries, comorbidities, family

issues, psychological issues, broader social issues, and economic issues.
- Mechanism and date of injury, structures involved, type and extent of medical and surgical intervention, concomitant injuries, and future treatment planned.
- Physical assessment including the following:
  - Baseline physical evaluation/interview to assess limitations not related to the surgery.
  - Pain (e.g., location, type, quality, and intensity).
  - Edema (e.g., circumferential measurements).
  - Sensory and motor function.
  - Coordination.
  - A/PROM of adjacent/uninvolved joints.
  - Cognitive assessment.
  - Ability to participate in life roles.

Interventions

Occupational therapy treatment is similar throughout the various orthopedic conditions of the lower extremity with some variation. Occupational therapy treatment includes compensatory, preparatory, and remedial approaches. Compensatory approaches attempt to teach adaptive strategies or incorporate adaptive equipment in order to achieve functional outcomes, whereas preparatory activities seek to prepare individuals for occupational engagement and remediation seeks to improve performance.

Symptom Management

Physical agent modalities are utilized to decrease pain and swelling of the arthritic joint(s). Hot and cold packs are utilized to manage symptoms and improve the client's ability to perform their daily tasks. Edema reduction techniques are helpful to maintain joint mobility and decrease pain. Therapeutic exercises and activities are helpful to maintain joint mobility, endurance levels, and strength (Frost & Harmeyer, 2011).

Energy Conservation

Individuals with hip or knee arthritis should utilize the following energy conservation techniques in order to save energy for the most important tasks of the day. Energy conservation techniques consist of planning ahead to eliminate unnecessary steps, gather materials, and spreading activities throughout the day/week. Additional examples include pacing one's self, prioritizing the tasks for the day, sitting when possible, and maintaining good posture. Work simplification techniques are used to minimize the steps necessary throughout the day. Tasks are broken down into components and strategies are developed to eliminate unnecessary steps. Potential equipment/products that can further simplify the tasks are purchased and utilized (Poole, 2009).

Joint Protection

Incorporation of joint protection techniques into the client's day will help maintain joint integrity and slow the progression of the arthritis. Common principles include respecting pain, use of proper body mechanics, avoiding prolonged repetitive motions and holding positions for a long time, avoiding positions of deformity, use of the largest and strongest muscles and joints, balance rest and activity, and never beginning an activity that cannot be stopped (Poole, 2009).

Total Hip Arthroplasty

Description: Joint arthroplasty is the most effective treatment of advanced arthritis in most joints, including the hip (Mortazavu & Parvizi, 2011). In 2010, 310,800 THAs were performed among inpatients aged 45 and over in the United States, and between 2000 and 2010, the number of hip arthroplasties increased from 138,700 to 310,800, with a respective increased rate of 142.2–257.0

per 100,000 population (Wolford, Palso, & Bercovitz, 2015). Common indications for THA include displaced FN fractures, avascular necrosis, and developmental dysplasia of the hip (Goh, Samuel, Su, Chan, & Yeo, 2009; Kusuma & Garino, 2007). Currently, the failure rate for total hip replacements is less than 1% per year (Mortazavu & Parvizi, 2011). Many THAs utilize a femoral stem and acetabular component that do not need to be cemented and instead rely on bone growth and remodeling to secure the implant (Huo, Parvizi, Bal, & Mont, 2008). There are a variety of approaches to THA including muscle sparing and minimally invasive approaches; common THA procedures are described in **Table 17-3**. More common complications of THA include DVT, infection, and periprosthetic femoral fracture (Huo et al., 2008). Similarly, more common reasons for THA failure include periprosthetic infection, instability, aseptic loosening, osteolysis, periprosthetic fractures, and component failure (Sassoon & Haidukewych, 2014).

Clinical presentation: Clients require early mobilization following THA and are often seen on postoperative day one. Most clients will have no weight-bearing restrictions with use of a walker, but it is important to follow the surgeon's recommendation, as well as any precautions associated with the approach.

Common diagnostic tests: X-ray is used to assess proper placement of the hardware during surgery and postsurgically (Sassoon & Haidukewych, 2014).

Table 17-3 Common THA Procedures

Approach	Interval	Advantages	Disadvantages
Anterior	• TFL and sartorius	• True internervous interval • Less pain • No muscle takedown	• Steep learning curve • Risk of fracture • Risk of nerve injury (e.g., lateral femoral cutaneous nerve injury)
Anterolateral (Watson–Jones)	• Tensor fasciae latae and gluteus medius	• Minimally invasive and beneficial for clients with high dislocation risk	• Weakens abductors and can cause limping
Posterolateral	• Gluteus maximus split and takedown of external rotators	• The abductors are intact • The technique is easier to perform	• Potentially higher rate of dislocation
Lateral	• TFL and gluteus maximus and then gluteus medius split • May be done with greater trochanter osteotomy	• Good exposure • A potentially lower dislocation rate	• Potential for gluteus medius gate (i.e., Trendelenburg gait)

TFL, tensor fascia lata.
Modified from Aoi and Toshida, 2009

Common medical and surgical procedures: There are many approaches to THA including posterolateral, transtrochanteric, lateral, anterior (i.e., muscle sparing), Watson–Jones or anterolateral, and minimally invasive procedures (Aoi & Toshida, 2009). Minimally invasive approaches involve a smaller incision than the traditional procedures; however, they are more difficult to perform due to limited exposure of the joint (Aoi & Toshida, 2009). The most common THA approaches are posterolateral and anterolateral (Aoi & Toshida, 2009).

Precautions and contraindications: Clients should avoid the position of hip adduction, internal rotation and flexion, and crossing the midline into adduction or flexion beyond 90° for the first six weeks postoperatively. Additionally, clients should not sleep on the operative side or cross their legs.

Screening and Assessments

Screening and assessments are similar throughout the various orthopedic conditions of the lower extremity with some variation. There are various top-down and bottom-up approaches to evaluation in orthopedics. Below is a list of top-down approaches that not only address the symptoms but also address the impact of the symptoms on the person's roles, contexts, and environments, followed by bottom-up approaches that are symptom specific. They are as follows:

- Client history including the client's age, hand dominance, occupational and avocational responsibilities, prior injuries, comorbidities, family issues, psychological issues, broader social issues, and economic issues.
- Mechanism and date of injury, structures involved, type and extent of medical and surgical intervention, concomitant injuries, and future treatment planned.
- Physical assessment including the following:
  - Baseline physical evaluation/interview to assess limitations not related to the surgery.
  - Observations of pain and fear with rest and movement (Lawson & Murphy, 2013).
  - Color, temperature, and signs of compromised circulation or compartment syndrome.
  - Edema (e.g., circumferential measurements).
  - Sensory and motor function.
  - Coordination.
  - Skin integrity and wound assessment:

  - *Wound or surgical incision*: Note location, size, integrity of closure, exposure of pins or hardware, and signs of infection.
  - *Scar*: Note location, size, adherence, hypertrophy, blanching with motion, pliability, and sensitivity.
  - A/PROM of adjacent/uninvolved joints.
  - Cognitive assessment.
  - Ability to participate in life roles.
  - Assessment of basic and instrumental ADLs.
  - Functional mobility (Lawson & Murphy, 2013).

Interventions

The OT team should address ROM, strengthening, and symptom management. OT practitioners are primarily responsible for ADL management performed within restrictions and precautions established by the physician (e.g., abduction braces for clients at high risk for dislocation).

- *Compensatory methods*: Treatment includes training in the use of assistive devices including a dressing stick, long-handled sponge, long-handled shoe horn, reacher, elastic shoelaces, leg lifter, elevated toilet seat, three-in-one commode, shower chair, and walker bags for walkers. Training in proper transfer techniques, ADLs and instrumental ADLs while maintaining hip and weight-bearing precautions.
- *Client education*: Education classes are important, especially if the client is planning on having a hip replacement. Attendance to a class is prepared by an OT to educate people at risk of falls and/or candidates for lower extremity joint replacement in the following topics:
  - Home modifications and removal of tripping hazards.
  - Transfer techniques.
  - Public transportation education.
  - Community mobility tips.
  - Presurgical education that covers topics, such as:
    - Surgical procedure education.
    - Precautions.
    - Potential assistive devices.
    - Therapy.
    - Recovery period (Lawson & Murphy, 2013).
- *Hip precautions*: It is critical to educate clients and their families on the positions of hip instability following hip joint replacement, which

is dependent on the specific surgical procedure performed:

- Posterolateral approach, which includes positions of instability such as adduction, internal rotation, and flexion greater than 90° (Lawson & Murphy, 2013).
- Anterolateral approach contains positions of instability such as adduction, external rotation, and excessive hyperextension (Lawson & Murphy, 2013).

- *Sleeping position*: It is important to provide client education on proper sleeping positions, which includes lying supine with an abduction pillow (i.e., recommended); side-lying sleepers are likely most comfortable lying on the noninvolved side with an abduction pillow to avoid adduction and rotation (Lawson & Murphy, 2013).
- *Bed mobility*: In terms of bed mobility, when clients are supine or in a seated position, it is important to prop them up on their elbows and move their legs incrementally to the side of the bed prior to getting up. Progress toward lowering legs out of bed using hip and knee extension (Lawson & Murphy, 2013).
- *Chair use*: The use of a stable chair with armrests is encouraged. Instruction should focus on stand to sit and sit to stand techniques. If the client is tall, the chair can be built up; however, all low/soft/reclining/rocking chairs should be avoided (Lawson & Murphy, 2013).
- *Commode chair*: Three-in-one commode chairs should be adjusted so the front legs are lower than the back legs. This helps avoid excessive hip flexion with posterolateral approach precautions. Clients with an anterolateral approach may be able to use a regular toilet. Wiping should take place between the legs while seated or from behind while standing (Lawson & Murphy, 2013).
- *Shower stall*: Nonskid strips, shower chair or stool, and grab bars are recommended. When entering the shower the walker or crutches should enter first, followed by the operated leg and then the nonoperated leg (Lawson & Murphy, 2013).
- *Tub shower* (*without shower door*): Baths should be avoided, although tub chairs or transfer benches are recommended. Client education must include how to back up to the tub chair, extend the leg and lower the body into a sitting position, and use an assistive device to extend the involved leg and lower it into the tub (Lawson & Murphy, 2013).

- *Car*: Bucket seats are not recommended. The seat should be prereclined prior to entry into the vehicle to avoid excessive hip flexion. The client should back up to the seat, extend the involved leg, and sit into the vehicle. Sitting in the backseat with the leg supported in extension is another option (Lawson & Murphy, 2013).
- *Lower body dressing*: Seated performance is recommended. Adherence to precautions is encouraged. Education on using a reacher or dressing stick for donning and doffing pants and shoes, and dressing the involved leg first is encouraged, as is the use of a reacher or dressing stick, and a sock aid for donning socks (Lawson & Murphy, 2013).
- *Lower body bathing*: Tub bathing on a tub bench or sponge baths are necessary for the first 7–10 days postop. With the physician's approval, the client can begin showering. A long-handled sponge can be used for washing the lower legs, soap on a rope is encouraged, and a towel wrapped around a reacher is recommended for drying lower extremities (Lawson & Murphy, 2013).
- *Hair shampoo*: Assistance is essential with hair washing until the client is cleared for showering by the surgeon. If unable to receive assistance, showering at the kitchen sink with a handheld sprayer is encouraged while following hip precautions (Lawson & Murphy, 2013).
- *Homemaking*: Heavy housework is contraindicated until cleared by the physician. Frequently used items should be placed on countertops or an easily accessed location (e.g., stovetop cooking and using the top shelf of the dishwasher). Use of adaptive aids or compensatory techniques for material handling should include sliding when possible, using a cart, attaching a carrying device to a walker, and using a reacher as needed (Lawson & Murphy, 2013).
- *Caregiver training*: The client's home caregivers should be educated on the precautions for the procedure performed, as well as education on all home activities listed above (Lawson & Murphy, 2013).

Knee Arthritis

Description: Arthritis of the knee may be degenerative (i.e., noninflammatory), inflammatory, or posttraumatic. OA is the most prevalent arthropathy of the knee and is most common in obese females and clients with past trauma (Brower & Flemming, 2012). The knee is the most affected joint in OA with a 45% lifetime risk of developing symptoms in at least one knee (Farrokhi, Voycheck, Tashman, & Fitzgerald, 2013). Degenerative joint space narrowing, spur formation, articular and meniscal cartilage degeneration, and cystic changes can occur globally or in a single compartment of the knee, such as the medial compartment or the patella femoral joint (Brower & Flemming, 2012). Inflammatory arthritis tends to involve the whole compartment and is characterized by aggressive articular destruction (Brower & Flemming, 2012).

Clinical presentation: Clients may present with pain, effusion, limited ROM, as well as mechanical symptoms such as crepitus, catching, and locking. OA will often lead to varus deformity of the knee (Brower & Flemming, 2012).

Common diagnostic tests: Weight-bearing and nonweight-bearing films to visualize the tibiofemoral and patellofemoral joints, as well as lower extremity alignment are needed for diagnosis and surgical planning. Anterior–posterior standing and flexed lateral view films are the most accurate (Brower & Flemming, 2012). As with hip arthritis, the extent of radiographic findings is not correlated with clinical symptoms (Mortazavu & Parvizi, 2011).

Common medical and surgical procedures: Nonsurgical therapy includes NSAID therapy and cortisone injections which are useful for mild-to-moderate degenerative changes (Mortazavu & Parvizi, 2011). Total knee arthroplasty (TKA) is used for severe arthritic changes and ongoing pain. Other procedures such as arthritic debridement, microfracture, and chondrocyte implantation have been implicated in the treatment of knee OA; however, evidence is very limited (Golish & Diduch, 2009).

Precautions and contraindications: Certain precautions will be indicated depending on procedures (e.g., weight-bearing restrictions). Clients should be educated on the benefits of exercise in the treatment of OA but care should be taken to maintain the safety of the older individual during exercise interventions (Goodman, 2009).

Screening and Assessments

Screening and assessments are similar throughout the various orthopedic conditions of the lower extremity with some variation. There are various top-down and bottom-up approaches to evaluation in orthopedics. Below is a list of top-down approaches that not only address the symptoms but also address the impact of the symptoms on the person's roles, contexts, and environments, followed by bottom-up approaches that are symptom specific (Lawson & Murphy, 2013). They are as follows:

- Client history including the client's age, hand dominance, occupational and avocational responsibilities, prior injuries, comorbidities, family issues, psychological issues, broader social issues, and economic issues.
- Mechanism and date of injury, structures involved, type and extent of medical and surgical intervention, concomitant injuries, and future treatment planned.
- Physical assessment including the following:
  - Baseline physical evaluation/interview to assess limitations not related to the surgery.
  - Pain (e.g., location, type, quality, and intensity).
  - Edema (e.g., circumferential measurements).
  - Sensory and motor function.
  - Coordination.
  - A/PROM of adjacent/uninvolved joints.
  - Cognitive assessment.
  - Ability to participate in life roles (Lawson & Murphy, 2013).

Interventions

Occupational therapy treatment is similar throughout the various orthopedic conditions of the lower extremity with some variation. Occupational therapy treatment includes compensatory, preparatory, and remedial approaches. Compensatory approaches attempt to teach adaptive strategies or incorporate adaptive equipment in order to achieve functional outcomes, whereas preparatory activities seek to prepare individuals for occupational engagement and remediation seeks to improve performance.

- *Symptom management*: Physical agent modalities are utilized to decrease pain and swelling of the arthritic joint(s). Hot and cold packs are utilized to manage symptoms and improve the client's ability to perform their daily tasks. Edema reduction techniques are helpful to maintain joint mobility and decrease pain. Therapeutic exercises and activities are helpful to maintain joint mobility, endurance levels, and strength (Frost & Harmeyer, 2011).
- *Energy conservation*: Individuals with hip or knee arthritis should utilize the following energy conservation techniques in order to save energy for the most important tasks of the day. Energy

conservation techniques consist of planning ahead to eliminate unnecessary steps, gather materials, and spread activities throughout the day/week. Pacing oneself, prioritizing the tasks for the day, sitting when possible, and maintaining good posture. Work simplification techniques are used to minimize the steps necessary throughout the day. Tasks are broken down into components and strategies are developed to eliminate unnecessary steps. Potential equipment/products that can further simplify the tasks are purchased and utilized (Poole, 2009).

- *Joint protection*: Incorporation of joint protection techniques into the client's day will help maintain joint integrity and slow the progression of arthritis. Common principles include respecting pain, using proper body mechanics, avoiding prolonged repetitive motions and holding positions for a long time, avoiding positions of deformity, using the largest and strongest muscles and joints, balancing rest and activity, and never beginning an activity that cannot be stopped (Poole, 2009).

Total Knee Arthroplasty

Description: TKA is often indicated in advanced arthritis. Approximately 655,000 primary TKAs and approximately 64,000 TKA revisions were performed in 2010, which are expected to increase to roughly 1,300,000 and 88,000 procedures by 2020, respectively (Kurtz, Ong,

Lau, & Bozic, 2014). By 2030, the demand for primary TKA is projected to increase by roughly 673%, representing roughly 3,480,000 procedures (Kurtz, Ong, Lau, Mowat, & Halpern, 2007). In comparison, the failure rate for primary TKA is less than 1% per year (Mortazavu & Parvizi, 2011). Risk factors for morbidity and complications following primary TKA include a body mass index $\geq$ 40 kilograms per square meter, operative times > 135 minutes, age 80 years and older, and cardiac disease, with diabetes and obesity identified as the predominate risk factors (Belmont, Goodman, Waterman, Bader, & Schoenfeld, 2014; Levine & Liporace, 2014).

Clinical presentation: Today, most TKAs are cemented and therefore can be weight-bearing as tolerated with care taken to protect the quadriceps incision more than the stability of the implant. Clients require early mobilization following TKA and are often seen on postoperative day one for ambulation.

Common diagnostic tests: X-ray is used to assess proper placement of the hardware during surgery and postsurgically (Levine & Liporace, 2014).

Common medical and surgical procedures: The most common TKA procedure is cemented fixation with a medial parapatellar approach (Hanssen & Scott, 2009; Thompson & Pellegrini, 2009). It is important to know what was disrupted in surgery to adequately protect the repair. Recently, minimally invasive procedures have been developed, but evidence shows minimal advantage over conventional procedures (Deirmengian & Lonner, 2014). Advantages and disadvantages of common TKA surgical procedures are described in **Table 17-4**.

Table 17-4 Advantages and Disadvantages of Common TKA Surgical Procedures

Approach	Advantages	Disadvantages
Medial parapatellar	- Easy to perform and visualize the joint	- Disrupts the extensor mechanism
Subvastus	- The extensor mechanism is preserved - Diminished postoperative pain	- Difficult to expose in revisions - Not indicated for individuals over 200 pounds
Midvastus	- The extensor mechanism is essentially preserved - May better preserve the blood supply of the knee	- Splits the vastus medialis - The potential for neurovascular damage
Trivector	- Spares all muscles that create a balanced force on the patella	- Not common
Lateral parapatellar	- Used in valgus knee deformities to release lateral tissue - More rapid rehabilitation due to sparing of the medial quadriceps	- More involved than medial approaches - Not common

Modified from Thompson and Pellegrini, 2009.

Precautions and contraindications: All total joint surgery comes with the risk of DVT and pulmonary embolism. Signs and symptoms of DVT must be addressed immediately. Also, with the use of lower extremity regional anesthesia, care needs to be taken to avoid falls and related injury during the postoperative period (e.g., rupture of the quadriceps repair or periprosthetic fracture) (Thompson & Pellegrini, 2009). Internal and external hip rotation and knee flexion beyond comfort are to be avoided (Lawson & Murphy, 2013).

Screening and Assessments

Screening and assessments are similar throughout the various orthopedic conditions of the lower extremity with some variation. There are various top-down and bottom-up approaches to evaluation in orthopedics. Below is a list of top-down approaches that not only address the symptoms but also address the impact of the symptoms on the person's roles, contexts, and environments, followed by bottom-up approaches that are symptom specific. They are as follows:

- Client history including the client's age, hand dominance, occupational and avocational responsibilities, prior injuries, comorbidities, family issues, psychological issues, broader social issues, and economic issues.
- Mechanism and date of injury, structures involved, type and extent of medical and surgical intervention, concomitant injuries, and future treatment planned.
- Physical assessment including the following:
  o Baseline physical evaluation/interview to assess limitations not related to the surgery.
  o Observations of pain and fear with rest and movement.
  o Color, temperature, and signs of compromised circulation or compartment syndrome.
  o Edema (e.g., circumferential measurements).
  o Sensory and motor function.
  o Coordination
  o Skin integrity and wound assessment:
    ▪ *Wound or surgical incision*: Note location, size, integrity of closure, exposure of pins or hardware, and signs of infection.
    ▪ *Scar*: Note location, size, adherence, hypertrophy, blanching with motion, pliability, and sensitivity.

- o A/PROM of adjacent/uninvolved joints.
- o Cognitive assessment.
- o Ability to participate in life roles.
- o Assessment of basic and instrumental ADLs.
- o Functional mobility (Lawson & Murphy, 2013).

Interventions

The OT team should address ROM, strengthening, and symptom management. OT practitioners are primarily responsible for ADL management performed within restrictions and precautions established by the physician (Lawson & Murphy, 2013). Common intervention considerations are as follows:

- *Bed mobility*: Sleeping in supine or on the involved side is recommended. Sleeping with the leg in elevation using balanced suspension or pillows is recommended to decrease edema and prevent contractures. An abduction wedge can be used if the client is on their noninvolved side (Lawson & Murphy, 2013).
- *Transfers*: Decreased knee flexion may make commode and car transfers difficult. Techniques used with hip replacement will assist with performance. Grab bars or shower chairs are recommended for tub transfers (Lawson & Murphy, 2013).
- *Lower extremity dressing and bathing*: This task can be problematic if the client cannot touch their toes; techniques used for hip replacement are recommended if the client has difficulty. The client should avoid rotation on the involved leg while dressing and bathing. Once healed, the client can shower (Lawson & Murphy, 2013).
- *Caregiver training*: Client's home caregivers should be educated on the precautions for the procedure performed, as well as educated on all home activities listed above (Lawson & Murphy, 2013).

Referrals and Discharge Considerations

Throughout the course of occupational therapy, the client is reassessed and progressed to increase ROM, strength, endurance, speed, confidence, and functional use of their involved upper extremity. The physician, OT, and caregiver ultimately work together with the client for a full return to meaningful activities and full participation in their vocational and avocational roles. Once the client has met his or her goals in therapy, or reached a plateau, the OT ensures the client's competence in completing a home exercise program to maintain or further promote their autonomy.

Management and Standards of Practice

In any setting, it is important for OT practitioners to participate in professional development and continuing education. This not only ensures continued certification, but also helps OTs and occupational therapy assistants to maintain and enhance knowledge of musculoskeletal disorders and injuries. Maintaining open communication with physicians and staff involved with client care is also necessary in this area of practice. Many issues that arise in orthopedic practice could have been addressed if communication between the OT and the physician was open and clear. It is also crucial here, and in any other area of practice, to maintain clear and concise medical records of all treatment provided, as well as planned treatment.

Chapter 17 Self-Study Activities (Answers Are Provided at the End of the Chapter)

1. Why should weight-bearing restrictions be followed strictly following hip fracture fixation?
2. Match the following weight-bearing restrictions to their appropriate descriptions.

Restriction	Description
A. Nonweight-bearing	1. No weight-bearing on the affected lower extremity. Utilize walker or crutches.
B. Toe-touch weight-bearing	2. 30–50% of weight on the involved lower extremity.
C. Partial weight-bearing	3. Affected toe can be used for balance, 85–90% of weight is placed on the uninvolved lower extremity. The client utilizes a walker or crutches.
D. Weight-bearing at tolerance	4. 75–100% weight-bearing allowed. Cane utilized as necessary.
E. Full weight-bearing	5. Weight-bearing on the involved lower extremity with minimal pain. The client utilizes a cane.

3. List the movement restrictions for an individual following hip surgery via a posterolateral approach.
   A. _____
   B. _____
   C. _____
4. List the movement restrictions for an individual following hip surgery via an anterolateral approach.
   A. _____
   B. _____
   C. _____
5. Hip and knee osteoarthritic clients should be instructed in what concepts?
   A. _____
   B. _____
   C. _____
6. The most common joint disease of men and women over 65 is:
   A. Rheumatoid arthritis
   B. Gout
   C. Osteoarthritis
   D. Pseudogout
7. Which of the following is not an acceptable sleeping position following THA?
   A. Sleeping supine with an abduction pillow.
   B. Side-lying on noninvolved side.
   C. Side-lying on noninvolved side with an abduction pillow.
   D. Side-lying on involved side.
8. Name two pieces of adaptive equipment that is often used for lower extremity dressing following hip surgery?
   A. _____
   B. _____
9. Describe the necessary steps for an individual following THA to safely get out of bed.
   A. _____
   B. _____
   C. _____

10. Name three joint protection techniques commonly provided to clients with OA.
    A. _____
    B. _____
    C. _____

11. What advancement in TKA surgery has allowed for near-immediate weight-bearing?
    _____

12. What motions are to be avoided following a TKA?
    A. Full extension
    B. Full flexion beyond comfort
    C. Internal hip rotation
    D. External hip rotation
    E. A, C, and D
    F. B, C, and D

Chapter 17 Self-Study Answers

1. Weight-bearing restrictions should be followed as strictly as possible to facilitate tissue healing and to help reduce hardware-related complications.
2. Weight-bearing restrictions matching choice.

Term	Response
A. Nonweight-bearing	1
B. Toe-touch weight-bearing	3
C. Partial weight-bearing	2
D. Weight-bearing at tolerance	5
E. Full weight-bearing	4

3. Posterolateral approach movement restrictions include no hip flexion greater than 90°, no internal rotation, and no adduction.
4. Anterolateral approach movement restrictions include no external rotation, no adduction, and no extension.
5. Symptom management, energy conservation, and work simplification. Clients with arthritis should be educated on symptom management techniques, including physical agent modality use, edema reduction techniques, therapeutic exercise to maintain joint mobility, and endurance and strength. Energy conservation techniques are utilized to save energy for the most important tasks of the day. Joint protection

techniques are utilized to help maintain joint integrity.
6. Osteoarthritis.
7. D.
8. A reacher, dressing stick, and sock aid are adaptive equipment that may assist with lower extremity dressing.
9. A. Clients should be supine and propped up on their elbows, B. move their legs incrementally to the side of the bed prior to getting up, C. progress toward lowering the legs out of the bed using hip and knee extension.
10. Joint protection techniques: respect pain, use proper body mechanics, avoid prolonged repetitive motions and hold positions for a long time, avoid positions of deformity, use the largest and strongest muscles and joints, balance, rest and activity, and never beginning an activity that cannot be stopped.
11. Most TKAs are cemented and therefore can be weight-bearing as tolerated with care taken to protect the quadriceps incision.
12. F.

References

Aoi, T., & Toshida, A. (2009). *Hip replacement: Approaches, complications and effectiveness.* New York, NY: Nova.

Belmont, P. J., Goodman, G. P., Waterman, B. R., Bader, J. O., & Schoenfeld, A. J. (2014). Thirty-day postoperative complications and mortality following total knee arthroplasty. Incidence and risk factors among a national sample of 15,321 patients. *The Journal of Bone and Joint Surgery, 96*(1), 20–26. doi:10.2106/jbjs.m.00018

Brower, A., & Flemming, D. (2012). Approach to the knee. In A. Brower & D. Flemming (Eds.), *Arthritis in black and white* (3rd ed., pp. 109–126). Philadelphia, PA: Elsevier.

Deirmengian, C., & Lonner, J. H. (2014). What's new in adult reconstructive knee surgery. *The Journal of Bone and Joint Surgery American Volume, 96*(2), 169–174. doi:10.2106/jbjs.m.01255

Farrokhi, S., Voycheck, C. A., Tashman, S., & Fitzgerald, G. K. (2013). A biomechanical perspective on physical therapy management of knee osteoarthritis. *The Journal of Orthopaedic and Sports Physical Therapy, 43*(9), 600–619. doi:10.2519/jospt.2013.4121

Fpoa, R. P. A. (2014). *Orthopedic emergencies: Extremity and pelvic trauma.* Ashland, OH: Ruben P. Arafiles.

Frost, L., & Harmeyer, F. (2011). *Occupational therapy's role in managing arthritis* (p. 2). Bethesda, MD: American Occupational Therapy Association. Retrieved from https://www.aota.org/-/media/Corporate/Files/AboutOT/Professionals/WhatIsOT/PA/Facts/Arthritis fact sheet.pdf

Goh, S. K., Samuel, M., Su, D. H., Chan, E. S., & Yeo, S. J. (2009). Meta-analysis comparing total hip arthroplasty with hemiarthroplasty in the treatment of displaced neck of femur fracture. *The Journal of Arthroplasty, 24*(3), 400–406. doi:10.1016/j.arth.2007.12.009

Golish, S. R., & Diduch, D. (2009). Arthroscopic debridement of the arthritic knee. In T. Brown, Q. Cui, W. Mihalko, & K. Saleh (Eds.), *Arthritis and arthroplasty: The knee* (1st ed., pp. 3–8). Philadelphia, PA: Elsevier.

Goodman, C. (2009). Soft tissue, joint, and bone disorders. In C. Goodman & K. Fuller (Eds.), *Pathology: Implications for the physical therapist* (pp. 1235–1317). St. Louis, MO: Elsevier.

Hanssen, A., & Scott, N. (2009). *Operative techniques: Total knee replacement*. Philadelphia, PA: Elsevier.

Huo, M. H., Parvizi, J., Bal, B. S., & Mont, M. A. (2008). What's new in total hip arthroplasty. *The Journal of Bone and Joint Surgery American Volume, 90*(9), 2043–2055. doi:10.2106/jbjs.h.00741

Kurtz, S. M., Ong, K. L., Lau, E., & Bozic, K. J. (2014). Impact of the economic downturn on total joint replacement demand in the United States. Updated projections to 2021. *The Journal of Bone and Joint Surgery, 96*(8), 624–630. doi:10.2106/jbjs.m.00285

Kurtz, S., Ong, K., Lau, E., Mowat, F., & Halpern, M. (2007). Projections of primary and revision hip and knee arthroplasty in the United States from 2005 to 2030. *The Journal of Bone and Joint Surgery, 89*(4), 780–785. doi:10.2106/jbjs.f.00222

Kusuma, S., & Garino, J. (2007). Total hip arthroplasty. In J. Garino & P. Beredjiklian (Eds.), *Adult reconstruction and arthroplasty: Core knowledge in orthopedics* (pp. 108–146). Philadelphia, PA: Elsevier.

Lawson, S., & Murphy, L. F. (2013). Hip fractures and lower extremity joint replacement. In L. W. Pedretti, H. M. Pendleton, & W. Schultz-Krohn (Eds.), *Pedretti's occupational therapy: Practice skills for physical dysfunction* (7th ed., pp. 1074–1090). St. Louis, MO: Elsevier.

Levine, B. R., & Liporace, F. A. (2014). Knee reconstruction and replacement. In L. K. Cannada (Ed.), *Orthopaedic knowledge update 11* (11th ed., pp. 579–604).

Rosemont, IL: American Academy of Orthopaedic Surgeons.

Maher, C. M. (2014). Orthopaedic conditions. In M. V. Radomski & C. A. T. Latham (Eds.), *Occupational therapy for physical dysfunction* (7th ed., pp. 1103–1128). Philadelphia, PA: Wolters Kluwer Health/Lippincott Williams & Wilkins.

Mak, J., Cameron, I., & March, L. (2010). Evidence-based guidelines for the management of hip fractures in older persons: An update. *Medical Journal of Australia, 192*(1), 37–41.

Mortazavu, S. J., & Parvizi, J. (2011). Arthritis. In J. Flynn (Ed.), *Orthopaedic knowledge update* (10th ed.). Rosemont, IL: American Academy of Orthopaedic Surgeons.

Poole, J. (2009). Musculoskeletal factors. In H. S. Willard, E. B. Crepeau, E. S. Cohn, & B. A. B. Schell (Eds.), *Willard & Spackman's occupational therapy* (11th ed., pp. 658–680). Philadelphia, PA: Wolters Kluwer Health/Lippincott Williams & Wilkins.

Sassoon, A., & Haidukewych, G. J. (2014). Hip and pelvic reconstruction and arthroplasty. In L. K. Cannada (Ed.), *Orthopaedic knowledge update 11* (11th ed., pp. 489–507). Rosemont, IL: American Academy of Orthopaedic Surgeons.

Scherger, J. E., & Mak, J. C. S. (2010). First consult: Hip fracture and dislocation. In *ClinicalKey*. Philadelphia, PA: Elsevier BV. Retrieved from https://www.clinicalkey.com/#!/content/medical_topic/21-s2.0-1014966

Stoneback, J. W., & Ziran, B. H. (2014). Hip trauma. In L. K. Cannada (Ed.), *Orthopaedic knowledge update 11* (11th ed., pp. 473–487). Rosemont, IL: American Academy of Orthopaedic Surgeons.

Thompson, S., & Pellegrini, V. (2009). Surgical approaches for primary total knee arthroplasty. In T. Brown, Q. Cui, W. Mihalko, & K. Saleh (Eds.), *Arthritis and arthroplasty: The knee* (pp. 81–89). Philadelphia, PA: Elsevier.

Wold, L., Unni, K., Sim, F., Sundaram, M., & Adler, C.-P. (2008). *Atlas of orthopedic pathology* (3rd ed.). Rochester, MN: Mayo Foundation for Medical Education and Research. Retrieved from ClinicalKey https://www.clinicalkey.com/#!/content/book/3-s2.0-B9781416053286500199

Wolford, M. L., Palso, K., & Bercovitz, A. (2015). *Hospitalization for total hip replacement among inpatients aged 45 and over: United States, 2000–2010*. NCHS Data Brief No. 186. Hyattsville, MD: National Center for Health Statistics.

Local, Regional, and Systemic Disorders

Christine Watt and Rita Troxtel

Learning Objectives

- Identify primary clinical features, signs and symptoms, pathology, and stages of clinical presentation of rheumatoid arthritis (RA), osteoarthritis, fibromyalgia (FM), complex regional pain syndrome (CRPS), juvenile rheumatoid arthritis (JRA), and psoriatic arthritis (PsA).
- Compare and contrast common diagnostic tests used to differentiate RA, osteoarthritis, FM, CRPS, JRA, and PsA from other conditions with similar signs and symptoms.
- Compare and contrast between medical procedures and surgical procedures used in the treatment of RA, osteoarthritis, FM, CRPS, JRA, and PsA.
- Recognize appropriate assessments and interventions used by occupational therapists to evaluate and treat clients with RA, osteoarthritis, FM, CRPS, JRA, and PsA.

Key Terms

- *Arthritis*: Inflammation of joints, often accompanied by pain, swelling, stiffness, and deformity.
- *Boutonniere deformity*: A finger position marked by extension of the metacarpophalangeal and distal interphalangeal joints and flexion of the proximal interphalangeal joint.
- *Edema*: An accumulation of fluid in the interstitial spaces of tissues that may indicate inflammation of a joint.
- *Hyperalgesia*: An excessive sensitivity to pain.

- *Nodules*: Painful masses that occur at weight-bearing joints in arthritic conditions.
- *Swan-neck deformity*: A finger deformity marked by flexion of the distal interphalangeal joints and hyperextension of the proximal interphalangeal joints.
- *Tenosynovitis*: Tendon sheath inflammation.

Rheumatoid Arthritis

Description

Rheumatoid arthritis (RA) is a systemic rheumatic illness believed to be caused by an autoimmune response to an unknown trigger (Deshaies, 2013; Vaughn, 2014). There is believed to be a genetic predisposition to the condition (Arnett & Asassi, 2009). The key symptom of this condition is bilateral destruction of connective tissue and inflammation of synovial joints, resulting in decreased range of motion (ROM) and strength in the affected joints (Hammond, 2014).

Etiology and Pathology

RA occurs in 1–2% of the U.S. population. Typical age of onset is between 40 and 60 years of age (Deshaies, 2013). Females are three times more likely to be diagnosed, with researchers looking at hormonal influence as a possible cause of the gender discrepancy. Initial onset may include symptom development over the course of weeks or months. The condition then continues with episodes of exacerbation and remission for approximately 80% of those affected. Approximately one in five will experience no further exacerbations for years after initial onset. Joints typically affected by RA include hips, knees, ankles, shoulders, jaw, and the joints of the hands. Rather than lubricating fluid, synovial joints produce enzymes that lead to the destruction of the connective tissue. Over time, the joint capsule thickens, the synovium becomes enlarged, and excess synovial fluid is produced. These conditions lead to enlarged joints. A pannus may form that eventually leads to permanent immobility of affected joints. The systemic nature of this condition may lead to inflammation of other areas of the body, including the blood vessels, eyes, heart, and lungs. The trigger of the immune system response leading to RA is unknown, but females who have a close relative diagnosed with the condition may have an increased risk (Deshaies, 2013). The stages of RA with associated symptoms are described in **Table 18-1**.

Descriptions and possible findings of common diagnostic tests for RA are described in **Table 18-2**.

Table 18-2 Common Diagnostic Tests for RA

Test	Possible Findings
Physical examination	Diagnosis is confirmed with the presence of four of the seven criteria for RA developed by the American College of Rheumatology.
Plain film radiograph	May only reveal soft tissue inflammation initially; but within 2 years most clients will develop observable joint changes.
Erythrocyte sedimentation rate	Used to indirectly determine the rate of inflammation present in the body and is useful in ruling out other conditions, such as osteoarthritis.
RF test	Although not conclusive in diagnosis, approximately 85% of those with RA have a positive result for this antibody.

RF, rheumatoid factor.
Data from Deshaies, 2013.

Table 18-1 Stages of RA

Stage	Description	Symptoms
1	Stage I (mild) RA: Initial onset of symptoms. Swelling of joints is present. No signs of damage present on x-ray.	Onset of symptoms in affected joints. Swelling, pain, and redness may be present. Client may feel fatigue and weakness.
2	Stage II (moderate) RA: Synovium begins to thicken. Articular cartilage destruction begins. Joint space begins to narrow. Muscle atrophy begins.	Client is experiencing exacerbations and remission episodes with destruction of joint dependent on degree of inflammation present in synovial tissue.
3	Stage III (severe) RA: Pannus formation occurs and joint mobility is permanently decreased. Subchondral bone begins to be affected. Significant muscle atrophy is present.	Joint deformities are visible. Cartilage loss is diagnosable via x-ray.
4	Stage IV (end stage) RA: Inflammation wanes, joint function is lost. Multiple systems may be affected.	In addition to criteria for Stage III, client will experience ankylosing of affected joints.

Data from Shiel, 2015

Table 18-3 Common Medical and Surgical Procedures for RA

Procedure	Description
Synovectomy	Surgical removal of synovial membrane of affected joints.
Tenosynovectomy	Surgical removal of diseased tendon sheaths.
Tendon realignment	Surgical intervention to move tendons that are shifted due to joint deformity into positions that will increase function of affected joints.
Arthroplasty	Surgical replacement of diseased joints to relieve pain and increase function.

Data from Deshaies, 2013.

Descriptions of common medical and surgical procedures for the treatment of RA are described in **Table 18-3**.

Precautions and Contraindications

Unstable joints due to weakened ligaments are a contraindication for passive stretching. All interventions must be performed within client tolerance regarding pain and fatigue. Progressive resistive exercise is contraindicated during period of exacerbation. Sensory perception and skin integrity should be addressed before use of splinting or modalities. These may be related to condition or age (Deshaies, 2013).

Osteoarthritis

Description

Osteoarthritis is the most common form of arthritis diagnosed in the United States. It is also referred to as degenerative joint disease. This condition is the third most prevalent health condition in modern societies. Pain, joint stiffness, decreased ROM, and formation of osteophytes in affected joints with resulting loss of function characterize osteoarthritis (Deshaies, 2013).

Etiology and Pathology

Twenty-seven million U.S. adults are affected by osteoarthritis, which has an unknown origin, but is believed to be influenced in part by secondary inflammation occurring due to cartilage loss in individual joints. Softening of articular cartilage is the first phase of this condition (Deshaies, 2013). A decreased joint space occurs as cartilage is lost (Vaughn, 2014). Bone-on-bone contact occurs, leading to remodeling of bony tissue through development of osteophytes and fluid-filled cysts (Hammond, 2014). Weight-bearing joints are commonly affected and obesity is thought to be a factor. Hands and spinal joints may also develop the condition. Predisposing factors to osteoarthritis include repetitive motion, genetics, age, trauma, and metabolic disease (Hammond, 2014; Vaughn, 2014). The condition is more commonly seen in males until age 50, at which time females develop an increased likelihood of diagnosis (Deshaies, 2013). The stages of osteoarthritis, with associated symptoms, are described in **Table 18-4**.

Descriptions and possible findings of common diagnostic tests for osteoarthritis are described in **Table 18-5**.

Descriptions of common medical and surgical procedures for the treatment osteoarthritis are described in **Table 18-6**.

Precautions and Contraindications

Osteoarthritis does not have periods of exacerbation and remission; progressive resistive exercise may be indicated, but should always be done with caution and within client tolerance (Deshaies, 2013).

Table 18-4 Stages and Symptoms of Osteoarthritis

Stage	Description	Symptoms
Early (mild)	Articular cartilage begins to soften and lose elasticity. Subchondral bone protection decreases and clefts form between cartilage cells.	Onset of symptoms in affected joints. Client may experience pain with use.
Moderate	Articular cartilage destruction continues. Joint space begins to narrow. Cysts containing fluid may develop on bone surface.	Client continues to experience pain with use and now may have stiffness when joint is at rest for extended periods of time.
Late (severe)	Large portions of cartilage are destroyed and osteophytes develop as bone-on-bone contact occurs within joint.	Cartilage loss and reduced joint space is diagnosable via x-ray. Joint deformity begins to occur due to osteophyte development. Loss of ROM and reduced function is present.

Data from Iliades, 2015.

Table 18-5 Common Diagnostic Tests for Osteoarthritis

Test	Possible Findings
Physical examination	Pain is rated via pain scale. ROM and MMT baselines are taken. Physical indications of inflammation are investigated (e.g., redness, swelling, and heat).
Plain film radiograph	May reveal narrowing of joint space. Changes in bony tissue—including osteophyte formation.
CBC	Used to rule out other rheumatologic disorders, particularly if multiple joints are affected or significant inflammation is present.
Arthrocentesis	Joint fluid is analyzed for evidence of cartilage and bone particles that have deteriorated and are freely floating within joint capsule.
Magnetic resonance imaging	Gives a more detailed view of joint to examine for osteophytes, bone surface damage, and deterioration of soft tissue.

MMT, manual muscle test; CBC, complete blood count.
Data from Deshaies, 2013.

Table 18-6 Common Medical and Surgical Procedures for Osteoarthritis

Procedure	Description
Joint debridement	Arthroscopic procedure for removal of osteophytes to relieve pain.
Subchondral bone resection	Removal or puncture of bone may stimulate soft tissue for increased cartilage cushion between articulating bones.
Joint fusion	Surgical binding of articulating bones in a joint with hardware or cement to prevent movement and increase stability.
Arthroplasty	Surgical replacement of damaged joints to relieve pain and increase function.

Data from Deshaies, 2013.

Complex Regional Pain Syndrome

Description

Complex regional pain syndrome (CRPS) is the term given to a variety of disorders in which pain occurs in a manner more severe or longer than would typically be expected from the initial insult (Engel, 2013). A variety of soft tissue changes occur along with intractable pain. This condition has both physical and psychological aspects that need to be addressed during treatment (Engel, 2013; National Institute of Neurological Disorders and Stroke, 2015). In an attempt to better classify the condition, three types have been identified. Type I follows an injury that does not include a peripheral nerve. Type II occurs in response to an injury that involves nerve tissue. Type III is designed to include clients who experience the same symptoms as Types I and II, but do not have an injury that would classify them in one of those types (Hammond, 2014).

Etiology and Pathology

There is no clear consensus of the underlying pathology of this disorder. Some theorize that a vasoconstriction/vasodilation cycle occurs, which leads to tissue anoxia and fibrosis following an injury (Engel, 2013). Approximately 0.03% of the population will be diagnosed with

Table 18-7 Stages and Symptoms of CRPS

Stage	Description	Symptoms
1	Acute or traumatic stage: Occurs within the first 3 months following injury.	Pain greater than is expected occurs following injury. Color changes in the skin and pitting edema may also be seen. Clients may begin to display guarding behaviors.
2	Dystrophic stage: This stage occurs between 3 and 6 months post-injury. Some sources indicate that it could last up to a year postinjury.	Client will continue to experience pain. Edema may become brawny and stiffness begins. Discoloration continues and skin may have a shiny appearance. Muscle wasting may begin to occur. Osseous demineralization, trophic and pilomotor changes may be present.
3	Atrophic stage: This stage may last an unlimited time if the condition becomes chronic.	Pain that has peaked in Stage II now may subside. Stiffness persists and edema may not be reversible. Joint capsule thickening decreases ROM and impairs function. Skin is typically cool, white, and dry.

Data from Engel, 2013; Hammond, 2014.

CRPS each year (deMos et al., 2006). Some studies have indicated a gender difference of four to one, with women being more likely to receive the diagnosis (Sandroni, Benrud-Larson, McClelland, & Low, 2003). Typical symptoms seen with all types of CRPS include pain, edema, hyperhidrosis, skin color changes, stiffness, and temperature changes in the skin over the affected area. The condition occurs in a series of three stages, with symptoms varying between them (Engel, 2013). The stages of CRPS with associated symptoms are described in **Table 18-7**.

Descriptions and possible findings of common diagnostic tests for CRPS are described in **Table 18-8**.

Descriptions of common interventions for CRPS are described in **Table 18-9**.

Table 18-8 Common Diagnostic Tests for CRPS

Test	Possible Findings
Physical examination	No single factor confirms diagnosis. A practitioner must make careful diagnosis and consider client's medical history. Symptoms consistent with the condition are present and lead to diagnosis.
Blood panel	Used to rule out other conditions such as RA or Lyme disease. No conclusive blood tests exist for diagnostic confirmation.
Magnetic resonance imaging	May indicate bone-metabolism changes that indicate CRPS.

Data from National Institute of Neurological Disorders and Stroke, 2015.

Table 18-9 Common Medical and Surgical Interventions for CRPS

Intervention	Description
Sympatholytic medication	This class of drugs reduces the sympathetic nervous system hyper reaction that exacerbates pain.
Neurontin	This medication modulates nerve impulse conduction and may reduce pain and normalize skin temperature of affected area.
Calcium channel blockers	May help break the noxious vasoconstriction/vasodilation process that damages tissue.
Pain medications	Opioids may be helpful in reducing pain for increased use of affected body part.
Stellate ganglion block	Injection to block sympathetic nervous system activity may allow increased mobilization during therapy.

Data from Engel, 2013; Hammond, 2014; National Institute of Neurological Disorders and Stroke, 2015.

Precautions and Contraindications

All interventions should be performed in the context of client education for self-management of the condition (Hammond, 2014). Failure to respond to treatment as anticipated is reason for referral for further diagnostic procedure. Return to work or other functional activity is recommended for addressing any underlying psychosocial issues. Casting, passive stretching, and dynamic splinting are to be avoided due to decreased circulation to the affected area and the possibility of further injury (Hammond, 2014).

Fibromyalgia

Description

Fibromyalgia (FM) is a condition resulting in widespread neurogenic pain lasting more than three months and having no specific cause (Centers for Disease Control and Prevention [CDC], 2015). Factors believed to be involved in the development of FM are genetic predisposition, trauma, physical and psychological stressors, and autoimmune dysfunction (Engel, 2013; Hammond, 2014).

Etiology and Pathology

Estimates of persons in the United States with FM vary, depending on the source of information. Generally, it can be said that approximately 5 million persons in the United States have this diagnosis at any given time (CDC, 2015). The condition is much more prevalent in females, with estimates being four to seven times the rate of occurrence in males (CDC, 2015; Hammond, 2014). Typically, diagnosis occurs during middle age, but children can also have the condition. Increasing age is considered a risk (CDC, 2013). A dysfunction in the brain's response to stress may be a predisposing factor to development. Clients diagnosed with the condition have shown unusual levels of neurotransmitters along the body's pain pathways. Increased levels of substance P and reduced levels of serotonin and endorphins likely increase pain perception and interfere with sleep and cognition. A process known as "pain wind-up" occurs due to repeated exposure of C-fibers to painful stimuli, leading to excessive substance P production (Hammond, 2014). The type of FM with associated symptoms is described in **Table 18-10**.

Descriptions of common diagnostic tests used for evaluation of FM are described in **Table 18-11**.

Descriptions of common interventions used in the treatment of FM are described in **Table 18-12**.

Table 18-10 Types of FM with Associated Symptoms

Type	Description	Symptoms
Primary	Primary FM has no clear-cut cause. It may be precipitated by traumatic events, repetitive injury, viral infection, obesity, or genetic predisposition.	Widespread pain in 19 pain locations. Clients also experience sleep disturbance, cognitive symptoms, hyperalgesia, sensory disturbances in extremities, headaches, migraines, morning stiffness, memory deficits, trouble concentrating, and digestive system disturbances.
Secondary	This type of FM is thought to occur due to the pain wind-up effect in clients previously diagnosed with osteoarthritis or rheumatoid arthritis.	Symptoms of type II FM are as above, but begin after long-term pain related to an arthritic condition.

Data from Hammond, 2014.

Table 18-11 Common Diagnostic Tests for FM

Test	Possible Findings
Physical examination	Past tests included firm palpation over 19 designated pain locations, with diagnosis requiring pain in greater than nine of these. A current diagnostic criterion does not require this standard. Widespread pain greater than 3 months with no known cause may be sufficient for diagnosis.
Client medical history	History of trauma or repetitive injury may be present in client medical or social history. Reports of pain for more than 3 months are indicative of this condition.
Blood panel test	Various blood tests, such as erythrocyte sedimentation rate test and thyroid function test, may be done to rule out other conditions with similar symptomatology.

Data from Mayo Clinic, 2015a.

Table 18-12 Common Medical Interventions for FM

Intervention	Description
Pregabalin	This reduces substance P and improves sleep.
Milnacipran Duloxetine	These two drugs are used to prevent reuptake of serotonin and norepinephrine, which improves fatigue and reduces pain, thereby improving overall function.
Tramadol	Pseudo-opioid medication that reduces overall pain.

Data from Hammond, 2014; Mayo Clinic, 2015a.

Precautions and Contraindications

All interventions must be performed within client tolerance. Pain and fatigue may be increased with overexertion. Clients should be encouraged to take part in social and meaningful activities to the greatest extent possible (i.e., without causing undue stress) to counteract the depression associated with this condition (Engel, 2013).

Juvenile Rheumatoid Arthritis

Description

Juvenile rheumatoid arthritis (JRA) is the most commonly diagnosed type of arthritis in children (CDC, 2013). It is also commonly referred to as juvenile idiopathic arthritis. The CDC uses the broader heading of childhood arthritis. Readers need to be aware that multiple terms for similar conditions may be used throughout the medical literature. The information included in this chapter refers to the specific classification used most commonly in the United States. JRA is defined as arthritis lasting longer than 6 weeks in a child under 16 years of age, who has no history of any other type of arthritis (Rogers, 2015). The condition has three subtypes: systemic (10% of cases), polyarticular (40% of cases), and pauciarticular (50% of cases) (CDC, 2013).

Etiology and Pathology

Because classifications of arthritis vary greatly, so do estimates of prevalence. To date, no national study has

Table 18-13 Subtypes of JRA with Associated Symptoms

Type	Description	Symptoms
Systemic	The most severe type of JRA. Multiple joints may be affected. Organ inflammation and an elevated white blood cell count may occur.	Initial symptoms typically include a high fever and rash. Depending on the body systems affected, pericarditis, hepatitis, weight loss, tenosynovitis, anorexia, peptic ulcer disease, and skeletal changes are seen. This subtype of JRA was once referred to as Stills disease.
Polyarticular	This subtype affects five or more joints. Smaller joints are more commonly affected. Progression of the disease may be influenced by whether a client is RF positive or RF negative.	This subtype causes the same type of bilateral joint degeneration in the hands, feet, and cervical spine as seen in adult RA. In extreme cases, nodules are also seen. Other symptoms include fatigue, low grade fever, and morning stiffness.
Pauciarticular	This subtype affects fewer than five joints. The larger joints such as hips, knees, shoulders, and elbows are typically affected.	This subtype affects joints in a unilateral manner. There is not a systemic presentation of the condition with this subtype. Joint deformities may occur. The long bones may have overgrowth, resulting in limb discrepancy and possible flexion contracture of the knee or elbow.

RF, rheumatoid factor.
Data from Genetics Home Reference, 2015; Rogers, 2015.

been done to accurately determine the prevalence of JRA among American children. The most commonly noted estimates in the literature state that between 1 and 4 children out of 1,000 will be diagnosed each year in the United States. The onset of this condition is typically between the ages of 2 and 4 years—with females being more likely than males to be diagnosed. As with adult RA, JRA is a systemic autoimmune disorder with no known specific cause. Multiple organs and joints may be affected and synovial joint destruction occurs. The systemic subtype is often diagnosed when children are taken to the pediatrician with a fever and widespread rash (Rogers, 2015). Onset of this subtype in children younger than 6 years results in shortened stature for 50% of cases (CDC, 2013; Rogers, 2015). The prognosis for JRA varies greatly, depending on factors such as age of onset and subtype. The majority of children with pauciarticular subtype recover in 1–2 years. Children with the other subtypes may also enter remission; however, it is estimated that one-third will have functional deficits 10 years after diagnosis. Approximately 15% of children diagnosed will be disabled as adults (Rogers, 2015). The subtypes of JRA with associated symptoms are described in **Table 18-13**.

Descriptions of common diagnostic tests used for JRA are described in **Table 18-14**.

Descriptions of common interventions used in the treatment of JRA are described in **Table 18-15**.

Table 18-14 Common Diagnostic Tests for JRA

Test	Possible Findings
Plain film radiograph	Imaging to determine extent and degree of damage to specific joints. Fractures, infection, and other joint trauma may be discovered.
Client medical history	A review of symptoms is done to determine age of onset, duration and pattern of symptoms, and involvement of other body systems.
Complete blood chemistry panel	Various blood tests such as erythrocyte sedimentation rate, complete blood chemistry, antinuclear antibody, RF, and anti-ccp test may be done to rule out other conditions.
Erythrocyte sedimentation rate	Used to indirectly determine the rate of inflammation present in the body and is useful in ruling out other conditions, such as osteoarthritis.
RF test	A test positive for this antibody may help determine the severity and course of the condition.

RF, rheumatoid factor.
Data from Children's Hospital of Wisconsin, 2015.

Table 18-15 Common Medical Interventions for JRA

Intervention	Description
NSAIDs	These are used to reduce overall inflammation; however, aspirin is typically not used due to possibility of children developing Reye's syndrome with aspirin use.
Methotrexate and other DMARDs	This classification of drugs slows the progression of JRA; but may take months to produce symptom relief. Methotrexate is the most common DMARD used in children.
Corticosteroids	Help stop inflammation in the systemic subtype, particularly around the heart. These may be given by injection or orally. Steroids in this category may stunt a child's growth and are used only in severe cases of JRA.
Biologic drugs	Genetically engineered medications may be designed for specific children when no other medications are effective in slowing the progress of the condition.

NSAIDs, nonsteroidal antiinflammatory drugs; DMARDs, disease-modifying antirheumatic drugs.
Data from Arthritis Foundation; Beukelman et al., 2011; Children's Hospital of Wisconsin, 2015.

Precautions and Contraindications

All interventions must be performed within client tolerance. As with adult RA, joint instability and weakened ligaments make stretching contraindicated. Skin integrity and functional use of extremities should be considered with any splinting or orthotic interventions. The impact of social development on a child with a serious disability needs to be taken into consideration during all interventions. Therapy interventions should be geared toward helping the child move through typical developmental milestones.

Psoriatic Arthritis

Description

Psoriatic arthritis (PsA) is a form of joint inflammation that affects some people who have the chronic skin condition known as psoriasis. On rare occasions, it can occur in persons without the skin condition, but typically this is a precursor to later development of the skin condition (Gladman, Antoni, Mease, Clegg, & Nash, 2005). It is believed the condition is caused by a combination of genetic and environmental factors resulting in the body's immune system attacking healthy cells. There is no known cure. Treatment emphasis is on managing symptoms and preventing further joint damage in those with the condition (Mayo Clinic, 2015b).

Etiology and Pathology

Psoriasis occurs in approximately 2–3% of people (Gladman et al., 2005). It is characterized by red, patches of skin covered with white, flaking scales. Estimates of persons in the United States with PsA vary; but most studies indicate that between 5 and 10% of persons with psoriasis will be diagnosed with PsA (Genetics Home Reference, 2015). There are five types of PsA with distinct clinical presentation. In all types, symptoms may resemble those of RA, including pain in the affected joints, warmth in the surrounding tissues, and generalized fatigue. Typical involvement occurs in feet, fingers, toes, and spine. Onset is usually between 30 and 50 years of age, but the condition can occur at any age (Mayo Clinic, 2015b). The types of PsA with associated symptoms are described in **Table 18-16**.

Descriptions and possible findings of common diagnostic tests for PsA are described in **Table 18-17**.

Descriptions of common medical and surgical interventions used in the treatment of PsA are described in **Table 18-18**.

Precautions and Contraindications

As with RA, unstable joints due to weakened ligaments are a contraindication for passive stretching. All interventions must be performed within client tolerance regarding pain and fatigue. Progressive resistive exercise may be contraindicated if significant joint deformity has occurred. Often this condition results in significant joint damage within a few years; therefore, the psychosocial impact on lifestyle and role must be taken into consideration. Sensory perception and skin integrity should be addressed before use of splinting or modalities (Deshaies, 2013).

Table 18-16 Types of Psoriatic Arthritis with Associated Symptoms

Type	Description	Symptoms
DIP predominant	This type of PsA affects the DIP joints (i.e., most distal in fingers and toes). These joints are closest to the nails, and nail changes frequently occur with this type of arthritis.	This type of PsA results in painful swelling of the DIP joints in fingers and toes. Digits may have a "sausagelike" appearance known as dactylitis. Nails may have pitted appearance or separate from the nail bed as is seen in a fungal infection. Swelling and pain may occur over tendons.
Asymmetric arthritis	In this type of PsA, different joints are affected on each side of the body. Often joint involvement will follow a "ray" pattern with all joints of a single digit affected.	One to three joints on each side of the body will have symptoms of pain, swelling, and/or redness. The small number of joints involved leads to this form sometime being referred to as asymmetric oligoarticular arthritis. This type of PsA is one of the mildest forms.
Symmetric arthritis	Bilateral involvement of (same) joints occurs with this type of PsA.	Typically multiple joints are involved (i.e., five or more on each side). For this reason, this type is often referred to as symmetric polyarticular arthritis.
Spondylitis	Inflammation in the joints of the spine is the key markers of this type of PsA.	The joints of the spine (i.e., including cervical area) will be painful and stiff. Other joints in the extremities may also be affected.
Arthritis mutilans	This is the most severe type of PsA. It primarily affects the proximal joints of the fingers and toes. Osteolysis of these joints causes joint collapse.	The proximal joints of the digits are destroyed and may have resorption or fusion, both leading to a lack of function in the affected extremity.

DIP, distal interphalangeal.
Data from Genetics Home Reference, 2015.

Table 18-17 Common Diagnostic Tests for Psoriatic Arthritis

Test	Possible Findings
Plain film radiograph	Imaging to determine if bony proliferation or erosion has occurred. A classic "pencil in cup" x-ray results from resorption of bone and is typically a confirming finding.
Magnetic resonance imaging	Detailed radio wave imaging may be used to reveal changes in soft tissue structures of the tendons and ligaments in the lumbar area or the feet.
Client medical history	Through gathering a thorough medical history, positive findings related to the Classification Criteria for Psoriatic Arthritis (CASPAR) may be discovered. These criteria, published in 2006, are becoming more widely used. Diagnosis is confirmed when 3 points are found to be present along with current inflammatory arthritis. The scale is: • Current or history of psoriasis or family history (2 points) • Nail psoriasis (1 point) • Lack of RF (1 point) • Current or history of dactylitis (1 point) • Periarticular new bone formation confirmed via x-ray (1 point)
Joint fluid test	Samples of fluid may be removed from the joint to look for uric acid crystals. A positive finding indicates the condition is gout, rather than PsA.
RF test	This test typically produces no sign of the RF antibody in persons with PsA.

RF, rheumatoid factor.
Data from National Institute of Arthritis and Musculoskeletal and Skin Diseases, 2014.

Table 18-18 Common Medical and Surgical Interventions for Psoriatic Arthritis

Intervention	Description
NSAIDs	This classification of medications may reduce inflammation and pain associated with milder forms of the condition. Typical medications include naproxen, ibuprofen, and aspirin.
DMARDs	Drugs in this classification include methotrexate and leflunomide. These may slow the progression of the disease and prevent further joint damage.
Immunosuppressants	Drugs such as azathioprine and cyclosporine are used to lower the immune system response, which may be helpful in autoimmune conditions such as PsA.
TNF-alpha inhibitors	TNF-alpha is produced by the human body and results in inflammation. Drugs such as etanercept and infliximab reduce the production often resulting in decreased inflammation and pain.
Steroid injections	Steroid medications are injected into affected joints and often reduce inflammation quickly, resulting in decreased pain.
Joint replacement surgery	Artificial prostheses formed of metal and plastic may be used to replace joints that have significant damage from PsA. Typically, these are done to reduce pain and restore function to affected extremities.

NSAIDs, nonsteroidal antiinflammatory drugs; DMARDs, disease-modifying antirheumatic drugs; TNF, tumor necrosis factor.
Data from Mayo Clinic, 2015b; National Institute of Arthritis and Musculoskeletal and Skin Diseases, 2014.

Screening and Assessments

Top-down and bottom-up assessments are appropriate for these conditions; **Table 18-19** lists top-down assessments and **Table 18-20** lists bottom-up assessments appropriate for local, regional, and systemic disorders discussed in this chapter.

- CRPS has a small body of scholarly work on assessment tools. Assessments with asterisk indicate that the instrument has been found to be reliable and valid for assessment of pain. May be used as appropriate to assess pain related to this condition.
- In addition to the assessment above, the following assessments are specifically designed to assess the impact of JRA on children:
    - The Juvenile Arthritis Quality of Life Questionnaire
    - Juvenile Arthritis Self-Report Index
    - The Juvenile Arthritis Assessment Scale

Interventions

Each of the diagnoses covered in this chapter is a multifaceted condition with symptomatology that impacts both physical functioning and social participation. The psychosocial impact is significant for these conditions, and the resulting stress may exacerbate physical symptoms such as pain and fatigue (Hammond, 2014; Vaughn, 2014). A comprehensive evaluation process that utilizes both standardized and nonstandardized assessments to produce a client-centered occupational profile is essential to determining the roles a client finds most important. Analysis of occupational performance for activities related to those roles will result in the highest degree of patient compliance and the best functional outcomes (Vaughn, 2014). These conditions are managed with a multidisciplinary approach, so systematic implementation of interventions that does not overwhelm the client is essential. Client education and frequent review of implementations are indicated as some interventions, such as splints, may need revision to facilitate the best client function (Engel, 2013).

Expected Functional Outcomes

Research indicates that occupational therapy intervention can reduce pain, stress, and improve overall function for the conditions in this chapter (Hammond, 2014; Vaughn, 2014). Early intervention has shown to provide the greatest benefit. Interventions such as joint protection, client education, and task modification can produce improved activities of daily living (ADLs) performance and increased social participation for clients. Functional

Table 18-19 Top-Down Assessments for Local, Regional, and Systemic Disorders

Assessment Name	Description	RA	OA	CRPS	Fibro	JRA	PsA
AMPAC	Assesses mobility, ADLs, and cognition to measure outcomes related to treatment.	*					
Arthritis Hand Function Test	Assesses bilateral hand strength, dexterity and function in ADL activities for RA and OA clients.	*	*				
AMPS	Utilizes familiar tasks to assess the motor and processing skills involved to complete them.	*					
COPM	Assesses client's interpretation of his abilities in self-care, leisure, and productive activities.	*	*	*			
Community Integration Questionnaire II	Assesses ADLs across several domains.	*	*				
DASH Outcome Measure	Assesses pain, along with abilities in ADL and IADL tasks. Suitable for a variety of UE conditions.	*	*	*			
Fatigue Severity Scale	Assesses how fatigue affects important life activities.	*			*		
Global Fatigue Index	Measures overall fatigue.	*	*				
Health Assessment Questionnaire	A self-report instrument that looks at overall disability. Suitable for a variety of conditions.	*					
Hospital Anxiety and Depression Scale	Assesses depression and anxiety in hospital clients who are dealing with physical illness.	*					
Impact of Participation and Autonomy Questionnaire	Assesses social participation of an individual	*			*		
Medical Outcomes Study Short Form 36	Assesses client's perception of quality of life as it relates to health issues.	*					
McGill Pain Measure	Assesses perception of pain and effect on life activities.		*		*		
Occupational Performance History Interview	Assesses how client choices, routines, and roles have changed over time.	*					
PASS	Measures abilities of self-care, mobility, and home management in the clinic and home environments.	*					
Role Checklist	This is used for assessment of important life roles and client's desire to return to the involved tasks.	*					
Sollerman Hand Function Test	Assesses grip and pinch patterns using 20 common tasks.	*	*				
WOMAC	This self-report item assesses how function is affected in clients with RA and FM among other conditions.	*	*	*	*	*	

AMPAC, Activity Measure for Post-Acute Care; AMPS, Assessment of Motor and Process Skills; COPM, Canadian Occupational Performance Measure; DASH, Disabilities of Arm, Shoulder, and Hand; IADL, instrumental activities of daily living; PASS, Performance Assessment of Self-Care Skills; WOMAC, Western Ontario and McMaster Universities Osteoarthritis Index; UE, upper extremity.
An asterisk (*) indicates that the instrument has been found to be reliable and valid for assessment of the following conditions.
Data from Boop, 2014; Rehabilitation Institute of Chicago, 2010.

Table 18-20 Bottom-Up Assessments for Local, Regional, and Systemic Disorders

Assessment Name	Description	RA	OA	CRPS	Fibro	JRA	PsA
Jebsen Hand Function Test	Simple task performed and scored according to speed. Quality is not assessed.	*					
Manual Muscle Testing	Individual muscles are tested per pre-established positioning and methodology.	*	*				
Pain Assessment Scale	Pain is rated 0 (no pain) to 10 (worst pain). May be accompanied by visual representation of levels.	*	*	*			
Pinch Strength	Using a pinch gauge, pure strength of a variety of pinches is measured in pounds.						
ROM	Full movement of body parts is measured in degrees, based on anatomic charts. May be measured with or without assistance of therapist.	*					

An asterisk (*) indicates that the instrument has been found to be reliable and valid for assessment of the following conditions.
Data from Boop, 2014; Rehabilitation Institute of Chicago, 2010.

outcomes may vary greatly, based on the client's ability to manage symptoms. Developing new routines and modifying activities can be challenging, and some interventions produce only 50% compliance after discharge (Hammond, 2014). An emphasis on client education to manage preparatory methods, use adaptive equipment, and balance occupations and rest will produce the best functional outcomes (Deshaies, 2013).

Impact on Occupational Performance

Although the conditions discussed in this chapter may be progressive in nature, clients can participate in meaningful occupations and achieve a high degree of satisfaction when they are proficient with self-management techniques (Hammond, 2014). To promote the best self-management of one's condition, education on overall wellness is essential (Vaughn, 2014). Many of these conditions have periods of remissions and exacerbations, so clients will also benefit from education about the typical disease progression, with emphasis on how they can continue to perform meaningful occupations throughout the life span. Interventions will be selected based on the

stage of condition and client's goals (Deshaies, 2013). **Table 18-21** lists common therapeutic interventions appropriate for all conditions discussed in this chapter.

Referrals and Discharge Considerations

Many resources are available, both in the local community and nationally, for the conditions discussed in this chapter. It is essential that clients are provided with information regarding these resources. Referral information for clients and their caregivers will provide the greatest benefit (Deshaies, 2013). Initiating contact prior to discharge is helpful in preventing a lapse in support. Compliance with interventions after discharge is dependent on the client's understanding of how to implement them and the value seen in them. Ensuring that a client has a thorough understanding of interventions and is proficient in implementation will produce higher compliance and better outcomes. Follow-up with the client after discharge to provide encouragement and help them remain focused on how self-management can improve compliance, which may lead to a better quality of life (Hammond, 2014).

Table 18-21 Common Occupational Therapy Interventions for Local, Regional, and Systemic Disorders

Condition	Intervention	Goal or Purpose	Description
OA RA CRPS JRA PsA	Joint protection	Decrease pain, prevent further joint damage, control inflammation, and maintain strength, mobility, and function.	Change movement patterns that increase force on affected joints, use larger joints, and correct body mechanics.
OA RA CRPS FM JRA PsA	Ergonomics	Maximize function of systems based on human performance. Decrease pain, and maintain strength.	Design or modify tools, equipment, and the way tasks are performed. Design environments to reduce maladaptive postures.
OA RA FM JRA PsA	Energy conservation	Conserve energy for meaningful tasks. Client education on performing activities safely.	Preplan activities, divide tasks into stages, use appropriate tools for each task, take rest breaks, position body and required items to decrease fatigue and increase efficiency. Techniques may include pursed lip breathing, and altering the way basic and instrumental activities of daily living (IADL) are performed.
OA RA CRPS FM JRA PsA	Splinting, orthotics	Preparatory technique to protect affected joints and allow them to rest, reduce pain, and promote function.	Common splints include finger splints to block deforming joint positions, thumb spica splint and wrist cock-up splint to promote functional positioning, and resting hand splint.
OA RA FM JRA PsA	Adaptation, adaptive equipment, compensatory strategies	Adaptation involves strategies to change the way tasks are performed in order to reduce pain or joint damage. Adaptive equipment devices are used to perform a task with reduced stress on affected joints.	Compensatory strategies focus on using techniques and equipment to compensate for deficits in ROM or strength. Adaptation depends on purpose and personal need. Common adapted equipment includes built-up handles, extended handles to increase reach, and nonslip plates. Adaptation can include changing physical demands such as altering the height of counters.
OA RA CRPS FM JRA PsA	ADL and IADL modification	Decrease joint stress and painful movement. Increase activity tolerance.	Modified techniques for bathing, dressing, grooming, toileting, home management, and functional mobility.
OA RA CRPS FM PsA	Work modification and work rehabilitation	Modify work tasks for immediate benefit, along with worker education for long-term results that prevent further injury.	Simplify work tasks, avoid or decrease repetitive motions, design or modify tools and equipment for reduced joint stress, decrease risk of work injury by altering unsafe behaviors.

(continues)

Table 18-21 Common Occupational Therapy Interventions for Local, Regional, and Systemic Disorders (*continued*)

Condition	Intervention	Goal or Purpose	Description
OA RA CRPS FM JRA PsA	Client education	Increase client knowledge regarding condition and improve client confidence in managing symptoms.	Self-management education, problem-solving strategies, and home programs.
OA RA CRPS FM JRA PsA	Therapeutic exercise	Increase strength of muscles to protect affected joints, increase fitness level, and overall endurance.	Aquatic exercise, gentle active ROM exercise, progressive resistive exercise, and cardio exercise.
OA RA FM CRPS JRA PsA	Alternative modalities	Reduce pain, increase flexibility and mobility, reduce stress, and increase client self-efficacy in managing condition.	Yoga, diaphragmatic breathing exercises, meditation, visualization, and biofeedback.
OA RA FM PsA	Physical agent modalities	Reduce pain, increase function, and decrease inflammation.	Thermotherapy such as paraffin dip, hot pack, and fluidotherapy. Iontophoresis for local corticosteroids. Studies found pulsed shortwave diathermy may be beneficial for knee and cervical OA.
CRPS	Physical agent modalities	Reduce pain, and increase function.	Contrast bath, transcutaneous electrical nerve stimulation, and biofeedback.
OA RA CRPS PsA	Scar management	Remodel collagen fibers, decrease appearance of scar, and increase ROM following surgical interventions.	Deep tissue massage, myofascial release, lymph drainage, and soft tissue mobilization.
OA RA FM CRPS JRA PsA	Functional activities	Increase client awareness of damaging positions during functional activity.	Therapeutic performance of ADL while addressing biomechanical goals.

Data from Cameron, 2013; Deshaies, 2013; Engel, 2013; Hammond, 2014; Rogers, 2015; RSDSA, 2014.

Management and Standards of Practice

The conditions of concern in this chapter all require interdisciplinary intervention for the best outcome.

Management of services will be of utmost importance as other services will be providing interventions to the patient simultaneously with occupational therapy. It is imperative that practitioners from each discipline coordinate care in a manner that provides the most comprehensive quality of care, and does not overwhelm the client (Engel, 2013).

Studies indicate that occupational therapy interventions are effective in providing clients with improved quality of life (Hammond, 2014). Practitioners are required to keep abreast of best practices to provide efficient and effective interventions. Ethical practice requires that education regarding the diagnosis and interventions needs to be presented in a manner the client can understand. Practitioners need to be aware of all privacy concerns when a client is unable to independently manage the condition and interaction with caregivers is required. The use of physical agent modalities is appropriate as a preparatory method for occupational performance. State regulatory agencies may govern their use. It is the responsibility of each practitioner to complete the required training and follow the practice act of the state they reside in (Engel, 2013).

Chapter 18 Self-Study Activities (Answers Are Provided at the End of the Chapter)

1. **Correctly Answer the Multiple-Choice Questions based on the Following Case Study:**
   Sally is the only occupational therapist in a small outpatient clinic at a rural hospital. She is asked to evaluate Ms. Bottmeyer for bilateral hand pain. Ms. Bottmeyer is a 70-year-old widow who lives alone in a small mobile home. She reports that she is responsible for all of the indoor care of her home, but she pays a neighbor to take care of her lawn and outside maintenance. Sally notices during the initial interview with Ms. Bottmeyer that both of her hands have enlarged metacarpophalangeal joints. She has a swan-neck deformity on her left index finger and a boutonniere deformity on her right long finger. Both hands have a slight ulnar drift of the digits, with the dominant right hand being more pronounced than the left. Ms. Bottmeyer states that she has undergone extensive testing over the years, but she has never had a positive result for a rheumatoid factor test.

   Answer the following questions based on the case above:

   1. Given the treatment diagnosis on the therapy order and Sally's clinical observations, which is the most likely cause of Ms. Bottmeyer's hand pain?
      A. Rheumatoid arthritis
      B. Osteoarthritis
      C. Complex regional pain syndrome
      D. Fibromyalgia
   2. What assessment is most appropriate to use first with this client?
      A. Hospital Anxiety and Depression Scale
      B. Assessment of Motor and Processing Skills
      C. Disabilities of the Arm, Shoulder, and Hand Outcome Measure
      D. Fatigue Severity Scale

2. Based on the information provided below, fill out the primary areas of concern Sally will address during an occupational therapy evaluation.

Occupation	Treatment Setting and Client Demographics	
	26-year-old male who works full time as a roofer. You are seeing him in an acute rehabilitation setting following a fall off a roof and multiple fractures in his right arm and leg. The client is nonweight-bearing on his affected leg. He has developed CRPS in his dominant right hand following ORIF for a wrist fracture.	82-year-old female who is quite active in her community and lives alone in an accessible apartment. She still drives and volunteers 2 days per week at a local food pantry. You are seeing her in a long-term care facility following hip replacement for severe OA.
ADL		
Functional mobility in the home		
Community access		
Leisure		
Important life roles		

ORIF, open reduction internal fixation.

Chapter 18 Self-Study Answers

1. **Case Study Multiple-Choice Question Answers:**
   1. A: Rheumatoid arthritis. This condition typically presents with bilateral involvement of the hands as seen in this client. The enlarged metacarpophalangeal joints, additional joint deformities, and ulnar drift are all consistent with this condition. Osteoarthritis typically presents in a unilateral fashion, making this choice less likely. CRPS and Fibro both present with pain, but the pronounced joint abnormalities seen here are not typical of those conditions.
   2. C: Disabilities of the Arm, Shoulder, and Hand (DASH) Outcome Measure. This instrument is specifically designed for assessment of upper extremity (UE) dysfunction and has evidence relating to its effectiveness in adults with UE disorders in addition to those specifically with arthritis. Ms. Bottmeyer is not being seen inpatient, so the Hospital Anxiety and Depression Scale is not appropriate. The Assessment of Motor and Process Skills (AMPS) test may be an appropriate tool, but requires specialized training. It should not be used by untrained personnel. The evaluation order cites pain as her primary complaint; therefore, an assessment that looks at pain and function would be preferable to one that looks at the construct of fatigue, making the Fatigue Severity Scale an inappropriate choice.

2. Treatment setting and client demographics answers

Occupation	26-year-old male who works full time as a roofer.	82-year-old female who is quite active in her community and lives alone in an accessible apartment.
ADL	Initial concern would be activities of personal care. A typical order is: feeding oneself, performing simple grooming, management of a urinal, don/doff clothing. More advanced tasks would include washing and drying one's body and managing clothing during toileting.	Given that this client was independent with ADLs at home and only has lower body involvement with her current diagnosis, most simple self-care tasks should be occurring at a level where assistance is required to gather items. Quickly checking container opening, grooming, self-feeding, and upper body dressing will confirm this. Beyond that, the emphasis will be on lower body activities. The client will need to perform lower body activities while maintaining any hip precautions or weight-bearing restrictions she has been given. She will benefit from education regarding adaptive equipment to perform lower body dressing, and clothing management with toileting and bathing.
Functional mobility in the home	Mobility to perform the above duties would be the first area of concern. The client will need to access the kitchen, bedroom, and bathroom. Safety in transfer to the bed, wheelchair, commode, and shower are typical goals.	Bed mobility, transfers to bed, wheelchair, commode, and shower would be of primary importance during evaluation. These will allow maximum independence for self-care. This is presuming that the room, bath, and dining areas are accessible in this facility.

Occupation	26-year-old male who works full time as a roofer.	82-year-old female who is quite active in her community and lives alone in an accessible apartment.
Community access	Safe exit from the home in the event of an emergency is imperative. The client will also need to transfer into and out of an automobile for accessing the community for doctor appointments and other important tasks.	It is possible the client will attend physician appointments via personal family vehicle, so transfer in and out on the passenger side needs to be addressed along with wheelchair management on an uneven surface. These can be addressed as goals, though they may not be addressed during the initial evaluation.
Leisure	Determining what quiet leisure tasks the client can take part in will be of primary importance. Given the fact that he is nonweight-bearing on one leg and has poor use of his dominant hand, it is likely he will spend a considerable amount of time at home initially. Finding ways he can enjoy leisure tasks will help reduce the sense of isolation this may bring. If tasks can incorporate the dominant hand in ways it can be desensitized through use as a functional assist, this will help address the CRPS.	The client appears to have an active lifestyle for a person of her age. It is not clear from the case if she enjoys active leisure in addition to the listed activities. Ascertaining what types of leisure she currently enjoys will be a starting point. The volunteering she does indicates she wants to perform duties that are of service to others. Allowing her to participate (i.e., as appropriate) in visiting, assisting, or working with other (i.e., possibly more impaired) residents may give her a sense of purpose while she resides in this facility.
Important life roles	The case study does not address the client's marital status or if he has children. These will be important things to ascertain in setting goals for him. It will be important that he is able to fulfill important family roles as fully as possible while he is recovering. The role of worker/employee will be temporarily on hold during recovery and the financial impact of this will need to be addressed.	The client's family status is not addressed in the case study. One area to address in the evaluation will be any family roles the client currently fills. It is clear she fills homemaker, volunteer, and active community member roles. Discovering the occupations and meaningful activities related to these roles will need to be addressed during the evaluation.

References

Arnett, F. C., & Asassi, S. (2009). *Heredity and arthritis. American College of Rheumatology Patient and Caregiver Resources.* Retrieved from http://www.arcarthritisclinic.com/Documents/heredity.pdf

Arthritis Foundation. (2011). *Juvenile idiopathic arthritis treatment.* Retrieved from http://www.arthritis.org/about-arthritis/types/juvenile-idiopathic-arthritis-jia/treatment.php

Beukelman, T., Patkar, N. M., Saag, K. G., Tolleson-Rinehart, S., Cron, R. Q., DeWitt, E. M., . . . Ruperto, N. (2011). 2011 American College of Rheumatology recommendations for the treatment of juvenile idiopathic arthritis: Initiation and safety monitoring of therapeutic agents for the treatment of arthritis and systemic features. *Arthritis Care & Research (Hoboken), 63*(4), 465–482. doi:10.1002/acr.20460

Boop, C. L. T. (2014). Appendix II: Table of assessments. In M. E. Scaffa, B. A. B. Schell, G. Gillen, & E. S. Cohn (Eds.), *Willard and Spackman's occupational therapy* (12th ed., pp. 1109–1112). Philadelphia, PA: Lippincott Williams & Wilkins.

Cameron, M. H. (2013). *Physical agents in rehabilitation: From research to practice* (4th ed.). St. Louis, MO: Elsevier.

Centers for Disease Control and Prevention. (2013). *Childhood arthritis*. Retrieved from http://www.cdc .gov/arthritis/basics/childhood.htm

Centers for Disease Control and Prevention. (2015). *Fibromyalgia*. Retrieved from http://www.cdc.gov /arthritis/basics/fibromyalgia.htm

Children's Hospital of Wisconsin. (2015). *Juvenile rheumatoid arthritis*. Retrieved from http://www .chw.org/medical-care/rheumatology/conditions /juvenile-rheumatoid-arthritis/

deMos, M., de Bruijn, A. G., Huygen, F. J., Dielman, J. P., Stricker, B. H., & Sturkenboom, M. C. (2006). The incidence of complex regional pain syndrome: A population-based study. *Pain, 103*(1–2), 12–20.

Deshaies, L. (2013). Arthritis. In L. W. Pedretti, H. M. Pendleton, & W. Schultz-Krohn (Eds.), *Pedretti's occupational therapy: Practice skills for physical dysfunction* (7th ed., pp. 1003–1036). St. Louis, MO: Elsevier.

Engel, J. M. (2013). Evaluation and pain management. In L. W. Pedretti, H. M. Pendleton, & W. Schultz-Krohn (Eds.), *Pedretti's occupational therapy: Practice skills for physical dysfunction* (7th ed., pp. 718–728). St. Louis, MO: Elsevier.

Genetics Home Reference. (2015). *Psoriatic arthritis*. Retrieved from http://ghr.nlm.nih.gov/condition /psoriatic-arthritis

Gladman, D. D., Antoni, C., Mease, P., Clegg, D. O., & Nash, P. (2005). Psoriatic arthritis: Epidemiology, clinical features, course, and outcome. *Annals of the Rheumatic Diseases, 64*(Suppl 2), ii14–ii17. doi:10.1136/ard.2004.032482

Hammond, A. (2014). Rheumatoid arthritis, osteoarthritis, and fibromyalgia. In M. V. Radomski & C. A. T. Latham (Eds.), *Occupational therapy for physical dysfunction* (7th ed., pp. 1215–1243). Philadelphia, PA: Lippincott Williams & Wilkins.

Iliades, C. (2015). *The stages of osteoarthritis progression*. Retrieved from http://www.everydayhealth.com /osteoarthritis/stages-of-progression.aspx

Mayo Clinic. (2015a). *Diseases and conditions: Fibromyalgia*. Retrieved from http://www.mayoclinic.org/diseases -conditions/fibromyalgia/basics/definition/con-20019243

Mayo Clinic. (2015b). *Diseases and conditions: Psoriatic arthritis*. Retrieved from http://www.mayoclinic .org/diseases-conditions/psoriatic-arthritis/basics /definition/con-20015006

National Institute of Arthritis and Musculoskeletal and Skin Diseases. (2014). *Psoriatic arthritis overview*. Retrieved from http://www.niams.nih.gov/health _info/psoriatic_arthritis/psoriatic-arthritis.pdf

National Institute of Neurological Disorders and Stroke. (2015). *Complex regional pain syndrome: Fact sheet*. Retrieved from http://www.ninds.nih.gov/disorders /reflex_sympathetic_dystrophy/detail_reflex _sympathetic_dystrophy.htm

Rehabilitation Institute of Chicago. (2010). *Rehabilitation measures database: The rehabilitation clinician's place to find the best instruments to screen patients and monitor their progress*. Retrieved from http://www .rehabmeasures.org/rehabweb/allmeasures .aspx?PageView=Shared

Rogers, S. L. (2015). Common conditions that influence children's participation. In J. Case-Smith & J. C. O'Brien (Eds.), *Occupational therapy for children and adolescents* (7th ed., pp. 146–192). St. Louis, MO: Elsevier.

RSDSA. (2014). *Coping strategies*. Retrieved from http://rsds.org/coping-strategies/

Sandroni, P., Benrud-Larson, L. M., McClelland, R. L., & Low, P. A. (2003). Complex regional pain syndrome type I: Incidence and prevalence in Olmsted county, a population-based study. *Pain, 103*(1–2), 199–207. Retrieved from http://www.ncbi.nlm.nih.gov /pubmed/12749974

Shiel, W. C., Jr. (2015). *Rheumatoid arthritis classification*. Retrieved from http://www.emedicinehealth.com /rheumatoid_arthritis/page8_em.htm

Vaughn, P. (2014). Appendix I: Common conditions, resources and evidence—Arthritis. In M. E. Scaffa, B. A. B. Schell, G. Gillen, & E. S. Cohn (Eds.), *Willard and Spackman's occupational therapy* (12th ed., pp. 1098–1189). Philadelphia, PA: Lippincott Williams & Wilkins.

Amputations

Section I: Upper Limb Amputation and Prosthetics

Bambi Lombardi and Joyce Tyler

CHAPTER 19

Learning Objectives

- Identify the upper limb amputation levels and the clinical presentation of each level.
- Identify the standardized and nonstandardized assessments used in the preprosthetic evaluation of a person with an upper limb amputation.
- Construct a preprosthetic intervention plan for a person with an upper limb amputation.
- Construct a postprosthetic intervention plan for a person with an upper limb amputation.
- Describe the benefits and limitations of prosthetic options for a person with an upper limb amputation.

Key Terms

- *Activity-specific prosthesis*: Customized for a specific function or recreational activity. This allows the person with an upper limb amputation to resume meaningful and exciting activities that typical prosthetic options do not allow.
- *Amputation levels*: The upper limb amputation levels are finger, transcarpal, wrist disarticulation, transradial, elbow disarticulation, transhumeral, shoulder disarticulation, and interscapulothoracic amputation.
- *Bimanual skills training*: Training with both hands. This will occur with two prostheses if the person is missing two limbs or with one prosthesis and the contralateral limb if the person is missing one limb.
- *Body-powered prosthesis*: A prosthesis operated by a harness system and control cable that activates a terminal device by using exaggerated body movements.
- *Controls training*: The stage of prosthetic training that encourages mastery of the basic control of the prosthesis.

- *Electrically powered prosthesis (myoelectric)*: A prosthesis that is powered by a battery system. One type of an electrically powered prosthesis is a myoelectric prosthesis controlled by electromyography signals generated during muscle contractions.
- *Hybrid prosthesis*: A prosthesis that combines the use of body power and external power for function of the prosthesis.
- *Myocyte assessment*: Two opposing Myocytes are selected for control of a myoelectric prosthesis using surface electrodes and a biofeedback unit.
- *Passive functional prosthesis*: A lightweight prosthesis that has no active prehension, but provides opposition and aids in balancing and carrying.
- *Postprosthetic intervention*: The stage of prosthetic rehabilitation that incorporates the prosthesis in activities of daily living (ADLs).
- *Preprosthetic intervention or* preprosthetic phase: The stage of prosthetic rehabilitation that prepares the person with an upper limb amputation to accept the use of a prosthesis.
- *Repetitive drills training*: The stage of postprosthetic intervention that encourages practice with activities that incorporate grasping and releasing of various objects in different planes and axes.

Description

Upper limp amputation and prosthetics are an important part of occupational therapy practice. Occupational therapy practitioners must understand basic knowledge related to the various amputation levels along with each corresponding clinical presentation. Further, occupational therapy practitioners need to be able to choose and distinguish between the different screenings and assessments

Prosthesis: artifical body part.

available to yield an appropriate treatment plan. Treatment plans are critical throughout all facets of care; however, specific to amputation and prosthetics, it is crucial for the occupational therapist (OT) to review the benefits and limitations associated with each unique individual.

Etiology and Pathology

According to the most recent estimates concerning the prevalence of limb loss in the United States, there are approximately 541,000 people living with upper limb loss in the United States (Ziegler-Graham, MacKenzie, Ephraim, Travison, & Brookmeyer, 2008). An estimated 92% of people living with an upper extremity (UE) amputation lost their limb due to trauma (Ziegler-Graham et al., 2008). Other causes of upper limb amputation include tumor, disease, and congenital anomalies. As of January 2012, over 200 military service members have sustained upper limb loss as a result of the wars in Iraq and Afghanistan (Harvey et al., 2012). Each year an estimated 1,454 children are born in the United States with a congenital anomaly affecting the development of their upper limbs (Parker et al., 2010). In 2012, it was estimated that there were 9,840 upper limb amputation procedures performed in the United States (HCUP National

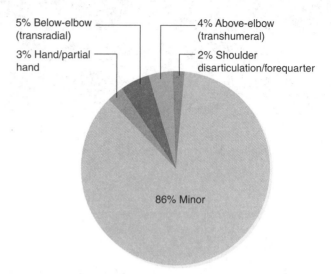

Figure 19-1 Incidence of acquired upper limb amputation.
Data from HCUP National Inpatient Sample (NIS) (2012) and Courtesy of the Amputee Coalition.

Inpatient Sample, 2012). See **Figure 19-1** for the incidence of acquired upper limb amputations.

Clinical Presentation

The levels of upper limb amputation are illustrated in **Figure 19-2** and described in **Table 19-1**. The higher

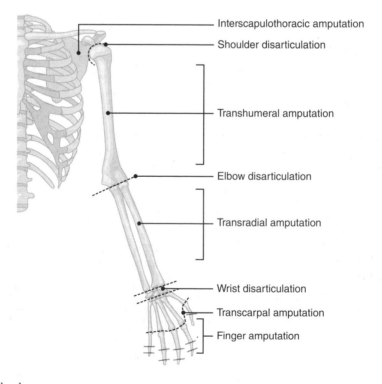

Figure 19-2 UE amputation levels.
Data from Westcoast Brace and Limb (2011).

the upper limb amputation, the more difficult it may be to use a prosthesis (e.g., activity-specific, body-powered, electrically powered, hybrid, passive functional) because fewer joints and muscles are available to control the prosthesis and the weight of the prosthesis is greater. For these and a variety of other reasons, a client may choose not to be a full-time prosthetic user in his or her daily activities (Biddiss & Chau, 2007). See Figure 19-2 for a depiction of upper limb amputation levels and **Table 19-1** for depictions and descriptions of the various amputation levels.

Surgical Considerations

Amputation surgery should be viewed as reconstructive surgery with the thought that the residual limb will be less painful and more functional than the limb prior to

Table 19-1 Amputation Levels	
Finger and Transcarpal Amputation	
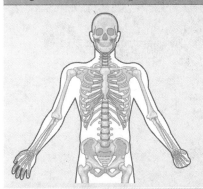	• Amputation through various bones of the hand. • Complete loss of the thumb results in 40% loss of hand function and 36% loss of the entire upper limb.* • This amputation level lends itself well to the use of a passive/nonprehensile prosthesis. • It is difficult to fabricate an aesthetically pleasing prosthesis that restores grasp.
Wrist Disarticulation	
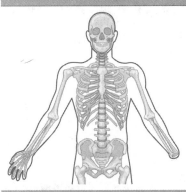	• The wrist joint is separated at the styloid process. • Very functional level for prosthetic usage. • The intact muscles provide full pronation and supination of the residual limb. About 50% of this ROM can be captured in a prosthesis.
Transradial Amputation	
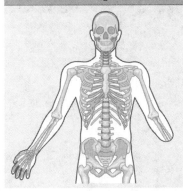	• Also known as below elbow amputation. • Amputation occurs through the radius and ulna. • Pronation and supination are maintained with longer residual limbs. • Complete loss of pronation and supination with proximal transradial amputations.

(continues)

Table 19-1 Amputation Levels (*continued*)

Elbow Disarticulation

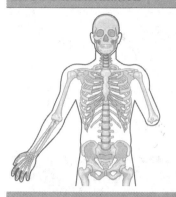

- The lower arm is removed at the elbow joint. The entire humerus is maintained.
- If the epicondyles are maintained, the prosthesis can capture active internal and external rotation and suspend the prosthesis.
- Due to the anatomic length, there is limited prosthetic componentry that can maintain elbow center equivalent to the unaffected side.

Transhumeral Amputation

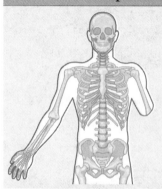

- Also known as above elbow amputation.
- Amputation occurs through the humerus. The elbow is no longer present.
- Loss of active humeral rotation in prosthesis.

Shoulder Disarticulation

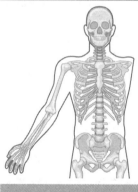

- In this procedure, the humerus is surgically removed from the scapula, clavicle, and the glenohumeral joint. The scapula remains. The clavicle may or may not be removed.
- No bones are cut during surgery.
- Muscle flaps can be used to maintain shoulder contour.

Interscapulothoracic Amputation

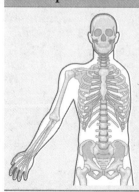

- Also known as a forequarter amputation.
- Often performed due to malignancy.
- The humerus, scapula, and clavicle are removed.
- Most mentally and physically debilitating UE amputation.
- Disfigurement is easily apparent through clothing if no prosthesis or shoulder cap is worn.

*Calculated from American Medical Association's Guides to the Evaluation of Permanent Impairment, fifth edition.
Modified with permission from Otto Bock Healthcare LP, Austin, TX

the amputation (Schnur & Meier, 2013). When amputation is necessary, conservation of residual limb length and uncomplicated wound healing are important. Before performing surgery, the surgeon should consult with the healthcare team, including the OT and prosthetist, to maximize a person's functional outcome. Functional goals are used to determine the most appropriate type of prosthesis; residual limb length directly affects the type of prosthesis that the limb can support (Keenan & Glover, 2013). Revision surgery may be considered to provide better prosthetic fit and function. Two indications for revision surgery are to improve the physical characteristics of the residual limb and to treat a painful stump. Removing excess soft tissue or providing better soft tissue coverage often improves the physical characteristics of the limb.

Screening and Assessments

The preprosthetic evaluation helps to establish a baseline of care for the person with a new amputation of the upper limb. Preprosthetic evaluation begins as soon as possible after surgery and identifies goals for preprosthetic intervention. Areas of treatment that are addressed include the following: psychological impact of injury, activities of daily living (ADLs), change of hand dominance, edema, hypersensitivity, range of motion (ROM), strength, and Myocyte selection. Once the prosthesis is received, therapeutic intervention shifts to operation and control of the prosthesis and its use in ADLs. **Tables 19-2** and **19-3** provide a summary of the screening and assessment process using standardized and nonstandardized approaches, respectively.

Table 19-2 Standardized Screening and Assessment Process

Assessments	Description
ROM/goniometry*	• Performance measure using a goniometer to measure joint ROM. • Important tool for establishing baseline information and documenting progress in rehabilitation. • Measurements of both the unaffected limb and the residual limb that do not fall in the normal range should be documented. Note ROM of trunk. • Note chest expansion and scapular mobility which are important with a cable-controlled system.
Manual muscle testing	• Performance measure that assesses muscle length and strength. • Integral part of a physical examination of the musculoskeletal and nervous systems. • Guides the prescription of a therapeutic exercise program. • The OT applies pressure in a specific direction. A score between 0 and 5 is assigned depending on how much the client is able to resist the pressure being applied by the OT.
COPM	• Self-reported outcome to assess an individual's perceived occupational performance in the areas of self-care, productivity, and leisure. • Semistructured interview with ordinal scale.

AM-ULA	• Performance measure for adults with upper limb amputation.
	• Eighteen items, clinician-rated assessment of multistep, functional tasks.
	• 0 to 4 rating scale is used to rate five aspects of performance:
	  ◦ Extent of completion
	  ◦ Speed
	  ◦ Quality of movement
	  ◦ Skillfulness of prosthetic use
	  ◦ Independence

ACMC	• Performance measure of a child or adult's capacity to *control* a myoelectric prosthesis. • Four-point capability scale is used to rate 24 prosthetic control items in areas of gripping, holding, releasing, and coordinating between hands. • A 2-day training course is required to become an ACMC rater.

(continues)

Table 19-2 Standardized Screening and Assessment Process (*continued*)

Assessments	Description
BBT of Manual Dexterity	• Performance measure of unilateral gross manual dexterity. • Transference of individual blocks within a partitioned box for 60 s. • Timed test. • The score is the number of blocks carried from one compartment to the other in 1 min. Each hand is scored separately.
JTHF	• Performance measure of unilateral hand function required for ADLs. • Timed test. Assesses speed, not quality of performance. • Lower score equals greater function. • Seven subtests performed on both the nondominant and dominant hands including the following: writing a letter, card turning, picking and placing small common objects, stacking checkers, simulated feeding tasks, and moving light and heavy objects.
OPUS-UEFS	• Self-reported outcome. • Twenty-eight-item questionnaire pertaining to an individual's performance of self-care and instrumental ADLs.
SHAP	• Performance measure to determine effectiveness of a terminal device. • Focuses on unilateral prosthetic performance. • Online scoring using SHAP software. Twenty-six timed tasks (i.e., 12 abstract object tasks and 14 ADLs). • Portable kit with standardized administration protocol.

DASH and *Quick*DASH	• Self-reported outcome to evaluate musculoskeletal disorders of the upper limb.
	• Thirty-item self-report questionnaire in the categories of upper limb physical function, symptoms, and social and role functioning.
	• A shortened 11-item version, known as the *Quick*DASH.
	• Two optional, four-item modules:
	  ◦ Work
	  ◦ Sports or performing arts
	• Scoring on a 5-point Likert scale with a lower score indicating less disability.

TAPES-R	• Self-reported outcome.
	• Fifty-four-item health-related quality of life questionnaire.
	• Measures the following:
	  ◦ Three items of psychosocial adjustment:
	    ▪ General adjustment
	    ▪ Social adjustment
	    ▪ Adjustment to limitation and activity restrictions
	  ◦ Two aspects of satisfaction:
	    ▪ Aesthetic
	    ▪ Functional satisfaction
	  ◦ Experience of phantom limb pain and residual limb pain
	  ◦ Frequency
	  ◦ Duration of each episode
	  ◦ Intensity of pain (*i.e., excruciating, horrible, distressing, discomforting, or mild*)
	  ◦ Interference with daily life (*i.e., a lot, quite a bit, moderately, a little bit, or not at all*)

*Lower extremity, trunk, and neck ROM should be evaluated in people with bilateral upper limb amputations. Good flexibility allows the client to use their feet if possible for greater functional independence (Mitsch, Walters, & Yancosek, 2014).

ACMC, Assessment of Capacity for Myoelectric Control; AM-ULA, Activities Measure for Upper Limb Amputees; BBT, Box and Block Test; COPM, Canadian Occupational Performance Measure; JTHF, Jebsen–Taylor Test of Hand Function; OPUS-UEFS, Orthotics and Prosthetics Users' Survey Upper Extremity Functional Status; SHAP, Southampton Hand Assessment Procedure.

Data from Department of Veterans Affairs & Department of Defense, 2014; Smith, Michael, and Bowker, 2004; Vaughn, 2014; and Wright, 2009.

Table 19-3 Nonstandardized Screening and Assessment Process

Assessments	Description
Interview	• Information about a person's occupational roles and tasks and the environment in which he or she lives.
Examination of Residual Limb	
Pain	• Check for phantom limb pain, phantom limb sensation, residual limb pain, and residual limb sensation.
	• Document the position of the phantom limb and the ability to move the phantom limb.
	• Assess the residual limb for light and deep touch, temperature, and proprioception. Diminished sensation indicates that a client may have trouble feeling pressure areas in the socket. The socket is the part of the prosthesis that encases the residual limb and connects the prosthesis to the body.
Hypersensitivity	• Palpate the residual limb and note any areas of hypersensitivity.
	• A hypersensitive limb may not be able to tolerate a prosthesis.
Shape	• Describe the shape of the residual limb.
	• After surgery, the shape of the residual limb will be bulbous (i.e., larger at the end than in the middle). Ace wraps or stump shrinkers are used to gradually shrink the limb to a conical shape.
	• A picture can be used to document shape.
Edema	• Document edema using a tape measure.
	• From a fixed point, measure the length and circumference of the residual limb.
	• Depending on residual limb length, circumference measurements are taken at 1–2 inches intervals.
Scar tissue	• Evaluate skin and joint flexibility.
	• Describe the presence of any scar tissue.
	• Adherent scar tissue restricts motion of the residual limb. When donning and doffing a socket, traction across a restricted scar can lead to skin breakdown.
Circulation	• Check the temperature of the residual limb and look for hair growth.
	• Warm temperature and hair growth indicates good circulation.
	• Good circulation is necessary for wound healing.
Skin integrity	• Thin skin, redness, and blisters indicate potential for skin breakdown when wearing a prosthesis.
Functional activity checklist	• Treatment is client directed.
	• An activity checklist is used to help the client identify activities that he or she would like to perform using a prosthesis.
	• Independence in these activities using a prosthesis becomes the goal of therapy.

Data from Department of Veterans Affairs & Department of Defense, 2014; Smith, Michael, and Bowker, 2004; Vaughn, 2014; and Wright, 2009.

Myocyte assessment and training should also be performed during the preprosthetic evaluation if a myoelectric prosthesis is being considered for the client. This should be a collaborative effort between the prosthetist and the OT (Tyler, 2014). Considerations include the following:

- Two opposing Myocytes are selected if the client has two muscles available for control.
- Adequate separation of two opposing Myocytes is the main objective when identifying the muscles to be used.
- Muscle strength and endurance should be considered to effectively operate a myoelectric prosthesis.

- One muscle site can be used with some types of prostheses if that is all the client has available for control due to scarring, grafts, and/or nerve damage. The prosthetist, OT, and client should collaborate to determine the best option.

Socket electrodes are hooked to a biofeedback unit, such as the MyoBoy (Ottobock) (**Figure 19-3**), Virtu-Limb (Touch Bionics Inc.), or MyoLab II (Motion Control, Inc.). The electrodes are placed over the muscle to identify the best Myocyte. Ideally, a flexor muscle site is used for pronation and closing of the terminal device of a prosthesis; an extensor muscle site is used for supination and opening of the terminal device. A signal is not

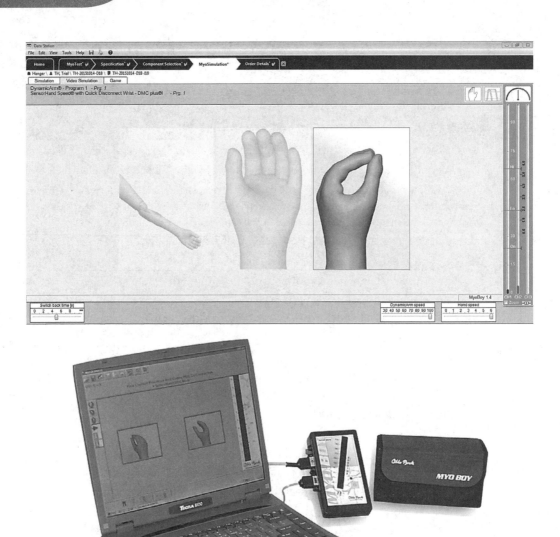

Figure 19-3 MyoBoy Virtual Evaluation and Training Tool.
Reproduced with the permission of Otto Bock HealthCare LP, Austin, TX.

easily transmitted through scars and grafts. It is best to place the entire electrode on the same type of skin (i.e., either all on the graft or scar area or all on unaffected skin) if possible. Independent activation of each muscle is practiced first and then the client progresses to adequate separation of opposing muscles. Cocontraction of two opposing muscles can be practiced as one alternative for use as a switching method in the prosthesis when there is more than one component to operate, such as a hand and wrist rotator. Myocyte training should begin with the upper limb in a relaxed position at or near midline. Once control is achieved at midline, training is completed with the limb in various positions to simulate reaching overhead, across midline, and to the floor.

Caution: Watch for signs of fatigue. Begin with 10- to 15-minute sessions and gradually increase time as strength and endurance increases (Tyler, 2014).

Interventions

Preprosthetic Intervention

Preprosthetic intervention is oftentimes a missed stage in the rehabilitation of a person with an upper limb amputation. It should be looked on as the time to prepare the client to accept the use of a prosthesis and become a good prosthetic user. The following should be considered during the preprosthetic phase of rehabilitation (Swanson, Atkins, & Tingleaf, 2003b).

Edema control and residual limb shaping: It is important to decrease volume to prepare for wearing the prosthesis. Compression bandaging such as figure-of-eight wrapping, a compressogrip sleeve or Tubigrip can be used to shape a limb, reduce edema, and begin limb desensitization. Initially, compression is worn 24 hours a day (Tyler, 2014).

Desensitization and scar management of the residual limb: Hypersensitivity may make it impossible for a client to tolerate a prosthesis. Techniques to decrease hypersensitivity include fabrics, particles (e.g., beans, rice, and macaroni), textures (e.g., felt, denim, and terry cloth), tapping, vibration, fluidotherapy, massage (i.e., light and deep), and weight-bearing. Skin flexibility and joint mobility can be improved with scar tissue management to decrease the risk of pressure from the prosthesis (Swanson et al., 2003b).

Residual limb care: Washing and drying the residual limb on a daily basis will encourage daily care and inspection of the limb. This will assist with awareness of changes to the residual limb and help the client to become comfortable with the new image of the limb. A lotion that is water based and not oil based should be used to toughen the skin and improve tolerance of the prosthetic socket (Swanson et al., 2003b).

Management of phantom limb pain: Mirror therapy can be used to alleviate phantom limb pain. A study of mirror therapy in clients with unilateral limb loss and phantom limb pain was conducted by Ramachandran and Rogers-Ramachandran (1996). Clients looked at a mirror image of their intact limb inside a mirror box. They were asked to slowly move the intact limb and to slowly mimic this movement with their residual limb. Eight out of ten subjects reported significant improvement with phantom limb pain, and in one case, repeated practice with the mirror box led to a permanent disappearance of the phantom arm and the hand became telescoped into the stump near the shoulder (Ramachandran & Rogers-Ramachandran, 1996).

Improve and maintain joint ROM: After injury, clients tend to hold their residual limbs in a protected position. It is important that a person performs ROM exercises for all motions of the residual limb to prevent soft tissue contractures from developing. Initially, low load prolonged stretching can be completed in supine. A general guideline is to hold each stretch for 30 seconds and repeat a minimum of five repetitions. Clients can gradually increase the duration of each stretch and eventually decrease the number of repetitions. Clients should attempt to complete a stretching program two to three times per day. If self-stretches are not successful, passive stretching in therapy or splinting may be required. After limb loss, a client frequently compensates with shoulder elevation on the affected side. It is important to emphasize proper body mechanics and body symmetry during activities to minimize incorrect postures that can lead to overuse and cumulative trauma injuries (Tyler, 2014).

Increase muscle strength: An individual must rely on core strength where arms were once used for support and balance. Completing activities in therapy while sitting on a therapy ball can help with trunk stability and core strengthening (Tyler, 2014). In addition to core strengthening, scapular stabilization and shoulder and elbow strengthening should be encouraged depending on the level of amputation. Amputee weight cuffs, a pulley system, and exercise bands can help increase muscle strength. The biofeedback units mentioned earlier can be used to reeducate muscles and increase the muscle strength of isolated muscles that will be used in the control of a myoelectric prosthesis.

Physical conditioning and endurance training: An important preprosthetic intervention that is a prerequisite for prosthetic training is achieving optimal physical conditioning. Exercises such as low-impact aerobics, aquatics, walking, and jogging are activities that can improve endurance, body image, and the physical condition of the body.

ADL training: ADLs during preprosthetic intervention should focus on the suggestion of adaptive techniques to promote self-care. Minimal use of adaptive devices is encouraged because once the client receives their prosthesis, it becomes a tool for completion of self-care tasks and the adaptive equipment may not be necessary. One-handed techniques can be introduced for the person with a unilateral upper limb amputation but it is important not to develop one-handedness. There can be a rejection of the prosthesis during prosthetic training if the client takes the attitude that they can do most things with one hand. ADL training for the person with a bilateral amputation during preprosthetic intervention should focus on adaptive equipment and techniques that can assist with independence prior to receiving a prosthesis. The person with a bilateral amputation is typically dependent on someone for their personal and basic needs prior to receiving their prostheses. This person can benefit from specialized rehabilitation to explore ways to approach self-care using adaptive equipment and foot skills for basic activities with the intent to perform these tasks with and without a prosthesis.

Change of dominance: The person with a unilateral amputation of the dominant side must undergo training to change hand dominance. The goals of this training should be to increase radial digit coordination and develop separation of the radial and ulnar sides of the hand. Activities such as checkers, dot-to-dot activity worksheets, printing name and address, and picking up marbles and dropping them one by one out of the small finger side of the hand can develop the fine motor skills necessary for handwriting and change of dominance (Yancosek & Gulick, 2012).

Psychological Support in the Grieving Process

Psychosocial healing is difficult and should not be overlooked because the remaining areas of treatment will not be adequately addressed. Since a person cannot be cured of their amputation, they need assistance to accept the amputation in order to heal. The five stages of grieving (i.e., denial, anger, bargaining, depression, and acceptance) should be considered throughout the intervention process (Tyler, 2014).

Postprosthetic Intervention

Primary concerns of individuals with amputations were reported as "fear of the unknown, loss of self-esteem, loss of self-confidence, fear of rejection, and loss of occupational roles" (Smurr, Gulick, Yancosek, & Ganz, 2008). Each of these concerns is within the scope of occupational therapy practice. All members of the rehabilitation team should provide psychological support (Smurr et al., 2008); however, occupational therapy practitioners are especially well suited to incorporate psychosocial support into treatment given the OT's holistic view of the client. **Table 19-4** provides a summary of the benefits and limitations with each prosthetic option.

Table 19-4 Benefits and Limitations of Prosthetic Options

Prosthetic Option	Benefits	Limitations
Passive functional • Similar in appearance to the unaffected limb	• Provides opposition and aids in balancing and carrying • Lightweight • Simple • Little maintenance • Realistic appearance • Good option for partial hands	• No active prehension • Limited function • High cost for custom design • Decreased durability
Body powered • Operated by a harness system	• Moderately lightweight • Durable • Environmentally resistant • Proprioception through the harness system (i.e., kinesthetic feedback) • Reduced cost and maintenance	• Limited pinch force • Uncomfortable harness • Axilla anchor (i.e., possible nerve entrapment syndrome) • Limited functional ROM due to harness system • Gross limb movement • Increased energy expenditure to operate terminal device • Poor static and dynamic cosmesis
Electrically powered • Powered by a battery system. One type is an electrically powered myoelectric controlled by electromyography signals generated during muscle contractions	• Stronger grip force • Moderate or no harnessing • Improved comfort • Increased functional envelope (ROM) • Minimal energy expenditure • Less body movement to operate • Moderate aesthetics	• Can be heavy • Expensive • Limited sensory feedback • Extensive therapy training

Table 19-4 Benefits and Limitations of Prosthetic Options (*continued*)

Prosthetic Option	Benefits	Limitations
Hybrid • Combines the use of body power and external power	• Reduced weight compared to all electric • Simultaneous control of the elbow and terminal device	• Less pinch with cable-controlled terminal device • Difficult to lift battery-powered terminal device
Activity specific • Customized for a specific function or recreational activity	• Designed for a specific activity when typical prosthetic options are not sufficient • Improves quality of life by allowing clients to resume meaningful and exciting activities • Helps people feel "normal"	

Data from Keenan and Glover (2013) and Mitsch et al. (2014)

Prosthetic Training

A client should complete preprosthetic treatment before moving on to prosthetic training with their prosthesis. In order to integrate the prosthesis into ADLs, the client must have knowledge of the operation and performance of the prosthesis and initiate learning to control the prosthesis, practice repetitive drills, and perform bimanual tasks (Smurr et al., 2009). Start with basic operation and performance of the prosthesis. The prosthetist and the OT team should work closely together at this early stage of prosthetic training to assure proper fit and operation of the prosthesis.

Donning and doffing: The client should be independent in donning and doffing the prosthesis. This should be thoroughly reviewed with the prosthetist at the time of fitting and practiced during each therapy session. There are several methods used for donning a prosthesis depending on the level of amputation and complexity of the prosthesis. Methods used are push-in, pull-in using a donning sock, or a silicone liner-assisted method (Tyler, 2014). Once the prosthesis is donned, a prosthetic wear and care schedule should be discussed with the client. A wearing schedule that gradually increases the wear time so the residual limb can develop a tolerance to the socket is suggested. Should there be any issues with skin concerns, encourage the client to visit the prosthetist to make adjustments in the socket. Cleaning and caring for the prosthesis should be discussed with the client. Using a mild soap and water to clean the inside of the socket is suggested. Inspection of the prosthesis should be encouraged to make sure that it is functioning properly as well. Continued limb hygiene is recommended now that the limb is enclosed in a socket (Swanson, Atkins, & Tingleaf, 2003a).

Controls training: The client should first master basic control of the prosthesis. The client can sit facing the OT practitioner and mirror (i.e., mimic) their actions while moving the terminal device, wrist rotator, or elbow of the prosthesis to match the OT practitioner. Incorporate movements away from the body such as overhead, out to the side, across the body, and straight down toward the floor. Once mastered in the sitting position, repeat the procedure in a standing position (Tyler, 2014). In addition, many of today's prosthetic devices have the ability to see the biofeedback of muscle activity by Bluetooth programming and computer software when a myoelectric option is chosen. This provides visual feedback of a client's ability to control muscle signals and can be great feedback for the prosthetist on socket fit if there are any issues with function.

Practice repetitive drills and activities: Once the client has an understanding of basic control, activities that incorporate grasp and release of various objects in different planes and axes can begin. Practice with objects of various shapes, sizes, weights, densities, and textures. Begin with solid objects where no adjustment of grip force is required, then switch to lighter, softer objects. Work first in sitting and progress to standing and walking. Learning proportional control will give precise control of the prosthesis. Proportional control means the stronger the muscle contraction, the faster the overall grasp. A lighter muscle contraction produces a slower, more delicate grasp. Placing the terminal device in the most optimal position before initiating grasp/release (e.g., prepositioning) minimizes compensatory movements and reduces unnecessary or awkward movements (Tyler, 2014). To master proportional control and prepositioning, the following objects can be used:

- One-inch wood squares
- Cotton balls
- Ping pong balls
- Styrofoam cups (e.g., empty and with water)
- Potato chips
- Transferring objects from one hand to the other (e.g., in different planes)

Bimanual skills training: This is the longest and most challenging phase of prosthetic training. Practice, repetition, and training are the keys to success in this phase. The use of a functional activity checklist can assist in determining which tasks are most useful and meaningful to the client. Demonstration of tasks by an experienced prosthetic user can assist the new user in identifying ways to accomplish a task more efficiently. Credible Internet sites can be a great resource for videos that show accomplished users. Here is a list of common activities to practice:

- Cutting food
- Tying shoelaces
- Opening a tube of toothpaste
- Using scissors to cut paper
- Zipping a jacket
- Donning socks
- Buckling a belt
- Stirring (e.g., in a bowl)
- Using a fork and knife
- Folding tasks (e.g., towels and clothes)
- Buttering bread
- Hammering a nail
- Assembly tasks using a screwdriver
- Opening and closing various types of packages, boxes, containers, and jars

There are other areas that therapy should focus on with a person with an upper limb amputation who is using a prosthesis; these include:

- *Recreational activities*: Speak with the prosthetist about recreational or sport adaptations to the prosthesis.

- *Return to work issues*: Will the prosthesis be functional back in the client's work environment or is a job change necessary?
- *Energy conservation*: A prosthetic user expends more energy and must learn to minimize efforts when using their prosthesis.

Referrals and Discharge Considerations

Reevaluation should be ongoing in the prosthetic training process. It is important for the OT to continually assess the abilities of the client with upper limb loss to determine if goals have been reached or if the client has plateaued. Functional outcome measures and activity checklists can be used to determine the progress of the client. The timeline can vary depending on the motivation of the client, the level of amputation, the healing of skin grafts and wounds, the OT and prosthetist's skill level, and of course, the insurance coverage.

Management and Standards of Practice

The OT and occupational therapy assistant (OTA) collaborate using clinical reasoning, activity analysis, and outcome measures to implement the most effective and comprehensive intervention plan that will ultimately promote optimal independence, safety, and quality of life. The OT must also work closely with the prosthetist in determining the most appropriate prosthetic option for the person with an upper limb amputation. Realistic expectations for function must be established from the beginning when discussing these options. The OT's primary concern for the person with an upper limb amputation should be using the prosthesis to increase independence with ADLs and improved quality of life.

Section II: Lower Limb Amputation and Prosthetics

Kristina Reid and Ken Eick

Learning Objectives

- Identify the lower limb amputation levels and the clinical presentation of each level.
- Identify the immediate postoperative needs of the client with a lower limb amputation.
- Describe the main prosthetic components of a lower extremity prosthesis.
- Discuss occupational therapy implications regarding rehabilitation of the lower extremity amputee.

Key Terms

- *Amputation levels*: The lower extremity amputation levels are partial foot, Symes, transtibial, knee disarticulation, transfemoral, and hip disarticulation.
- *Early rehabilitation phase*: During this phase, the amputee may be receiving home care, outpatient services, or care in a skilled nursing or rehabilitation center. Considerations during this four- to six-week period include residual limb care, shrinkage, healing without complications, and pregait.
- *Foot/ankle assemble*: The distal component of the prosthesis and type of foot determines both stability during gait and the ability to walk on uneven surfaces. Gait training should be customized based on the characteristics of the foot.
- *Immediate postoperative phase*: This phase typically lasts three to five days beginning after surgery and including the client's acute care hospital stay.
- *Knee*: A prosthetic knee must offer both stability and normal gait characteristics relating to the knee (i.e., flexion at the knee and timing during swing).
- *Pylon*: The component that connects the foot/ankle assembly to the socket. It can be either endoskeleton (i.e., made of an adjustable inner skeleton) or exoskeleton (i.e., a rigid outer shell of composite material containing no adjustability but extremely durable).
- *Rehabilitation phase*: Typically involves training with a preparatory prosthesis, which includes donning the prosthesis, monitoring proper sock ply, ambulation with the proper assistive device and setting, and moving toward goals of independence.
- *Residual limb*: The section of the intact extremity after amputation surgery.
- *Shrinker*: A sock-like garment usually made up of elastic or rubber-reinforced cotton and used for volume control and edema. Shrinkers come in a variety of sizes to create the proper compression.
- *Socket*: The component of the prosthesis that supports and contains the residual limb.
- *Suspension*: The mechanism that links the prosthesis to the residual limb.

Description

Rehabilitation of the individual with lower limb amputation requires collaboration among the entire rehabilitation team. This team typically consists of the client, surgeon, physician, prosthetist, OT, and physical therapist (PT). The role of the OT team in assisting the individual with a lower limb amputation typically involves instruction on ADLs, residual limb care, and prosthetic donning and doffing. This is instrumental in the immediate postoperative care of the client with a lower limb amputation. The OT practitioners must understand the prosthetic components and the rehabilitation process of individuals with lower limb amputation to maximize functional outcomes. Input from the OT in UE strength and dexterity can have an impact on the selection of prosthetic components and ultimately the level of independence.

Etiology and Pathology

The prevalence of lower extremity amputations in the United States far exceeds that of UE amputations. Although we have seen a decline in nontraumatic lower limb amputations in the diabetic population, peripheral vascular disease is still considered the most common secondary cause with a rate of 3.9 per 1,000 (Li, Burrows, Gregg, Albright, & Geiss, 2012). According to the literature, the main cause among those living with limb loss is vascular disease (54%), which includes diabetes and peripheral arterial disease, trauma (45%), and cancer (<2%) (Ziegler-Graham et al., 2008). Lower extremity amputations are performed by vascular or orthopedic surgeons with the goal of surgery being to provide a viable residual limb that has optimal biomechanical function with the prosthesis and mobility. The ultimate goal for training and prosthetic prescription is to return the client back to prior function, and provide components to enhance mobility and support for an energy efficient gait. See **Figure 19-4** for a depiction of lower extremity amputation levels.

Clinical Presentation

The higher the level of amputation, the more energy required for mobility and ambulation. In addition, clients who have received their amputation as a result of peripheral vascular disease associated with smoking and diabetes have lower activity tolerance due to secondary cardiovascular conditions, which may result in additional complications (Keenan & Glover, 2013). Clients with unilateral transtibial amputations typically have a good prognosis for rehabilitation and functional ambulation with a prosthesis. Individuals with bilateral transtibial amputations typically have higher energy expenditure but are likely to perform functional ambulation with the proper prosthetic components. Individuals with transfemoral amputations require higher energy expenditure, which suggests that young and/or healthy individuals

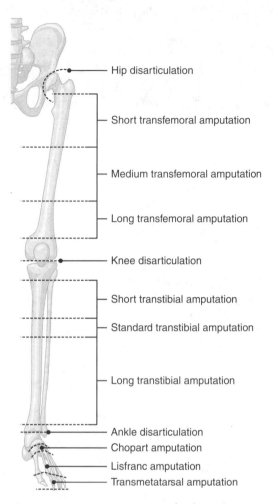

Figure 19-4 Lower extremity amputation levels.

have a higher chance of functional ambulation. For older individuals or those with additional health issues, achieving functional independence with a prosthesis may be more difficult. Clients with bilateral transfemoral amputations may have the greatest difficulty achieving functional independence using a prosthesis and many will choose wheelchairs for functional mobility (O'Sullivan & Schmitz, 2007). **Table 19-5** provides a summary of the types of lower extremity amputation levels.

Preprosthetic Screening and Assessments

The person with a lower extremity amputation will be seen by both physical therapy and occupational therapy immediately postoperatively. Communication within the rehabilitation team is essential in the coordination of care. The initial postoperative focus is on the condition

Table 19-5 Lower Extremity Amputation Levels and Descriptions

Level	Description
Partial foot	• Chopart—amputation at the talonavicular and calcaneocuboid joints • Lisfranc—amputation at the tarsometatarsal joint • Transmetatarsal—transection amputation at the level of the metatarsals
Ankle disarticulation	• Loss of the foot at the level of the ankle joint • Symes-ankle disarticulation in which the heel pad is preserved and used at the base of the residual limb for weight-bearing
Transtibial	• Transection of the tibia/fibula resulting in an amputation below the knee • Short transtibial—when greater than 80% of the calf is removed • Standard transtibial—when between 80% and 50% of the calf is removed • Long transtibial—when less than 50% of the calf is removed
Knee disarticulation	• Loss of the entire lower segment (i.e., tibia and fibula) at the level of the knee
Transfemoral	• Transection of the femur resulting in an amputation above the knee • Short transfemoral—when greater than 65% of the femoral length is removed. Creating a short lever arm for prosthetic function. • Medium transfemoral—between 65% and 40% of the femoral length is removed • Long transfemoral—less than 40% of the femoral length is removed
Hip disarticulation	• Loss of the entire femur • Pelvis remains fully intact

Data from Seymour, 2002.

of the residual limb and safe mobility. Many individuals who have undergone amputation surgery will have preexisting conditions that may further reduce mobility (Keenan & Glover, 2013). **Table 19-6** provides a summary of postoperative assessments for individuals of lower limb amputations.

Interventions

The initial focus of interventions in the immediate postoperative phase for the person with an amputation is on care of the residual limb, and independence with mobility and ADLs. As the time between amputation and prosthetic fitting decreases, less likely complications may develop, which promotes improved functional outcomes (May & Lockard, 2011). Both the PT and OT practitioners will provide family education on wound care, limb wrapping, bed mobility, transfers, and wheelchair propulsion (Mitsch, Walters, & Yancosek, 2014). Determining the client's ability to balance and sit at the side of the bed, as well as transferring safely to protect the residual

limb, is critical during this phase (May & Lockard, 2011). In addition, maintaining a clean environment for healing of the sutures is essential, as well as prepping the residual limb for prosthetic utilization. Immediate postoperative infection control involves care of the postoperative bandages, protection of the residual limb, and client education. A variety of postoperative dressings are used for edema control; **Table 19-7** provides a summary of postoperative dressings.

Contracture management during the postoperative phase may decrease the delay in prosthetic fitting and allow for a more functional gait during the prosthetic training phase. Intervention for contracture management begins with proper positioning in an acute care setting and continues with stretching into the early rehabilitation and rehabilitation phases.

Early rehabilitation should focus on bed mobility, sitting, transfers, residual limb shaping, and early gait training without the use of a prosthesis. Continuation of preparing the limb for the prosthesis involves the use of a shrinker to shape the limb. The residual limb will need to go through significant reductions

Table 19-6 Assessment Process for Individuals with Lower Limb Amputations

Assessment	Description
PEQ—Standardized assessment	• Self-reported questionnaire used to assess perceived quality of life and functional abilities.
Manual muscle testing	• Assessment of UE strength and dexterity to assist with determination of prosthetic components (e.g., management of suspension donning and doffing) and use of appropriate assistive devices.
Residual limb examination	• To decrease the exposure to environmental pathogens, removal of postoperative bandages is unessential by rehab support staff for the first 3 to 5 days postoperatively. Management and monitoring healing of the suture line should be the role of the nursing staff and physician, with exposure of the suture line kept to a minimum. • Check for phantom limb pain, phantom limb sensation, residual limb pain, and residual limb sensation. • The residual limb may have an initial increase in size due to surgical trauma, edema, and muscle size. The limb must be wrapped to encourage shrinking of the residual limb tissue (i.e., as the muscle atrophies). Then, the limb can be prepared for socket fit.
ROM	• Assessment of common joint contractures based on amputation level (e.g., hip flexion and adduction for transfemoral and knee flexion for transtibial).
Functional status	• ADLs • Bed mobility • Transfers
Cognitive function and emotional status	• Assessment of cognitive function may be required to evaluate the client's ability to properly don and doff the prosthesis and edema control appliances. • Acceptance and body image to determine referral to support system.
Home evaluation	• Home modifications such as a transfer tub bench and toilet grab bars may be required for safety early in prosthetic training and when not wearing the prosthesis.

PEQ, Prosthesis Evaluation Questionnaire.
Data from Keenan and Glover (2013), Mitsch, Walters, and Yancosek (2014), and O'Sullivan and Schmitz (2007).

Table 19-7 Summary of Lower Limb Amputation Postoperative Dressings

Postoperative Dressing	Advantages	Disadvantages
Soft dressing	• Easily applied with no trauma to the limb during application • Covers the suture line	• Offers minimal protection to the limb • No edema control • No shaping • Limited desensitization of the limb
Elastic wrap	• Easy to remove to allow for inspection of the suture • No trauma to the limb during application • Helps to prevent swelling	• Must be trained to apply • If donned improperly may cause uneven compression and a tourniquet effect • Does not stay in place • Offers minimal limb protection • Potential for contractures
*Shrinker**	• Easily applied • Able to be removed to allow for inspection of the suture • Helps to prevent swelling and helps shape the residual limb	• Offers minimal protection to the limb • May be difficult to don without assistance and may cause shearing of skin if "pulling" on • Potential for contractures

Table 19-7 Summary of Lower Limb Amputation Postoperative Dressings (*continued*)

Postoperative Dressing	Advantages	Disadvantages
Rigid removable dressing[†]	• Removable to inspect the limb • Desensitizes the limb • Controls swelling • Excellent protection to the limb and the suture line • May use a pylon system for early weight-bearing up to but not exceeding 20 pounds	• Cannot be used on a bulbous limb • May be difficult to apply after removal • Must be closely monitored for volume changes • Potential for contractures
Adjustable postoperative preparatory prosthetic system (APOPPS) Bivalve plastic brace that acts as a knee immobilizer besides providing ridged protection to residual limb[†]	• Protects the residual limb • Prevents knee flexion contracture • Easy to apply • Potential for early weight-bearing • Protects the residual limb	• No volume or edema control • Not custom (i.e., off the shelf sizing)
Immediate postoperative prosthesis (IPOP) Cast extending above the knee usually made of fiberglass or plaster	• Applied in surgery, which greatly reduces the amount of postsurgical edema • Custom fit to the client • Excellent protection to the limb and the suture line • Volume control • Potential for weight-bearing • Nonremovable, therefore less exposure to infection	• Difficulty in ability to inspect the limb • Costly cast changes • Specialized/trained staff is necessary • Weight-bearing is unpredictable

*Clients with transfemoral amputations may use this earlier as application of elastic wrap of the residual limb is difficult due to the length and differences in soft tissue.

[†]Only used for clients with transtibial amputations.

Data from May and Lockard (2011), O'Sullivan and Schmitz (2007), and Seymour (2002).

in size until it stabilizes. When the residual limb volume stabilizes and the suture line is well healed, the individual can be fit for a preparatory prosthesis. **Table 19-8** provides a summary of postoperative management and intervention for individuals of lower limb amputations.

Referrals and Discharge Planning

Input from the OT may be used to select proper components for the prosthesis. Considerations such as strength for ambulation with and without an assistive device, functional ADLs, recreational hobbies, cognition, and safety will play a role. Once the individual is fit with their prosthesis, prosthetic training will occur. The OT team continues to address ADLs, and education of prosthetic management application, wearing schedule, and proper donning and doffing techniques. It will be even more critical for the individual to inspect the condition of the residual limb daily once they begin ambulation. The fit of the prosthetic socket directly affects the biomechanical alignment and successful prosthetic outcomes. UE and intact cognition is required for donning and doffing some types of suspension. Inadequate strength and dexterity may be a concern with the safety of improperly donning the prosthesis. Proper donning and doffing of the prosthesis is also critical for minimizing gait deviations and risk of falls; therefore, it is imperative that

Table 19-8 Intervention and Management for Individuals with Lower Limb Amputations

Intervention and Management	Description
Residual limb care and wrapping*	• Instruction on residual limb care and proper hygiene. • Edema management.
Positioning and contracture management	• Proper positioning should be emphasized to decrease flexion contractures. • Supine—both legs extended and in neutral abduction. Pillows should not be used under the residual limb. • Side-lying—the residual limb should be positioned on the top; resting with 0° of hip and knee flexion with a pillow placed between the knees. • Prone—the prone position should be encouraged if tolerated. • Sitting—clients with a transtibial amputation should have the residual limb resting on a straight surface to prevent the limb from hanging down into knee flexion and use of an extension board should be encouraged when sitting in a wheelchair.
ADLs	• Bed mobility with and without the prosthesis. • Sitting balance at the end of the bed. • Safe transfers from the wheelchair to the bed, toilet, furniture, and car; with and without the prosthesis. • Self-maintenance skills (e.g., housekeeping and cooking).
Mobility	• Basic wheelchair mobility may be taught prior to use of the prosthesis. • Individual may use a standard or wheeled walker prior to use of prosthesis (i.e., depending on strength). Once a prosthesis begins to be worn, a rolling walker is recommended to encourage a more normal gait pattern. • During standing, attention must be on safety and balance in single limb support prior to prosthetic use, and to equal weight-bearing once the prosthesis is worn.
Strengthening	• UE strengthening will aid in mobility with an assistive device. • Core strengthening is important in all phases to promote normal gait with the prosthesis. • Functional activities of UE are used to encourage sitting balance (e.g., tossing and catching). • Encouraging normal weight shifting activities in sitting will assist in preparing the individual for prosthetic training later in rehabilitation.
Instruction of donning and doffing lower extremity prosthesis	• Proper application of the prosthesis is critical for safety when ambulating (e.g., individuals must understand the proper application of liners, socks, and suspension systems).
Client education	• Care of the residual limb and prosthetic wear time. • Diabetic management and care of the intact lower extremity may be required for many of our clients. Providing a long handled mirror may assist the client with foot inspection.

*Ideal residual limb shape for a client with a transfemoral amputation is conical and transtibial is cylindrical.
Data from Keenan and Glover (2013), Mitsch et al. (2014), and O'Sullivan and Schmitz (2007).

the individual is instructed on proper socket fit and application. The client will continue to manage volume fluctuations through the use of prosthetic socks during the day and a shrinker at night. Volume changes need to be monitored by the client and rehabilitation team. In addition, the OT team members should instruct the individual on safety and fall recovery. Clients are ready for discharge after they reach independence and safety in ADLs and mobility, which typically involves follow-up with a prosthetist for continuation of prosthetic needs and monitoring. Follow-up is necessary to recognize changes in both fit and gait as the limb matures.

Management and Standards of Practice

Occupational therapy practitioners working in the area of amputations and prosthetics need to ensure that they are maintaining an open line of communication with the surgeon, physicians, PT, and prosthetist. This will ensure safe and appropriate therapeutic recommendations and treatment. This will also facilitate communication with the OTA, who, if involved, will carry out specific interventions.

Chapter 19 Self-Study Activities: Upper Limb Amputation and Prosthetics (Answers Are Provided at the End of the Chapter)

Matching Amputation Level to Description of Amputation Level: (Levels May Be Used More Than Once)	
Amputation Level	**Description of Amputation Level**
A. Finger and transcarpal amputation B. Wrist disarticulation C. Transradial amputation D. Elbow disarticulation E. Transhumeral amputation F. Shoulder disarticulation G. Interscapulothoracic amputation	1. _____ Removal of the humerus, scapula, and clavicle. 2. _____ Amputation occurs through the humerus. The elbow is no longer present. 3. _____ Amputation is performed where the humerus meets the clavicle, scapula, and glenohumeral joint. 4. _____ Amputation occurs through the radius and ulna. 5. _____ Amputation through various bones of the hand. 6. _____ The wrist joint is separated at the styloid process. 7. _____ The lower arm is removed at the elbow joint. The entire humerus is maintained. 8. _____ Most mentally and physically debilitating upper limb amputation. 9. _____ This amputation level lends itself well to the use of a passive/nonprehensile prosthesis. 10. _____ Muscle flaps can be used to maintain the contour of the shoulder at this level of amputation. 11. _____ The intact muscles provide full pronation and supination of the residual limb at this level. 12. _____ Loss of active humeral rotation in the prosthesis at this level. 13. _____ Due to the anatomic length, there is limited prosthetic componentry that can maintain the elbow center equivalent to the unaffected side at this level. 14. _____ Also known as "below elbow."

Matching Standardized and Nonstandardized Assessments with the Descriptions of Each Assessment

Assessment	Description of Assessment
A. Circulation **B.** TAPES-R **C.** ROM/goniometry **D.** JTHF **E.** Manual muscle testing **F.** ACMC **G.** BBT of Manual Dexterity (BBT) **H.** Pain **I.** DASH **J.** Interview **K.** Scar tissue **L.** Functional activity checklist **M.** Edema **N.** Skin integrity	**1.** _____ Timed test for transference of individual blocks within a partitioned box for 60 s. **2.** _____ Documents the length and circumference of the residual limb from a fixed point using a tape measure. **3.** _____ Evaluates skin and joint flexibility. **4.** _____ Performance measure that assesses muscle length and strength. **5.** _____ Checks for hair growth and temperature of the residual limb. **6.** _____ Performance measure using a device to measure joint ROM. **7.** _____ Used to identify which tasks are most useful and meaningful to the client when using their prosthesis. **8.** _____ Fifty-four-item self-report questionnaire measuring psychosocial adjustment and satisfaction with a prosthesis. **9.** _____ Thin skin, redness, and blisters indicate potential for skin breakdown when wearing a prosthesis. **10.** _____ Seven subtests performed with both the nondominant and dominant hand including the following: writing a letter, card turning, picking and placing small common objects, stacking checkers, simulated feeding tasks, and moving light and heavy objects. **11.** _____ Assesses phantom limb pain, phantom limb sensation, residual limb pain, and residual limb sensation. **12.** _____ Information about a person's occupational roles and tasks and the environment in which he or she lives. **13.** _____Thirty-item self-report questionnaire in the categories of upper limb physical function, symptoms, social, and role functioning. **14.** _____ Performance measure for control of a myoelectric prosthesis using a four-point capability scale to rate 24 prosthetic control items in the areas of gripping, holding, releasing, and coordinating between hands.

ACMC, Assessment of Capacity for Myoelectric Control; BBT, Box and Block Test; DASH, Disabilities of the Arm, Shoulder, and Hand; JTHF, Jebsen–Taylor Test of Hand Function; ROM, range of motion; The Trinity Amputation and Prosthesis Experience Scales-Revised (TAPES-R).

Matching Pre and Postprosthetic Interventions with the Strategies for Each Intervention

Pre and Postprosthetic Intervention	Strategies
A. Donning and doffing **B.** Residual limb care **C.** Edema control and residual limb shaping **D.** Change of dominance **E.** ADL training **F.** Bimanual skills training **G.** Controls training **H.** Psychological support in the grieving process **I.** Physical conditioning and endurance training **J.** Practice repetitive drills (i.e., repetitive drills training) **K.** Increase muscle strength **L.** Management of phantom limb pain **M.** Improve and maintain joint ROM **N.** Return to recreation and leisure activities	**1.** _____ The five stages of grief (i.e., denial, anger, bargaining, depression, and acceptance) should be considered throughout this intervention process. **2.** _____ This is the longest and most challenging phase of prosthetic training. Practice, repetition, and training are the keys to success in this phase. **3.** _____ Exercises such as low-impact aerobics, aquatics, walking, and jogging are activities that can improve body image and the physical condition of the body during this intervention. **4.** _____ Methods used in this process are push-in, pull-in using a donning sock or a silicone liner-assisted method. **5.** _____ Weight cuffs, an exercise pulley system and exercise bands can be used during this intervention. **6.** _____ Washing and drying the residual limb will assist with awareness of changes to the limb and help the client to become comfortable with their new body image. **7.** _____ This preprosthetic intervention should focus on the suggestion of adaptive techniques to promote self-care until the client receives their prosthesis. **8.** _____ It is important to decrease volume to prepare the client for wearing the prosthesis. **9.** _____ The intervention has the client facing the occupational therapy practitioner and mirror (i.e., or mimic) their actions while moving the terminal device, wrist rotator, or elbow of the prosthesis to match them. **10.** _____ The goals of this training should be to increase radial digit coordination and develop separation of the radial and ulnar sides of the hand. **11.** _____ Prevention of soft tissue contractures from developing in the residual limb is important during this intervention. **12.** _____ Activities that incorporate grasping and releasing of various objects in different planes and axes can begin during this postprosthetic intervention. **13.** _____ Activity-specific or sport adaptations to the prosthesis are discussed during this intervention. **14.** _____ Mirror therapy is often used during this intervention.

ADL, activities of daily living; ROM, range of motion.

Chapter 19 Self-Study Activities: Lower Limb Amputation and Prosthetics (Answers Are Provided at the End of the Chapter)

Please read the following case study and answer the provided questions.

You have arrived in a clinic and have a pending order for occupational therapy for a 64-year-old female who had a transtibial amputation secondary to gangrene from diabetic ulcers yesterday. She lives at home with her husband who is in good health and is 67 years old. They live in a ranch style home with the bedroom located across the hall from the bathroom. They have four grown children, two who live locally and help out whenever needed. Upon entering the room your client is in bed with the head of the bed raised and the residual limb is wrapped in soft wrap of gauze and Kerlix, and resting elevated on a pillow.

Develop a plan of care for this individual in the following areas:

- ROM/strengthening
- Residual limb care
- Functional activities

What additional occupational therapy interventions could be performed after the individual with a lower extremity amputation receives their prosthesis?

Chapter 19 Self-Study Answers—Upper Limb Amputation and Prosthetics

Amputation level answers:

1. G
2. E
3. F
4. C
5. A
6. B
7. D
8. G
9. A
10. F
11. B
12. E
13. D
14. C

Screening and assessment answers:

1. G
2. M
3. K
4. E
5. A
6. C
7. L
8. B
9. N
10. D
11. H
12. J
13. I
14. F

Intervention strategy answers:

1. H
2. F
3. I
4. A
5. K
6. B
7. E
8. C
9. G
10. D
11. M
12. J
13. N
14. L

Chapter 19 Self-Study Answers—Lower Limb Amputation and Prosthetics

The initial discussion for this client should focus on immediate postoperative needs. The first area to address is the care of the residual limb. Focus on infection control, edema, and positioning.

Residual Limb Care

Many clients who have status postamputation surgery will elevate the residual limb on a pillow. While elevation may assist with edema control, clients with transtibial amputations are predisposed to flexion contractures due to the musculoskeletal changes of the amputation. The residual limb should rest in extension on the bed, or if a pillow is used, the pillow should be placed lengthwise extending from mid femur past the distal end of the limb.

Attention should be made not to remove the dressing for inspection unless a nurse or physician is present. Every effort should be made to limit exposure to environmental pathogens. Most commonly, the limb is wrapped only in soft dressing following the surgery. It is beneficial to begin appropriate compression as soon as possible. An ace wrap will offer compression without compromise to the suture line and can be initiated with approval of the surgeon. Only properly trained staff should apply the ace wrap as an improperly donned ace wrap could cause a tourniquet effect. As soon as the suture line is healed, residual limb compression should be continued with a shrinker to help shape and prepare the limb for the prosthesis.

The client may initiate desensitization by gently touching the residual limb over the bandages. This may also assist with acceptance. If the client is struggling with looking at or dealing with the amputation, it may be helpful to ask the prosthetist if there is a support group available.

ROM/Strengthening

The client can be given general UE ROM and strengthening exercises for home use. Activities that strengthen both the UE and trunk are beneficial for the individual with a lower extremity amputation. Sitting while performing a ball toss and catch will assist with core strength and balance.

Clients should be instructed to keep the knee extended, and if possible, the prone position could be used for stretching.

Functional Activities

The primary concern here is on the safety of movement and balance during all transfer and mobility activities. The OT should communicate regularly on the treatment plan. Initially, sitting balance and standing stability will need to be assessed. Due to the change in the center of mass and weight distribution, sitting balance may be impaired and time should be spent on sitting at the edge of the bed, reaching out from their base of support, and safely returning to their original position.

The use of a walker for transfers and mobility will be necessary. Proper transfer training is critical for safety during single limb transfers.

Home modifications may be necessary to decrease risk of falls including a shower chair, toilet grab bars, and a reacher. The client may also benefit from a wheelchair if the use of a standard walker is too difficult.

Additional Considerations

Diabetic referral may be necessary to assist the client in gaining improved control of their diabetes. Many individuals with transtibial amputation due to gangrene develop ulcers on the nonamputated side. It is imperative to instruct clients on proper foot care and inspection of the intact foot. A long handled mirror may assist. Communication and coordination of care with the treatment team will benefit the client and prevent duplication of services.

Additional occupational therapy interventions could be performed after the individual with a lower extremity amputation receives their prosthesis. Occupational therapy care of the individual with a lower extremity amputation does not have to stop the day they receive their prosthesis. The OT practitioner can continue to work on bipedal standing with equal weight-bearing and weight shifting for balance and safety of household activities such as housekeeping, making the bed, cooking (e.g., small steps and crossover steps in the kitchen), and fall recovery.

References

Biddiss, E. A., & Chau, T. T. (2007). Upper limb prosthesis use and abandonment: A survey of the last 25 years. *Prosthetics and Orthotics International, 31*(3), 236–257. doi:10.1080/03093640600994581

Department of Veterans Affairs & Department of Defense. (2014). *VA/DoD clinical practice guideline for the management of upper extremity amputee rehabilitation.* Washington, DC: Author.

Harvey, Z. T., Loomis, G. A., Mitsch, S., Murphy, I. C., Griffin, S. C., Potter, B. K., & Pasquina, P. (2012). Advanced rehabilitation techniques for the multi-limb amputee. *Journal of Surgical Orthopaedic Advances, 21*(1), 50–57.

HCUP National Inpatient Sample. (2012). *Healthcare cost and utilization project (HCUP).* Rockville, MD: Agency for Healthcare Research and Quality. Retrieved from http://www.hcup-us.ahrq.gov/nisoverview.jsp

Keenan, D. D., & Glover, J. S. (2013). Amputations and prosthetics. In L. W. Pedretti, H. M. Pendleton, & W.

Schultz-Krohn (Eds.), *Pedretti's occupational therapy: Practice skills for physical dysfunction* (7th ed., pp. 1149–1193). St. Louis, MO: Elsevier.

Li, Y., Burrows, N. R., Gregg, E. W., Albright, A., & Geiss, L. S. (2012). Declining rates of hospitalization for nontraumatic lower-extremity amputation in the diabetic population aged 40 years or older: U.S., 1988–2008. *Diabetes Care, 35*(2), 273–277. doi:10.2337/dc11-1360dc11-1360

May, B. J., & Lockard, M. A. (2011). *Prosthetics & orthotics in clinical practice: A case study approach.* Philadelphia, PA: F.A. Davis.

Mitsch, S., Walters, L. S., & Yancosek, K. (2014). Amputations and prosthetics. In M. V. Radomski & C. A. T. Latham (Eds.), *Occupational therapy for physical dysfunction* (7th ed., pp. 1266–1299). Philadelphia, PA: Wolters Kluwer Health/Lippincott Williams & Wilkins.

O'Sullivan, S. B., & Schmitz, T. J. (2007). *Physical rehabilitation* (5th ed.). Philadelphia, PA: F.A. Davis.

Ottobock. (2013). *Information for upper limb amputees and their families.* Retrieved from http://www.ottobock .co.uk/prosthetics/info-for-amputees/information-for -upper-limb-amputees-and-their-families/

Parker, S. E., Mai, C. T., Canfield, M. A., Rickard, R., Wang, Y., Meyer, R. E., . . . Correa, A. (2010). Updated national birth prevalence estimates for selected birth defects in the United States, 2004–2006. *Birth Defects Research Part A: Clinical and Molecular Teratology, 88*(12), 1008–1016. doi:10.1002/bdra.20735

Ramachandran, V. S., & Rogers-Ramachandran, D. (1996). Synaesthesia in phantom limbs induced with mirrors. *Proceedings of the Royal Society of London B: Biological Sciences, 263*(1369), 377–386. doi:10.1098/rspb.1996.0058

Schnur, D. S., & Meier, R. H. (2013). Amputation surgery. In R. Meier (Ed.), *Physical medicine and rehabilitation clinics of North America: Amputee rehabilitation* (pp. 35–43). Philadelphia, PA: Elsevier.

Seymour, R. (2002). *Prosthetics and orthotics: Lower limb and spinal.* Philadelphia, PA: Lippincott Williams & Wilkins.

Smith, D. G., Michael, J. W., & Bowker, J. H. (2004). *Atlas of amputations and limb deficiencies: Surgical, prosthetic,* *and rehabilitation principles* (3rd ed.). Rosemont, IL: American Academy of Orthopaedic Surgeons.

Smurr, L., Yancosek, K., Gulick, K., Ganz, O., Kulla, S., Jones, M., & Esquenazi, A. (2009). Occupational therapy for the polytrauma casuality with limb loss. In P. F. Pasquina & R. A. Cooper (Eds.), *Care of the combat amputee, textbooks of military medicine* (pp. 493–533). Washington, DC: Borden Institute, Walter Reed Army Medical Center.

Smurr, L. M., Gulick, K., Yancosek, K., & Ganz, O. (2008). Managing the upper extremity amputee: A protocol for success. *Journal of Hand Therapy, 21*(2), 160–176. doi:10.1197/j.jht.2007.09.006

Swanson, S., Atkins, D., & Tingleaf, L. (2003a). Postprosthetic training. *Advance for Directors, 12*(11), 61.

Swanson, S., Atkins, D., & Tingleaf, L. (2003b). Preprosthetic management of the upper limb amputee. *Advance for Directors, 12*(10), 69.

Tyler, J. (2014). *Principles of myoelectric prosthetic training of the upper limb amputee: The therapist's guide, unilateral transradial amputation.* San Antonio, TX: Hanger Clinic.

Vaughn, P. (2014). Appendix 1: Common conditions, resources and evidence. Amputations. In M. E. Scaffa, B. A. B. Schell, G. Gillen, & E. S. Cohn (Eds.), *Willard & Spackman's occupational therapy* (12th ed., pp. 1101–1103). Philadelphia, PA: Wolters Kluwer Health/Lippincott Williams & Wilkins.

Westcoast Brace & Limb. (2011). *Upper extremity prosthetics.* Retrieved from http://www.wcbl.com /prosthetics-2/upper-extremity-prosthetic-services/

Wright, V. (2009). Prosthetic outcome measures for use with upper limb amputees: A systematic review of the peer-reviewed literature, 1970–2009. *Journal of Prosthetics and Orthotics, 21*(Suppl. 4), P3–P63. Retrieved from http://www.oandp.org/jpo /library/2009_04S_003.asp

Yancosek, K., & Gulick, K. (2012). *Handwriting for heroes: Learn to write with your non-dominant hand in six weeks.* Ann Arbor, MI: Loving Healing Press.

Ziegler-Graham, K., MacKenzie, E. J., Ephraim, P. L., Travison, T. G., & Brookmeyer, R. (2008). Estimating the prevalence of limb loss in the United States: 2005 to 2050. *Archives of Physical Medicine and Rehabilitation, 89*(3), 422–429. doi:10.1016/j.apmr.2007.11.005

Burn Rehabilitation

Jennie Gilchrist McGillicuddy

Learning Objectives

- Describe medical intervention following a burn injury.
- Describe the role of the occupational therapy (OT) practitioner with the client following a burn injury.
- Identify phases of burn care and the role of the occupational therapist during each phase.
- Describe the assessment of the burn client during the OT evaluation process, including the identification of challenges, formulation of goals, and selection of interventions.
- Describe specific burn OT interventions for incorporation into treatment sessions.
- Identify methods for the assessment of functional progress with the burn population.
- Describe strategies to progress the burned client between each phase of burn recovery.
- Explain how the intervention plan can be updated based on functional progress or decline.
- Identify OT strategies specific to the pediatric population following a burn injury.
- Identify methods of incorporating families and caregivers into OT intervention with the burn population.
- Identify the need for evidence-based practice with burn OT interventions.
- Describe options for incorporating compassionate care into OT treatment specific to the burn population.
- Identify the rehabilitation need and long-term follow-up with the burn population.

Key Terms

- *Allogeneic skin graft (i.e., allograft)*: Cadaver skin, which serves as a temporary, durable biologic covering that is applied in the operating room and allows for the underlying structures to stabilize and become prepared for eventual permanent skin graft placement.
- *Autogeneic skin graft (autograft)*: Human autograft is a permanent surgical graft of tissue from a nonburned area of the client's body to the burn wound.
- *Donor site*: The nonburned area from which the tissue is taken for an autograft surgery.

Description

Due to medical advances with wound care and infection control, an increased number of individuals are surviving burn injuries that in the past would have proven fatal. Rehabilitation therapies are an important part of the multidisciplinary burn treatment team. Healthcare professionals involved in the treatment of the burned client should demonstrate knowledge and compassionate care in the clinical environment, with the common goal of restoring meaningful lives. Burn rehabilitation practitioners specifically focus on movement and functional activity throughout the burn sequela for initial contracture prevention, with a long-term goal of restoring quality of life.

Etiology and Pathology

It has been estimated that 486,000 individuals receive medical treatment for burn injuries each year in the United States, with a 96.7% survival rate (American Burn Association, 2015). This improvement in survival increases the need for comprehensive rehabilitation, with the goals of restoring occupation and improving the quality of life of the burn population (Reeves &

Deshaies, 2013). Thermal damage to the skin may be caused by fire, scald, contact with a hot surface, radiation, chemicals, or electricity (Pessina & Orroth, 2014). Select statistics based on 2003–2012 admissions to burn centers show that the majority of burns in adults occur in males (60%) and the most common cause is flame/fire (43%) (American Burn Association, 2015). The data also show that the majority of burn injuries occur at home (70%) (American Burn Association, 2015). Children are most commonly hospitalized for burn injuries with scald burns (65%), contact burns (20%), and flame burns (15%); the criteria for hospital admission due to major burn injury are described in **Table 20-1** (American Burn Association, 2015; Pruitt, Wolf, & Mason, 2012).

The time from initial injury to approximately 72 hours after the burn is considered to be the medically emergent phase (Pessina & Orroth, 2014). During this critical time, the medical team will initiate lifesaving resuscitation interventions and determine the extent of burn damage. An important consideration in the emergent phase is the possibility of damage to the upper airway from smoke inhalation, or inhalation injury (Pessina & Orroth, 2014). Clients with significant inhalation injuries are intubated for airway protection and treatment. In addition, systemic edema may develop following large body surface area cutaneous burns. If there is a risk that the edema may involve the airway and constrict breathing, these clients are intubated for airway protection as well. During the emergent phase, rehabilitation therapies are delayed to prioritize medical stabilization. Once the client is medically stable, rehabilitation therapies are initiated with a referral from the physician.

Clinical Presentation

Anatomy of the Skin

The skin is the largest organ of the body. Skin provides a water-resistant barrier, acting as a physical barrier for an individual to the outside world. The skin also protects against infection and helps to regulate body temperature. The epidermis is the thinner top layer of the skin. The dermis is the thicker second layer, which contains the nerve endings that feel pain and vasculature essential for tissue regeneration. The dermis also contains sweat glands and hair follicles, which contain reservoirs of specialized stem cells for regeneration of epidermal cells. The subcutaneous tissue is the next layer, a fat layer that helps the body to maintain temperature. Underneath the subcutaneous layer is muscle and bone (Williama, 2002). **Figure 20-1** demonstrates a cross section of skin.

Burn Classification

Historically, burns were classified as first, second, and third degree. However, healthcare providers are moving away from this scheme, and the modern classification system describes the depth of the burn injury: superficial, superficial partial-thickness, deep partial-thickness, and full-thickness (Pessina & Orroth, 2014).

Superficial Burns

Cell damage to the epidermis is referred to as a superficial burn. These injuries are pink, dry, and painful. The most common type of superficial burn is sunburn, which is caused by ultraviolet radiation. With a well-nourished, intact epithelial bed, these injuries heal within approximately seven days and generally do not scar (Pessina & Orroth, 2014). Individuals with superficial burns are not usually admitted to burn centers and do not require rehabilitation therapies.

Superficial Partial-Thickness Burns

Cell damage to the epidermis and the upper level of the dermis is referred to as a superficial partial-thickness

---

Table 20-1 Major Burn Injury Criteria

American Burn Association Major Burn Injury Criteria
• Second- and third-degree burns greater than 10% of the total body surface
• Third-degree burns
• Burns that involve the face, hands, feet, genitalia, or perineum and those that involve skin overlying major joints
• Chemical burns
• Electrical burns including lightning injuries
• Any burn with concomitant trauma in which the burn injuries pose the greatest risk to the client
• Inhalation injury
• Clients with preexisting medical disorders that could complicate management, prolong recovery, or affect mortality
• Hospitals without qualified personnel or equipment for the care of critically burned children

Modified from Pruitt, Wolf, and Mason, 2012.

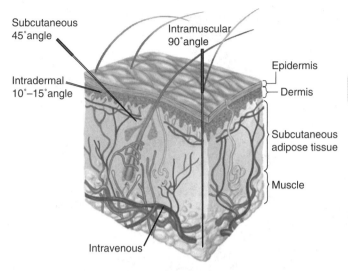

Figure 20-1 Cross-sectional anatomy of the skin.

burn. These burns may occur from flame, scald, or contact with a hot surface. The temperature of the item, which the skin contacted, and the length of contact determine the extent of the burn. An intact blister over the injured area is a common sign of a superficial partial-thickness burn (Pessina & Orroth, 2014). Burns to the upper dermal layer are painful because of irritation of nerve endings in this layer of the skin. Superficial partial-thickness burns heal with conservative management, without surgery, within 7–21 days (Pessina & Orroth, 2014). Depending on the extent, anatomic location, and context of the injury, individuals with superficial partial-thickness burns may be admitted to the burn center for medical management (e.g., a child with a large superficial partial-thickness burn over the entire lower body with suspected child abuse). These burns leave minimal and sometimes no scarring and require rehabilitation therapies only during inpatient hospitalization.

Deep Partial-Thickness Burns

Cell death of the epidermis and severe damage to the dermal layer are referred to as a deep partial-thickness burn. Because of damage to the nerve endings in the dermal layer of the skin, light touch sensation is diminished. Deeper dermal burns appear blotchy with areas that are pale in color due to damage of the blood vessels in the dermal layer of skin. Due to damage of the nerve endings and vasculature required for wound healing, deep partial-thickness burns require skin-grafting surgeries for healing and to minimize scarring (Pessina & Orroth, 2014). Individuals with deep partial-thickness burns are

admitted to the hospital for burn care and require rehabilitation during the inpatient hospitalization and often outpatient therapies for follow-up.

Full-Thickness Burns

Tissue death to both the epidermal and dermal layers is referred to as a full-thickness burn. Full-thickness burn injuries appear white or tan in color and are insensate because of the extent of damage to the dermal nerves. Due to dermal nerve and vasculature compromise, individuals with full-thickness burns are admitted to the burn center for wound management and surgical interventions. Some full-thickness burns result in damage to the structures below the dermal layer, including subcutaneous fat, muscle, or bone (Pessina & Orroth, 2014). Individuals with full-thickness burn injury to this depth may require amputation due to the extent of tissue damage. Rehabilitation is important following full-thickness burn injuries, both during the inpatient hospital stay and for long-term outpatient follow-up.

Rule of Nines

Burns are described by the size of the total body surface area (TBSA) involved. The rule of nines method divides the body surface area into percentages, allowing for an estimated percentage of body surface area involvement. The rule of nines is a quick method used by medical professionals to calculate the extent to which the body has been burned (LeBorgne, 2014). Due to the difference in body proportions of children, the percentage breakdown is adjusted, resulting in a modified rule of nines. **Figure 20-2** demonstrates an estimation of burn size using the rule of nines in both the adult and pediatric populations (Micak, Buffalo, & Jimenenz, 2012).

Medical and Surgical Management of the Burn Wound

The medical team will begin wound management, including surgeries, once the burn wound has declared itself and once the eschar (i.e., burned tissue) has been removed. Burn injuries that involve the deep dermal layer require surgical skin graft intervention for healing. The initial purposes of skin grafts are protection of

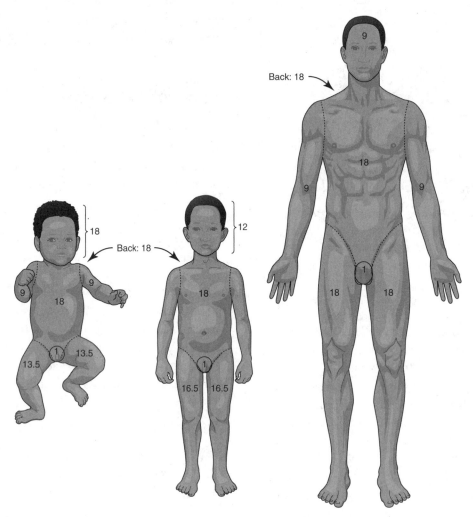

Figure 20-2 Rule of nines.

the wound bed, prevention of infection, facilitating pain control, and hydration of the wound bed. The long-term purposes of skin grafts include burn wound coverage and healing, optimizing cosmetic appeal, and maximizing the range of motion (ROM).

Escharotomy

An escharotomy is a surgical procedure in which incisions are made through the burn eschar, which is usually performed emergently for pressure relief. If a client has a burn that is circumferential on an extremity or the torso, then the circulation of the body segment should be closely monitored for compromise. Symptoms of compartmental pressure may include paresthesias, coldness, and decreased pulse or the absence of a pulse (Pessina & Orroth, 2014). Due to the inelasticity of the eschar, if a decrease or absence of a pulse is determined in an

extremity following a cutaneous burn injury and an increased internal pressure is suspected, an escharotomy is necessary. On the torso, eschar can act as a corset, which limits lung expansion and adequate respiration (Pessina & Orroth, 2014), resulting in the need for an emergent escharotomy for pressure relief.

Debridement/Excision

Upon admission to the burn center, the burn wound is debrided by the physician and nursing staff. In an attempt to remove eschar, burn wounds are cleaned, or debrided at the bedside with appropriate pain management interventions in place. A wound excision is performed in the operating room (OR) by a surgeon. While the client is under anesthesia, the eschar is removed from the wound surface using a handheld blade with a calibrated depth guard, until a viable tissue plane is reached (Rosenberg, 2012).

Allogeneic Skin Graft (Allograft)

Human allograft is obtained from organ donors. Viable allograft, or cadaver skin, is a temporary, durable biologic covering that is applied in the OR and allows for the underlying structures to stabilize and become prepared for eventual permanent skin graft placement. Allografts are temporary by nature and are eventually rejected by the host, usually within three to four weeks (Sheridan & Tompkins, 2012), and are removed in the OR by the surgeon for autograft placement.

Autogeneic Skin Graft (Autograft)

Human autograft is a permanent surgical graft of tissue from a nonburned area of the client's body to the burn wound. The area from which the tissue is taken is referred to as the donor site. The donor site is designed not to cross joints, when avoidable, and while the donor site is painful, it heals quickly with local, basic wound care. Because autograft involves grafting tissue from the same body, it does not incite the inflammatory response and has a much lower risk of rejection. It will also grow with the child if used in the pediatric population.

Upper layers of the skin, or split-thickness skin grafts (STSG), are harvested from the donor site and are applied to a clean, excised burn wound. STSG include the full epidermal skin layer and part of the dermal skin layer, and they may be meshed or unmeshed. A meshed STSG is used to increase body surface area coverage. After being harvested from the donor site, the STSG is perforated in the OR with a scalpel by a burn surgeon and then applied to the clean burn wound bed. Meshed skin grafts have a higher risk for contracture when used for burn coverage over a joint, as the tissue tends to revert to the original (i.e., preharvested) size. This, in combination with ill positioning of the extremities during periods of prolonged bed rest, requires meshed STSG to be carefully monitored for contraction. Unmeshed STSG, also referred to as sheet grafts, are not perforated and are placed directly on the wound bed following tissue harvest. Unmeshed skin grafts generally have more satisfactory cosmetic outcomes and also result in less risk for joint contracture. For these reasons, unmeshed STSG are commonly used for coverage of the hands and face following burn injury.

Full-thickness skin grafts (FTSG) consist of both the epidermal and the dermal layers of skin. FTSG tend to resemble normal skin better than STSG (Kamolz & Huang, 2012), offering good cosmetic outcomes and also less risk for contracture when used over a joint. When FTSG are harvested, the donor site requires surgical closure, as it cannot heal spontaneously since no skin appendages are left behind (Kamolz & Huang, 2012). FTSG are commonly used for coverage of small full-thickness burns.

INTEGRA

INTEGRA® is a synthetic dermal layer used prior to placement of an autograft to prepare a viable wound bed. It consists of a porous matrix of collagen fibers, with an epidermal substitute layer made of silicone to control moisture loss from the wound (INTEGRA®, 2010). It is used post excision in the treatment of deep partial-thickness and full-thickness burns where autografts are presently not available or not desirable due to the physiologic condition of the client (INTEGRA®, 2010). Areas with INTEGRA® require an eventual autograft for full burn wound healing.

The rehabilitation protocols following each surgical intervention are described in detail later in this chapter.

Rehabilitation Services

Rehabilitation services are an important component of the burn interdisciplinary team and are essential for burn clients to return to their prior levels of function. Rehabilitation therapies involved in the treatment of the burned client include physical therapy (PT), occupational therapy (OT), and speech and language pathology. OT is primarily concerned with the remediation of impairments and disabilities and the promotion of health and well-being through occupation. The primary goal of OT is to enable clients to regain participation in activities of daily living (ADLs) via examination, evaluation, and intervention planning in relation to occupations (American Occupational Therapy Association, 2015).

Regarding the burn population, acute OT often includes face and upper body ROM exercises, splinting, and upper body positioning. Intermediate OT focuses on assisting clients to reengage in ADLs, upper body strengthening and endurance training, and scar management interventions for the face and the upper extremities. OT interventions with the burn population may include specialized activities and/or goals for return to work and driving programs.

Rehabilitation therapists facilitate an interdisciplinary approach, and direct communication must be maintained among the OT, the physician, nursing staff, psychology staff, case managers, social workers, and dieticians. Direct communication between the healthcare disciplines and the client, as well as the family of the client, is vital to a smooth recovery.

Screening and Assessments

The rehabilitation process is initiated by an order from the physician. Following the order, each discipline will examine the client and begin the evaluation process. During the evaluation, each discipline will document the client's social and occupational profile, current concerns and priorities, and results of an initial assessment. Evaluation components include the date of injury, medical history, history of the client's prior level of function, and current assessment of the level of function following injury. This assessment gathers data regarding prior ADLs, ROM of joints, muscle strength, muscle endurance, fine and gross motor coordination, any sensory deficits, neurologic and psychological orientation, current communication abilities and level of cognition, client attitudes, and cultural factors. Rehabilitation practitioners evaluate clients following burn injury to assess which joints of the body the injury crosses and note this for the purposes of contracture prevention. Each rehabilitation team member will also assess and note the client's home environment, social and emotional support systems, occupation, and leisure interests prior to injury. The goals of the client and any family members in relation to therapy interventions should be recorded.

Challenges and strengths are noted, and based on the initial assessment, an intervention plan is formed. This formal plan includes a list of challenges following the injury, goals to target for each challenge, and intervention strategies or treatment activities to help achieve each goal. Each goal is described in functional, time-sensitive, observable, measureable, and action-oriented terms.

Interventions

Frequency of therapy with clients following burn injury varies. Rehabilitation evaluations occur once the initial burn resuscitation phase is complete and the client is deemed stable enough to tolerate passive range of motion (PROM) and initial splinting. During the acute phase, PT and OT practitioners usually see the client daily. Communication between the therapy team and the nurse is important to clarify if the client is able to tolerate PROM and splinting during the acute phase of rehabilitation. Frequency of therapy with the client in the burn intermediate care phase is usually daily to twice daily, based on the client's needs and deficits. Frequency of outpatient therapy is also based on the client's needs and is usually two to three times a week. A common goal of PT and OT throughout the burn sequelae is to progress the client toward the prior level of functioning or as close to this level as possible.

Expected Functional Outcomes

For purposes of instruction, this chapter divides the rehabilitation process into expected functional outcomes throughout the three phases. The acute phase directly following the burn injury involves working in an intensive care setting with the client often on mechanical ventilation with accompanying sedative and paralytic medications. The intermediate phase of healing is after transferring to a less-intensive medical setting, in which the client is allowed out of bed and is able to participate more in therapy; with a decreased level of sedation. The third phase is the outpatient phase, which requires long-term and at-home plans for rehabilitation, client motivation, and compliance.

Acute Phase

Areas of focus for burn rehabilitation in the acute phase of healing include initial ROM exercises, splinting, and positioning recommendations. Often ROM exercises in the burn intensive care unit (ICU) focus on PROM, where the OT passively stretches each joint as the client is intubated, sedated, or receiving paralytic medications, which prevent active ROM (AROM) stretching.

Splints are fabricated for each extremity or joint as necessary and optimal positioning for each joint of the body is established. Splinting and positioning decisions are based on the location and the depth of the burn. The involvement of nursing staff and family members is important at this stage, and their education is implemented in addition to daily rehabilitation treatment sessions. The nursing staff can facilitate the splint schedule and the PROM exercise routine. Prolonged positioning that achieves a passive stretch can be the most effective intervention at this stage for contracture prevention (Serghiou et al., 2012).

Table 20-2 Rehabilitation in the Burn Acute Phase			
Example Injury	**Challenges**	**Goals**	**Interventions**
Full-thickness burn crossing the axilla	• Risk of joint contracture • Risk of functional limitation	• Full PROM for shoulder forward flexion for future overhead reach • Family demonstration of independence in providing PROM to the client's arm	• Daily PROM exercises • Prolonged positioning sessions between PROM exercises • Family education regarding methods of providing PROM
Deep partial-thickness burn crossing the joints of the dominant hand	• Risk of joint contracture • Risk of functional limitation	• Full PROM of the hand for future grasp on fork and toothbrush • Full digit opposition for future hand use with fine motor coordination activities • The daily nurse will independently implement the splinting schedule, as directed by the OT	• Daily PROM for the hand • Implement the hand splinting protocol between ROM sessions
Full-thickness burn crossing the creases of the hand in a pediatric client	• Risk of palmar contracture • Risk of functional limitation	• Full PROM of the palm and hand for future functional grasp with an age-appropriate play task • The daily nurse will independently implement the splinting schedule, as directed by the OT	• Daily PROM for the hand with a focus placed on the palm • Implement the palmar splinting protocol between ROM sessions

Challenges, goals, and interventions are often categorized by the location and depth of the burn injury in relation to joints of the body and the resulting risks of joint contracture. Common challenges, goals, and intervention strategies in the burn acute phase are listed in **Table 20-2**.

Intermediate Phase

When the client reaches the intermediate phase of healing after a burn, sedation is usually decreased and the client is cleared by the physician to transfer out of bed. Areas of focus for rehabilitation in the burn intermediate healing phase include teaching the client an AROM exercise program, retraining a client how to complete ADLs incorporating the injured extremities into activity, reinforcing the splinting and positioning schedules at night with functional activity during the day, initial intervention for scar management, functional mobility training, and muscle strengthening and endurance activities. Goals at this stage are often geared toward preparing the client for discharge to home (e.g., home exercise program, safety training with standing ADLs, and functional mobility). Common

challenges, goals, and intervention strategies in the burn intermediate care phase are listed in **Table 20-3**.

Outpatient Phase

Following discharge from the hospital, the client may be followed on an outpatient basis for rehabilitation if needed. Areas of focus for rehabilitation in the outpatient stage continue to target ROM, muscle strengthening, functional mobility training, and endurance activities. In addition, a main focus of rehabilitation in the outpatient stage is scar management. Also, the rehabilitation professional may work with the client to teach the optimal home exercise stretch program, customized as needed based on the location of any skin grafts, in relation to function. A primary goal of the OT in the outpatient phase is to teach the client to continue rehabilitation interventions throughout the maturation phase of the scar. Scars continue to remodel for up to 1 year (Kirsner, 2008); therefore, interventions should be continued for up to 12 months. Common challenges, goals, and intervention strategies in the burn outpatient stage are listed in **Table 20-4**.

Table 20-3   Rehabilitation in the Burn Intermediate Care Phase

Example Injury	Challenges	Goals	Interventions
40% TBSA burn to the upper extremities and torso	• Decreased independence with ADLs, self-care, and functional mobility	• Complete dressing and bathing with independence • Ambulate to the sink and complete grooming tasks standing with a walker • Ambulate to the restroom with a walker	• Functional mobility training • ADL training • Mobility device safety training for use of the walker with ADLs • Safety training during functional mobility and standing tasks
Autologous skin graft over the antecubital fossa and circumferentially around the elbow	• Contracture of the elbow soft tissue • Decreased functional use of the arm with ADLs	• The client will demonstrate full elbow flexion for functional use of the arm with self-feeding and oral hygiene • The client will demonstrate self-feeding using the affected extremity without an adaptive feeding device	• AROM exercise program training for the elbow • Introduce daily activities incorporating functional use of the affected arm • Establish an optimal nightly elbow splinting schedule
Prolonged hospitalization due to burn sequelae (e.g., deeper burns/multiple surgeries)	• Decreased endurance with activity	• Tolerate a 20-minute functional standing activity without rest breaks	• Therapeutic endurance training • Daily endurance exercise program • Routine transfers out of bed for standing ADLs and functional mobility

Impact on Occupational Performance

Burn Rehabilitation Principles

Rehabilitation therapists follow the burn client from the time of hospital admission through the burn sequelae to following hospital discharge. The primary rehabilitation interventions include ROM, splinting, and positioning.

After reparative surgeries, a protocol must be followed to ensure caution with therapy in the postoperative period. After each visit to the OR, the physician's orders are necessary for the OT to begin or to resume treatment. Rehabilitation therapy protocols in relation to surgery type are described in **Table 20-5**. Occasionally, if a skin graft is fragile and requires an extra day of healing prior to therapy intervention, the physician will request OT on the appropriate postoperative day (POD). Conversely, if the graft is strong enough prior to the standard start date, then therapy may be resumed earlier. Splinting and positioning may begin or resume immediately following surgery, on the same POD. POD #0 indicates that the splinting, positioning, or ROM intervention may occur in the OR, prior to or immediately following the surgery. However, this is at the discretion of the physician, depending on the type of graft, fragility of the graft, and the necessity of the splint immediately postoperatively.

Range of Motion

ROM is the direction and distance that a joint may move. Each joint has a normal ROM that is expressed in degrees. Joint ROM is obtained using a goniometer, a tool used to measure the arc of motion of a joint angle (Meriano & Latella, 2008). Examples of goniometers are reflected in **Figure 20-3**. During the evaluation, the initial ROM of each joint is determined and compared to the potential joint ROM. **Table 20-6** demonstrates normal ranges for each joint of the body. Achieving the potential joint ROM is the goal of the OT. Types of ROM include passive ROM, active ROM, and active assistive range of motion (AAROM). PROM is completed by the

Table 20-4 Rehabilitation in the Burn Outpatient Phase

Example Injury	Challenges	Goals	Interventions
Burn, skin graft, and scarring crossing the antecubital fossa	• Scarring limits full AROM of the elbow • Decreased elbow ROM for arm use	• Demonstrate independence with scar massage over the elbow joint • Demonstrate elbow ROM for independence with arm use • Decreased scar height and increased soft tissue elasticity of the scar over the elbow joint	• Education for scar massage technique • Establish an elbow AROM exercise program • Silicone devices and pressure therapy
Hypertrophic scarring of the face	• Scarring limits the client's ability to open the mouth • Decreased nutrition • Decreased oral hygiene • Decreased communication	• Demonstrate independence with ROM exercise program for the mouth • Demonstrate independence with scar massage techniques for the face • Demonstrate compliance with use of the silicone face mask	• Establish a mouth exercise program routine • Education for the scar massage technique • Fabrication of custom face silicone mask including client education regarding the purpose of the mask
Burn, skin graft, and scarring over the palmar creases of the hand in a pediatric client	• Decreased hand flexibility for grasp • Risk of further scar contracture due to the location and depth of the burn and skin graft	• The mother of the child will demonstrate independence with providing scar massage to the palm • The child will demonstrate full palmar flexibility for grasp of a toy • The mother of the child will demonstrate independence with assisting the child with palmar stretches	• Education of the child's mother for follow-up with a scar massage protocol at home • Age-appropriate play incorporating palmar grasp and release with the affected hand • Education of the child's mother for follow-up with the stretch routine at home

OT alone, while moving the extremity through the available arc of motion without the muscle assistance of the client. During AROM, the client moves the extremity through the arc of motion without the assistance of the OT. AAROM is a combination of AROM and PROM, with the client moving the extremity through the arc of motion as much as possible with the OT providing the more difficult end ROM passively. AAROM becomes necessary when pain, edema, bandages, or psychological factors become limiting factors to AROM.

During therapy in the acute stage, joint PROM is the focus, as limiting factors to AROM may include thick bandages, edema, and sedation of the client. Often during the acute stage of large burns, the client may

Table 20-5 Rehabilitation Intervention Start Dates Following Common Burn Surgeries

Surgery	ROM	Splinting	Positioning
Escharotomy	POD #0 or POD #1	POD #0 or POD #1	POD #0 or POD #1
Burn debridement	POD #0 or POD #1	POD #0 or POD #1	POD #0 or POD #1
Allograft	POD #3	POD #0 or POD #1	POD #0 or POD #1
Traditional autograft	POD #5	Varies	Varies
INTEGRA® synthetic dermal regeneration template	POD #7	Varies	Varies
Cultured epithelial autograft	POD #14	Varies	Varies

Table 20-6 Normal ROM Angles for Each Joint of the Body

Plane of Motion	Normal ROM (Degrees)	Plane of Motion	Normal ROM (Degrees)
Face		*Hand*	
• Mouth opening	Varies, depending on the size of the client	• Thumb MP joint flexion	0–90
Neck		• Thumb MP joint extension	90–0
• Cervical lateral rotation	0–60	• Thumb IP joint flexion	0–90
• Cervical lateral flexion	0–45	• Thumb IP joint extension	90–0
• Cervical flexion	0–45	• Digit MP joint flexion	0–90
• Cervical extension	0–45	• Digit MP joint extension	90–0
Torso		• Digit PIP joint flexion	0–100
• Spinal flexion	0–80	• Digit PIP extension	90–0
• Spinal extension	0–25	• Digit DIP joint flexion	0–90
• Spinal lateral flexion	0–35	• Digit DIP extension	90–0
• Spinal rotation	0–45	• Digit opposition	0 cm between fingertips
Axilla		• MP abduction	0–30
• Humeral flexion	0–180	• MP adduction	As compared to the unaffected side
• Humeral extension	0–60	*Hip*	
• Humeral abduction	0–180	• Flexion	0–120
• Humeral adduction	180–0	• Extension	0–30
• Humeral external rotation	0–90	• Abduction	0–45
• Humeral internal rotation	0–70	• Adduction	30–0
• Humeral horizontal abduction	0–45	• Internal rotation	0–45
• Humeral horizontal adduction	0–135	• External rotation	0–45
Elbow		*Knee*	
• Flexion	0–135	• Flexion	0–135
• Extension	135–0	• Extension	135–0
Forearm		*Ankle*	
• Supination	0–90	• Dorsiflexion	0–20
• Pronation	0–90	• Plantar flexion	0–50
Wrist		• Inversion	0–35
• Flexion	0–80	• Eversion	0–15
• Extension	0–70		
• Radial deviation	0–20		
• Ulnar deviation	0–30		

Data from (Latella & Meriano, 2003).

be sedated, receiving paralytic medications, and/or intubated for mechanical ventilation. PROM provided by the OT in the burn ICU usually consists of 2 sets of 20 repetitions, varying therapy sessions once to twice daily depending on the needs of the client and the severity of the burn.

During therapy in the intermediate phase, AROM becomes the focus as the client is more able to participate. Limiting factors to AROM may be pain and burn dressings. The OT provides AAROM as needed during the session to achieve full end ROM. It is important for the OT to initiate training for the client to engage in

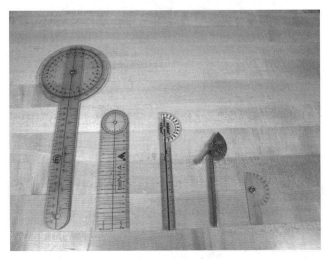

Figure 20-3 Examples of goniometers.
Courtesy of Jennie Gilchrist McGillicuddy

self-AAROM (i.e., by the client alone, using an unaffected extremity to move the affected extremity into the full end ROM). ROM is generally performed as 2 sets of 20 repetitions, 3 times a day. The therapy session may count as one of these sets with the client completing the other two sets on their own. Often, a combination of AROM and AAROM becomes the exercise program with which the client is discharged.

During the outpatient phase, if a scar band forms over a joint, both AROM and AAROM for a greater stretch become necessary and are incorporated into therapy sessions. Frequency of ROM exercises while the client is in the outpatient phase of healing, throughout the scar maturation process of several months, varies; however, a common protocol is 2 sets of 20 repetitions per session, with 3 sessions of ROM exercises daily. This varies based on the client's individual needs and circumstances. It may be noted that PT usually focuses on burns of the lower body, while OT focuses on burns of the upper body and the face.

Splinting

Besides ROM exercises, splinting is the most common type of therapy intervention in rehabilitation of the burn client and is equally important. A splint is a device used to secure, support, immobilize, or mobilize an anatomic structure. Different types of splints are used in burn rehabilitation. Articular splints cross joints, while nonarticular splints provide support or protection to a fragile

area that does not cross a joint. Static splints, or immobilization splints, do not allow motion of the joint to which they are applied. Static splints may be articular, crossing a joint to provide optimal stretch, or nonarticular, protecting a fragile skin graft, for example. Static splints have a firm, rigid structure (Jacobs & Austin, 2003). **Figure 20-4** demonstrates a static hand splint. Static progressive splints begin with a static base component and are molded to progress the stretching force over a joint. The stretch of the joint angle may be slowly progressed to end with a static splint with optimal stretch. Static progressive splints are also referred to as serial static splints (Jacobs & Austin, 2003). **Figure 20-5** demonstrates a static progressive elbow splint.

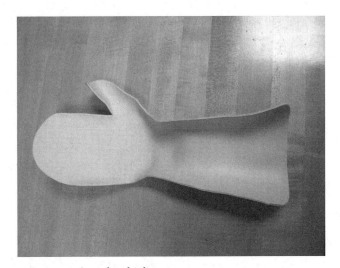

Figure 20-4 Static hand splint.
Courtesy of Jennie Gilchrist McGillicuddy

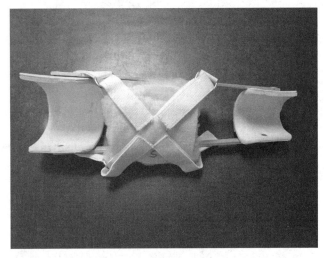

Figure 20-5 Static progressive elbow splint.
Courtesy of Jennie Gilchrist McGillicuddy

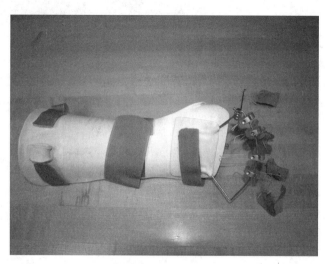

Figure 20-6 Dynamic hand splint.
Courtesy of Jennie Gilchrist McGillicuddy

Dynamic splints have a mobilizing component and exert force on a target tissue that results in passive ROM gains. Dynamic splints have a static component, which provides a foundation for a dynamic outrigger attachment. Controlled mobilizing forces are applied, which may be through the use of rubber bands, hydraulics, or spring attachments (Jacobs & Austin, 2003). **Figure 20-6** demonstrates a dynamic hand splint.

The most common type of splint material is a thermoplastic material, which may be heated to mold for shaping and adjustment to fit the client, as well as to achieve the optimal stretch. Each type of splint has its place during the burn sequelae.

During the acute phase, splinting is one of the first rehabilitation interventions introduced. During the initial evaluation, the OT notes which joints the burn crosses and the depth of the burn. Splints are introduced accordingly. The primary type of splint used in the acute burn stage is the static, articular, immobilization splint for joint immobilization or optimal stretch (e.g., use of an intrinsic plus splint for optimal hand stretching). Occasionally, the nonarticular splint is introduced if protection of the soft tissue is the goal (e.g., protection of a skin graft on the forearm). Splints may be padded to prevent skin breakdown, and edges of the splint may be flared for the same reason. The splint is easily cleaned as needed to maintain a hygienic environment. The wear schedule for splints during the acute phase commonly alternates the splint on and off for two-hour periods during the day and then worn all night. Because the client is commonly sedated during the acute stage, direct and daily communication with the nursing staff and the family of the client is imperative regarding the purpose of and the positioning of the splint. Written splint wear schedules and instructions may be helpful to maintain communication between the OT and the burn interdisciplinary team, as well as the family.

During the burn intermediate phase of healing, commonly the client's sedation decreases and the client is more alert and mobile. It is during this time that joint AROM, ADLs out of bed, mobility, and functional use of the affected extremity become the priorities. However, splinting is still important for a prolonged soft tissue stretch. For this reason, the splint use is decreased to nighttime wear with ROM exercises and functional use of the affected body part during the day. The client may require a period of time to work up to being able to tolerate the splint, as the physician in preparation for hospital discharge may concurrently decrease the pain medication regimen. Also, because the splint was initially worn during the ICU phase when the client was sedated, pain and psychological factors now come into play. Splint wear time may be incorporated into the naptime for children. Often, the splints are made larger to accommodate for postoperative bandages during the acute stage of healing and must be trimmed down for a better fit once the client reaches the intermediate phase. Also of note, extra padding may be required to increase the client's comfort with splint use and the probability that the client will wear the splint as directed. During this stage, direct communication with the client and family, as well as the nursing staff is important to ensure proper splint use. Prior to discharge from the burn hospital, the splint is adjusted for ease of placement and removal. Straps may be attached and extra padding may be provided. Written instructions are helpful to ensure that the client will continue with appropriate splint use and positioning at home.

Dynamic splints are most often introduced during the outpatient phase of burn care. Use of dynamic splints is common when a client has developed a joint contracture. The wear schedule for dynamic splints most commonly begins with 30 minutes twice daily and progresses to 60 minutes twice daily. However, the wear schedule for dynamic splint use varies greatly based on the type of contracture, the extent of the scar contracture, and the tolerance that the client has to the splint. Direct communication between the OT and the client, as well as support from the caregiver, is important. A period of time to allow the client to work up to the desired wear schedule may be beneficial. **Figure 20-7** demonstrates examples of patterns for the most common types of splints (e.g., ankle, elbow, wrist, and hand). These splints are described below.

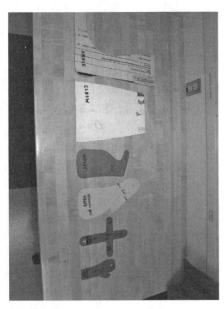

Figure 20-7 Examples of patterns for common types of splints.
Courtesy of Jennie Gilchrist McGillicuddy

Positioning

A prolonged soft tissue stretch achieved by consistent and correct joint positioning is the single most successful method of contracture prevention (Serghiou et al., 2012). Joint positioning is highly utilized in the acute phase of healing. Optimal positioning may be achieved with specialized structures, wedges, or positioning devices. Pillows may be used initially for optimal positioning, if the positioning device is not tolerated. Static splints may also be considered a form of positioning. The experience—alternating ROM exercises with a strong focus on static positioning—results in successful contracture prevention following prolonged immobilization and burn injury to the soft tissue surrounding the joints. Wear schedules for positioning devices vary; however, positioning devices should be worn as long as possible, that is, with consistent skin checks to prevent breakdown to achieve the best contracture prevention.

Therapeutic Interventions

Primary Interventions by Anatomic Site of Injury

Face

For ROM of the face, the focus is placed on the mouth. Functions of the mouth include communication, oral

hygiene, and nutrition. Available planes for the mouth include horizontal stretch, vertical stretch, and circumferential stretch. Measurements are obtained with a small goniometer. The oral commissures are used for a horizontal measurement landmark; and the centers of the nares (i.e., nostrils) are used for vertical measurement landmarks. The most common regions of the mouth for contracture are the commissures, limiting opening of the mouth; however, this is dependent on the location of the burn and any skin grafts. Another target for therapy of the face is the nares. Focus is placed on prevention of closing of the nares following a burn injury.

Mouth splints are used for contracture prevention. Using thermoplastic material, vertical, horizontal, and circumferential splints may be made. Splints are alternated with consistent repetitions of ROM exercises throughout the day. Mouth splints may be worn during set periods throughout the day and/or at night, based on the recommendation/guidance of the OT and depending on the age of the client, the depth of the burn, the location of the autograft, and the tolerance of the client to the splint (Gilchrist, Potenza, & Tenenhaus, 2013). Mouth splinting usually begins with static splints and the splints may be adjusted to become static progressive mouth splints if needed. Direct supervision is required if mouth splints are used with children due to the risk of aspiration. The mouth splints may be padded to prevent skin breakdown. If mouth splints are used during the acute and intermediate stages of healing, while the client is in the hospital, the nursing staff may assist to monitor for skin breakdown. If the splints are used as an intervention in the outpatient phase, the client and/or caregiver should be taught how to monitor for skin breakdown.

Nasal splints may be made with small circular pieces of thermoplastic material, with the edges flared to prevent the splints moving proximally into the nares. The splints must be removed twice daily to allow for skin checks for the prevention of skin breakdown. The portion of the splint that comes in contact with the skin may be padded.

Neck

Functional ROM of the neck is important for turning the head to navigate the environment during daily mobility and during tasks such as driving a motor vehicle. Planes of motion of the neck include lateral rotation, lateral flexion, cervical flexion, and cervical extension. The common landmark for goniometry is the external

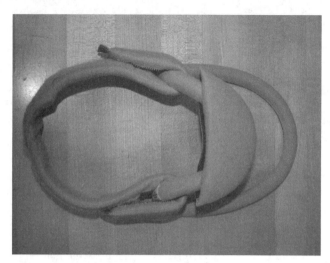

Figure 20-8 Headmaster™ Collar neck splint.
Courtesy of Jennie Gilchrist McGillicuddy

auditory meatus. Cervical lateral flexion is measured in relation to the spinous process of the C7 vertebra. The landmark for measuring cervical rotation is the vertical axis over the middle of the crown of the head. A flexion contracture is one of the more common contractures of the neck following burn injury.

Static thermoplastic neck splints are fabricated to prevent neck contractures. During the burn acute stage, neck splints are most commonly fabricated to hold the neck in a neutral position. Splints are worn over the burn dressings and may be padded to prevent skin breakdown. A common wear schedule for the neck splint is three one-hour sessions daily (e.g., the client works up to this gradually); however, this varies depending on the tolerance of the client, the age of the client, and the severity of the contracture. During the outpatient stage, static progressive neck splints are most commonly used. **Figure 20-8** demonstrates a common neck splint called the Headmaster Collar.

The anticontracture position for the neck is with the neck in neutral. During the acute phase of burn healing, prolonged bed rest and immobility are common. It is important to remove the pillow behind the head of the client during this time, as the pillow promotes the client to be positioned for a prolonged time with the neck in flexion. A small towel roll may be used instead or nothing may be placed behind the head.

Torso

Functional ROM of the spine is important for daily tasks such as lower body dressing and bathing. Planes of motion for the spine include spinal flexion, extension, lateral

flexion, and rotation. The landmarks for measuring spinal ROM are the spinous processes of C7 and S1 for spinal flexion, extension, and lateral flexion, and the vertical axis of the crown of the head for spinal rotation. A more common contracture in clients with torso burns is the pectoralis muscles, which tighten; causing the shoulders to shift anteriorly. This contracture results from prolonged supine bed rest or from burns and skin grafts over the anterior torso. However, with prolonged bed rest during the acute stage, generalized spine stiffness is common. Spinal ROM is important during the intermediate phase of healing during the therapy sessions after the client has been cleared to sit up. AAROM may be required to assist the client with achieving end ROM of the torso. During this stage, it is important to incorporate torso ROM into ADLs (e.g., spinal flexion for a pregait exercise to shift the center of gravity and spinal flexion in preparation for lower body dressing).

Splinting is rarely used for the torso. Rather, a variety of positioning strategies are implemented, as described below.

Positioning of the torso is important during the acute stage of healing if the client is supine with prolonged bed rest. Positioning strategies may be implemented using common items such as a rolled towel or a foam wedge. The positioning device is placed vertically behind the spine, along the spinal column. This position results in an optimal anterior body and chest stretch. Another common positioning technique for the torso during the acute stage of healing is using gauze or other dressings to wrap the shoulder joint in a "figure-of-8" direction, with the direction of traction pulling the shoulder posteriorly. OT education may be necessary to educate the nursing staff so that as the burn dressings are placed during each dressing change, they may be placed for optimal positioning.

Axilla

Functional ROM of the axilla, or the glenohumeral region, results in appropriate use of the arm with daily tasks such as dressing and reaching into cabinets. Full ROM at the glenohumeral joint results in functional use of the arm. Available planes of motion for this joint include flexion, extension, abduction, adduction, external rotation, internal rotation, horizontal abduction, and horizontal adduction. Regarding landmarks for measurement, the axis of the goniometer is placed on the glenohumeral joint, with anterior or posterior placement depending on the plane being measured. Regions for contracture of the axilla depend on the depth and the location of the burn in relation to the joint. Anterior, medial, and posterior axilla contractures are more common than a contracture over the superior aspect of the shoulder, due to the arms resting in adduction in anatomic position. As soon as the client is able to participate in therapy sessions, strategies for self-AAROM for the affected extremity may be taught. For example, using the unaffected arm to clasp hands with the affected arm and lift it. Another method may be to use the wall, with the client facing the wall, and guide the client to slide a small piece of fabric (e.g., a towel) up the wall, while facing the wall (i.e., shoulder forward flexion) and while perpendicular to the wall (i.e., shoulder abduction). These stretches allow for the client to control the speed of ROM exercises and the end ROM within pain barriers.

Axillary splints can be fabricated from thermoplastic material for the desired angle during the acute phase of healing. The wear schedule for a shoulder splint when used in the acute phase is continuous postoperatively, with removal for skin checks and for consistent ROM exercises. However, often the softer axillary positioning wedge, that is, as described below, is used in the acute setting instead of a splint. When the client moves to the intermediate phase of healing, the splinting is relegated to nighttime only, with ROM exercises and functional use of the extremity prioritized during the day. The most common splint used for the glenohumeral region is the airplane splint (**Figure 20-9**). This is a static progressive splint with a harness around the midsection and an

outrigger holding the shoulder in the desired degrees of stretch for abduction. Airplane splints are most often utilized as an outpatient intervention. They are commercially available, and do not have to be fabricated in-house. A common goal for the wear schedule for an airplane splint is three one-hour sessions daily; however, this varies depending on the splint tolerance of the client, the age of the client, and the severity of the contracture. The static progressive airplane splint as demonstrated in the photograph is rarely used during the acute stages of healing due to the risk of skin breakdown.

The anticontracture position for the axilla is with the extremity in abduction. For a burn in the axilla during the acute stage, the positioning wedge is the preferred device over a splint as it is easier to clean and has less risk for causing skin breakdown. **Figure 20-10** shows a positioning wedge which may be used to position the joint at 75°, 90°, or 120° for a prolonged stretch. The wear schedule for the positioning wedge is two hours on, two hours off, during the day, with ROM exercises when the wedge is not in place, and continuous wear at night. The wedge may be alternated between the bilateral axillae. During the intermediate stage of healing, the wedge is worn at night, with ROM exercises and functional use of the extremity during the day. If an axillary wedge is not available, a more commonly found hip abduction wedge or standard pillows may be used for positioning the shoulder in abduction. Figure 20-10 also demonstrates an axillary positioning wedge, most commonly used in the burn ICU.

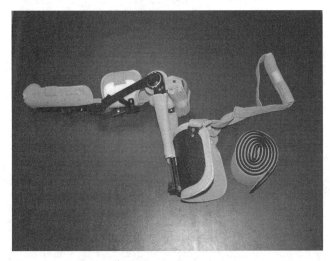

Figure 20-9 Airplane splint.
Courtesy of Jennie Gilchrist McGillicuddy

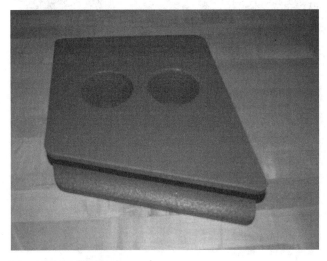

Figure 20-10 Positioning wedge.
Courtesy of Jennie Gilchrist McGillicuddy

Elbow

Functional ROM for the elbow is important for daily activities, such as self-feeding, grooming, and hygiene. Elbow planes of motion include flexion and extension. The landmark for measuring elbow joint ROM is the lateral epicondyle of the humerus. The most common type of elbow contracture is a flexion contracture (Kung, Jebson, & Cederna, 2012), due to the increased strength of the flexor muscle group compared to the extensor muscles. When a beginning contracture over the antecubital fossa is noted, ROM exercises and aggressive splinting are imperative. Strategies for elbow AAROM include using the unaffected extremity to stretch the affected extremity for both flexion and extension. For clients with beginning flexion contractures, a 1–3 pound weight may be used with the client holding the elbow in extension with the weight in the hand for a prolonged period of time. It may be helpful to have a towel roll under the elbow joint for support.

During the acute stage of healing, a static elbow extension splint is used. The purpose of the splint is to prevent elbow flexion contracture and often for protection of a skin graft in this area. **Figure 20-11** demonstrates a static elbow extension splint. The edges may be flared to prevent proximal and distal skin breakdown. Extra padding may be applied over the medial and lateral epicondyles. The wear schedule for this splint is alternating two hours on, two hours off during the day with ROM exercises between wear sessions and continuous wear at night. During the burn intermediate phase of healing, the splint use is decreased to night wear with ROM exercises and

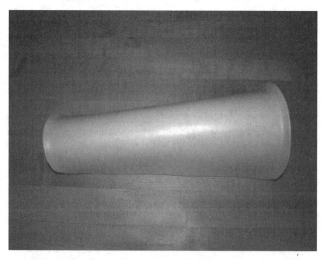

Figure 20-11 Static elbow extension splint.
Courtesy of Jennie Gilchrist McGillicuddy

functional use of the affected extremity during the day. During the outpatient stage of healing, a dynamic elbow flexion or extension splint may be introduced, if needed for a forming elbow contracture or for contracture management. Dynamic elbow flexion splints are more common than dynamic elbow extension splints because elbow flexion is required for functional use of the extremity. Research shows that functional elbow flexion is 130° (Sardelli, Tashjian, & MacWilliams, 2011).

The anticontracture position of the elbow is with the elbow in extension. During the acute stage of healing, prolonged optimal positioning with the use of the elbow extension splint is important for a stretch over a period of time. If a splint is not available or if splinting is not possible, an elbow anticontracture position may be achieved with pillows by positioning the arm with the elbow in extension.

Forearm

Functional ROM of the forearm is important for common daily tasks such as opening doorknobs and for holding and carrying items. Forearm planes of motion include supination and pronation. The landmark for measuring supination and pronation is the volar surface of the distal forearm. The most common type of forearm contracture results in deficits in supination. During the acute stage of healing, clients are commonly positioned in bed with the forearms in pronation; it is important to utilize positioning and the strategies described below to prevent supination deficits. Supination is prioritized over pronation, as it is a more important plane of motion in regard to functional use of the extremity.

Forearm supination—pronation mobilization splints are introduced if needed during the outpatient stage. Forearm supination—pronation mobilization splints use torsion stress to increase supination of the forearm (Jacobs & Austin, 2003). The wear schedule for this splint varies based on the severity of the contracture formation and on the tolerance of the client. A common goal is a wear time of three times daily for one hour each.

The anticontracture position for the forearm is supination. A supination strap (**Figure 20-12**) may be fabricated from material with elastic properties. Weight is applied for a dynamic force; most commonly, a 2 pound weight is used. This strap is often used in addition to an elbow splint and may be used without increasing the risk for skin breakdown due to its nonrigid nature.

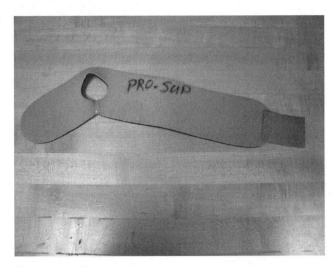

Figure 20-12 Supination strap.
Courtesy of Jennie Gilchrist McGillicuddy

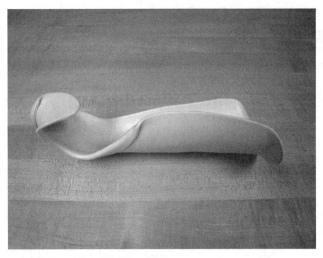

Figure 20-13 Wrist cock-up splint.
Courtesy of Jennie Gilchrist McGillicuddy

A common wear schedule for the supination strap is similar to a splint wear schedule: two hours on, two hours off, during the day with ROM exercises while it is off, and continuous wear at night.

Wrist

Functional ROM of the wrist joint is important for daily tasks such as bathing and opening doors. Planes of motion for the wrist include flexion, extension, radial deviation, and ulnar deviation. The most common contracture seen of the wrist is a flexion contracture. The axis for joint measurement is the base of the third metacarpal, where it meets the wrist. A common method to teach the client for AAROM is the "prayer stretch" with the use of the unaffected extremity to assist the affected extremity to achieve greater wrist extension; the hands meet together and the client moves the elbows parallel to the floor to achieve wrist extension.

Splinting the wrist during the acute stage is important for contracture prevention. Oftentimes, if the hand is burned in addition to the wrist, the custom-fabricated hand splint may include a wrist component. For example, a common hand splint, the intrinsic plus splint (as discussed later in this chapter), includes a wrist component which positions the wrist in 30° of extension. If only the wrist is affected with no hand involvement, a wrist cock-up splint can be fabricated. A wrist cock-up splint is a static articular splint with a forearm component with the angle of the splint holding the wrist in 30° of extension, with the metacarpophalangeal (MP) joints and the distal palmar crease of the hand free to allow hand motion and some functional use of the hand while the splint is in place. **Figure 20-13** demonstrates a wrist cock-up splint. The intrinsic plus splint and the wrist cock-up splint may be padded and worn during the acute stage of healing. Similar to other splints, a common wear schedule is alternating two-hour periods on and off during the day, with ROM exercises while off and continuous wear at night. During the intermediate stage of healing, the wrist splints are worn at night only, with ROM exercises and functional use of the affected extremity during the day. During the outpatient stage of healing, if needed due to contracture formation of the soft tissue or joint, static progressive and dynamic wrist splints are fabricated. An example of a static progressive splint would be a wrist cock-up splint starting with the wrist in neutral, gradually increasing the wrist joint angle during every other visit and sending the client home with the altered splint. Dynamic wrist splints are fabricated by adding a dynamic component to the static splint. The wear schedule for static progressive and dynamic wrist splints varies based on the severity of the contracture and on the client's tolerance. As mentioned with other splinting, a client may require a period to work up to being able to tolerate the splint.

The anticontracture position for the wrist is a neutral position or slight wrist extension (e.g., 10°). During the acute stage of healing, this position may be achieved with the use of pillows to prop the hand ventrally if the forearm is in pronation. As mentioned earlier, common hand splints with a wrist component help with optimal wrist anticontracture positioning.

Hand

ROM of the hand is important for a functional grasp. Hand grasp is necessary for almost every ADL, from basic tasks such as grasping a fork or a toothbrush to complex occupation-related tasks. Planes of motion for hand ROM include composite fist, intrinsic plus, intrinsic minus, opposition, digit abduction, and digit adduction. Landmarks for measurements vary, but most commonly are taken with the axis of the goniometer placed over the joint capsule. The most common type of hand contracture seen following burn injury is the intrinsic minus position (i.e., a "claw" deformity). Clients in acute care without splints or positioning interventions are often positioned with the forearm in pronation with the MP joints in extension and the interphalangeal (IP) joints in flexion, the intrinsic minus position. The intrinsic minus position is considered the position of contracture and does not allow for functional use of the hand (Serghiou et al., 2012); for this reason, ROM in the intrinsic plus plane is important. Intrinsic plus is considered a functional hand position and may be described as the MP joints in 90° of flexion and the IP joints in extension. However, full flexion and extension for each joint of the hand is important to contribute to functional grasp. The second most common type of hand contracture is a contracture of the palmar creases of the hand. The palmar creases of the hand are viewed as high risk for joint contracture. The palmar creases of the hand should be stretched throughout the healing process if the client has a palmar burn. Palmar burns are most commonly seen in children. A third common type of hand contracture is a contracture in the web space between the thumb and the second finger. Syndactyly is a webbing or a soft tissue fusion of the joint space between the digits. Syndactyly between the thumb and second finger results in limited abduction of the thumb, which results in functional limitations in grasp. Opposition of the index finger and the thumb is important for fine motor coordination activities; therefore, if this type of contracture is developing, it is important to engage the client in thumb and index abduction stretches. Ultimately, the type of contracture formation is dependent on the depth and the location of the burn in relation to the joints of the hand. It is important to teach the client how to complete self-AAROM of the affected hand with the use of the unaffected hand. It may be beneficial to get the family of the client involved with providing ROM exercises. Educating the family on the importance of ROM in relation to contracture

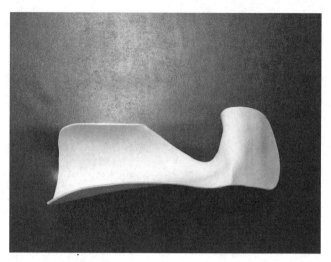

Figure 20-14 Intrinsic plus splint.
Courtesy of Jennie Gilchrist McGillicuddy

prevention may be beneficial and result in optimal contracture prevention.

The type of splint utilized with hand burns depends on the depth and the location of the burn. The intrinsic plus splint is the most common type of splint used with the burned hand (**Figure 20-14**). The intrinsic plus splint has a forearm component with the wrist extended at 30°, the MP joints at 90° of flexion, and the IP joints extended. When applying the intrinsic plus splint, the curve of the splint is positioned securely in the thumb web space. A roll of gauze bandage (e.g., KERLIX) is commonly used to wrap the splint to secure it in place. The gauze is wrapped around the splint, starting at the wrist and is wrapped through the thumb web space to the dorsum of the hand. The wrap then proceeds around the fingers so they are extended at the digit proximal IP (PIP) and digit distal IP (DIP) joints and are flexed at the MP joints.

The second most common type of hand splint used with the burned hand is the palmar pancake splint (**Figure 20-15**). This splint is used following a burn to the palm of the hand if the burn crosses the palmar creases of the hand. The splint includes a wrist component to help stabilize the splint and for a more equal distribution of pressure. It may be worn during the immediate postoperative phase and is alternated with ROM exercises for the palm. The palmar pancake splint is commonly used with children due to the prevalence of contact burns.

A third common splint used with the burned hand is the C-bar splint (**Figure 20-16**). The C-bar splint is a fabricated cross-shaped splint, which is molded into

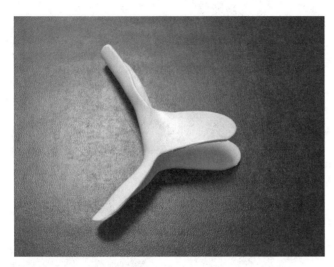

Figure 20-15 Palmar pancake splint.
Courtesy of Jennie Gilchrist McGillicuddy

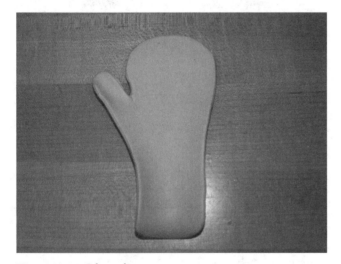

Figure 20-16 C-bar splint.
Courtesy of Jennie Gilchrist McGillicuddy

the hand to fit in the web space between the thumb and second finger. The anchors for the splint wrap around the palmar and dorsal sides of the hand. A common wear schedule for splints during the acute phase is alternating two hours on, two hours off during the day, with the removal for ROM exercises and skin checks, and continuous wear at night.

Splints are secured with a burn bandage dressing (e.g., KERLIX) during the acute stage, which may be discarded and replaced when it becomes soiled. During the intermediate state of healing, splint use may be transitioned to nighttime use only, with ROM exercises and functional use of the hand during the day. During the intermediate stage and the outpatient stage, the OT may apply VELCRO straps to the splint for ease of donning and removing. Dynamic hand splints are introduced if

needed for the management of hand joint contractures. A wrist cock-up splint may be made into a dynamic hand splint by adding a finger cuff with a dynamic component (i.e., rubber band) placed between the finger cuff and the wrist splint (i.e., to target MP joint flexion). The anticontracture position for the hand is the intrinsic plus position. This position may be achieved with the use of an intrinsic plus splint throughout all stages of burn healing.

Besides splinting, additional interventions can be used to achieve functional hand ROM throughout the stages of healing. One modality, used during the acute and intermediate stages of healing, is use of a self-adherent compression bandage wrap (e.g., Coban) to hold the fingers in flexion, and the client maintains this position as long as tolerated, usually for a period of 30–45 minutes. This modality is most commonly used once the autograft over the hand has healed enough to withstand such a wrap. Use of a compression wrap to stretch the fingers in flexion is particularly applicable if the IP joints are stiff or restricted, and this intervention helps to balance the use of an intrinsic plus splint.

A similar intervention is the use of a flexion glove, a fitted glove with a dynamic component, which holds the fingers in flexion by using rubber bands attaching the fingertips to the proximal palm or wrist, pulling the MP and IP joints into flexion. This intervention is also used once the autograft has healed enough to not be damaged during placement or removal of the glove.

A third adjuvant to increase hand flexion is the continuous passive motion device, which is a mechanized method of constantly moving the joints through a controlled ROM with set parameters for force and time. This device can be particularly useful when the client has physiologic and/or psychological barriers to active therapy.

Use of the above three interventions to induce flexion is the most common practice when conventional interventions mentioned above are not effectively producing functional joint ROM.

Hip

ROM of the hip is imperative for lower body mobility. Functional ROM of the hip is also important for dressing and bathing the lower body. Planes of motion for the hip include hip flexion, extension, abduction, adduction, internal rotation, and external rotation. For measuring flexion and extension of the hip, the greater trochanter is the landmark. For measuring hip abduction and adduction, the anterior superior iliac spine is the landmark. For measuring hip internal and external rotation, the axis for the goniometer is the patella. The most common type of hip contracture following burn injury is a hip flexion contracture, due to the position of comfort during the acute stage of healing. Posture will be modified if the hip is contracted in any degree of flexion. Bilateral hip contractures increase lumbar lordosis; an asymmetric contracture may result in scoliosis (Serghiou et al., 2012). During the acute stage of healing, soft mattresses should be avoided because they promote hip flexion. During the intermediate and outpatient stages of healing, small hip flexion contractures can be easily corrected when the client begins functional mobility training following the burn.

An anterior hip spica splint is used to correct a hip flexion contracture. This type of splint is particularly helpful with more extreme hip flexion contractures and is most commonly used with clients in the outpatient stage of healing.

The anticontracture position for the hip is with the hip positioned in neutral. Optimal positioning is achieved during the acute stage of healing while the client is supine in bed. Hip abduction pillows are used to avoid hip rotation. If the client is turned for pressure relief, the hip should be maintained in a neutral position in line with the torso.

Knee

Functional ROM at the knee joint is important for functional standing tasks and for mobility. Planes of motion for the knee include flexion and extension. The landmark for measurement is the lateral epicondyle of the femur. Contracture at the knee most commonly results in deficits of extension. Deep anterior burns may expose and damage the patellar tendon. Deep posterior burns may result in scar formation in the popliteal fossa and will result in functional ROM deficits.

A knee extension splint may be fabricated out of thermoplastic material. More often, however, a commercially available knee immobilizer brace (**Figure 20-17**) is used. The wear schedule is two hours on, two hours off during the day and ROM exercises when the brace is off, with continuous wear at night during the acute stage. During the intermediate stage, the knee extension device is most commonly used at night with mobility encouraged during the day. Knee extension splints are not as commonly

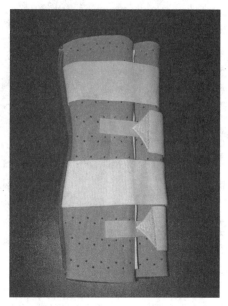

Figure 20-17 Knee extension splint fabricated out of thermoplastic material.
Courtesy of Jennie Gilchrist McGillicuddy

used in the outpatient stage, as the primary focus is placed on mobility.

The anticontracture position for the knee is extension. A knee extension immobilization brace is the most common device used for knee positioning. During the acute stage, pillows under the lower extremities between the knee and ankle are not used as this position would promote hip flexion.

Ankle and Foot

Functional ROM of the ankle is important for mobility and ADLs. Planes of motion for the ankle include dorsiflexion, plantar flexion, inversion, and eversion. Landmarks for measuring ankle ROM is at the joint, midway between the malleoli. Each plane of functional foot ROM is important for posture and gait. Ankle equinus is the most common type of ankle contracture following burn injury, where dorsiflexion is limited (Serghiou et al., 2012), which results in a condition called foot drop and is problematic with mobility. Ankle equinus occurs when the Achilles tendon shortens and the tendon of the tibialis anterior muscle lengthens secondary to prolonged bed rest without proper positioning (Hur et al., 2013).

Due to the prolonged period of bed rest following a large burn, and the gravity with the common supine position, proper ankle splinting is important for prevention of contracture and foot drop. Prefabricated splints may

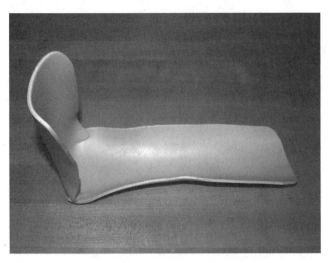

Figure 20-18 Custom-made thermoplastic foot drop splint.
Courtesy of Jennie Gilchrist McGillicuddy

be utilized. However, custom-made thermoplastic foot drop splints (**Figure 20-18**) are commonly fabricated for the protection of lower body grafts and for the proper positioning of the ankle. Wear schedule for the ankle splint is on at all times, with removal only for ankle ROM exercises, for cleaning the extremity, and for skin checks. This type of splint is used primarily in the burn acute stage of healing. During the burn intermediate stage, splinting is primarily at night with mobility and joint ROM exercises during the day. The use of ankle splints is not as common once the client reaches the outpatient stage, unless needed for contracture management. In this case, the splint is primarily worn at night.

Anticontracture positioning for the ankle is with the ankle in neutral. A neutral position of the ankle is a 90° angle at the malleolus. Optimal ankle positioning is achieved with the use of ankle splints. Aggressive positioning is important during the burn acute stage of healing to prevent foot drop due to the prolonged period of bed rest during the surgical, sedated, and intubated stage of burn healing.

Regarding the burn population, PT often includes intervention for the lower body. However, it is important to note that PT and OT services may overlap during rehabilitation of the burned client. An example would be an individual with complex lower body burns. PT interventions for this client may include lower body ROM, positioning, mobility, and gait training. OT interventions may include standing ADLs, lower body self-care, and functional transfers to the restroom and the sink. Physical and OT practitioners play distinct but overlapping

roles in the rehabilitation of clients following burn injuries. Rehabilitation practitioners collaborate to achieve the highest level of function with the burn population.

Activities of Daily Living

ADLs are defined as daily tasks, which are oriented toward caring for one's own body (American Occupational Therapy Association, 2015). Basic ADLs include self-feeding, dressing, grooming and hygiene, bathing, and functional transfers to the shower and toilet. Higher level ADLs include childcare, cooking, and driving. Clients with burn injuries having prolonged hospitalization, which may have included endotracheal intubation and periods of sedation, will experience ADL deficits. OT with the burn population focuses on the functional use of the affected extremities following the burn. In the ICU the focus is placed on initial ROM, splinting, and positioning strategies and interventions, all with the target goal of preventing contracture for increasing future functional use of the affected extremity with daily tasks. During the initial OT sessions following a period of prolonged bed rest, OT practitioners begin to engage clients in ADL retraining, and work with clients at bedside on basic self-care. Upper body joint ROM, strength, endurance, balance, pain, and the client's psychological status are all factors that influence the success of initial ADL retraining.

Clients in the intermediate stage of recovery are more able to actively participate in retraining for ADLs, which becomes the focus in order to increase the client's independence in preparation for hospital discharge. ADL retraining increases the client's ability to care for himself or herself, thus increasing quality of life after burn injury. ADL retraining begins with the OT engaging the client in basic self-care tasks with the client sitting at the edge of the bed and progresses to working with the client out of bed for ADLs. For example, the client may progress to ambulating to the sink to complete grooming and hygiene while standing at the sink. This targets endurance, balance, functional use of the upper extremities, grip strength, coordination, and task sequencing.

During the outpatient stage, ADL retraining may include higher level, more difficult self-care tasks, which have been affected as a result of the burn injury; for example, an OT may work with a client to retrain the use of a dominant, burn-affected upper extremity in the activity of childcare. If the ADL is permanently affected by a joint contracture or amputation, OT practitioners teach clients compensatory strategies for increasing the client's efficiency with daily tasks, for example, teaching the client how to use a new upper extremity prosthetic for self-feeding. Prosthetic training is described in detail later in this chapter. Adaptive equipment commonly used with OT following nonburn injury is not often utilized with clients following burn injury. For example, a built-up eating utensil may be appropriate for a client following a cerebrovascular accident; however, for clients with a hand burn and an autograft, a common goal is increasing hand AROM, rather than providing adaptive eating utensils, which would encourage the client to permanently use the tool and to limit regaining a full composite fist of the affected hand. Daily functional use of the affected hand is a valuable tool in encouraging ROM of the affected hand, rather than allowing the client to permanently compensate. Addressing the client's ADL deficits helps the client to regain purpose and quality of life.

Functional Mobility

Rehabilitation therapists focus on functional mobility with clients following burn injury. Initial interventions such as lower body ROM exercises, positioning, and splinting with clients in the burn ICU are attempts to prevent lower body contractures in preparation for future ambulation. In recent burn rehabilitation research, studies found that early mobilization of clients overall results in greater functional gains (Taylor, Manning, & Quarles, 2013). In the ICU, OT practitioners work with clients to make them sit at the edge of the bed for ADLs and to begin initial pregait training as soon as the client is cognitively able to participate, as these clients are often recovering from prolonged periods of sedation. Early mobility is also facilitated by a tracheostomy placement, as opposed to an endotracheal tube. Some controversy exists regarding whether OT practitioners should avoid progressing the client to an upright-seated position before any femoral intravenous (IV) lines or arterial lines are removed. Early mobility is promoted in clients with small femoral IV lines. However, great caution is advised in mobilizing clients with IV vascular catheters for dialysis and with arterial lines or sheaths. While displacement and occlusion of the lines and catheters are a risk, the most feared complication is perforation of the blood vessel by intravascular lines or sheaths. Therefore, early

mobilization by OT practitioners of clients with femoral intravascular lines should only be undertaken under strict physician orders and supervision.

Early mobilization is an interdisciplinary approach; the nurse is present to monitor the vital signs, telemetry wires, nasogastric tube, and peripheral IV lines of the client. The respiratory OT is present to monitor the ventilator and the client's breathing patterns during exertion. The rehabilitation therapist, nurse, and respiratory therapist monitor the tracheostomy site and oxygen lines. "Figure-of-8" bandage wrapping is a therapy intervention for the lower body to aid in pain management by increasing venous return from the lower extremities during the initial stages of healing (Serghiou et al., 2012). Figure-of-8 wrapping is used over lower body skin graft donor sites and over lower body autograft sites. An elastic compression bandage is commonly used for figure-of-8 wrapping. The OT starts on the top of the foot near the base of the toes; the wrap is pulled for slight tension. The bandage is wrapped at a 45° angle horizontally across the back of the leg and/or foot, keeping slight tension on the bandage. The wrap is angled upward on the foot and brought horizontally across the back of the leg, and angled downward toward the front medial foot. The bandage is then brought horizontally across the back of the leg and angled upward to wrap up the leg toward the groin. The bandage is overlapped on the previous wrap by one-third only, completing additional wraps up the remaining portion of the leg. The extremity should be monitored for comfort and blood flow during use of this wrapping technique, as wrapping too tightly is contraindicated and may affect circulation.

Pregait strategies are initiated at the edge of the bed. During the first few therapy sessions sitting the client upright at the edge of the bed, the focus is placed on proper positioning of the upper extremities and lower extremities to assist with balance in a seated position. The OT will target hip and knee flexion to allow for a sitting position for ADLs at the edge of the bed. Proper placement of the upper extremities in support also assists the client in an upright posture as part of pregait exercises. Initial spinal and extremity ROM exercises begin during the first few therapy sessions at the edge of the bed, in preparation for sit-to-stand, standing ADLs, and functional mobility. During the acute stage of healing, it may be noted that during the initial therapy sessions, clients present with torso and extremity stiffness and ROM deficits due to early contracture formation and muscle atrophy resulting from nonuse and prolonged periods of bed rest. Therapy sessions progress according to the client's tolerance and with the client's safety always in mind. Functional mobility and weight-bearing through the lower extremities can typically begin on POD #3 if the client does not have skin grafts over any joints of the lower extremities. If skin grafts cross any lower extremity (LE) joints, functional mobility training will begin on POD #5. It should be noted that if a client has a skin graft on the plantar surface of the foot, LE weight-bearing precautions should be specified by the physician. As with ADLs, many factors have an effect on the functional mobility of the client. OT practitioners take into account the many components necessary for functional mobility and address each deficit accordingly to progress the client to an ambulatory state. A front-wheeled walker is commonly used with initial gait following a burn injury and prolonged immobility. If the client has upper body weight-bearing precautions as a result of a fracture or an amputation, a single point cane or a quad cane may be utilized. If a client has lower body weight-bearing precautions, crutches may be introduced. **Figure 20-19** shows mobility device options: front-wheeled walker, single point cane, crutches, and wheelchair. OT practitioners may introduce a mobility device to use temporarily to aid in ambulation during healing of a lower body skin graft donor site or to manage pain during initial standing ADLs and functional mobility.

With clients in the intermediate stage of recovery, the rehabilitation therapists will continue to progress the functional mobility status of the client. Like the use of

adaptive equipment for ADLs, durable medical equipment mobility devices are primarily used in the acute and intermediate stages of healing for initial gait training and to manage pain with standing and improve overall strength and endurance deficits. A goal of OT practitioners in the outpatient setting is to progress the client away from the use of mobility devices and to encourage independent ambulation by continuing to target lower body ROM, strength, and endurance training. However, if ambulation is permanently affected, the rehabilitation therapists will begin to teach the client how to permanently implement the mobility device for use with daily routines in the home and community and on a variety of surfaces. For example, training a client to use a wheelchair for mobility may include operation of the wheelchair, upper body strengthening for chair self-propulsion, techniques for controlling the wheelchair during uphill/downhill motion, and use of the wheelchair in a public community setting for instrumental ADLs.

Rehabilitation therapists strive to communicate and coordinate with the client's family, nursing staff, social workers, and psychology staff with progressions in ADLs and functional mobility. The OT team depends on the family and nurses to follow through between therapy sessions, for example, getting the client out of bed three times daily and avoiding total assistance with client grooming. Rehabilitation therapists are consulted initially for contracture prevention and also later in recovery if needed for functional mobility or ADL deficits. It is important to note that while rehabilitation therapists target ADLs and functional mobility, the primary focus on all rehabilitation sessions continues to be on ROM and prevention and/or management of contractures.

Endurance

Following periods of prolonged immobilization, endurance limitations are common. Aerobic deconditioning is common in clients following major burn injuries. Clients often become easily fatigued with basic ADLs during initial functional mobility training. During the acute stage of healing, endurance exercise is as basic as assisting a client out of bed for ADLs two to three times per day. During the intermediate stage of healing and the outpatient stage, endurance training therapy sessions may include repetitive use of the affected extremity with an intense endurance exercise program (de Lateur et al., 2007). Aerobic training

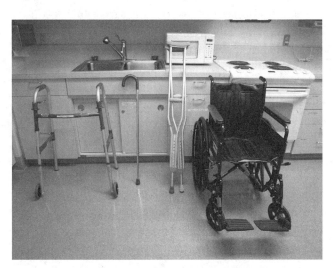

Figure 20-19 Examples of common mobility devices.
Courtesy of Jennie Gilchrist McGillicuddy

is important to improve muscle endurance, as well as muscle strength and aerobic capacity.

Strengthening

Strength limitations and muscle atrophy have been observed in clients following major burns and prolonged periods of bed rest (St-Pierre, Choiniere, Forget, & Garrel, 1998). The overload principle states that to improve strength, the client must be provided with and perform tasks exceeding those of the client's baseline. Because of deconditioning and muscle weakness following major burn injury and prolonged immobilization, the overload principles can be easily fulfilled and achieved for strength training. During the acute stage of healing, strength training overlaps with endurance training; daily consistent low-load exercises and daily out-of-bed activity target both muscle strengthening and endurance.

During the intermediate stage of healing, aerobic conditioning, treadmill exercises, low-load exercise bands or free weights, and the recumbent bicycle can be used. Additional forms of exercise introduced during the outpatient stage include swimming, upright cycling, and team sports (Baldwin & Li, 2013). Strength training activities can be graded, and intensity should be increased based on the client's tolerance and with the goal of assisting the client back to the pre-traumatic baseline. Caution should be taken to avoid muscle overload.

Scar Management

A primary role of rehabilitation therapists working with burn clients is scar management. Scar management may begin as soon as there are no open wounds (Serghiou et al., 2012). Scar management interventions are effective up to 12 months postinjury, during the maturation phase of the scar (Kirsner, 2008); the deeper the burn, the greater the risk of scarring. Superficial epidermal burn wounds that heal within 7–14 days are least likely to scar. Partial-thickness dermal burns that heal within 14–21 days most likely will not produce scar tissue that limits function; however, clients should be monitored for scar management needs prophylactically. Deeper dermal burns, which affect the vasculature and nerves (i.e., full-thickness burns), will result in scarring that may require intervention. Factors that contribute to scarring include age, genetics, wound infections, ethnicity, and location of injury (Serghiou et al., 2012). A hypertrophic scar is characterized by thick, raised collagenous tissue at the site of the injury. Hypertrophic scars crossing joints may result in functional limitations. Rehabilitation therapists focus primarily on scar management for functional reasons, but also for optimal cosmetic outcomes.

Intervention for scar management is most effective if implemented during the remodeling phase of scar healing (Kirsner, 2008). The effectiveness of scar management interventions may be measured by scar assessment. The Vancouver Scar Scale is a tool to objectively record hypertrophic scarring over time. This scale targets burn scar pigmentation, pliability, height, and vascularity (Sullivan, Smith, Kermode, McIver, & Courtemanche, 1990). Conservative interventions for scar management from a rehabilitation perspective include scar massage, pressure therapy, and topical silicone dressings as primary interventions. Additional conservative physician-performed interventions include intralesional steroid injections, or fractional CO_2 laser therapy can also be used in difficult cases. Follow-up clinic visits are necessary to monitor the client's compliance with scar management interventions.

Scar Massage

Once all open wounds have healed and the skin can withstand sheering, scar massage is introduced. The purpose of scar massage is skin mobilization, increasing blood flow, and decreasing bands of fibrous tissue. Types of scar massage include skin rolling while lifting the skin and subcutis away from underlying structures, and parallel pressure massage over the scar band. With the skin rolling type of massage, scar tissue may be lifted between the thumb and index finger, using a lubricant, mobilizing the tissue from the underlying tissue. This is a useful type of massage for scar formation over the dorsal hand, for example. It is important to separate the fibrous tissue from the underlying structures (e.g., extensor tendons) to prevent tendon adherence and functional limitations. Parallel pressure massage is performed using a lubricant and motions parallel to the scar band, massaging in combination with the end ROM exercises. The joint is stretched to the point of blanching, with scar massage provided in combination with end ROM stretching. This type of massage may be effective with scar formation in the axilla, for example. Frequency for scar massage varies, but is typically for twenty minutes, three times a day. The skin should be monitored for breakdown and irritation.

Pressure Therapy

Another primary intervention for the management of hypertrophic scarring is pressure therapy. Use of pressure therapy for scar management has been documented since the 1970s (Reid, Evans, Naismith, Tully, & Sherwin, 1987). Studies show that 10 mmHg of pressure is effective in the prevention of hypertrophic scarring, while pressure greater than 40 mmHg may be harmful to tissue healing and may result in sensation deficits (Serghiou et al., 2012). Constant moderate pressure can help reduce collagen synthesis in a hypertrophic scar and cause re-alignment of existing collagen fibers (Costa et al., 1999). Pressure therapy should begin during the maturation process of the healing burn scar, for optimal results as soon as all open wounds have healed. The most common form of pressure therapy during the burn intermediate stage of recovery includes use of Tubigrip and Coban wrappings. Tubigrip is a disposable, circumferential tube-shaped dressing, which is available in a variety of sizes (**Figure 20-20**). Tubigrip is most commonly used on the extremities for early pressure. Caution must be taken to ensure the adequate amount of pressure, enough to be effective; however, too much pressure may result in edema of the hands or feet. Coban wrapping (**Figure 20-21**) is used for initial scar management of the hands. To wrap the fingers, strips approximately twice the length of the finger are cut and should be stretched to 25% or one-fourth of the elasticity (Serghiou et al., 2012). Wrapping for the digits begins distally and proceeds from the nail surface to the web space; Coban should overlap half the width of the previous pass when wrapping distal to proximal over each digit. After the

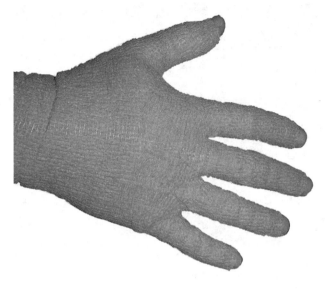

Figure 20-21 Example of Coban™ wrapping.
Courtesy of Jennie Gilchrist McGillicuddy

digits are wrapped, the hand is wrapped from finger web space to just past the wrist also with one-half the width overlap and with a 25% tension stretch. Additional strips of Coban are cut and used in the web space between each digit. With the exception of the fingertips, no skin should be showing. The full hand should be wrapped for adequate and equal-pressure therapy. Caution should be taken to prevent wrapping too tightly, which could result in deformity of the healing structures. On the contrary, wrapping that is too loose may result in promotion of edema of the hand, especially when used in combination with Tubigrip over the arm (Serghiou et al., 2012). When wrapped correctly, Coban provides effective pressure therapy, which has been shown to be an effective early scar management intervention (Costa et al., 1999).

Tubigrip and Coban are the most effective if worn 23 hours per day and should be changed daily, with removal only for showering, or as needed if soiled. Once possible, measurements are obtained and custom pressure garments are fabricated for the client. Custom pressure garments may be made for all parts of the body (**Figure 20-22**), and are a widely accepted treatment intervention for the management of hypertrophic scarring (Serghiou et al., 2012). Custom pressure garments take the place of Tubigrip and Coban wrapping for the hand or extremity. Garments are generally worn up to 24 months following surgery, during scar maturation. Garments should only be removed for exercise and showering. Clients are provided with two sets of garments, one garment to wear while the other is being cleaned. Garments are replaced approximately every

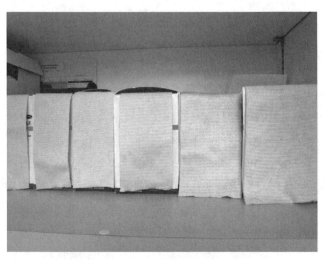

Figure 20-20 Examples of Tubigrip™ in a variety of sizes.
Courtesy of Jennie Gilchrist McGillicuddy

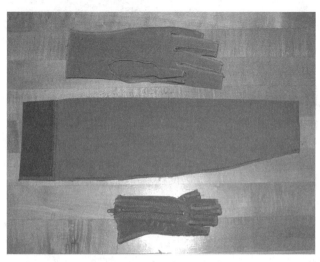

Figure 20-22 Examples of custom pressure garments.
Courtesy of Jennie Gilchrist McGillicuddy

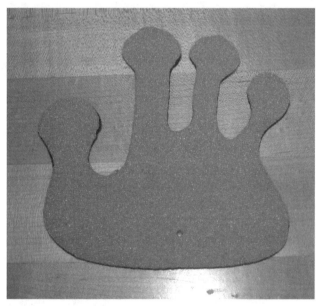

Figure 20-23 Example of a web space insert fabricated out of soft
foam.
Courtesy of Jennie Gilchrist McGillicuddy

12 weeks (Serghiou et al., 2012; Williams, Knapp, &
Wallen, 1998), in order to ensure maximal elasticity and
continued pressure. Williams et al. (1998) found 90 days
to be the mean from the time of garment provision to the
time of garment replacement, with factors for replacement being deterioration of the garment, garments being
too large, garments being too small, or other reasons.
Children with pressure garments should be monitored
for proper fit, due to periods of growth.

Inserts are used under garments to provide additional
pressure over areas that may be difficult to compress
with garments alone (e.g., concave areas of the body such
as the sternum). **Figure 20-23** demonstrates a web space

insert fabricated out of soft foam to be used to prevent
syndactyly of the web spaces. Additional inserts are
made, based on the client's need in relation to scarring.

Silicone

Silicone gel sheets are one of the most commonly used
scar inserts. Silicone is available commercially in gel
sheets and is used in combination with pressure therapy
for optimal scar management. Research has found that
silicone is effective when used alone; however, it works
best when used in combination with pressure therapy
(Momeni, Hafezi, Rahbar, & Karimi, 2009). Silicone
therapy has been proven effective in increasing pliability and decreasing erythema of hypertrophic scars
(Momeni et al., 2009). Silicone is commonly used on the
skin of the hands and the face for cosmetic reasons, as
they are visible and socially important areas of the body.
The mechanism of silicone is not clearly understood;
however, hypothetical mechanisms include hydration
and occlusion, leading to local hypoxemia and neovascularization (Hoeksema, DeVos, Verbelen, Pirayesh, &
Monstrey, 2013; Momeni et al., 2009; Sawada & Sone,
1992). Commonly used silicone gel sheets include CICA-
CARE® and NOVAGEL. The silicone gel sheet is placed
between the garment and the skin. The silicone should
be changed and cleaned as often as the burn garments.
Caution should be taken to prevent skin maceration with
silicone use as the gel sheets are occlusive to moisture.
Figure 20-24 shows the types of silicone that are commonly used with hypertrophic scarring following skin
autografts.

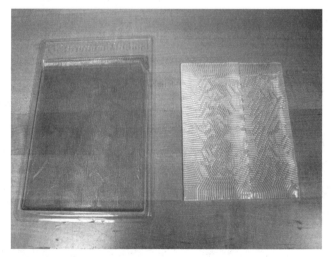

Figure 20-24 Examples of silicone commonly used with
hypertrophic scarring.
Courtesy of Jennie Gilchrist McGillicuddy

Scar Management of the Face

For cosmetic, as well as functional, reasons, the face is a target for intense scar management following burn injury. Early use of facial scar management interventions and exercise has been shown to improve scar vascularity and pigmentation outcomes (Parry, Sen, Palmieri, & Greenhalgh, 2013). Elastic pressure burn garments have been used in the past; however, a current trend in scar management of the face is the use of pressure masks (Powell, Haylock, & Clarke, 1985). Custom-made silicone masks are the most recent advance in scar management for the face. Total Contact is a company that fabricates burn scar masks and neck orthotics for the application of pressure and silicone (Total Contact, 2008). The process for obtaining a mask begins with a three-dimensional scan of the face using a specialized scanning device, which is connected to a software program (**Figure 20-25**) (Total Contact, 2008). Hundreds of images are obtained from each scan, and the data are organized and merged into one clear three-dimensional image of the face with limited to no noise from motion during the scan series. From the composite image, trim lines are delineated to mark where the mask should begin and end in relation to the scar. From the data, a mold of the face or neck is fabricated. From the mold, the custom silicone-lined mask is made. During the initial fitting session of the mask, straps are attached to allow the device to provide adequate pressure. Straps and anchors comprise a harness system and a variety of harness designs are available to secure a face mask for adequate pressure (Parry et al., 2013). Head pressure garments

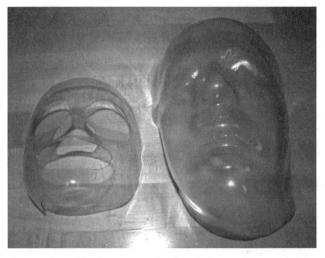

Figure 20-26 Clear custom-made silicone face mask.
Courtesy of Jennie Gilchrist McGillicuddy

may be used in place of straps to hold the mask in place. The edges of the mask are inspected to prevent signs of skin breakdown. The edges may be padded with moleskin if needed to increase comfort and compliance with use. The client and family should be educated on the purpose of the mask, how to clean the mask, and on the importance of monitoring for skin breakdown. The mask is clear, compared to some older methods for facial scar management, and may be more cosmetically appealing to clients during mask use, thus resulting in increased compliance. **Figure 20-26** shows a clear custom-made silicone face mask. The wear schedule for the mask is 23 hours per day, with removal for facial exercise, scar massage, eating, and showering. As with other scar management options, clients may take a period of time to build up tolerance with mask use. Handheld models are available for the scanning device, which results in ease of and increased speed of measurement for fabrication of the facial mask or neck splint. Accompanying software is used to measure millimeters of change in the hypertrophic scar height, and pigmentation may be tracked as well.

Additional Rehabilitation Interventions

Serial Casting

Serial casting is a therapy intervention used over any joint following burn injury, as a method of a low-load, prolonged stretch. Hypertrophic scar tissue requires a greater amount of energy to stretch than normal skin

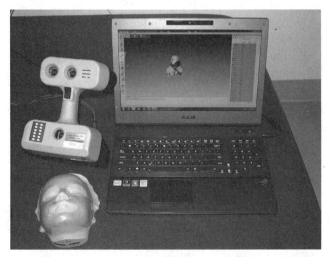

Figure 20-25 Three-dimensional scanning device used to create burn scar masks.
Courtesy of Jennie Gilchrist McGillicuddy

(Dunn, Silver, & Swann, 1985). Serial casting allows prolonged positioning with the goal of increasing ROM of a contracted joint. In a study of 35 clients, Bennett, Helm, Purdue, and Hunt (1989) found a 30% increase (i.e., 56–86% of normal) in joint ROM after serial casting. Serial casting has been shown to result in functional gains (Bennett et al., 1989). Indications for serial casting include clients who are noncompliant with traditional interventions (e.g., active ROM exercises, splinting, and positioning). For example, serial casting can be a good choice in children when traditional interventions are not effective and in clients with burns involving multiple joints (e.g., the hands) with a need for a low-load prolonged stretch. In addition to being used for joints, serial casting is also used for contractures of the palmar crease, such as on a child's hand. While the most common use for serial casting is to increase joint ROM by a prolonged stretch of soft tissue, serial casting may also be used for graft protection or for postoperative immobilization. The most common joints for serial casting include the wrist, the hand in the intrinsic plus position, the ankle, the axilla, and the elbow. Joints are most commonly casted in the anticontracture positions described earlier in this chapter. Joint ROM is documented prior to each cast placement and following each cast removal.

Depending on where one works, casts can be applied by rehabilitation therapists. Supplies required for serial casting include a tubular stockinette for an under layer against the skin, cast padding, water-immersed cast material, a bucket of water, casting gloves, scissors, a cast saw, and cast spreaders. The extremity is cleaned, and the client is positioned in maximal stretch. The cast is placed with the stockinette and padding first, followed by the cast material. Padding is placed over the bony prominences, such as the epicondyles of the elbow, the malleoli of the ankle, the ulnar styloids of the wrist, and the MP and IP joints of the hand. Serial casts remain in place from a period of three days to one week and are changed and replaced according to the needs of the client. Routine cast assessment includes monitoring the fit of the cast for changes due to edema, capillary refill, temperature, movement, sensation of the distal extremity, and skin breakdown (e.g., pressure marks, cuts, and/or bruises). The serial casting process may go on for months, with consistent cast changes and progressive increases in joint angle. The cast may be cut on either side, or bivalved, to be easily removed and replaced at home, and to allow regular skin checks and ROM exercises. Serial casts can be effective after 24 hours; yet, they can be kept on up to one week. A series of casts may be used for a gradual, slow increase in joint ROM.

A cast saw and cast spreaders are used to remove a serial cast. Clients are taught to monitor for edema, skin breakdown, or sensory deficits (e.g., numbness or tingling) of the distal extremity, and are instructed to contact the therapy clinic, emergency room, or local fire station, if the cast requires immediate removal. Contraindications to serial casting include clients with known nerve injury, infection, open wounds, and clients with sensory deficits at baseline. If a serial cast is used with a child, education of the caregivers is important so that the cast and the child's extremity may be properly monitored. Following a series of casting, a splint is often introduced and implemented for follow-up.

Paraffin Wax

Paraffin wax is a heat modality used to warm the soft tissue in preparation for joint or soft tissue mobilization. If used according to the proper protocol, paraffin has several functional benefits. Indications for use include joint contracture and pain with ROM. Paraffin works well when used in combination with a low-load, prolonged stretch. Paraffin wax heats the collagen fibers of the scar in preparation for stretching and is most commonly used at the beginning of outpatient therapy sessions. It can help relieve superficial stiffness and minor aches, and it contains mineral oil, which moisturizes the epidermis overlying the scar, decreasing the chances of fissures during motion (Rocky Mountain Model System for Burn Injury Rehabilitation, 2015). Paraffin is most commonly used on the hands and feet. It is important to note that caution must be taken when using heat modalities on clients with burn injuries. Areas with hypertrophic scars have impaired sensation and an altered vascular system. When using a heat modality over a burn hypertrophic scar, caution should be taken to avoid causing an additional burn injury, as the scarred region will have difficulty dissipating heat. For this reason, paraffin wax is not used with clients in the acute or intermediate stages of healing following burns.

During use, the skin should be checked for blistering or burning, and the client should be able to self-monitor and report pain or sensation abnormalities. Additional contraindications include known infection, open wounds, ischemia, bleeding disorders, inability to communicate or respond to pain, edema, and acute trauma and inflammation (Prentice, 2003).

Materials required for paraffin use include a heating pot, paraffin wax, a thermometer, plastic wrap, and towels. The procedure for paraffin is as follows. The paraffin wax is heated to 118°F–120°F (Prentice, 2003), measured carefully by a thermometer. The target extremity is placed in the stretched position and dipped into the paraffin bath six to eight times. The extremity is wrapped in a plastic wrap, and two towels are layered on top. The paraffin is left on for 15 to 20 minutes. It is removed sooner if the client reports pain or sensation abnormalities. Following paraffin removal, the client is engaged in ROM exercises and scar management interventions.

Ultrasound

Ultrasound is a modality commonly used in the outpatient setting to target soft tissue contractures, including those crossing joints. Ultrasound consists of waves that transmit energy at greater than 20,000 Hz (i.e., cycles per second). Generally, therapeutic ultrasound has a frequency between 0.7 and 3.3 MHz in order to achieve energy absorption into soft tissue. In the burn population, goals of ultrasound include increased soft tissue elasticity and extensibility, increased circulation, decreased pain, and reduction in joint stiffness and joint contractures by increasing the tissue temperature of deep tissues (Prentice, 2003). Contraindications for ultrasound use include ischemia, bleeding disorders, impaired sensation, inability to communicate pain or abnormal sensation, malignancy, or acute trauma or inflammation. As with other heat modalities, caution should be taken prior to the use of ultrasound with hypertrophic scarring and joint contracture following burn injury. Because of possible sensation deficits and the altered vascularity characteristic of hypertrophic scarring, the heat may not dissipate appropriately and the client can sustain an additional burn injury easily. The OT should be familiar with the ultrasound protocol. Caution should be taken and intensities lowered to err on the side of caution with the use of ultrasound for therapeutic intervention in burn clients.

Evidence is mixed regarding the effectiveness of therapeutic ultrasound to increase soft tissue elasticity of hypertrophic scarring following burns and autografts (Cambier & Vanderstraeten, 1997; Sar et al., 2013). Of note, ultrasound has been shown to be effective in increasing soft tissue elasticity when applied with the joint positioned in maximal tissue elongation (i.e., stretched to the point of blanching). More research exists in support of the use of therapeutic ultrasound to reduce deep joint stiffness and pain and to increase circulation by heating the deep tissues (Prentice, 2003; ter Haar, 1999).

The ultrasound frequency depends on the targeted depth: 3 MHz is used for superficial heat and 1 MHz is used for deep heat. The intensity depends on the desired amount of heat. In the burn population, an intensity range is 0.9 to 1.0 W/cm^2. Conservatively, intensity should never be greater than 1.0 W/cm^2 for use in the burn population. The duration is calculated using the size of the sound head and the size of the targeted treatment area, usually 5 to 10 minutes on average. The duration should not exceed ten minutes. Common, commercially available sound head sizes include 1, 5, and 10 cm. Use of ultrasound to treat burn scarring and contractures is continuous and is never pulsed.

It is imperative that OT practitioners using ultrasound, paraffin wax, or any other heat modality are familiar with the protocol, indications, and contraindications prior to use. Most institutions are under regulations that require specialized training and certification prior to the OT's use of heat modalities with clients.

Rehabilitation of Children Following Burns

Pediatric clients may pose a challenge to implementation of standard, routine burn therapy interventions. Therapy begins with a developmental assessment of the child to screen for preexisting developmental delay or baseline disorders. For burn-related intervention, creativity is utilized to implement proper stretching, splinting, positioning, and functional mobility protocols. The basic principles are identical to those discussed above; however, alternate strategies are required to work with children. Distraction techniques can be valuable (Miller, Rodger, Bucolo, Greer, & Kimble, 2010). It is important to obtain involvement of the family or caregivers of the child for the comfort of the child during therapy and for appropriate follow-up with therapy interventions between professional sessions.

During the acute stage of injury, the child may undergo periods of sedation with the medical team for bandage changes. If the child is sedated during the bandage change, the OT is able to provide thorough PROM, visualize which joints the burn crosses, and assess burn location in relation to function. When not under sedation, the child is engaged in age-appropriate play incorporating functional use of the affected extremity.

Use of video games has been shown to be an effective intervention for increasing the child's participation and motivation with rehabilitation therapy sessions (Carbullido et al., 2013; Parry et al., 2012). For functional mobility training, the child is taught to begin with gentle weight onto the affected LE in preparation for mobility. Functional mobility is progressed accordingly. As with adults, initial functional mobility training may include gait with an assistive device.

Family education regarding the technique of ROM and strategies for assisting the child with ROM exercises, and education regarding the importance of functional use of the affected extremity is implemented. Strategies for splinting are utilized to prevent the child from self-removing, for example, use of a mitten to secure the splint when worn at night. Scar management strategies such as massage with young children are usually the responsibility of the caregiver. A reward system may be helpful to encourage active participation of the child and to progress the child toward established rehabilitation goals. Coordination with a staff child life specialist is helpful to monitor for developmental regression as a result of trauma, pain, or fear during the healing stages.

Amputations and Prosthetic Training Following Burn Injury

Full-thickness thermal injuries resulting in amputation are not common; however, in some instances, amputation can reduce the rate of mortality and thereby become a necessity to save the client's life. Following amputation, the OT completes an assessment of the residual limb and of the client's total body function. Initial preprosthetic care begins with assessment of the residual musculature, nerves, vascular supply, sensation, ROM, strength, and endurance. Scar massage, positioning, edema control, desensitization techniques, and strength and endurance training are implemented for the residual limb. Extra caution should be taken if the residual limb was also involved in the burn injury.

The potential for a client to obtain a prosthetic device following burn injury is improved with thorough preprosthetic care, client motivation, the social support system in place for the client, and the client's access to a qualified medical team following amputation, including the medical and rehabilitation teams, the psychology staff, and an orthotist.

Types of prosthetics include body-powered, myoelectric, hybrid body-powered and myoelectric, and passive devices (i.e., cosmetic only) (Smurr, Gulick, Yancosek, & Ganz, 2008). Often, a client may prefer to own a variety of prosthetics and will select the device based on the planned activity level for the day. Rehabilitation therapists work with clients for prosthetic training, including use, cleaning, and operation of the device.

Following upper extremity amputations, the type of prosthetic is chosen based on residual nerves and musculature, type of activity, and available ROM of the residual joints. Types of upper extremity prosthetics include components for the hand, devices for below the elbow, and devices for above the elbow. Upper extremity body-powered prosthetic devices (e.g., hook prosthetic devices) are the less expensive option, are lighter in weight, and accommodate for residual limb changes. This type of device offers visual and tactile feedback. Due to the figure-of-8 harness attachment, pressure is more equally distributed, and as a result, the device is able to be used for heavier activities compared to a myoelectric device. The myoelectric device utilizes the voluntary muscle contraction of the residual musculature. The myoelectric device requires stable residual limb musculature and appropriate strength. Myoelectric devices are more expensive than body-powered devices; however, they are more cosmetically appealing because they mimic the lost extremity in appearance.

Training for upper extremity prosthetic use begins with the OT teaching the client operational knowledge. The OT works with the client for initial maintenance and care for the prosthetic and its components, as well as how to apply and remove the prosthetic device. The OT teaches the client how to control the device, operations as basic as turning it on and off to as complex as the use of the prosthetic to achieve more natural movements. Care for the residual limb is taught and reinforced throughout the process. ADL training is targeted with the prosthetic device, and a common goal is to initiate the movement prior to contact with the ADL item, for example, hand opening while the arm is en route to a cooking pot handle, opening prior to contacting the handle with gradual hand grasp once the hand is near and has come in physical contact with the pot handle (Smurr et al., 2008).

Evidence-Based Practice

The consistent introduction of new techniques and materials, especially with scar management devices, and consistent research publications lead to ever-changing burn rehabilitation options. It is important to select the best intervention based on the needs of the client, utilizing devices, strategies, and interventions that research has shown effective. However, when new, less-known interventions are tried and lead to functional success with clients, rehabilitation therapists should consider further studies or, at least, case report publications in order to potentially develop and share new knowledge.

Referrals and Discharge Considerations

Many support groups and outreach programs exist for clients following burns. One of the most well-known and successful programs in the United States is Survivors Offering Assistance in Recovery (SOAR) (The Phoenix Society for Burn Survivors, 2014). This is a program designed to provide training and social support to burn survivors and family members by utilizing volunteers who return to hospital burn units to tell their stories in hopes of helping other burn survivors. The SOAR program can be beneficial to PT and OT sessions, as it can provide the client with motivation needed to continue with therapy and to not give up.

Return to work (e.g., work hardening) programs exist in rehabilitation clinics for adults reentering professional roles. In collaboration with child life specialists, analogous return to school programs exist for children following burn injury. Burn summer camps can also be a helpful experience for a child to socialize with other children his or her age, who have undergone similar experiences, and it may help the child to process feelings and to progress emotionally (Maslow & Lobato, 2010; Rimmer et al., 2007).

During this period of return to work, school, or other social and occupational roles the client had prior to burn injury, it is important to reinforce that thorough burn care follow-up is imperative. This may be achieved with consistent therapy clinic visits and with routine follow-up visits to outpatient physician burn clinics. The client must be educated on what to expect regarding scar and functional outcomes. The client is routinely educated on the recommended length of time to wear devices such as pressure garments and splints and how long the daily ROM, strength, and endurance home exercise programs should be followed. In addition, the client is taught to monitor for specific signs of skin breakdown, joint contracture, or for decreasing functional use of areas of concern during the

long-term healing process. Parents or caregivers of children are educated on methods of monitoring the scar as the child grows and when to seek medical attention. Clients with prosthetics know whom to contact if the device malfunctions. As the endurance improves, gym membership and participation in sporting teams are encouraged. Yoga can be particularly effective in recovery, including managing chronic persistent pain (Dauber, Osgood, Breslau, Vernon, & Carr, 2002) following burn injury and skin graft surgery due to the amount of static stretching and breathing throughout the routine. Throughout this follow-up and throughout the long-term burn sequelae, it is most important that clients return to meaningful occupations and to the highest quality of life possible.

Compassionate Care and Social Reintegration

Each small step in the rehabilitation process is important, as the client may psychologically benefit from achieving small milestones during the early healing process. However, most clients develop concerns about their comprehensive recovery, particularly regarding issues such as returning to prior roles, occupations, and routines. Clients also express the desire to return to the quality of life that was known to them prior to the burn injury. As a healthcare clinician working with burn survivors, it is important to practice with compassionate care. This may include practices such as appreciation of the client as a human being, demonstration of one's respect for and sensitivity to the client, viewing the client as an individual, and speaking with, as well as authentically listening to, the client (Badger & Royse, 2012; Brunton & Beaman, 2000). Compassionate care is facilitated by communication and finding common ground through empathy (Sanghavi, 2006).

During the acute stage of healing, it is important to allow the client as much control as possible. For example, allowing the client to select the time of day for therapy sessions, as opposed to surprising the client with drop in therapy visits, can allow the client a degree of empowerment. Another example is to allow the client a choice in the number of repetitions for the exercises during therapy (e.g., "Would you like to complete 2 sets of 20, or 1 set of 40?"). Practicing with compassionate care is beneficial because it may lead to establishment of a stronger working relationship between the OT and the client, with greater client trust in the competence of the OT practitioner. This may lead to the client feeling more comfortable surrendering control of the rehabilitation process to others during what is often an otherwise vulnerable time. As a result, the client is often more willing to work with the OT team toward the established mutual goals. During this time, the OT practitioner may have to validate the client's feelings of inadequacy, frustration at dependence on others, and sadness when improvements are gradual. As the client progresses, he or she may express fear over return to work, school, or prior roles. It is the job of the OT team to imbue confidence in the client's capabilities and to progress the client toward functional goals in preparation for return to society. If the client has permanent morbidity, OT practitioners teach compensatory strategies for clients to lead functional, meaningful lives. It is important for rehabilitation therapists to have an interdisciplinary approach to client care and to know when to consult a psychologist, physician, or social worker when appropriate.

Management and Standards of Practice

Due to the complexity of the burn sequela, all disciplines involved in care of the burned client should demonstrate some level of training and competency. National certifications and competencies are being developed for burn rehabilitation therapists. Certified OT assistants involved in the treatment of the burned client should maintain direct communication with the primary burn OT. In addition, all OT assistants should be familiar with burn rehabilitation strategies and protocols specific to burn care prior to practice in this clinical environment.

In an ever-changing healthcare world, it is important that all medical practitioners uphold ethical standards. Severe burn injuries often leave clients temporarily incommunicative, which may create complex ethical situations (Cole, Stal, & Hollier, 2008). As a result, client autonomy and the ability to make decisions become of concern. Though family involvement is encouraged and appreciated, only thorough and thoughtful application of ethics can provide maximal respect for client autonomy during the medical management and rehabilitation of individuals following burn injury. Providing compassionate and thorough care while upholding ethical standards is imperative for OT practitioners to assist clients who have recovered from burn injury reintegrate into society and meaningful lives.

Chapter 20 Self-Study Activities (Answers Are Provided at the End of the Chapter)

Please select the best choice for each scenario. Please note each phase of burn healing with each question.

Client Scenario	Answer Choices
1. Client A.G. was admitted to the burn ICU with full-thickness burns crossing all metacarpophalangeal and all interphalangeal joints on the dorsal side of the right hand. This client is currently intubated and sedated. Surgeries for skin grafting are pending; however, initial burn rehabilitation interventions may begin. What type of interventions for the right upper extremity would client A.G. benefit from during this phase of healing?	A. ADLs and functional transfer training with a focus on safety, endurance, and light strengthening
	B. Use of video games to encourage participation, motivation, and functional use of the right upper extremity
	C. ADL training to encourage functional use of the right upper extremity during the day, with use of a static elbow extension splint at night
2. Client M.J. is currently POD #7 status post placement of autograft to the right elbow on both the anterior and posterior sides. The client is cleared for occupational therapy without ROM or activity restrictions. What interventions would you prioritize as his or her OT at this phase of healing?	D. Use of a shoulder positioning wedge for abduction of the right upper extremity, alternated with torso, shoulder, and elbow joint PROM
	E. Fabrication of a right-hand palmar pancake splint for use at night, family education regarding age-appropriate play incorporating functional use of the right hand, and both passive and active hand ROM

Client Scenario	Answer Choices
3. Client J.S. has been in the burn ICU with 9% TBSA burns to the right upper extremity, which have healed without skin grafting. However, J.S. also sustained an inhalation injury during the accident requiring a prolonged period of bedrest. She is cleared for therapy without restrictions. What types of interventions would you focus on during this phase in her recovery?	**F.** Fabrication of a right intrinsic plus splint for use at night and alternating periods throughout the day, right-hand passive ROM, and family education regarding OT interventions at this phase of healing
4. Client T.Y. sustained a full-thickness burn to the palm of his right hand following contact with a hot iron. T.Y. went to surgery for placement of autograft to the right hand. The graft crosses the creases of the hand. OT intervention began on POD #5. He is currently POD #7 and was cleared to go home with his parents. T.Y. was referred to your outpatient OT clinic for follow-up. What types of interventions would you target as his OT during this phase of healing?	**G.** Assessment of nerves, musculature, and available joint ROM of the residual right upper extremity; followed by training for use of the device with natural, anticipatory movements during ADLs involving functional hand grasp
5. Client P.W. is status post deep partial-thickness burns to her right upper extremity, crossing the elbow, forearm, wrist, and all joints of her right hand. She is currently POD #25 for placement of autograft to all areas of burn. She was discharged home and is being followed by your outpatient OT clinic. What interventions would you target for scar management of her right upper extremity during this phase of healing?	**H.** Provide the client with an explanation of achievement of small goals and milestones, specifically regarding the right upper extremity; introduction of compensatory strategies for functional use of the right upper extremity with returning to prior roles, routines, and occupations
6. Client T.U. is currently POD #30 for placement of autograft to his right antecubital fossa following a full-thickness scald burn. He is right arm dominant. He is being followed by your outpatient OT clinic and is compliant with all recommended OT interventions, including use of a static elbow splint, daily consistent AROM, and functional use of his right upper extremity with work-related activity. However, his functional elbow ROM progress has plateaued. What types of interventions would you select to target further progression of his right elbow ROM?	**I.** Fabrication of a right elbow static progressive splint with a night time wear schedule, with simulated daily work-related activities incorporating functional use of the right upper extremity
7. Client I.D. sustained a full-thickness electrical burn injury to the right upper extremity, extending from the mid forearm area down to the finger tips. Unfortunately, the extremity had extensive tissue death and an amputation was required. You are working with the client for OT training targeting functional use of a right arm body-powered prosthetic for ADLs. What types of interventions would you target for I.D.?	**J.** Right upper extremity scar massage, use of compression, and silicone placement

Client Scenario	Answer Choices
8. Client E.R. was admitted to the burn unit with 25% TBSA deep partial-thickness burns to her upper body, involving the right axilla. E.R. is currently POD #3 for placement of allograft to the right upper extremity, covering the anterior, medial, and posterior axilla. She is currently intubated and sedated in the burn ICU. Per physician orders, OT interventions may resume within the postoperative protocol for this phase of healing following placement of allograft. What types of interventions would you select based on the location of the injury, as well as the phase of healing?	
9. Client W.D. is a four-year-old male admitted to the burn unit with 70% TBSA superficial and deep partial-thickness flame burns to the face, neck, torso, and bilateral upper extremities. All surgical needs are pending. You are following this child for OT with a focus on functional use of the upper extremities and traditional contracture prevention interventions. W.D. is compensating with his left upper extremity and is refusing to use his right upper extremity. What might be a successful intervention to try at this phase of healing and may also be an intervention to help establish rapport with the child?	
10. Client B.K. sustained a deep partial-thickness burn to 96% of her body following a work-related explosion. B.K. has been in the burn unit for 14 mo, both intensive and intermediate care units during recovery. You have been following B.K. for OT interventions throughout each phase of recovery for contracture prevention and ADL training. B.K. will be discharged soon; however, she mentions feeling discouraged about progress during an OT session regarding her dominant right upper extremity. What approach should you take to target compassionate care at this phase of her recovery?	

Answer the following questions based on this case scenario and the stated phase of healing.

R.W. is a 60-year-old male who was admitted to the burn unit with 9% TBSA deep partial-thickness flame burns to his right upper extremity. He is right arm dominant. The client has a high risk for joint contracture, as the burn crosses the elbow, forearm, wrist, and all joints of the hands.

Acute Phase of Healing

He is currently in the ICU, sedated and intubated due to an inhalation injury. Physician orders were received to begin initial OT interventions for burn rehabilitation during the acute phase of healing.

1. Write three appropriate goals for R.W. during this phase of recovery.
2. List three therapy interventions to target the goals for R.W. during this phase of recovery.

Intermediate Phase of Healing

R.W. underwent surgery and now has autograft on the entire right upper extremity. He is POD #10, extubated, and the physician has cleared him for therapy without ROM or activity restrictions. He is now in the intermediate phase of healing.

3. Write three appropriate goals for R.W. during this phase of recovery.
4. List three therapy interventions to target the goals for R.W. during this phase of recovery.

Outpatient Phase of Healing

R.W. is now discharged home and is being followed in your outpatient OT clinic. He has full AROM of his right upper extremity; however, has developed hypertrophic scarring over the antecubital fossa and the dorsal wrist. He also has significant strength and endurance limitations. He is having trouble using his right arm with work-related activities.

5. Write three appropriate goals for R.W. during this phase of recovery.
6. List three therapy interventions to target the goals for R.W. during this phase of recovery.

Please match each anatomic site of injury with the anticontracture position

Location of Burn	Anti-Contracture Position
1. Hand	Extension
2. Wrist	Extremity abduction
3. Elbow	Neutral
4. Neck	Intrinsic plus position
5. Axilla	Neutral or slight extension
6. Forearm	Supination

Chapter 20 Self-Study Answers

Matching Answers

1. F
2. C
3. A
4. E
5. J
6. I
7. G
8. D
9. B
10. H

Case Study Answers

1. Goals should focus on initial elbow, forearm, wrist, and hand PROM, splinting, and positioning.
2. Possible interventions: elbow, forearm, wrist, and hand PROM, splinting, positioning, education with the nurse and family.
3. Goals should focus on AROM, use of the splint at night, and ADLs incorporating functional use of the right upper extremity, and functional transfer training.
4. Possible interventions: AROM home exercise program training, education for splint use, ADL training incorporating functional use of the right upper extremity (e.g., grooming), self-feeding, and functional transfers to the sink, restroom, or shower.
5. Goals should focus on scar management interventions, endurance training, strength training, and further work-related activities targeting functional use of his right upper extremity.
6. Possible interventions: scar management (e.g., pressure), silicone, massage, endurance training, strength training, and simulated work-related activities incorporating right arm use.

Anti-Contracture Position Answers

1. Hand – Intrinsic plus position
2. Wrist – Neutral or slight extension
3. Elbow – Extension
4. Neck – Neutral
5. Axilla – Extremity abduction
6. Forearm – Supination

References

American Burn Association. (2015). *Burn incidence and treatment in the United States: 2015*. Retrieved from http://www.ameriburn.org/resources_factsheet.php

American Occupational Therapy Association. (2015). *About occupational therapy*. Retrieved from http://www.aota.org/About-Occupational-Therapy.aspx

Badger, K., & Royse, D. (2012). Describing compassionate care: The burn survivor's perspective. *Journal of Burn Care & Research, 33*(6), 772–780. doi:10.1097/BCR.0b013e318254d30b

Baldwin, J., & Li, F. (2013). Exercise behaviors after burn injury. *Journal of Burn Care & Research, 34*(5), 529–536. doi:10.1097/BCR.0b013e31827a2bcd

Bennett, G. B., Helm, P., Purdue, G. F., & Hunt, J. L. (1989). Serial casting: A method for treating burn contractures. *Journal of Burn Care & Rehabilitation, 10*(6), 543–545.

Brunton, B., & Beaman, M. (2000). Nurse practitioners' perceptions of their caring behaviors. *Journal of the American Academy of Nurse Practitioners, 12*(11), 451–456.

Cambier, D. C., & Vanderstraeten, G. G. (1997). Failure of therapeutic ultrasound in healing burn injuries. *Burns, 23*(3), 248–249.

Carbullido, C., Parry, I. S., Kawada, J., Sen, S., Greenhalgh, D. G., & Palmieri, T. L. (2013). *A comprehensive guide for using interactive video games as a tool to achieve burn rehabilitation goals.* Paper presented at the American Burn Association Annual Meeting, Palm Springs, CA.

Cole, P., Stal, D., & Hollier, L. (2008). Ethical considerations in burn management. *Journal of Craniofacial Surgery, 19*(4), 895–898. doi:10.1097/SCS.0b013e318175b485

Costa, M. A., Peyrol, S., Porto, L. C., Comparin, J. P., Foyatier, J. L., & Desmouliere, A. (1999). Mechanical forces induce scar remodeling. Study in non-pressure-treated versus pressure-treated hypertrophic scars. *American Journal of Pathology, 155*(5), 1671–1679. doi:10.1016/S0002-9440(10)65482-X

Dauber, A., Osgood, P. F., Breslau, A. J., Vernon, H. L., & Carr, D. B. (2002). Chronic persistent pain after severe burns: A survey of 358 burn survivors. *Pain Medicine, 3*(1), 6–17. doi:10.1046/j.1526-4637.2002.02004.x

de Lateur, B. J., Magyar-Russell, G., Bresnick, M. G., Bernier, F. A., Ober, M. S., Krabak, B. J., . . . Fauerbach, J. A. (2007). Augmented exercise in the treatment of deconditioning from major burn injury. *Archives of Physical Medicine and Rehabilitation, 88*(12, Suppl 2), S18–S23. doi:10.1016/j.apmr.2007.09.003

Dunn, M. G., Silver, F. H., & Swann, D. A. (1985). Mechanical analysis of hypertrophic scar tissue: Structural basis for apparent increased rigidity. *Journal of Investigative Dermatology, 84*(1), 9–13.

Gilchrist, J. S., Potenza, B., & Tenenhaus, M. (2013, March 22–26). *Occupational therapy intervention for the mouth following traumatic facial burns.* Paper presented at the American Burn Association Annual Meeting, Palm Springs, CA.

Hoeksema, H., DeVos, M., Verbelen, J., Pirayesh, A., & Monstrey, S. (2013). Scar management by means of occlusion and hydration: A comparative study of silicones versus a hydrating gel-cream. *Burns, 39*(7), 1437–1448.

Hur, G. Y., Rhee, B. J., Ko, J. H., Seo, D. K., Choi, J. K., Jang, Y. C., & Lee, J. W. (2013). Correction of postburn equinus deformity. *Annals of Plastic Surgery, 70*(3), 276–279. doi:10.1097/SAP.0b013e31827a6c83

INTEGRA®. (2010). *What is INTEGRA® template?* Retrieved from http://www.ilstraining.com/idrt/faq.asp#q1

Jacobs, M. L., & Austin, N. (2003). Splint classification. *Splinting the hand and upper extremity principles and process* (pp. 2–18). Baltimore, MD: Lippincott Williams & Wilkins.

Kamolz, L. P., & Huang, T. (2012). Reconstruction of burn deformities. In D. N. Herndon (Ed.), *Total burn care* (4th ed., pp. 571–580). Edinburgh, NY: Saunders Elsevier.

Kirsner, R. S. (2008). Wound healing. In *Dermatology* (2nd ed., pp. 2147–2158). Atlanta, GA: Mosby Elsevier.

Kung, T. A., Jebson, P. J., & Cederna, P. S. (2012). An individualized approach to severe elbow burn contractures. *Plastic and Reconstructive Surgery, 129*(4), 663e–673e. doi:10.1097/PRS.0b013e3182450c0c

Latella, D., & Meriano, C. (2003). *Occupational therapy manual for evaluation of range of motion and muscle strength.* Clifton Park, NY: Delmar Learning.

LeBorgne, A. (2014). Burns. In M. E. Scaffa, B. A. B. Schell, G. Gillen, & E. S. Cohn (Eds.), *Willard & Spackman's occupational therapy* (12th ed., pp. 1117–1119). Philadelphia, PA: Wolters Kluwer Health/Lippincott Williams & Wilkins.

Maslow, G. R., & Lobato, D. (2010). Summer camps for children with burn injuries: A literature review. *Journal of Burn Care & Research, 31*(5), 740–749. doi:10.1097/BCR.0b013e3181eebec4

Meriano, C., & Latella, D. (2008). *Occupational therapy interventions: Function and occupations.* Thorofare, NJ: SLACK.

Micak, R. P., Buffalo, M. C., & Jimenenz, C. J. (2012). Pre-hospital management, transportation and emergency care. In D. N. Herndon (Ed.), *Total burn care* (4th ed., pp. 93–102). Edinburgh, NY: Saunders Elsevier.

Miller, K., Rodger, S., Bucolo, S., Greer, R., & Kimble, R. M. (2010). Multi-modal distraction. Using technology to combat pain in young children with burn injuries. *Burns, 36*(5), 647–658. doi:10.1016/j.burns.2009.06.199

Momeni, M., Hafezi, F., Rahbar, H., & Karimi, H. (2009). Effects of silicone gel on burn scars. *Burns, 35*(1), 70–74. doi:10.1016/j.burns.2008.04.011

Parry, I., Hanley, C., Niszczak, J., Sen, S., Palmieri, T., & Greenhalgh, D. (2013). Harnessing the transparent face orthosis for facial scar management: A comparison of methods. *Burns, 39*(5), 950–956. doi:10.1016/j.burns.2012.11.009

Parry, I., Sen, S., Palmieri, T., & Greenhalgh, D. (2013). Nonsurgical scar management of the face: Does early versus late intervention affect outcome? *Journal of Burn Care & Research, 34*(5), 569–575. doi:10.1097 /BCR.0b013e318278906d

Parry, I. S., Bagley, A., Kawada, J., Sen, S., Greenhalgh, D. G., & Palmieri, T. L. (2012). Commercially available interactive video games in burn rehabilitation: Therapeutic potential. *Burns, 38*(4), 493–500. doi:10.1016/j .burns.2012.02.010

Pessina, M. A., & Orroth, A. C. (2014). Burn injuries. In M. V. Radomski & C. A. T. Latham (Eds.), *Occupational therapy for physical dysfunction* (7th ed., pp. 1244–1265). Philadelphia, PA: Wolters Kluwer Health/Lippincott Williams & Wilkins.

The Phoenix Society for Burn Survivors. (2014). *Survivors offering assistance in recovery.* Retrieved from http:// www.phoenix-society.org/programs/soar/

Powell, B. W., Haylock, C., & Clarke, J. A. (1985). A semi-rigid transparent face mask in the treatment of postburn hypertrophic scars. *British Journal of Plastic Surgery, 38*(4), 561–566.

Prentice, W. E. (2003). *Laboratory manual to accompany therapeutic modalities for sports medicine and athletic training* (5th ed.). Boston, MA: McGraw-Hill.

Pruitt, B. A., Wolf, S. E., & Mason, A. D. (2012). Epidemiological, demographic, and outcome characteristics of burn injury. In D. N. Herndon (Ed.), *Total burn care* (4th ed., pp. 15–45). Edinburgh, NY: Saunders Elsevier.

Reeves, S. U., & Deshaies, L. (2013). Burns and burn rehabilitation. In L. W. Pedretti, H. M. Pendleton, & W. Schultz-Krohn (Eds.), *Pedretti's occupational therapy: Practice skills for physical dysfunction* (7th ed., pp. 1110–1147). St. Louis, MO: Elsevier.

Reid, W. H., Evans, J. H., Naismith, R. S., Tully, A. E., & Sherwin, S. (1987). Hypertrophic scarring and pressure therapy. *Burns, Including Thermal Injury, 13*(Suppl), S29–S32.

Rimmer, R. B., Fornaciari, G. M., Foster, K. N., Bay, C. R., Wadsworth, M. M., Wood, M., & Caruso, D. M. (2007). Impact of a pediatric residential burn camp experience on burn survivors' perceptions of self and attitudes regarding the camp community. *Journal of Burn Care & Research, 28*(2), 334–341. doi:10.1097 /bcr.0b013e318031a0f4

Rocky Mountain Model System for Burn Injury Rehabilitation. (2015). An easy guide to outpatient burn rehabilitation. Retrieved from http://www.researchutilization .org/matrix/resources/burn/burnguide.html

Rosenberg, L. (2012). Enzymatic debridement of burn wounds. In D. N. Herndon (Ed.), *Total burn care* (4th ed., pp. 131–135). Edinburgh, NY: Saunders Elsevier.

Sanghavi, D. M. (2006). What makes for a compassionate patient-caregiver relationship? *The Joint Commission Journal on Quality and Patient Safety, 32*(5), 283–292.

Sar, Z., Polat, M. G., Ozgul, B., Aydogdu, O., Camcoglu, B., Acar, A. H., & Yurdalan, S. U. (2013). A comparison of three different physiotherapy modalities used in the physiotherapy of burns. *Journal of Burn Care & Research, 34*(5), e290–e296. doi:10.1097 /BCR.0b013e3182789041

Sardelli, M., Tashjian, R. Z., & MacWilliams, B. A. (2011). Functional elbow range of motion for contemporary tasks. *Journal of Bone & Joint Surgery, American Volume, 93*(5), 471–477. doi:10.2106/jbjs.i.01633

Sawada, Y., & Sone, K. (1992). Hydration and occlusion treatment for hypertrophic scars and keloids. *British Journal of Plastic Surgery, 45*(8), 599–603.

Serghiou, M. A., Ott, S., Whitehead, C., Cowan, A., McEntire, S., & Suman, O. E. (2012). Comprehensive rehabilitation of the burn patient. In D. N. Herndon (Ed.), *Total burn care* (4th ed., pp. 517–549). Edinburgh, NY: Saunders Elsevier.

Sheridan, R. L., & Tompkins, R. G. (2012). Alternative wound coverings. In D. N. Herndon (Ed.), *Total burn care* (4th ed., pp. 209–214). Edinburgh, NY: Saunders Elsevier.

Smurr, L. M., Gulick, K., Yancosek, K., & Ganz, O. (2008). Managing the upper extremity amputee: A protocol for success. *Journal of Hand Therapy, 21*(2), 160–175; quiz 176. doi:10.1197/j.jht.2007.09.006

St-Pierre, D. M., Choiniere, M., Forget, R., & Garrel, D. R. (1998). Muscle strength in individuals with healed burns. *Archives of Physical Medicine and Rehabilitation, 79*(2), 155–161.

Sullivan, T., Smith, J., Kermode, J., McIver, E., & Courtemanche, D. J. (1990). Rating the burn scar. *Journal of Burn Care & Rehabilitation, 11*(3), 256–260.

Taylor, S., Manning, S., & Quarles, J. (2013). A multidisciplinary approach to early mobilization of patients with burns. *Critical Care Nursing Quarterly, 36*(1), 56–62. doi:10.1097/CNQ.0b013e31827531c8

ter Haar, G. (1999). Therapeutic ultrasound. *European Journal of Ultrasound, 9*(1), 3–9.

Total Contact. (2008). *Information for therapists.* Retrieved from http://www.totalcontact.com

Williama, W. G. (2002). Pathophysiology of the burn wound. In D. Herndon (Ed.), *Total burn care* (2nd ed., pp. 514–522). London, UK: WB Saunders.

Williams, F., Knapp, D., & Wallen, M. (1998). Comparison of the characteristics and features of pressure garments used in the management of burn scars. *Burns, 24*(4), 329–335. doi:10.1016/S0305-4179(98)00026-6

Occupational Functioning: Selected Medical Conditions Days 15-17

Cardiopulmonary

Thomas J. Birk and Moh H. Malek

Learning Objectives

- Describe etiology and pathology, common diagnostic tests, and common medical and surgical procedures for chronic obstructive pulmonary disease (COPD), myocardial infarction (MI), and chronic heart failure (CHF).
- Describe screenings and assessments for COPD, MI, and CHF.
- Compare and contrast therapeutic interventions for COPD, MI, and CHF.
- Construct basic intervention programs for adults with cardiovascular and pulmonary diseases.

Key Terms

- *Cardiovascular disease*: Also referred to as coronary artery disease, it is a narrowing of the small blood vessels that supply blood and oxygen to the heart.
- *Chronic obstructive pulmonary disease*: A lung disease characterized by chronic obstruction of lung airflow that interferes with normal breathing and is not fully reversible.
- *Congestive heart failure*: A condition in which the heart's function as a pump is inadequate to meet the body's needs.
- *MET*: Metabolic equivalent ratio. One MET is defined as 1 kilocalorie per kilogram per hour.

Chronic Obstructive Pulmonary Disease

Etiology and Pathology

Chronic obstructive pulmonary disease (COPD) is a chronic and progressive disease of the lungs, which is the fourth leading cause of death (American Thoracic Society, 1999a, 1999b; Keaney, Kay, & Taylor, 2009; Olfert, Malek, Eagan, Wagner, & Wagner, 2014). Within the United States, it has been projected that the medical cost of COPD will increase from $32.1 billion in 2010 to approximately $49 billion by 2020 (Ford et al., 2015). The pathophysiology of COPD is due, in part, to damage of the alveoli, which is the site of gas (i.e., O_2 and CO_2) exchange (Coburn & Malek, 2012). This damage may be the result of repeated exposure to toxins such as those observed with chronic smokers. It should be noted; however, that a small percentage of clients with COPD are alpha-1-antitrypsin deficient. This condition is an inherent genetic disorder in which individual's exhibit symptoms associated with COPD (Olfert et al., 2014).

Common Diagnostic Tests

The guidelines for treatment of clients diagnosed with COPD are set by a committee of physicians and scientists called the Global Initiative for Chronic Obstructive Lung Disease (GOLD) (Vestbo et al., 2013).

The GOLD stages range from 1 (mild) to 4 (very severe) in the severity of COPD, and are based on the client's pulmonary function test (Vestbo et al., 2013). Specifically, the percentage of the client's FEV1 (i.e., forced expiratory volume in one second) relative to normative data is used to categorize clients into the different GOLD stages (Vestbo et al., 2013). For example, a client with an FEV1 of 30–50% of predicted normative values would be in GOLD Stage 3. For a more comprehensive review of the GOLD stages and the various pulmonary function indices, refer to Vestbo et al. (2013).

Common Medical and Surgical Procedures for COPD

Medical procedures in treating COPD are typically noninvasive and include:

- Smoking cessation
- Medications
- Oxygen therapy
- Pulmonary rehabilitation

Surgical procedures for treating COPD include:

- *Lung volume reduction surgery*: Removes part of one or both lungs and increases space for the rest of the lung to work better. This procedure is indicated for certain types of severe *emphysema*.
- *Lung transplant*: Replaces a diseased lung with a healthy lung from a person who has just died.
- *Bullectomy*: Removes the part of a lung that has been damaged by the formation of large, air-filled sacs called bullae. This surgery is rarely performed.

Precautions and Potential Complications for COPD

Exercise precautions for individuals with COPD include:

- Shortness of breath (SOB), fatigue, dizziness, nausea, pain, weakness, and rapid heart rate.
- Exercising outside in extreme temperatures may result in early-onset SOB.

Relative exercise contraindications for individuals with COPD include:

- Using certain types of inhalation therapy, a recent myocardial infarction (MI), severe arrhythmias, and/or severe heart failure.

Potential complications from COPD include:

- Respiratory infections
- Heart problems
- Lung cancer
- High blood pressure (BP)
- Depression

Screening and Assessments

There are numerous screenings and assessments that may rule out COPD, but there is no one single test which confirms the diagnosis.

1. *Standardized assessments*: A thorough medical history and physical examination is paramount. These assessments will provide important information about overall health and the pulmonary system.
   - Lung function tests, including an FEV1 test, are needed. These tests measure the amount of air in your lungs and the speed at which air moves in and out.
   - Chest x-ray is another test, which helps to rule out other conditions with similar symptoms (e.g., lung cancer).
   - An arterial blood gas test is an invasive test used to measure how much oxygen, carbon dioxide, and acid is in the blood. The assessment helps to determine whether oxygen therapy is needed.
   - Oximetry is a noninvasive test used to measure oxygen saturation in the blood. Oximetry provides less information than an arterial blood gas test, but can also be used to determine if oxygen treatment is needed (Senior & Silverman, 2007).
2. *Semistandardized assessments*: Checking and asking about the presence, severity, and length of time of the following symptoms can be an accurate means of screening for COPD:
   - Wheezing (i.e., a breathing sound that is higher pitched) suggests breathing difficulty.
   - Excessive and/or discolored sputum suggests fluid and/or infection in the lungs.
   - Breathing difficulties at rest, which manifest in an elevated and expanded chest cavity (i.e., thorax).
   - A chronic cough is another symptom of COPD. The cough signifies that irritants in the lungs, which may result in breathing problems, need to be expelled.

- Cyanosis (i.e., a lack of oxygen in the blood) exhibits a bluish hue to the skin, fingernails, lips, and mucous membranes.
- A chronic cough and cyanosis associated with a history of smoking (Senior & Silverman, 2007).
- SOB during mild or usual daily activities as rated by a four-point dyspnea scale (American College of Sports Medicine, 2006).

3. *Nonstandardized assessment*: These assessments and symptoms may be associated with COPD or may be associated with another pathology, and should be considered in the overall evaluation. Fatigue and low energy during activities of daily living (ADLs), instrumental ADLs, and vocational and prevocational activities can be a sign and/or symptom of COPD. Observation of difficulty during eating can also be a sign of COPD and depression may manifest during COPD (Huntley, 2014). Exposure to tobacco smoke is a significant risk factor for COPD; the amount a person has smoked (e.g., packs per day) over a long period of time (i.e., years or packs/years) equates to greater risk. Similarly, people who smoke pipes, cigars, and marijuana are at risk, as are people exposed to large amounts of secondhand smoke. People with asthma who smoke are also at greater risk of developing COPD. Correspondingly, the combination of factors such as asthma, a chronic airway disease, and smoking increases the risk of developing COPD. Occupational exposure to dusts and chemicals (e.g., long-term exposure to chemical fumes, vapors, and dusts) can irritate and inflame the lungs and increase the risk of COPD. Because COPD develops slowly over years and with advancing age, most people are at least 35–40 years old when symptoms of COPD occur. Genetics can be another COPD risk factor (e.g., alpha-1-antitrypsin deficiency) and likely makes certain smokers more susceptible to the disease (Senior & Silverman, 2007).

4. *Criterion-referenced*: The six-minute walk test is a clinical assessment that measures the functional impairment of COPD. When conducting the test, the occupational therapy practitioner encourages clients to walk the maximum distance that can be covered within six minutes, while documenting symptoms and signs of intolerance. The six-minute walk test, used in conjunction with lung function and blood gas tests, is quite accurate in determining the extent and severity of COPD (Chhabra, Gupta, & Khuma, 2009). When used independently as a clinical assessment for COPD, the six-minute walk test has demonstrated good reliability and reproducibility (Coburn & Malek, 2012).

Interventions

A comprehensive plan for a client with COPD should focus on lifestyle changes, adjusting daily activities, overcoming the fear of extreme SOB, and combating hopelessness and depression (Huntley, 2014).

Impact on Occupational Performance

Therapeutic use of occupations and activities, including group interventions when applicable, should comprise instruction and training in proper breathing techniques with ADLs. Appropriate breathing during ADLs will facilitate greater tolerance and functional endurance (Huntley, 2014).

Interventions

1. *Preparatory methods and tasks*: These tasks should include warm-up periods of at least 10 minutes of slow physical activities, emphasizing major muscle groups. Breath holding should be discouraged and rhythmic breathing should be emphasized (American College of Sports Medicine, 2006).

2. *Education and training*: Client and family/caregiver education and training in a pulmonary rehabilitation program is highly encouraged. Besides the use of large muscle group exercises emphasizing both endurance and strength enhancement, using a short duration of up to two minutes to start followed by up to eight intervals with one to two minutes of rest between intervals, work simplification, and energy conservation should be included. These activities should include optimal bathing conditions (e.g., light, temperature, ventilation, and humidity), use of a tub bench or shower chair, and the type of bathrobe to use, as applicable. Also, support of the upper extremity while combing hair, shaving, and putting on makeup should be included in work simplification and energy conservation education and training. Other techniques should include

the use of a long handled shoehorn and reacher for bending, which will conserve energy and allow for more complete inspiration and expiration secondary to decreased bending of the thorax (Huntley, 2014).

3. *Reevaluation and plan modification or discontinuation*: Reevaluation is ongoing and should be considered during every therapeutic session in order to respond to changes directed by ADLs and exercise intolerance. If the client has not shown progress over a two-week span, discharge should be considered, especially if there has been an adverse exacerbation of the lungs. Symptoms and signs of problems, as well as indications for a physician referral, include increased fatigue, decreased appetite, lack of response to oxygen supplement, increased dyspnea, cyanosis, and a persistent chest cold or cough. Client plans should eventually include continuous large muscle activities for up to five minutes, followed by subsequent intervals of the same length. Cardiopulmonary rehabilitation activities, although not increasing survival, have reduced the number of hospital days per year. Treatment plan goals may need to be modified if the client contracts a cold or develops other upper respiratory tract problems (Huntley, 2014). Generally, when the client returns to rehabilitation, the treatment plan will decrease intensity to accommodate for deconditioning that typically occurs during time off from therapy, followed by a safe and gradual increase in intensity as tolerated (American College of Sports Medicine, 2006). Reevaluation of the client should take place at the start of each rehabilitation session and at two-week intervals (i.e., minimally), unless symptoms and adverse signs arise.

Referrals and Discharge Considerations

Referral and discharge considerations from a pulmonary rehabilitation program are generally made to a home program. The home program should include ADLs and exercise intensity and duration guidelines. Also, as mentioned previously, work simplification, energy conservation, humidity, and temperature precautions should be included. Avoiding exposure to fumes, cigarette smoke, and other respiratory irritants should also be part of the home program. Other components of a comprehensive home program include adapted leisure activities and evaluation for adaptive equipment. If education and training in stress management and relaxation has not occurred, a referral should be made. Also, any precautions in the use of oxygen therapy and supplementation should be made known (e.g., written instructions) and understood by the client. Finally, any side effects from pulmonary medications should be overtly identified and understood by the client (Huntley, 2014).

Myocardial Infarction

Etiology and Pathology

MI is characterized by irreversible death or necrosis of the heart muscle due, in part, to a lack of oxygen (i.e., hypoxia). Myocardial tissue that is hypoxic for more than four minutes becomes necrotic. Tissue necrosis eventually leads to scarring and nonfunctional cardiac tissue. Nonfunctional cardiac tissue is unable to contribute to inotropic contraction, reducing the efficacy and efficiency of the left and right ventricles (Birk & Talley, 2015).

Common Diagnostic Tests

It should be noted that the use of electrocardiogram (ECG) can provide insight into whether a client has an MI. Specifically, the ST segment of the ECG trace is associated with ventricular repolarization (i.e., relaxation of the ventricles after contraction). Therefore, the amount of ST elevation from the normal baseline determines the presence of MI. Recently, the American College of Cardiology Foundation and the American Heart Association provided guidelines for management of ST-elevation MI (for a detailed review, see American College of Emergency Physicians and Society for Cardiovascular Angiography and Interventions et al., 2013). When the MI is stable, recommended interventions may include a cardiac rehabilitation program, dietary changes, smoking cessation, exercise, and risk factor management (Birk & Talley, 2015).

Common Medical and Surgical Procedures for MI

Medical procedures in treating MI are typically noninvasive and include:

- Resting ECG
- Angiogram
- Stress testing ECG
- Medications
- Cardiac rehabilitation

Surgical procedures for treating MI include:

- Cardiac catheterization
- Angioplasty and stenting
- Coronary artery bypass surgery

Precautions, Contraindications, and Complications

Precautions for MI may include:

- Signs of overexertion (e.g., SOB during exercise, dizziness, nausea, weakness, fatigue, and a rapid heart rate).
- Temperature extremes (i.e., may result in early-onset fatigue and weakness).

Contraindications prior to exercise for individuals with MI include:

- Unstable angina
- Resting systolic BP (SBP) > 200 mm Hg or resting diastolic BP (DBP) > 110 mm Hg that should be evaluated on a case-by-case basis
- Orthostatic BP drop of >20 mm Hg with symptoms
- Acute systemic illness or fever
- Uncontrolled atrial or ventricular dysrhythmias
- Uncontrolled sinus tachycardia (i.e., heart rate >120 beats per minute)

Potential complications that result from an MI may include:

- Left ventricular wall rupture
- Left ventricular aneurysm
- Ischemia of heart muscle
- Arrhythmias or abnormal beats of the heart
- Cardiogenic shock
- Early pericarditis or inflammation of the heart
- Late pericarditis

Screening and Assessments

There are invasive and noninvasive tests and assessments, which are utilized for determining whether an MI has occurred and to what extent. The standardized assessments listed below include invasive and noninvasive examples.

1. *Standardized*:
   - Blood tests are invasive and may include cardiac enzymes (e.g., troponin and creatine kinase), C-reactive protein, fibrinogen, homocysteine, lipoproteins, triglycerides, brain natriuretic peptide, and prothrombin. These tests confirm that a heart attack has occurred and determines the extent of the damage, as well as information pertaining to future risk for coronary artery disease (Vaughn, 2014).
   - Prothrombin provides information on the time it takes for the blood to clot.
   - A catheterization is an invasive test to examine the inside of the heart's blood vessels using special x-rays called angiograms. A thin hollow tube called a catheter is threaded from a blood vessel in the arm, groin, or neck to the heart and the dye is injected from the catheter into blood vessels to make them visible by x-ray. A catheterization or coronary angiography takes two to three hours to perform and is typically used to evaluate chest pain by determining if plaque is narrowing or blocking coronary arteries. BP within the heart and oxygen in the blood can also be measured during catheterization, which aids in determining heart muscle and valve function (Chou & High Value Care Task Force of the American College of Physicians, 2015).
   - A thallium stress test or myocardial perfusion imaging is classified as a noninvasive assessment. A radioactive substance called thallium is injected into the bloodstream at a maximum level of exercise while the client performs an exercise stress test. The injected thallium in conjunction with a special gamma camera is used to render images of the heart muscle cells. The assessment helps to measure blood flow of heart muscle, the extent of coronary artery blockage, the extent of MI, and/or the cause of angina (Chou & High Value Care Task Force of the American College of Physicians, 2015).

- ECG is a noninvasive test, which records the electrical activity of the heart including the timing and duration of each electrical phase in your heartbeat, during rest and/or exercise. The test is used to help determine whether an MI has occurred, to help predict if a heart attack is developing, and to assess and monitor changes in heart rhythm (Birk & Talley, 2015).
- Pharmacologic stress testing is used when a client cannot exercise vigorously. A drug such as dobutamine or dipyridamole is commonly injected as the client lies supine on a table. ECG and/or echocardiographic measurements are recorded to determine whether there is ischemia and heart wall motion abnormalities (American College of Sports Medicine, 2006).

2. *Semistandardized*: An assessment of risk factors, which increase the chance of heart disease and an MI, include high cholesterol, hypertension, diabetes, cigarette smoking, obesity, and lack of physical activity. Determination of the presence and extent of these risk factors, while not diagnosing an MI, will more accurately predict whether an MI is more likely to occur in the future (Vaughn, 2014). Furthermore, coronary artery calcium assessment through noninvasive imaging may be used to determine the risk of developing heart disease and a possible subsequent MI. Calcium assessment of coronary arteries through tomography scanning has shown high predictability for the presence of heart disease (Zeb & Budoff, 2015).

3. *Nonstandardized*: Assessments such as a six-minute walk test and three-minute step test have been used to predict cardiovascular fitness, which in turn has some correlation with the heart's capacity to circulate blood without abnormal symptoms. For the six-minute walk test, a greater distance covered is more predictive of higher fitness. For the three-minute step test, a lower heart or pulse rate after three minutes on a 12-inch step at 24 steps per minute is more predictive of higher fitness (American College of Sports Medicine, 2006).

4. *Criterion-referenced*: A treadmill test, called the Bruce protocol, using a metabolic equivalent of task (MET)-based achievement has been a predictive measure of MI risk and subsequent damage. Each three-minute stage of the walking protocol on an elevated treadmill that is accomplished before fatigue, the greater the MET level of amount of oxygen consumed. Higher MET levels are predictive of a reduced risk of heart disease and MI. Further, if an MI has been sustained, the test can estimate the extent of muscle wall damage to the heart, with higher MET levels suggestive of lesser heart damage (American College of Sports Medicine, 2006).

Interventions

A comprehensive client program for someone who has experienced an MI should include goals and treatments or interventions. The goals should prevent muscle loss and deconditioning, assessing and monitoring physical function, and instruction on home activities, and risk factors. These goals and the subsequent treatment are generally implemented in a Phase I or inpatient cardiac rehabilitation program. If the client with an MI is stable, they are generally eligible for group treatment. Programs may vary but will generally have mild calisthenics or walking for a couple of minutes followed by rest breaks and then progress over the next weeks with increased minutes and fewer rest breaks. The program may also include a grid format, which includes ADLs, client and family education on nutrition, and discharge planning. Outcomes are evaluated to ensure a standard level of care and to document that the client with an MI is functioning adequately to be as independent as possible (Huntley, 2014).

Impact on Occupational Performance

Therapeutic use of occupations and activities, including group interventions when applicable, may include ADLs such as dressing, grooming, bed mobility, and sitting and standing from a chair. Incorporate activities such as walking and stationary bicycling (i.e., large mass muscle groups) beginning at a maximum of two to three METs. Activities and progressions must take the extent and severity of the MI and relevant client history into consideration (i.e., progression may be slow or more rapid) and signs, symptoms, BP, and pulse rate must be monitored during interventions, more frequently with symptomatic clients (American College of Sports Medicine, 2006; Huntley, 2014).

Interventions

1. *Preparatory methods and tasks*: Include warm-up periods of at least 10 minutes of slow physical activities, which should not include isometric or

static physical exertion that may compromise the heart (American College of Sports Medicine, 2006).

2. *Education and training*: While in a cardiac rehabilitation program, clients will be monitored during exercise using ECG and BP during both inpatient (i.e., Phase I) and outpatient (i.e., Phase II) rehabilitation. This will ensure a reasonable level of safety while exercising and also document that an effective intensity is followed. Also, education for secondary prevention of heart disease and subsequent MI will be featured, including instruction on diminishing risk factors and how to maximize psychosocial and vocational status (Huntley, 2014).

3. *Reevaluation and plan modification or discontinuation*: Referral to a physician should be made if symptoms result and progress is not made. If the client does not progress but has an absence of symptoms, discharge should be considered provided the client has been educated and can demonstrate proper physical activity monitoring safety knowledge and skills (American College of Sports Medicine, 2006). The cardiac rehabilitation plan for each client should be adjusted so that the client is eventually able to exercise continuously for 20 to 40 minutes, at an intensity that is safe and effective for increasing endurance. The evaluation of exercise tolerance should take place at each cardiac rehabilitation session. Discontinuation of the ECG monitored sessions should occur when there are no consistent heart abnormalities and there is no abnormal exercise intolerance or symptoms (Huntley, 2014).

Referrals and Discharge Considerations

Discharge from Phase II cardiac rehabilitation can be to a home program or a community-based cardiac rehabilitation program or Phase III program. The referral to a Phase III non-ECG monitored program should include activity and exercise intensity and duration guidelines. Additionally, work simplification, pacing, and temperature precautions should be included if the client can be involved in work hardening (i.e., if included in occupational goals). Social activity guidelines, sexuality, signs and symptoms of exercise intolerance, discussion of risk factors, and client and family-centered and focused activities can all be part of a Phase III comprehensive program. If referral is to home, all of the above referral guidelines should be included with the final session upon discharge from Phase II,

as well as family participation in understanding and activating the home program for the client (Huntley, 2014).

Congestive Heart Failure

Etiology and Pathology

Data from the American Heart Association indicate that congestive heart failure (CHF), within the United States, affects a large number of Americans (Roger et al., 2012). Moreover, each year there are over 600,000 new cases of CHF suggesting the prevalence of the disease (Roger et al., 2012). Although the factors resulting in CHF vary, the manifestation is the lack of adequate blood flow throughout the body to vital organs based on the energy demands of the body (Braunwald, 2013a, 2013b). Furthermore, because human circulation is a closed system, not only the blood flow to organs is compromised, but blood flow returning to the heart is also compromised. Thus, the amount of oxygenated blood leaving the left ventricular is limited and often results in the onset of fatigue from ADLs (Braunwald, 2013a, 2013b). These physiologic limitations must be considered when clients with CHF undergo rehabilitation so that the individual is not unduly stressed. Treatment and intervention should focus on improving symptoms and delaying disease progression. Lifestyle changes include diet modification, exercise, and stress management.

Common Diagnostic Tests

Magnetic resonance imaging is used to determine if the heart is enlarged. If the heart is enlarged, the extent of CHF is further investigated. Stress tests may be completed to see how well the heart performs under different levels of stress. These tests can be completed during exercise or with drug injections to assess the response of the heart. Blood tests can also be used to check for abnormal blood cells and to determine the cause of CHF (Yancy et al., 2013).

Common Medical and Surgical Procedures for CHF

Medical procedures in treating CHF are typically noninvasive and include:

- Medications
- Proper nutrition
- Cardiac rehabilitation

Surgical procedures for treating CHF include:

- Heart valve replacement
- Coronary artery bypass surgery
- Left ventricular assist device
- Cardiac pacemaker
- Implantable cardioverter defibrillator
- Heart transplant

Precautions, Contraindications, and Complications

Precautions for individuals with CHF include:

- Medications that could result in lowered cardiac function
- Signs of overexertion (e.g., SOB during exercise, dizziness, nausea, weakness, fatigue, and a rapid heart rate)
- Temperature extremes (i.e., may result in early-onset fatigue and weakness)

Contraindications before or during exercise include:

- Unstable angina
- Resting SBP > 200 mm Hg or resting DBP > 110 mm Hg that should be evaluated on a case-by-case basis
- Orthostatic BP drop of >20 mm Hg with symptoms
- Acute systemic illness or fever
- Uncontrolled atrial or ventricular dysrhythmias
- Uncontrolled sinus tachycardia (i.e., heart rate >120 beats per minute)

Potential complications from CHF include:

- Kidney damage or failure
- Heart valve problems
- Heart rhythm problems
- Liver damage

Screening and Assessments

1. *Standardized*: The following symptoms should be assessed prior to ADLs and physical activity. These symptoms are predictors of CHF involvement:
   - SOB during mild or usual daily activities can be assessed by having the client rate their SOB on a four-point dyspnea scale (American College of Sports Medicine, 2006).
   - Trouble breathing when lying down is a standard measure used to determine the inability of the heart to fill and empty, which could result in elevated blood vessel and lung pressures (Huntley, 2014).
   - Use of the four-point dyspnea scale (i.e., as mentioned previously) to objectively quantify the difficulty of breathing in a lying position (American College of Sports Medicine, 2006).
   - Asking the client if they are tired or feeling run-down to determine the extent of CHF symptoms such as fatigue.
   - Comparisons of the past seven days should be asked of the client and are useful in assessing progressive tiredness and fatigue.
   - Swelling in the feet, ankles, and legs may be used to predict the circulatory capability of the heart.
   - Increased edema or swelling is an indication that the return of the blood to the heart is compromised.
   - Measuring the ankle(s) at specific anatomic landmarks facilitates a relatively objective indicator of the extent of fluid buildup.
   - Weight gain from fluid buildup is a whole-body predictor of the amount of edema or fluid that has amassed.
   - The use of an accurate and reliable bathroom scale may be predictive of edema or fluid that has amassed. Measurements must be taken with similar clothing (e.g., clothing weight or clothing on or off) and at the same time of the day.
   - Confusion or trouble thinking clearly can be a result from the heart's inability to pump oxygenated blood adequately to the brain. This symptom or sign can be more objectively evaluated by asking the client orientation (i.e., person, place, time, and situation) questions. Increasing fatigue, worsening dyspnea, and/or feelings of palpitations in the chest are also signs of CHF and further screening and assessment is warranted (American College of Sports Medicine, 2006).

2. *Semistandardized*: These symptoms associated with the semistandardized assessments are not always unique and identifying with CHF. Hence, a "semistandardized" designation is used.
   - Claudication or pain with walking is a cramping and/or tightening of the lower posterior leg or calf. This condition is usually associated with reduced blood flow to the calf(s). There is a four-point assessment scale, which can be used to evaluate and demonstrate progress (American College of Sports Medicine, 2006).

- Cool extremities or cold and clammy hands are typically suggestive of a lack of blood circulation. Also, some anxiety disorders will cause skin to become cool and hands to become clammy.
- Dizziness can be the result of a lack of blood flow to the brain, caused by low BP. The hypotensive state of the person could result in a lack of balance and falls. Frothy sputum is usually a symptom of some form of respiratory distress but can occur in CHF due to lung congestion.
- Frothing occurs when *phlegm* or *mucus* in the lungs combines with fluid and air, and is then coughed up.
- Nocturia or urination during the night is the need to urinate two or more times during the night. It can occur at any age, but becomes more common with advancing age. Causes of nocturia can be as straightforward as drinking fluids just before bedtime to disorders such as CHF.
- Nocturnal cough is a cough, or tussis, that occurs primarily at night, typically when lying down (i.e., postural cough). A night cough may be a symptom of conditions specifically affecting the lungs and throat or a more generalized condition, such as a cold or flu (Huntley, 2014; Vaughn, 2014).

  The above symptoms are not specific to CHF but should be considered with the standardized symptoms and signs when screening for CHF (Yancy et al., 2013).

3. *Nonstandardized assessments*: Risk factors including high cholesterol, hypertension, diabetes, poor diet, cigarette smoking, physical activity, and alcohol use should be assessed when screened. However, these risk factors could be etiology for many other vascular diseases, and need to be associated with standardized screening results (Vaughn, 2014).

4. *Criterion-referenced assessments*: Gauging the severity of CHF can be assessed with an exercise or physical activity test. The higher the class of the New York Heart Association (NYHA) criteria, as included below, the more severe the disease. For example, class IV indicates symptoms at rest and very low or less than a two MET capacity for physical exertion. NYHA assessment is as follows:

   I. No symptoms with ordinary activity.
   II. Slight limitation of physical activity. Comfortable at rest, but ordinary physical activity results in fatigue, palpitation, dyspnea, or angina.
   III. Marked limitation of physical activity. Comfortable at rest, but less than ordinary physical activity results in fatigue, palpitation, dyspnea, or angina.
   IV. Unable to carry out any physical activity without discomfort with symptoms of cardiac insufficiency present at rest (Smirnova, 2015).

Interventions

A comprehensive program for a client with CHF should include goals and interventions. The goals should focus on preventing muscle loss and deconditioning, assessing and monitoring function and instructing clients in a home program, as well as managing risk factors. These goals and the subsequent interventions are generally implemented during a Phase I or inpatient cardiac rehabilitation program. Clients with stable CHF symptoms typically participate in group treatment programs. Programs may vary, but will generally include mild calisthenics or walking for a couple of minutes, followed by rest breaks with a progression of exercise and a reduction in rest breaks over ensuing weeks to months. The program may also include a grid format, which includes ADLs, client education on nutrition, and discharge planning. Outcomes are evaluated to ensure a standard level of care and to document that the client with CHF is as functional and independent as possible (Huntley, 2014).

Impact on Occupational Performance

Therapeutic use of occupations and activities may include ADLs such as dressing, grooming, bed mobility, and sitting and standing from a chair. However, activities that incorporate large mass muscle groups are incorporated (e.g., walking); initial activity should not exceed two to three METs. Additionally, BP and pulse rate must be monitored, particularly with symptomatic individuals (American College of Sports Medicine, 2006; Huntley, 2014).

1. *Preparatory methods and tasks*: Include warm-up periods of at least 10 minutes of slow physical activities that should not include isometric or static physical exertion, which could compromise the heart (American College of Sports Medicine, 2006; Huntley, 2014).

2. *Education and training*: Self-monitoring of vital signs, not holding breath, positioning when lying down for optimal breathing (i.e., head somewhat

elevated) should all be part of client training and education, and should include a family member or significant other (Smirnova, 2015).

3. *Reevaluation and plan modification or discontinuation*: Plans should be modified every session if warranted secondary to symptoms. A reevaluation should be minimally conducted every 30 days.

Referrals and Discharge Considerations

If symptoms persist and progress is not made, referral to a physician should occur. Discharge should be considered if the client does not progress and does not have symptoms. In either circumstance, client education and demonstration on proper physical activity monitoring and safety should occur. If a client progresses well and is safe to be discharged, a home program should include activity and exercise guidelines, work simplification, pacing, temperature precautions, social activity, sexual activity concerns, signs and symptoms of exercise intolerance, discussion of risk factors, and client-centered and focused activities (Huntley, 2014).

Management and Standards of Practice

The occupational therapist (OT) manages the care of a client with CHF by developing the intervention plan and overseeing the occupational therapy assistant (OTA) in the administration and execution of the plan. However, the OTA, while trained to carry out the plan, cannot interpret evaluation results. The evaluation of the client is performed by the OT and subsequent changes to the treatment plan are the responsibility of the OT. Also, discharge planning must be supervised and is the responsibility of the OT. While the OTA can assist in a home evaluation, the OT is responsible for the final discharge plan.

Chapter 21 Self-Study Activities (Answers Are Provided at the End of the Chapter)

1. What is an important, and usually initial standardized, assessment for an adult with COPD?

2. Physical training in a pulmonary rehabilitation program for an adult with COPD should include the use of what type of group exercises?

3. Name one type of noninvasive assessment for an adult with cardiovascular disease.

4. List three goals when planning interventions for an adult who has experienced an MI.

5. What are two symptoms that should be screened/assessed prior to ADLs for an adult with CHF?

6. When developing a home program before discharge for an adult with CHF, list the components that should be included.

7. Given the following case scenario, what should be the primary intervention in the OT treatment plan?
   - *Client*: 56-year-old male with diagnosis of COPD secondary to four packs per day cigarette smoking for the past 40 years.
   - *Problem*: Complains of increasing lack of overall and lower extremity (LE) endurance.
   - *Assess*: Six-minute walk test (criterion-referenced), using four-point dyspnea scale to determine SOB severity while measuring total walking distance achieved on a level surface to determine overall and LE endurance.
   - *Findings*: >3 (i.e., moderately severe, very uncomfortable) on a scale of 4 (i.e., most severe ever experienced), at the conclusion of a 1,100 foot walk.

8. When screening, explain what symptoms and signs are similar for both COPD and CHF?

9. In treating an adult with an MI, how many phases of cardiac rehabilitation should the OT be actively involved in?

Chapter 21 Self-Study Answers

1. Medical history and physical examination.
2. Group exercises that emphasize both endurance and strength enhancement and the use of short intervals of exercise up to two minutes at the beginning, eventually progressing to eight intervals.
3. ECG.
4. Planned goals should focus on: (1) preventing muscle loss and deconditioning, (2) assessing and monitoring function, and (3) instructing clients in a home program and risk factors.

5. SOB, especially during mild activities or ADLs and swelling or edema in the extremities, particularly the ankles and feet.

6. Activity and exercise guidelines, work simplification, pacing, temperature precautions when exercising or physically working, amount of social activity and sexual activity concerns, signs and symptoms present during exercise intolerance, and a discussion of heart disease risk factors.

7. The plan should include group ADL activities with proper breathing instruction to increase tolerance and functional endurance.

8. SOB and dyspnea during mild ADLs and exercise are similar signs and symptoms in both COPD and CHF.

9. An OT should be actively involved in Phase I and II, which include inpatient and outpatient coverage, respectively, and serve as a planner, developer, and consultant for Phase III.

References

American College of Emergency Physicians and Society for Cardiovascular Angiography and Interventions, O'Gara, P. T., Kushner, F. G., Ascheim, D. D., Casey, D. E., Chung, M. K., . . . Yancy, C. W. (2013). 2013 ACCF/AHA guideline for the management of ST-elevation myocardial infarction: A report of the American College of Cardiology Foundation/American Heart Association Task Force on Practice Guidelines. *Journal of the American College of Cardiology, 61*(4), e78–e140. doi:10.1016/j.jacc.2012.11.019

American College of Sports Medicine. (2006). *Guidelines for exercise testing and prescription* (7th ed.). Baltimore, MD: Lippincott Williams & Wilkins.

American Thoracic Society. (1999a). Pulmonary rehabilitation. *American Journal of Respiratory and Critical Care Medicine, 159*(5, Pt. 1), 1666–1682. doi:10.1164/ajrccm.159.5.ats2-99

American Thoracic Society. (1999b). Skeletal muscle dysfunction in chronic obstructive pulmonary disease. A statement of the American Thoracic Society and European Respiratory Society. *American Journal of Respiratory and Critical Care Medicine, 159*(4, Pt. 2), S1–S40. doi:10.1164/ajrccm.159.supplement_1.99titlepage

Birk, T. J., & Talley, S. A. (2015). Cardiovascular pathophysiology. In S. Levine (Ed.), *Clinical exercise electrocardiology* (pp. 9–25). Burlington, MA: Jones & Bartlett Learning.

Braunwald, E. (2013a). Heart failure. *JACC Heart Failure, 1*(1), 1–20. doi:10.1016/j.jchf.2012.10.002

Braunwald, E. (2013b). Heart failure: An update. *Clinical Pharmacology and Therapeutics, 94*(4), 430–432. doi:10.1038/clpt.2013.149

Chhabra, S. K., Gupta, A. K., & Khuma, M. Z. (2009). Evaluation of three scales of dyspnea in chronic obstructive pulmonary disease. *Annals of Thoracic Medicine, 4*(3), 128–132. doi:10.4103/1817-1737.53351

Chou, R., & High Value Care Task Force of the American College of Physicians. (2015). Cardiac screening with electrocardiography, stress echocardiography, or myocardial perfusion imaging: Advice for high-value care from the American College of Physicians. *Annals of Internal Medicine, 162*(6), 438–447. doi:10.7326/M14-1225

Coburn, J. W., & Malek, M. H. (2012). *NSCA's essentials of personal training* (2nd ed.). Champaign, IL: Human Kinetics.

Ford, E. S., Murphy, L. B., Khavjou, O., Giles, W. H., Holt, J. B., & Croft, J. B. (2015). Total and state-specific medical and absenteeism costs of COPD among adults aged ≥ 18 years in the United States for 2010 and projections through 2020. *Chest, 147*(1), 31–45. doi:10.1378/chest.14-0972

Huntley, N. (2014). Cardiac and pulmonary diseases. In M. V. Radomski & C. A. T. Latham (Eds.), *Occupational therapy for physical dysfunction* (7th ed., pp. 1305–1314). Philadelphia, PA: Wolters Kluwer Health/Lippincott Williams & Wilkins.

Keaney, N., Kay, A., & Taylor, I. (2009). Guidelines and the diagnosis of COPD. *American Journal of Respiratory and Critical Care Medicine, 179*(8), 734. doi:10.1164/ajrccm.179.8.734

Olfert, I. M., Malek, M. H., Eagan, T. M., Wagner, H., & Wagner, P. D. (2014). Inflammatory cytokine response to exercise in alpha-1-antitrypsin deficient COPD clients 'on' or 'off' augmentation therapy. *BMC Pulmonary Medicine, 14*, 106. doi:10.1186/1471-2466-14-106

Roger, V. L., Go, A. S., Lloyd-Jones, D. M., Benjamin, E. J., Berry, J. D., Borden, W. B., . . . Stroke Statistics Subcommittee. (2012). Heart disease and stroke statistics—2012 update: A report from the American Heart Association. *Circulation, 125*(1), e2–e220. doi:10.1161/CIR.0b013e31823ac046

Senior, R. M., & Silverman, E. K. (2007). Chronic obstructive pulmonary disease. In D. C. Dale & D. D. Feerman (Eds.), *ACP Medicine*. New York, NY: WebMD.

Smirnova, I. V. (2015). The cardiovascular system. In C. C. Goodman & K. S. Fuller (Eds.), *Pathology implications for the physical therapist* (pp. 538–660). St. Louis, MO: Elsevier.

Vaughn, P. (2014). Appendix I—Cardiac conditions. In B. A. B. Schell, G. Gillen, & M. E. Scaffa (Eds.), *Willard & Spackman's occupational therapy* (12th ed., pp. 1124–1127). Philadelphia, PA: Wolters Kluwer Health/Lippincott Williams & Wilkins.

Vestbo, J., Hurd, S. S., Agusti, A. G., Jones, P. W., Vogelmeier, C., Anzueto, A., . . . Rodriguez-Roisin, R. (2013). Global strategy for the diagnosis, management, and prevention of chronic obstructive pulmonary disease: GOLD executive summary. *American Journal of Respiratory and Critical Care Medicine, 187*(4), 347–365. doi:10.1164/rccm.201204-0596PP

Yancy, C. W., Jessup, M., Bozkurt, B., Butler, J., Casey, D. E., Jr., Drazner, M. H., . . . American Heart Association Task Force on Practice Guidelines. (2013). 2013 ACCF/AHA guideline for the management of heart failure: A report of the American College of Cardiology Foundation/American Heart Association Task Force on Practice Guidelines. *Journal of the American College of Cardiology, 62*(16), e147–e239. doi:10.1016/j.jacc.2013.05.019

Zeb, I., & Budoff, M. (2015). Coronary artery calcium screening: Does it perform better than other cardiovascular risk stratification tools? *International Journal of Molecular Sciences, 16*(3), 6606–6620. doi:10.3390/ijms16036606

Oncology

Sheila M. Longpré

Learning Objectives

- Describe the incidence and risk factors of cancer.
- Explain common physical and psychological conditions associated with cancer and its treatments.
- Identify appropriate occupational therapy assessments for individuals with cancer.
- List interventions that can be used to assist clients who have primary or secondary complications due to cancer and its treatment.
- Select appropriate interventions as a result of cancer staging and prognosis.

Key Terms

- *Cancer care continuum*: Delivery of care from diagnosis to death (National Cancer Institute, 2015).
- *Cancer survivor*: A person diagnosed with any form of cancer who is still living.
- *In situ*: Confined to the site of origin.
- *Late effects*: Side effects of cancer treatment that become apparent after your treatment has ended (Mayo Clinic, 2015a).
- *Metastatic cancer*: Cancer that has spread from the site of origin to another place in the body (National Cancer Institute, 2015).

Description

The term cancer is used to describe the abnormal growth of cells within a specific organ or tissue type (Cooper, 2006; Longpre & Newman, 2011). Cancer is

described, or identified, by the type of tissue in which they arise, such as carcinoma, sarcoma, chondroma, lymphoma, or leukemia (Burkhardt & Schultz-Krohn, 2013; Cooper, 2006) as well as whether the cancer is metastatic. If left untreated, the abnormal cells will continue to grow into a mass or tumor, which can impact vital organs (Cooper, 2006).

A specialist, generally an oncologist, is required to diagnose cancer. Additionally, tests completed with the DNA, RNA, and protein of the cell may also aid in diagnosing the presence of cancer. The results from the test will allow the specialist to determine the best course of treatment for the individual (American Cancer Society, 2015b).

Etiology and Pathology

Nearly 1.7 million new cases of cancer will be diagnosed and approximately 600,000 cancer deaths are anticipated in the United States this year (American Cancer Society, 2016). Men are more likely than women to develop cancer. Age and survivorship are proportionately related. The older an individual, the greater the risk of death (Vaughn, 2013). The most common types of cancer in men are prostate, lung, and colorectal. Similarly, the most common types of cancer in women are breast, lung, and colorectal (American Cancer Society, 2015a).

Pathology is used to determine the type of cancer and how aggressive it is. This is completed through grading and staging (National Cancer Institute, 2015; Radomski, Anheluk, Grabe, Hopkins, & Zola, 2014). Grading is a term used to describe how abnormal tumor cells look under the microscope, or how differentiated they are

Table 22-1 Cancer Staging

TNM Staging System		
T	Tumor size	TX: tumor cannot be evaluated
		T0: no evidence of primary tumor
		Tis: cancer in situ abnormal cells that have not spread to surrounding tissue
		T1, T2, T3, T4: the greater the number, the more invasive the tumor
N	Extend of tumor spreading to the lymph nodes	NX: lymph nodes cannot be evaluated
		N0: no lymph node involvement
		N1, N2, N3: the greater the number, the greater the lymph node involvement
M	Presence of metastasis	MX: metastasis cannot be evaluated
		M0: no known distant metastasis
		M1: distant metastasis is present

Stages of Cancer (0–IV)	
Stage	**Definition**
0	Carcinoma in situ for most cancers. A very early stage in which cancer is present only in the layer of cells which it began and has not spread
I	Cancer that is the next least advanced
II–III	Cancer involving more extensive disease as indicated by greater tumor size and/or spread of the cancer to nearby lymph nodes and/or organs
IV	Cancer has spread to other organs

Modified from Table 45-1 in Radomski, Anheluk, Grabe, Hopkins, & Zola, 2014.

(Hutson, 2004). Grading does vary across tumor types, but follows a general pattern: the lower the grade, the better the prognosis (Radomski et al., 2014). Staging is used to determine the extent of the disease (**Table 22-1**). The staging system used in oncology care is the TMN System. The TMN System indicates the tumor size (T), extent of the tumor spreading to the lymph nodes (N), and the presence of metastasis (M). Tumor size is similar to grading—the lower the stage of cancer, the better the prognosis.

Risk Factors

There are multiple risk factors associated with cancer, including hereditary, environmental, stress, obesity, exposure to sunlight, occupational exposure (i.e., asbestos), and infections such as human immunodeficiency virus/acquired immunodeficiency syndrome and human papilloma virus. Approximately one-third of all cancers are preventable through early intervention and lifestyle changes (Sharpe & Fenton, 2008).

Clinical Presentation

Signs and symptoms vary depending on the type of cancer present. Signs are indicators that can be seen by other people and symptoms are what is felt by the individual (American Cancer Society, 2015a). Individuals who experience signs and symptoms of cancer should seek medical attention to rule out cancer. See **Table 22-2** for a list of general signs and symptoms.

Table 22-2 General Signs and Symptoms of Cancer

- Unexplained weight loss
- Fever
- Fatigue
- Pain
- Skin changes

Data from American Cancer Society, 2015.

Diagnostic Tests

Early detection is key for a more favorable prognosis. Individuals with cancer may present in a variety of conditions based on tumor location. The disease can be both acute and chronic. The oncology specialist completes a comprehensive evaluation by gathering a clinical history, completing a physical examination, and by ordering specialized tests such as x-rays, computed tomography scans, magnetic resonance imaging, positron emission tomography, and laboratory tests, including tumor markers and cytology. A biopsy is typically used to provide the definitive pathology (Sharpe & Fenton, 2008; Vaughn, 2013).

Common Medical Procedures

There are three common types of medical treatment, which include surgery, chemotherapy, and radiation. Surgical procedures are performed in efforts to rid the body of the tumor mass and reconstruct any physical deficits to improve overall functional performance and appearance. Chemotherapy is a type of cancer treatment that uses a toxic chemical substance to rid the body of cancer cells. Radiation is a more precise medical treatment delivery that relies on radioactive materials that target the cancer cells in a specific area of the body. Unfortunately, radiation not only destroys the cancer cells, but it can also destroy surrounding healthy tissue as well, which can lead to future complications (Burkhardt & Schultz-Krohn, 2013; Cooper, 2006). See **Tables 22-3** and **22-4** for a list of common impairments.

Table 22-3 Common Impairments Occurring with Cancer

Weakness	Joint and soft tissue restrictions
Poor coordination	Bowel and bladder incontinence
Sensory loss	Pain
Loss of balance	Depression
Fatigue	Anxiety
Decreased endurance	Memory loss

Data from Cooper, 2006; Rankin, Robb, Murtagh, Cooper, & Lewis, 2008.

Table 22-4 Psychosocial Complications of Cancer

Loss of control	Depression
Altered body image	Disconnection from activities/routines
Separation from friends and loved ones	Helplessness
Loss of support of family and friends	Dependence

Data from Cooper, 2006; Rankin et al., 2008.

Precautions and Contraindications

Chronic Complications

Due to improved technologies and advancement in cancer treatment, there is an increasing number of individuals who are diagnosed with cancer but are living longer. Cancer is no longer thought of solely as a fatal disease. It can, however, present with chronic complications related to tumor involvement and medical treatment. **Table 22-5**

Table 22-5 Late Effects of Cancer Treatment

Chemotherapy	Radiation	Surgery
Cataracts	Cataracts	Lymphedema
Early menopause	Cavities/tooth decay	
Heart problems	Heart and vascular problems	
Increased risk of other cancers	Increased risk of other cancers	
Infertility	Infertility	
Liver problems	Lymphedema	
Lung disease	Lung disease	
Nerve damage	Memory problems	
Osteoporosis	Osteoporosis	
Reduced lung capacity	Hypothyroidism	
	Intestinal problems	
	Skin changes	

provides examples of late effects that individuals who are cancer survivors might experience.

Role of Occupational Therapy in Oncology

The role of occupational therapy in oncology is to facilitate and empower clients to achieve their maximum level of "functional performance, both physically and psychologically, in everyday living skills regardless of his or her life expectancy" (Cooper, 2006; Penfold, 1996, p. 75; Watterson, Lowrie, Vockins, Ewer-Smith, & Cooper, 2004). Through evaluation, intervention, and outcomes, the occupational therapy practitioner has the opportunity to provide best-practice standards across settings.

Screening and Assessments

The evaluation component of occupational therapy consists of the occupational profile and the analysis of occupational performance (American Occupational Therapy Association, 2014). As part of the initial evaluation, measurements for range of motion, edema, pain, and muscle strength are also appropriate to procure. In addition, observation and choosing the appropriate assessment to target client needs is an integral part of the evaluation (see **Table 22-6** for a list of assessments which can be utilized in an oncology setting).

Table 22-6 Occupational Therapy Assessments

Occupation-Focused	
COPM	Semi-structured, interview-based rating scale used to detect changes in a client's self-perception of occupational performance over time.
PASS	Observation-based performance rating of an individual's daily living skill performance (i.e., meant to be used as a baseline).
Role Checklist	Self-administered questionnaire and rating form used to assess a client's perception of participation in past, present, and future roles.
OSA	Self-report questionnaire based on the individual's self-perception of occupational competence.
ADL/IADL	
A-One	Rating scale and checklist used to identify neurobehavioral deficits that impact ADL performance as related to the specific site of the cortical lesion.
Cognition	
MoCA	Screening instrument used to detect mild cognitive impairments.
EFPT	Functional test used to identify impairments in executive functions in performing common daily occupations; IADL specific.
MET-R	Performance-based measure of executive function.
Client Factors	
SF-36	Self-report questionnaire in which the individual rates his/her physical and mental health.
DASH	Self-report questionnaire designed to measure physical functions and symptoms for musculoskeletal disorders of the upper extremity.
BFI	Questionnaire used to assess the severity and impact of cancer-related fatigue on daily functioning.
BDI-II	Self-report questionnaire used to measure the severity of depression.
QL Index	Questionnaire which requires an interview by the health professional administering it. It addresses ADLs, health, support, and outlook.

ADL, activities of daily living; A-One, Arnadottir OT-ADL Neurobehavioral Eval; BDI-II, Beck Depression Inventory; BFI, Brief Fatigue Inventory; COPM, Canadian Occupational Performance Measure; DASH, Disability of Arm, Shoulder, and Hand; EFPT, Executive Function Performance Test; IADL, instrumental activities of daily living; MET-R, Multiple Errands Test—Revised; MoCA, Montreal Cognitive Assessment; OSA, Occupational Self-Assessment; PASS, Performance Assessment of Self-Care Skills; QL Index, Quality of Life Index; SF-36, Short Form-36 Health Survey. Data from Asher, 2007; Radomski et al., 2014; Vaughn, 2013.

Interventions

Occupational therapy interventions can occur at many points along the cancer care continuum from prevention to hospice. Interventions in occupational therapy consist of planning, implementation, and review (American Occupational Therapy Association, 2014).

Expected Functional Outcomes

Providing a client-centered approach to the intervention planning will promote client involvement and increase well-being. See **Table 22-7** for common occupational therapy interventions throughout the various phases of oncology care.

Table 22-7 Intervention Considerations

Wellness	Prevention Programs
Acute care	• Postsurgical precautions/applications (i.e., indicative of tumor type) • Typical blood counts and laboratory values are the same as what followed for individuals without cancer. For these clients, their laboratory values will generally be lower and will require monitoring throughout the treatment session to ensure safety. • Positioning and splinting • Education • Coping • Breathing techniques • Caregiver training • Equipment training
Inpatient and outpatient rehabilitation	• Energy conservation • Exercise/movement • Progression occurs as the client can tolerate activity • Endurance • Education • Coping • Guided imagery • Breathing techniques • Caregiver training • Equipment training
Home health	• Home modifications • Caregiver training • Equipment training • Education (e.g., exercises, breathing techniques, anxiety management, and lymphedema management)
Community	• Survivorship groups • Yoga
Hospice/palliative care	• Comfort measures (e.g., symptom management and engagement in meaningful activities)

Data from Burkhardt & Schultz-Krohn, 2013; Cooper, 2006; Cramer, Lange, Klose, Paul, & Dobos, 2012; Radomski et al., 2014; Rankin et al., 2008; Roffe, Schmidt, & Ernst, 2005; Vaughn, 2013; Watterson et al., 2004; Yadav, 2007.

Referrals and Discharge Considerations

Outcome assessments are utilized in occupational therapy practice to determine client success in achieving desired goals, "plan future actions with the client," and evaluate services offered (American Occupational Therapy Association, 2014, p. S10). The information gathered in the outcomes component could aid in the preparation for discharge. Discharge can occur at any moment across the continuum of care. Safe discharge remains a priority in the oncology setting.

Management and Standards of Practice

In the area of oncology care, occupational therapy practitioners need to ensure that they are working closely with the other team members. This is important because any slight growth or a new episode of cancer may be related to the client's behavior or performance. When even slight changes are noticed, the occupational therapist (OT) must relay that information to the treatment team as soon as possible.

The communication between the OT and the occupational therapy assistant (OTA) is also critical. The OTA, if involved, can carry out specific interventions. Again, any changes in behavior, affect, or performance need to be communicated and addressed immediately. As with other diagnoses, a cancer diagnosis can leave clients feeling depressed and at times desperate. These psychosocial challenges can lead to clients facing additional challenges. Addressing these concerns and providing appropriate supportive resources is a critical aspect for both the client and any caregivers.

Chapter 22 Self-Study Activities (Answers Are Provided at the End of the Chapter)

1. Define cancer:_____
2. In the United States, who is more likely to develop cancer?
   A. Men
   B. Women
3. You are about to complete an initial evaluation with a man who has lung cancer. You review his medical records and it indicates that his staging was as follows: T1, N0, M0 Stage I. What is his prognosis?_____
4. Identify three common impairments derived from the medical treatment for cancer.

   _____

   _____

   _____

5. Identify three common psychosocial complications of cancer and its treatment.

   _____

   _____

   _____

Answer questions 6–10 using the following case scenario.

Mrs. Wu has just been referred to you by her oncologist. She has a history of left breast cancer and completed her last dose of radiation and chemotherapy two weeks ago. She is status post a mastectomy without reconstruction. She complains of a limited range of motion of the left upper extremity shoulder (e.g., flexion and abduction). She states she works at the United States Postal Services and is required to lift objects overhead that weigh 10 pounds. She is unable to return to work until she can perform all of her job duties. In addition, she tells you that she has a daughter in dance and a son in soccer and it is her role as a parent to take them to their after-school activities. She informs you that it is getting increasingly difficult as she gets very tired these days.

6. What is the first thing that you should do during your initial session with Mrs. Wu?
   A. Develop a home exercise program to increase the range of motion in her left shoulder.
   B. Complete a client-centered evaluation to include occupational profile and a standardized assessment.
   C. Complete the DASH.
   D. Educate her on the importance of going back to work to make money to support her children.
7. What late effects do you need to consider with Mrs. Wu?

   _____

   _____

8. Identify two occupational therapy assessments that would be appropriate for Mrs. Wu.

   _____

   _____

9. You have recommended continued outpatient therapy for Mrs. Wu, two times a week for four weeks. She is progressing well, but now that she is in the third week of treatment she expresses concerns with increased shortness of breath. How would you modify your treatment session, if at all, to address her concerns?

_____

_____

_____

_____

10. Mrs. Wu is now preparing for discharge. What is the best way you can determine that she is able to achieve her goals she has identified as important (i.e., reaching overhead and shortness of breath)?

_____

_____

_____

_____

Chapter 22 Self-Study Answers

1. An abnormal growth of cells
2. Men
3. Good
4. Possible common impairments include:
   - Weakness
   - Joint and soft tissue restrictions
   - Poor coordination
   - Bowel and bladder incontinence
   - Sensory loss
   - Pain
   - Loss of balance
   - Depression
   - Fatigue
   - Anxiety
   - Decreased endurance
   - Memory loss
5. See table below:
   - Loss of control
   - Depression
   - Altered body image
   - Disconnection from activities/routines
   - Helplessness
   - Separation from friends and loved ones
   - Dependence
   - Loss of support of family and friends
6. B
7. See the following table:

8. Any of the following: Canadian Occupational Performance Measure (COPM), Role Checklist, Occupational Self-Assessment (OSA), Short Form-36 Health Survey (SF-36), Disability of Arm, Shoulder, and Hand (DASH), Brief Fatigue Inventory (BFI).
9. You consider that this may be a late effect of cancer treatment and you modify it by addressing breathing techniques to improve overall lung function.
10. You can have Mrs. Wu complete a functional task of reaching overhead; you could also have her complete the same standardized assessment you used at the initial evaluation (e.g., DASH); you could also have Mrs. Wu review the home exercises provided for breathing techniques to see if she can recall them independently and have her complete a functional task to measure her overall shortness of breath.

Chemotherapy	Radiation	Surgery
• Cataracts • Early menopause • Heart problems • Increased risk of other cancers • Infertility • Liver problems • Lung disease • Nerve damage • Osteoporosis • Reduced lung capacity	• Cataracts • Cavities/tooth decay • Heart and vascular problems • Skin changes • Infertility • Lymphedema • Lung disease • Memory problems • Osteoporosis • Hypothyroidism • Intestinal problems • Increased risk of other cancers	• Lymphedema

References

American Cancer Society. (2015a). *Cancer signs and symptoms.* Retrieved from http://www.cancer.org/cancer/cancerbasics/signs-and-symptoms-of-cancer

American Cancer Society. (2015b). *Testing biopsy and cytology specimens for cancer.* Retrieved from http://www.cancer.org/treatment/understandingyourdiagnosis/examsandtestdescriptions/testingbiopsyandcytologyspecimensforcancer/testing-biopsy-and-cytology-specimens-for-cancer-how-is-cancer-diagnosed

American Cancer Society. (2016). *Cancer statistics center.* Retrieved from https://cancerstatisticscenter.cancer.org/?_ga=1.29656184.614500760.1457023411#/ http://www.cancer.org/acs/groups/content/@editorial/documents/document/acspc-044509.pdf

American Occupational Therapy Association. (2014). Occupational therapy practice framework: Domain and process (3rd edition). *American Journal of Occupational Therapy, 68*(Suppl. 1), S10–S48. doi:10.5014/ajot.2014.682006

Asher, I. E. (2007). *Occupational therapy assessment tools: An annotated index* (3rd ed.). Bethesda, MD: American Occupational Therapy Association.

Burkhardt, A., & Schultz-Krohn, W. (2013). Oncology. In H. M. Pendleton & W. Schultz-Krohn (Eds.), *Pedretti's occupational therapy: Practice skills for physical dysfunction* (7th ed., pp. 1215–1227). St. Louis, MO: Elsevier.

Cooper, J. (2006). *Occupational therapy in oncology and palliative care* (2nd ed.). West Sussex, UK: John Wiley & Sons.

Cramer, H., Lange, S., Klose, P., Paul, A., & Dobos, G. (2012). Yoga for breast cancer patients and survivors: A systematic review and meta-analysis. *BMC Cancer, 12*, 412. doi:10.1186/1471-2407-12-412

Hutson, L. M. (2004). Breast cancer. In C. G. Varricchio (Ed), *A cancer source book for nurses* (8th ed., pp. 173–186). Sudbury, MA: Jones and Bartlett Publishers.

Longpre, S. M., & Newman, R. (2011). *Fact sheet: The role of occupational therapy in oncology.* Retrieved from http://www.aota.org/-/media/Corporate/Files/AboutOT/Professionals/WhatIsOT/RDP/Facts/Oncology fact sheet.pdf

Mayo Clinic. (2015a). *Cancer.* Retrieved from http://www.mayoclinic.org/diseases-conditions/cancer/in-depth/cancer-survivor/art-20045524

National Cancer Institute. (2015). *Late effects of treatment for childhood cancer (PDQ).* Retrieved from http://www.cancer.gov/types/childhood-cancers/late-effects-pdq

Penfold, S. L. (1996). The role of the occupational therapist in oncology. *Cancer Treatment Reviews, 22*(1), 75–81. Retrieved from http://www.ncbi.nlm.nih.gov/pubmed/8625332

Radomski, M. V., Anheluk, M., Grabe, K., Hopkins, S. E., & Zola, J. (2014). Cancer. In M. V. Radomski & C. A. T. Latham (Eds.), *Occupational therapy for physical dysfunction* (7th ed., pp. 1368–1387). Philadelphia, PA: Wolters Kluwer Health/Lippincott Williams & Wilkins.

Rankin, J., Robb, N., Murtagh, N., Cooper, J., & Lewis, S. (2008). *Rehabilitation in cancer care.* Chichester, UK: Wiley-Blackwell.

Roffe, L., Schmidt, K., & Ernst, E. (2005). A systematic review of guided imagery as an adjuvant cancer therapy. *Psychooncology, 14*(8), 607–617. doi:10.1002/pon.889

Sharpe, G., & Fenton, P. A. (2008). Cancer and its management: An introduction. In J. Rankin, K. Robb, N. Murtagh, J. Cooper, & S. Lewis (Eds.), *Rehabilitation in cancer* (pp. 3–23). Chichester, UK; Ames, Iowa: Wiley-Blackwell.

Vaughn, P. (2013). Cancer. In B. A. B. Schell, G. Gillen, & M. E. Scaffa (Eds.), *Willard & Spackman's occupational therapy* (12th ed., pp. 1120–1124). Baltimore, MD: Lippincott Williams & Wilkins.

Watterson, J., Lowrie, D., Vockins, H., Ewer-Smith, C., & Cooper, J. (2004). Rehabilitation goals identified by inpatients with cancer using the COPM. *International Journal of Therapy and Rehabilitation, 11*(5), 219–224.

Yadav, R. (2007). Rehabilitation of surgical cancer patients at the University of Texas M.D. Anderson Cancer Center. *Journal of Surgical Oncology, 95*, 361–369.

Diabetes

Camille Dieterle

Learning Objectives

- Define the two main types of diabetes.
- Describe how diabetes impacts the body and occupational performance in all of its stages.
- Describe the incidence and risk factors of diabetes.
- Compare and contrast the different tests used to measure blood sugar.
- Describe the key elements of client education for a client with diabetes.
- Explain how medical treatment of diabetes can impact occupation.
- Describe safety precautions that are utilized when working with clients who have diabetes.
- Describe how secondary complications from diabetes impact occupation and disability.
- Identify appropriate occupational therapy (OT) assessments for clients with diabetes.
- Describe the role of the OT practitioner when working on a diabetes care team.
- Construct lifestyle interventions that can be used to help clients who have diabetes prevent secondary complications and disabilities.
- Construct interventions that can be used to help clients who have secondary complications and disabilities as a result of diabetes, prevent further disease progression.
- Describe interventions that reinforce the American Association of Diabetes Educators seven self-care behaviors (AADE7 Self-Care Behaviors).

Key Terms

- *Autoimmune disease*: An illness in which the body's immune system attacks and damages its own tissues.
- *Endocrinopathies*: A disease of an endocrine gland.
- *Gestational diabetes mellitus*: Any degree of glucose intolerance that begins or occurs during pregnancy.
- *Hyperglycemia*: High blood glucose.
- *Idiopathic*: A disease of unknown origin.
- *Insulin*: A hormone produced by the pancreas that regulates glucose metabolism by lowering the levels of glucose in the blood.

Description

Diabetes is a chronic metabolic disorder that causes abnormalities in carbohydrate, fat, and protein metabolism, which leads to hyperglycemia (American Association of Diabetes Educators [AADE], 2010). Systemic and progressive diabetes cause glucose in the bloodstream to elevate to dangerous levels (i.e., fasting blood glucose of 126 mg/dL or more) (Sotelo, 2014) and left uncontrolled can cause serious immediate and long-term effects on the body (Sokol-McKay, 2011). There are several types of diabetes, the most common of which are Type 1, Type 2, and gestational, with Type 2 being by far the most common. There are several other rare types, including genetic defects of beta cell foundation, exocrine pancreatic diseases, endocrinopathies, drug or chemically induced, and other rare forms (AADE, 2010).

Incidence

According to the American Heart Association, the incidence of diabetes has doubled in the last 30 years, similar to obesity (Huntley, 2014) and in 2012, a total of 29.1 million people (i.e., 9.3% of the population) in the United States had diabetes: 21 million diagnosed and 8.1 million undiagnosed (Centers for Disease Control and Prevention [CDC], 2014). The incidence of diabetes increases with age; of the total population of Americans suffering from diabetes, 25.9% are aged 65 years and older, 16.2% are in the age range 45–64 years, 4.1% are in the age range 20–44 years, and 0.25% are younger than 20 years (CDC, 2014). By ethnicity, American Indians/Native Alaskans have the highest incidence, followed by non-Hispanic blacks, Hispanics and Asians and non-Hispanic whites (National Diabetes Information Clearinghouse [NDIC], 2011). Diabetes is the seventh leading cause of death in the United States and is expected to rise by 25% over the next 10 years (CDC, 2014; Cooper & Geyer, 2009). In 2009–2012, 37% of U.S. adults aged 20 years or older had prediabetes and 51% of those were aged 65 years and older (CDC, 2014).

Pathogenesis

In Type 1 diabetes, which used to be called juvenile diabetes, there is complete insulin deficiency (AADE, 2010). Most often, Type 1 diabetes is caused by an autoimmune disease that initiates destruction of the beta cells in the pancreas, which produce insulin (i.e., a hormone that is required to convert sugar and other types of food into energy) (Homko, Sisson, & Ross, 2009). Type 1 diabetes is no longer called juvenile because there are now so many children with Type 2 diabetes. Type 2 diabetes, the most common type of diabetes, is caused by a combination of beta cell dysfunction, which creates a relative insulin deficiency, and insulin resistance, when the body is not able to use insulin efficiently. According to the American Diabetes Association (ADA), Type 2 diabetes, which is closely associated with obesity and physical inactivity (Sotelo, 2014), starts with insulin resistance (see **Table 23-1**). When the body becomes resistant to insulin, it causes the pancreas to release excessive amounts of insulin to maintain normal blood sugar

Table 23-1 Differences Between Type 1 and Type 2 Diabetes

	Type 1	**Type 2**
Etiology	Autoimmune (i.e., most common) and idiopathic	Obesity, family history, and lifestyle choices
Prevalence	0.4% and rising	9.3% and rising
Onset	Rapid and acute	Gradual and silent
Treatment	Insulin therapy: • Fixed regimen • Flexible regimen (i.e., multiple daily injections) • Insulin pump	Combination of: • Lifestyle change (e.g., weight loss, physical activity, and dietary changes) • Oral medication • Insulin therapy (see T1DM)

T1DM, type 1 diabetes mellitus.
Data from (CDC, 2014); O'Keefe, Bell, and Wyne (2009).

levels. As a result, beta cells in the pancreas, which produce the insulin, eventually wear out and are unable to produce insulin, so blood sugar levels elevate. This first causes prediabetes and then diabetes (Sotelo, 2014). Gestational diabetes mellitus is relative insulin resistance during pregnancy when insulin resistance is higher. Women who have had gestational diabetes have a 35–60% chance of developing diabetes in the next 10–20 years (CDC, 2011).

Clinical Presentation

People with Type 2 diabetes or prediabetes are often unaware that they have it. According to the ADA, symptoms of Type 2 diabetes include frequent urination, unusual thirst, extreme hunger, unusual weight loss, extreme fatigue and irritability, frequent infections, blurred vision, cuts and bruises that heal slowly, peripheral neuropathy (e.g., tingling and numbness), sensation loss in the hands or feet, and recurring skin, gum, or bladder infections (Sotelo, 2014).

Risk Factors for the Development of Diabetes

According to the American Heart Association, risk factors for Type 2 diabetes include family history, ethnic background, age, overweight or obesity, physical inactivity, hypertension, smoking, and excessive alcohol consumption (Sotelo, 2014). Obesity, or a body mass index (BMI) of 30 or higher, is the second leading preventable cause of death and increases the risk for developing diabetes (Huntley, 2014; Sotelo, 2014). Barriers to exercise are another significant risk factor for both children and adults regarding obesity and diabetes. Many communities in the United States are poorly designed for physical activity because of the built environment and safety. According to Wallis, Miranda, and Park (Hocking, 2009), a lack of safe walking and biking areas and parks, time, and boredom while exercising are the top reasons American adults say they are not exercising.

Acute Complications of Uncontrolled Diabetes

Hypoglycemia, the most prevalent acute complication of diabetes, can be life-threatening and requires immediate attention (Sokol-McKay, 2011). When a client is experiencing hypoglycemia (see **Table 23-2**), it is critical to administer fast-absorbing forms of sugar, such as orange juice, candy, or sports drinks (Homko et al, 2009).

Insulin-Related Illnesses

It is important for an occupational therapy (OT) practitioner to know the different signs and symptoms of the two main insulin-related illnesses: insulin reaction (i.e., insulin shock) when the client is experiencing hypoglycemia, or very low blood sugar, and ketoacidosis or

hyperglycemia, when the client is experiencing very high blood sugar (see Table 23-2) (George, 2013).

Chronic Complications of Uncontrolled Diabetes

The presence of diabetes is also a risk factor for other diseases and secondary complications (see **Table 23-3**).

Table 23-3 Chronic Complications of Uncontrolled Diabetes

Microvascular	Macrovascular	Other
Retinopathy, vision loss, and blindness	Peripheral arterial disease	Diabetic foot ulcers, which can lead to lower extremity amputations (i.e., secondary to peripheral arterial disease and sensation loss), are the leading cause of nontraumatic foot and leg amputations. Fifty percent of diabetic foot ulcers are preventable.
Peripheral neuropathy and sensation loss	Cardiovascular disease (e.g., MI and CHF)	Infections (e.g., UTI and skin infections).
Autonomic neuropathy	Cerebrovascular disease (e.g., stroke and TIA)	Impaired wound healing (e.g., diabetes can affect both the duration and potential of the rehabilitation process for fractures).

Nephropathy, kidney disease, and failure. Diabetes is the leading cause of kidney failure and dialysis. The mortality rate of people with diabetes and kidney disease is 50% within the first 2 years.

MI, myocardial infarction; CHF, congestive heart failure; UTI, urinary tract infection; TIA, transient ischemic attack.
Data from Homko, Sisson, and Ross, (2009); CDC (2014); Maher (2014); Sokol-McKay (2011); Sotelo (2014).

Table 23-2 Signs and Symptoms of Insulin-Related Illnesses

	Insulin Reaction (Insulin Shock) (Hypoglycemia)	Ketoacidosis (Diabetic Coma) (Hyperglycemia)
Onset	Sudden	Gradual
Skin	Moist and pale	Dry and flushed
Behavior	Excited and agitated	Drowsy
Breath odor	Normal	Fruity
Breathing	Normal to shallow	Deep and labored
Tongue	Moist	Dry
Vomiting	Absent	Present
Hunger	Present	Absent
Thirst	Absent	Present

Data from: George (2013).

For example, women with diabetes have a significantly higher risk for coronary artery disease (CAD) because diabetes diminishes their hormonal protection from CAD (Huntley, 2014). In order to reduce the risk of heart disease, clients with both Type 1 and Type 2 diabetes must control their blood sugar through medication, diet, and exercise (Huntley, 2014). This type of secondary prevention requires OT practitioners to spend a significant amount of time educating their clients on the risk factors and how to decrease them (Huntley, 2014). Because elevated blood sugar over time increases the deposit of fatty materials along blood vessels, heart disease and stroke are the leading causes of death in people who have diabetes (NDIC, 2014).

Diabetic Retinopathy

Almost 40% of people with diabetes develop diabetic retinopathy (Kaldenberg, 2014). In this complication, the small blood vessels of the retina become damaged by diabetes, including swelling and bleeding, and can cause serious vision loss (Kaldenberg, 2013). Because diabetic retinopathy is both progressive and degenerative, it is more common among the elderly and may eventually lead to total blindness, according to Hooper and Dal Bello-Haas (Bonder & Goodman, 2014). Functional complaints include difficulty discriminating contrast and color, impaired night vision, and fluctuations in vision (Kaldenberg, 2014). Medical treatments include surgery, laser treatment, and vitrectomy. OT may include color and contrast enhancement, glare control, magnification, lighting, visual skills training, sensory substitution, organizational strategies, mobility training, and potential referrals to optometry or ophthalmology (Kaldenberg,

2014). Proprioception may also be affected by loss of vision (Bonder & Goodman, 2014).

Diagnostic Tests

Diabetes is diagnosed when there are symptoms present in addition to one positive test from **Table 23-4**.

Prediabetes is diagnosed when there is any one of the following present (see Table 23-4): impaired fasting glucose (IFG), impaired glucose tolerance, or elevated hemoglobin A1C (HbA_{1c}).

Metabolic syndrome, which increases the risk for diabetes and heart disease, is diagnosed when at least three of the following are present: IFG, triglycerides $\geq$ 150 mg/dL, blood pressure $\geq$ 130/85, abdominal obesity (i.e., waist circ. >40 inches in men and >35 inches in women), or low high-density lipoprotein (HDL) cholesterol (i.e., <40 mg/dL in men and <50 mg/dL in women) (ADA, 2014).

Medical Treatment for Diabetes

According to the ADA, diabetes treatment includes close monitoring of blood glucose levels, medications (e.g., insulin, sulfonylureas, meglitinides, and biguanides), healthy lifestyle choices, including dietary choices, physical activity, adequate sleep, and maintaining regular medical care to prevent, identify, or treat secondary conditions (Sotelo, 2014). Intensive glucose control through medication, lifestyle changes, and consistent medical care

Table 23-4 Diagnosis Criteria			
	Fasting Plasma Glucose (FPG) • Amount of glucose in the blood after a 12-hr (i.e., overnight) fast • Abnormal = impaired fasting glucose (IFG)	**Oral Glucose Tolerance Test (OGTT)** • Amount of glucose in the blood after consuming high-glucose beverage	**A1C % (Hemoglobin A1C/HbA_{1c})** • Average blood glucose levels over approximately 6–12 weeks
Diabetes	>126 mg/dL	>200 mg/dL	<5.7%
Prediabetes	100–126 mg/dL	140–200 mg/dL	5.7–6.4%
Normal	<100 mg/dL	<140 mg/dL	>6.4%

Data from: ADA (2014).

can reduce the risk of eye disease by 76%, kidney disease by 50%, nerve disease by 60%, any cardiovascular disease event by 42%, and nonfatal heart attack, stroke, or death from cardiovascular causes by 57% (NDIC, 2013).

The Diabetes Prevention Program (DPP) demonstrated that people at risk of developing diabetes can prevent or delay the onset of diabetes by losing a modest amount of weight through diet and exercise. DPP participants in the lifestyle intervention group reduced their risk of developing diabetes by 58% during the study. The oral diabetes medication metformin also reduced their risk of developing diabetes, but not as much as those who participated in a lifestyle intervention (NDIC, 2013).

Surgical Treatment for Diabetes

It has been demonstrated widely that bariatric surgery treatment of morbid obesity can quickly resolve Type 2 diabetes in most cases, and significantly reduces mortality from diabetes (Keidar, 2011). Roux-en-Y and biliopancreatic diversion are the most effective procedures for diabetes and success rates have been so strong that surgeries are being indicated for clients who are obese or even overweight in order to control/resolve diabetes (Keidar, 2011).

Precautions for the Treatment for Diabetes

According to the ADA, Type 2 diabetes requires the following precautions: keeping feet clean, dry, and free of cuts/wounds, special attention to diet, engaging in physical activity, and adhering to the medication schedule (Sotelo, 2014). Additional precautions must be taken when exercising. People who take insulin or insulin secretagogues must plan to prevent hypoglycemia during and after (i.e., even several hours after) engaging in vigorous physical activity (Homko et al., 2009). This plan could be adding glucose by having a snack or by reducing insulin medication prior to exercise (Homko et al., 2009). Clients must always carry a quick hypoglycemia remedy such as candy, juice, or sports drinks (Homko et al., 2009). Clients with retinopathy have the following contraindications when exercising: avoiding lowering the head below the waist, avoiding vigorous bouncing, and avoiding strenuous upper extremity exercise. With

clients who have nephropathy, it is recommended to keep the heart rate at 40–60%, slightly lower than when nephropathy is not present (AADE, 2010). Clients who are instructed to monitor ketones by their physician, and test positive for ketones, should not engage in strenuous activity (AADE, 2010).

Screening and Assessments

In addition to observation, interview, and taking history, the following assessments may be appropriate for clients diagnosed with diabetes, prediabetes, or metabolic syndrome. OT assessments are described below for participation (see **Table 23-5**), basic and instrumental activity of daily living skills (see **Table 23-6**), and client factors (see **Table 23-7**).

Table 23-5 Participation and Activity

Instrument	Description
Canadian Occupational Performance Measure (COPM) (Law et al., 1990)	Self-report of occupational performance and satisfaction
Health Status Questionnaire (SF-36)	Assesses client perception of health and physical limitation
Activity Card Sort (ACS)	Assists client description of instrumental and social activities
Assessment of Occupational Functioning-Collaborative Version (AOF-CV)	Assesses how personal causation, values, roles, habits, and skills impact functional performance
Occupational Performance Interview II (OPHI II)	Assesses critical life events, daily routines, and occupational roles
Occupational Questionnaire (OQ)	Assesses time use

Data from: Sotelo (2014).

Table 23-6 Basic and Instrumental Activity of Daily Living Skills

Instrument	Description
Kohlman Evaluation of Living Skills (KELS)	Assesses safety and independence in the community including self-care, safety, work, and leisure
Assessment of Motor and Process Skills (AMPS)	Assesses motor and process skills in context

Data from: Sotelo (2014).

Table 23-7 Client Factors

Instrument	Description
Beck Depression Inventory-II (BDI-II)	Assesses the severity of depression
Visual acuity	The Early Treatment of Diabetic Retinopathy Study (ETDRS) Chart is considered the gold standard for visual acuity measurement, according to the International Council of Ophthalmology

Data from Sotelo (2014); Weisser-Pike (2014).

Interventions

OT interventions can be designed both to prevent and to manage diabetes for people with and without disabilities (Sokol-McKay, 2011). OT practitioners may work to accomplish primary, secondary, and tertiary prevention for diabetes and work together with the diabetes care team to emphasize "lifestyle modification, health promotion, remediation of physical and visual impairments, and maximize self-care independence" (Sokol-McKay, 2011, p. 2). OT practitioners may treat diabetes as a primary diagnosis, a secondary diagnosis, and can also treat the secondary complications to diabetes. OT practitioners also have the opportunity to help clients who are at risk of developing Type 2 diabetes.

Team-Based Approach

Diabetes requires that healthcare providers work collaboratively. In addition to OT, some providers who may be involved in a diabetes care team include primary care providers (e.g., physicians, nurses, and physician assistants), endocrinologists, occupational therapists, physical therapists, occupational and physical therapy assistants, optometrists, ophthalmologists, nutritionists/dieticians, certified diabetes educators, social workers, case managers, pharmacists, and others (Cohn, 2009; Sotelo, 2014). The American Association of Diabetes Educators have stated in their disabilities position statement that occupational therapists are part of the diabetes self-care team, according to Williams et al. (Sokol-McKay, 2011) and can become certified diabetes educators (AADE, 2010).

The treatment from the entire team focuses on the following two sets of recommendations for treating diabetes:

1. The Center for Disease Control's ABCs of diabetes care: A1C, blood pressure, and cholesterol. Reductions in each of these measures can reduce the risk for complications significantly (CDC, 2007).
2. AADE seven self-care behaviors (AADE, 2010):
   - Healthy eating
   - Being active
   - Monitoring
   - Taking medication
   - Problem solving
   - Healthy coping
   - Reducing risks

Most of the treatment for diabetes itself is self-care. OT practitioners can assist clients with the implementation of the AADE7 Self-Care Behaviors in order to achieve basic information (Sokol-McKay, 2011).

AADE7 Self-Care Behaviors

1. *Healthy eating*: When a person with diabetes engages in consistent healthy eating, they can improve glucose levels, "reduce risk for short-term emergencies and long-term complications, and improve overall health and quality of life" (Homko et al., 2009, p. 23). The nutritional content, amount of food, and the timing of eating all have a big impact on glucose levels. Cultural and family eating habits and patterns, food availability, and emotions related to food and eating all play a large role in a person's ability to maintain consistent healthy eating (Homko et al., 2009). Because different people have different metabolic responses to the same foods, meal planning for people with diabetes must be individualized (Homko et al., 2009). Dieticians are the most appropriate providers to create meal plans for individuals with diabetes and include a recommended ratio of carbohydrates, fats, and proteins. OT practitioners can help clients to adhere to meal plans and overcome barriers such as adapting preferences, shopping, and meal preparation.
2. *Being active*: Consistent physical activity can have the following benefits for people with diabetes:
   - Reduces blood glucose during and immediately after the activity

- Reduces HbA$_{1c}$
- Improves insulin sensitivity
- Helps with weight loss and weight maintenance
- Decreases cardiovascular risk factors
- Increases muscle mass and decreases body fat
- Improves strength and physical work capacity (Homko et al., 2009, p. 25)
- For people who have prediabetes, physical activity can be a critical component of preventing diabetes, and both aerobic and resistance exercises are recommended (AADE, 2009). OT practitioners are well equipped to help clients find sustainable and enjoyable physical activity routines.

3. *Monitoring*: Monitoring the body is critical to successful diabetes management. People with diabetes must monitor blood glucose, ketones, A1C, blood pressure, lipids/cholesterol, and microalbuminuria (Homko et al., 2009).

- Self-monitoring blood glucose is an occupation that occurs frequently throughout the day and clients benefit from noticing how food, activities, and medications impact their blood glucose. There are a variety of blood glucose meters available, including those with features for people with disabilities. The timings of checking blood glucose and record keeping are also important considerations (Homko et al., 2009).
- Ketone testing is done via blood or urine and is most commonly needed with Type 1 diabetes, though some people with Type 2 diabetes may require ketone testing too (Homko et al., 2009).
- HbA$_{1c}$ measures the amount of hemoglobin in the blood with glucose attached. It provides a reliable picture of blood glucose over the previous three months. It is a laboratory test and is recommended every three to six months. Typically, the A1C target for a person with diabetes is <6.5–7.0%, whereas the normal range for a person without diabetes is 4–6% (Homko et al., 2009).
- Because dyslipidemia is a greater risk factor for cardiovascular disease in people with diabetes, it is recommended to have a fasting lipid (i.e., measures low-density lipoprotein [LDL] and HDL cholesterol and triglycerides) profile laboratory test. Lipid goals for preventing cardiovascular disease are as follows: LDL < 100 mg/dL, HDL > 40 mg/dL for men, and > 50 mg/dL for women, and triglycerides < 150 mg/dL (Homko et al., 2009).
- An annual urinary screening can detect microalbuminuria, when there are low levels of albumin in the urine, which indicates early nephropathy (Homko et al., 2009).
- Additionally, people who have diabetes need to monitor their weight, blood pressure, and perform periodic foot inspections (Homko et al., 2009).

4. *Taking medications*: Clients with diabetes should know the names of their medications and understand when and how much to take and how they affect their bodies (Homko et al., 2009). Many diabetes medications are pills taken orally (e.g., alpha-glucosidase inhibitors, biguanides, DPP-4 inhibitors, meglitinides, sulfonylureas, and thiazolidinediones) (Homko et al., 2009). Noninsulin injectables are also sometimes prescribed. Insulin therapy is essential for Type 1 diabetes and common for Type 2 diabetes, especially after the disease has progressed. Insulin is delivered via syringe, pens, and insulin pumps. Pens can be especially helpful for people with vision impairment because they give auditory and tactile feedback regarding dose (Homko et al., 2009).

5. *Problem solving*: OT practitioners have a particularly important role to help clients problem-solve in their daily management of diabetes. The AADE defines problem solving as "a learned behavior that includes generating a set of potential strategies for problem resolution, selecting the most appropriate strategy, applying the strategy, and evaluating the effectiveness of the strategy" (Homko et al., 2009, p. 38). Training clients to problem-solve is a skill that all OT practitioners do on a regular basis, regardless of the practice setting. This process can range from direct instruction to collaboration with the client and training in assistive and adaptive tools and techniques. A few examples include large print or recorded handouts regarding diabetes information, talking blood glucose monitors, meters that do not require handling strips, insulin pens, insulin pumps that alarm with vibration, nonvisual foot inspection, and physical activity programs (Homko et al, 2009). Additionally, OT practitioners must be able to assess and address readiness to change and adherence to healthy self-care behaviors when

clients are struggling to implement their required habits and routines. Motivational interviewing is a useful tool when working with a client who is having difficulty increasing their self-care behaviors in order to properly manage diabetes and prevent complications, or a person with prediabetes who is having trouble making lifestyle changes to prevent the disease.

6. *Healthy coping*: Adjusting to a diagnosis of diabetes and managing the disease for a lifetime takes time and effort. People with diabetes are at greater risk of stress, decreased quality of life, and mental illness, including depression, anxiety disorders, and eating disorders (Homko et al., 2009). An OT should screen for signs and symptoms of mental illness and know where and how to refer to a mental health professional when necessary. To treat mental illness, occupational therapists can help clients identify social supports, manage stressors, and provide education regarding healthy daily routines and the prevention of depression. OT practitioners can also help with increasing self-care behaviors when depression is present (Sokol-McKay, 2011; Sotelo, 2014).

7. *Reducing risks*: People with diabetes need to be screened consistently for specific diabetes complications, including eye disease, foot problems, nephropathy, and neuropathy. The care team and the client need to be aware of the importance of these regular screenings and encourage clients to keep regular appointments and engage in lifestyle changes. Safety concerns for people with diabetes include proper disposal of sharp objects, wearing medical identification, safe driving for people who develop hypoglycemia, and managing diabetes during pregnancy (Homko et al., 2009). Special attention is required to prevent the complications of diabetes including hyperglycemia, hypertension, hyperlipidemia, being overweight, smoking, dental care, eye disease (e.g., cataracts, glaucoma, and optic neuropathies), foot problems, nephropathy, and neuropathy. To prevent foot problems, people with diabetes should wash and thoroughly dry feet every day, inspect feet daily for anything abnormal, moisturize dry skin to prevent cracking, cut toenails properly, inspect shoes for safety, and wear protective footwear (Homko et al., 2009).

Additional Common Occupational Therapy Interventions

1. *Client and caregiver education/training*: OT practitioners often must train clients and caregivers about healthy food choices, safe cooking methods, safe physical activity, sleep hygiene (Sokol-McKay, 2011), monitoring blood glucose levels, blood pressure, weight, and skin/foot health which includes foot inspections (Pyatak et al., 2014; Sotelo, 2014).

2. *Sleep hygiene*: Sleep quality and quantity is important for diabetes management. Inadequate sleep can have a detrimental impact on glucose tolerance, diabetes, hypertension, and cardiovascular disease, among many other harmful effects (Solet, 2014). To assess sleep, occupational therapists can rely on client self-report and questionnaires, but some clients may not be aware of impaired sleep. Occupational therapists do not diagnose sleep disorders, but they can screen using the *Epworth Sleepiness Scale* (Solet, 2014). Common barriers to sleep include environmental factors (e.g., noise, light, temperature, safety, and comfort) and behavioral factors, which include aligning routine with circadian rhythms, consistent sleep and wake times, and enough time in bed (Solet, 2014). OT practitioners can discuss sleep hygiene upon discharge or during outpatient treatment and in home evaluations to help clients make environmental and behavioral modifications, including blocking light from the sleeping environment, including bright screens or digital clocks, placing cords or equipment to prevent falls, ensuring temperature is cool enough for sleep (e.g., mid-high 60 °F), and controlling pets, other people, and other disturbances (Solet, 2014). Sleep apnea may be an issue since it is significantly more common in people who are obese (AADE, 2010). People with sleep apnea commonly have lower sleep duration, which leads to greater glucose intolerance (AADE, 2010).

3. *Medication management*: Medication management techniques include adaptations and strategies for people throughout all disabilities and stages of life (Pyatak et al., 2014; Sokol-McKay, 2011; Sotelo, 2014).

4. *Safety*: Protective or compensatory techniques for sensory loss in activities involving exposure to heat,

cold, sharp and other sensations that can cause potential harm (Sotelo, 2014).

5. *Secondary disability*: Interventions for secondary complications such as vision impairment, sensation loss, and amputations make up a significant portion of OT care for diabetes with older adults (Sotelo, 2014).

6. *Fine motor impairment*: Rehabilitation and compensatory strategies for any fine motor impairments to ensure the client can complete blood glucose monitoring and insulin injections when necessary (Sotelo, 2014).

7. *Weight management*: Occupational therapists can create an intervention to address weight loss (e.g., losing 10% of body mass improves metabolic abnormalities, such as blood glucose, hypertension, and dyslipidemias) (AADE, 2010).

Impact on Occupational Performance

Diabetes can impact occupational performance in many different ways across the various stages of the disease. A diagnosis of prediabetes or metabolic syndrome is usually a call for a change in occupational engagement and routines with regard to healthy lifestyle behaviors, such as eating choices and routines, engagement in physical activity, managing stress, getting adequate sleep and rest, and reaching or maintaining a healthy BMI. The disease itself may not have a significant impact on occupational performance, but preventing and managing diabetes often does, since it requires lifestyle changes and increased attention to, and engagement in, self-care behaviors.

After a diagnosis of diabetes, the disease requires frequent blood glucose monitoring, adherence to medication schedules, which includes acquisition and maintenance of supplies and equipment at all times when engaging in occupations and travel, etc., as well as the lifestyle modifications listed above to prevent secondary complications.

The long-term complications of chronic hyperglycemia when blood glucose is not well controlled create the most significant changes in occupational performance, including blindness, amputation, kidney failure, and heart disease, which can significantly impact mobility, endurance, and the ability to be physically active, and can lead to death. Depression and anxiety are also

frequent comorbidities, which can significantly impact occupational engagement (Sokol-McKay, 2011). When working with clients who have diabetes, there are so many occupations and activities to use both individually and in groups. Any activity relating to the seven self-care behaviors previously listed would be a useful intervention.

Functional and Community Mobility

Visual acuity is important for community mobility. OT practitioners working with people with diabetes need to screen for visual acuity deficits and then provide appropriate treatment for accomplishing activities of daily living (ADLs) and instrumental ADLs (IADLs) if deficits are identified. The OT starts by discussing the client's prior method for accomplishing ADLs and IADLs and then works through each step required to complete the occupation (Pierce, 2014).

Referrals and Discharge Considerations

OT practitioners are an important part of any diabetes care team and can work with people who have disabilities in order to help prevent morbidity and mortality. Additionally, occupational therapists are eligible to become certified diabetes educators. This certification process requires a course, examination, and clinical hours caring for clients with diabetes.

Discharge considerations include the following:

- Does the client understand all of the self-care behaviors that they need to perform, including their medications and how to administer them?
- Is the client or caregiver able to administer all medications according to schedule?
- Do they have a follow-up plan for future medical visits in place?
- Is the client able to problem-solve in their daily life to achieve optimal diabetes management?
- For clients whose mobility is impaired, all mobility considerations would be required.
- Common referrals may include optometry, ophthalmology, and mental health.

Management and Standards of Practice

When a client has several diagnoses, or when diabetes is not the primary reason for referral, it can be difficult to prioritize diabetes management or prevention, as part of treatment. Also, some occupational therapists and occupational therapy assistants (OTAs) have less experience treating diabetes because until more recently it was not always emphasized in OT education. A common perception is that other medical professionals will address diabetes. However, because the treatment of diabetes is mostly self-care and ADLs, it is critical for OT practitioners to address it, and to use their expertise in activity analysis, adaptation, and habit change to the client's advantage.

After an OT has identified diabetes management/prevention goals and deficits during an evaluation, in subsequent sessions, the OTA may monitor the client's progress, provide education and support related to the client's goals, train and engage the client in adaptive/compensatory techniques, and help motivate the client to increase engagement in self-behaviors and sufficient medical management of diabetes.

Chapter 23 Self-Study Activities (Answers Are Provided at the End of the Chapter)

1. At the beginning of a treatment session, you are preparing to begin physical activity with a client who recently had a total hip replacement. This client is a 75-year-old male who has Type 2 diabetes and takes insulin. Which of the following precautions do you need to take?
   A. Check to see that you have a fast-absorbing form of sugar at hand.
   B. Ask the client when is the last time he ate, took his insulin, and checked his blood sugar.
   C. Ask the client the last time he checked his feet.
   D. All of the above.
2. Ms. Johnson, a 67-year-old female client, has recently been admitted to a skilled nursing facility and is receiving OT. She has the following diagnoses: mild myocardial infarction (two weeks prior), obesity, Type 2 diabetes, hypercholesterolemia, hypertension, and weakness secondary to recent hospitalization. In the evaluation, the client also complains of knee pain when walking and you learn that her physical activity has been significantly reduced for many months because of it. You also notice that the client has several empty soda cans next to her bed. Which of the following items do you focus on in treatment?
   A. Engage the client in treatment to increase stamina, functional mobility, and pain management.
   B. Provide education about the link between soda, blood sugar, and secondary complications that could arise, such as peripheral neuropathy, retinopathy, nephropathy, and lower extremity amputation.
   C. Provide education about the number of carbohydrates she should be consuming each day.
   D. A. and B.
3. Match the following terms (left column) to the most appropriate definition (right column).

Term		Definition
A. Insulin		1. Caused by uncontrolled diabetes and can result in vision loss and blindness.
B. Type 1 diabetes		2. The leading cause of nontraumatic foot and leg amputations.
C. Type 2 diabetes		3. One of the diagnostic tests for diabetes which shows the average blood glucose levels over 6–12 weeks.
D. Hypoglycemia		4. Kidney disease often resulting in kidney failure or dialysis.
E. Hyperglycemia		5. Used to be called juvenile diabetes and occurs when there is complete deficiency in insulin.
F. Retinopathy		6. Healthy levels for the following: A1C, blood pressure, and cholesterol.

Term		Definition
G. Nephropathy		**7.** Risk factor for developing diabetes.
H. Diabetic foot ulcers		**8.** An acute complication of diabetes requiring immediate administration of fast-absorbing forms of sugar.
I. A1C		**9.** Hormone created by the pancreas that is required to convert sugar into energy.
J. ABCs of diabetes care		**10.** Is preventable.
K. Monitoring		**11.** Very high blood sugar.
L. Elevated BMI		**12.** A person with diabetes may require sensation or fine motor intervention because of this.
M. Peripheral Neuropathy		**13.** Critical and ongoing self-care behavior for someone who has diabetes.

4. What is the difference between Type 1 and 2 diabetes and which type is more common?

_____
_____
_____
_____

5. Briefly summarize the seven self-care behaviors for someone who has diabetes.

_____
_____
_____
_____
_____
_____
_____
_____

6. Name the four most common bio-measures that people with diabetes must track for their health.

1. _____
2. _____
3. _____
4. _____

7. What do you think could be potentially frustrating about working with someone who has Type 2 diabetes?

_____
_____
_____
_____
_____
_____
_____

8. Why is client education so critical for a disease like diabetes?

_____
_____
_____
_____

9. As an OT, who is not a nutritionist, and may have no background knowledge of nutrition, describe how you can support a client who has diabetes to eat healthier in order to better manage their diabetes.

_____
_____
_____
_____
_____

Chapter 23 Self-Study Answers

Question 1

- D

Question 2

- D

Question 3

1. F
2. H
3. I
4. G

5. B
6. J
7. L
8. D
9. A
10. C
11. E
12. M
13. K

Question 4

- Type 1 diabetes has a sudden onset and there is an absolute deficiency in insulin. It is usually caused by autoimmune destruction of beta cells in the pancreas. Type 2 diabetes, on the other hand, has a gradual onset, may go unnoticed, and is typically caused by a combination of unhealthy lifestyle factors, including diet, exercise, sleep, and stress. Family history can also have a significant impact. Type 1 diabetes requires insulin treatment immediately. Type 2 diabetes typically progresses more slowly and the treatment starts off with other medications and then progresses to insulin. Type 2 diabetes is typically preventable and Type 1 diabetes is not. Type 2 diabetes is significantly more common than Type 1 diabetes.

Question 5

- *Healthy eating*: The client needs to understand how various foods impact their blood glucose and be able to make daily choices that help to maintain healthy glucose levels.
- *Being active*: The client needs to understand how much physical activity can help them to maintain healthy blood glucose levels and be able to engage in healthy and safe physical activity on a daily or almost daily basis.
- *Monitoring*: The client needs to monitor blood glucose throughout the day. Additionally, they need to monitor blood pressure, cholesterol, skin integrity on feet, and, with some clients, ketones and microalbuminuria, as well.
- *Taking medications*: The client needs to understand what medications to take, how much, and how frequently to take them. They need to be able to obtain medications and supplies on a timely basis and bring them along when away from home. Some clients may need adaptations for administering medications.
- *Problem solving*: Clients need to have the skills to be able to adapt spontaneously to life situations that arise and impact their diabetes management. This includes planning and strategizing skills.
- *Healthy coping*: Clients with diabetes are at greater risk for mental health challenges and may need to increase their coping skills and support.
- *Reducing risks*: Clients need to be aware of the various medical screenings they need, and how frequently to obtain them. They need to be aware of their precautions and to pay particular attention to the early warning signs of secondary complications, including foot care.

Question 6

1. Blood glucose
2. A1C
3. Cholesterol/blood lipids
4. Blood pressure

Question 7

- Consistently engaging in the seven self-care behaviors is difficult for many clients. The lifestyle choices and ongoing persistence required may be undesirable for many clients. Also, humans often naturally have a resistance to change and may hold strongly to their preferred lifestyle habits that may be harmful.

Question 8

- Education is critical to prevent serious secondary complications. It is especially critical because secondary complications are preventable!

Question 9

- Shopping and meal preparation
- Support and reinforcement of recommendations from dietician/dietary habit changes
- Training and support for increasing problem-solving skills around healthy eating
- Support for the psychosocial impact of changing eating habits and routines

References

American Association of Diabetes Educators. (2010). *Core concepts: The art and science of diabetes education: Continuing education program for diabetes educators participant manual*. Chicago, IL: American Association of Diabetes Educators.

American Diabetes Association. (2014). *Diagnosing diabetes and learning about prediabetes*. Retrieved from http://www.diabetes.org/diabetes-basics/prevention/pre-diabetes/how-to-tell-if-you-have.html

Bonder, B. R., & Goodman, G. D. (2014). Preventing occupational dysfunction secondary to aging. In M. V. Radomski & C. A. T. Latham (Eds.), *Occupational therapy for physical dysfunction* (7th ed., pp. 974–998). Philadelphia, PA: Wolters Kluwer Health/Lippincott Williams & Wilkins.

Center for Disease Control and Prevention. (2007). *National diabetes fact sheet, 2007*. Retrieved from http://www.cdc.gov/diabetes

Centers for Disease Control and Prevention. (2011). *National diabetes fact sheet: National estimates and general information on diabetes and prediabetes in the United States, 2011*. Atlanta, GA: U.S. Department of Health and Human Services, Centers for Disease Control and Prevention. Retrieved from http://www.cdc.gov/diabetes/pubs/pdf/ndfs_2011.pdf

Centers for Disease Control and Prevention. (2014). *National diabetes statistics report: Estimates of diabetes and its burden in the United States, 2014*. Atlanta, GA: U.S. Department of Health and Human Services. Retrieved from http://www.cdc.gov/diabetes/pubs/statsreport14/national-diabetes-report-web.pdf

Cohn, E. S. (2009). Team interaction models and team communication. In E. B. Crepeau, E. S. Cohn, & B. A. B. Schell (Eds.), *Willard & Spackman's occupational therapy* (11th ed., pp. 396–402). Philadelphia, PA: Wolters Kluwer Health/Lippincott Williams & Wilkins.

Cooper, H. C., & Geyer, R. (2009). What can complexity do for diabetes management? Linking theory to practice. *Journal of Evaluation in Clinical Practice, 15*(4), 761–765. doi:10.1111/j.1365-2753.2009.01229.x

George, A. H. (2013). Infection control and safety issues in the clinic. In L. W. Pedretti, H. M. Pendleton, & W. Schultz-Krohn (Eds.), *Pedretti's occupational therapy: Practice skills for physical dysfunction* (7th ed., pp. 140–156). St. Louis, MO: Elsevier.

Hocking, C. (2009). Contribution of occupation to health and well-being. In E. B. Crepeau, E. S. Cohn, & B. A. B. Schell (Eds.), *Willard & Spackman's occupational therapy* (11th ed., pp. 72–81). Philadelphia, PA: Wolters Kluwer Health/Lippincott Williams & Wilkins.

Homko, C. J., Sisson, E. M., & Ross, T. A. (2009). *Diabetes education review guide: Test your knowledge* (2nd ed.). Chicago, IL: American Association of Diabetes Educators.

Huntley, N. (2014). Cardiac and pulmonary diseases. In M. V. Radomski & C. A. T. Latham (Eds.), *Occupational therapy for physical dysfunction* (7th ed., pp. 1300–1326). Philadelphia, PA: Wolters Kluwer Health/Lippincott Williams & Wilkins.

Kaldenberg, J. (2014). Optimizing vision and visual processing. In M. V. Radomski & C. A. T. Latham (Eds.), *Occupational therapy for physical dysfunction* (7th ed., pp. 699–724). Philadelphia, PA: Wolters Kluwer Health/Lippincott Williams & Wilkins.

Keidar, A. (2011). Bariatric surgery for type 2 diabetes reversal: The risks. *Diabetes Care, 34*(Suppl. 2), S361–S366. doi:10.2337/dc11-s254

Law, M., Baptiste, S., McColl, M., Opzoomer, A., Polatajko, H., & Pollock, N. (1990). The Canadian occupational performance measure: An outcome measure for occupational therapy. *Canadian Journal of Occupational Therapy, 57*(2), 82–87. Retrieved from http://www.ncbi.nlm.nih.gov/pubmed/10104738

Maher, C. M. (2014). Orthopaedic conditions. In M. V. Radomski & C. A. T. Latham (Eds.), *Occupational therapy for physical dysfunction* (7th ed., pp. 1103–1128). Philadelphia, PA: Wolters Kluwer Health/Lippincott Williams & Wilkins.

National Diabetes Information Clearinghouse. (2013). *DCCT and EDIC: The diabetes control and complications trial and follow-up study*. Retrieved from http://diabetes.niddk.nih.gov/dm/pubs/control/

National Diabetes Information Clearinghouse. (2014). *Diabetes, heart disease and stroke*. NIH Publication No. 13–5094. Retrieved from http://diabetes.niddk.nih.gov/dm/pubs/stroke/#connection

O'Keefe, J. H., Bell, D. S. H., & Wyne, K. L. (2009). *Diabetes essentials* (4th ed.). Sudbury, MA: Jones and Bartlett Publishers.

Pierce, S. L. (2014). Restoring functional and community mobility. In M. V. Radomski & C. A. T. Latham (Eds.), *Occupational therapy for physical dysfunction* (7th ed, pp. 804–843). Philadelphia, PA: Wolters Kluwer Health/Lippincott Williams & Wilkins.

Pyatak, E. A., Sequeira, P. A., Whittemore, R., Vigen, C. P., Peters, A. L., & Weigensberg, M. J. (2014). Challenges contributing to disrupted transition from paediatric to adult diabetes care in young adults with Type 1 diabetes. *Diabetic Medicine, 31*(12), 1615–1624. doi:10.1111/dme.12485

Sokol-McKay, D. (2011). *Occupational therapy's role for diabetes self-management*. Retrieved from http://www.homehealthquality.org/getattachment/UP/UP-Event-Archives/Diabetes-fact-sheet-ashx.pdf.aspx

Solet, J. M. (2014). Optimizing personal and social adaptation. In M. V. Radomski & C. A. T. Latham (Eds.), *Occupational therapy for physical dysfunction* (7th ed., pp. 925–954). Philadelphia, PA: Wolters Kluwer Health/Lippincott Williams & Wilkins.

Sotelo, D. (2014). Appendix 1 common conditions, resources, and evidence: Obesity, diabetes, & hypertension. In B. A. B. Schell, G. Gillen, & M. E. Scaffa (Eds.), *Willard & Spackman's occupational therapy* (12th ed., pp. 1159–1161). Philadelphia, PA: Wolters Kluwer Health/Lippincott Williams & Wilkins.

Weisser-Pike, O. (2014). Assessing abilities and capacities: Vision and visual processing. In M. V. Radomski & C. A. T. Latham (Eds.), *Occupational therapy for physical dysfunction* (7th ed. pp. 103–120). Philadelphia, PA: Wolters Kluwer Health/Lippincott Williams & Wilkins.

Human Immunodeficiency Virus and Acquired Immune Deficiency Syndrome

Michael A. Pizzi

Learning Objectives

- Describe and understand the pathogenesis and transmission of HIV.
- Compare and contrast the stages of HIV and the clinical presentations of each stage.
- Describe the public health model of prevention of HIV/AIDS.
- Recognize and identify occupational therapy assessment and interventions related to HIV/AIDS.
- Describe the role of the occupational therapy assistant in HIV occupational therapy service delivery.
- Recognize occupational therapy ethical issues related to HIV/AIDS.

Key Terms

- *Acquired immunodeficiency syndrome (AIDS)*: A disease caused by a retrovirus that increases susceptibility to infection, certain cancers, and neurologic disorders.
- *Human immunodeficiency virus (HIV)*: A virus that infects people for life, attacking and killing CD4 T-cells, which help fight infections.
- *Public health model*: Addresses health and/ or social challenges while considering possible sources of harm in order to identify the cause and possible interventions.
- *Universal precautions*: A universal approach to infection control by treating all people and bodily fluids in a consistent manner.

Description

Human immunodeficiency virus (HIV) is a retrovirus initially discovered in 1981 (Greene, 2007). A retrovirus is a virus that replicates in a host cell through a process called reverse transcription (Sharp & Hahn, 2011). This means that the usual DNA–RNA sequence is reversed to be an RNA–DNA sequence (National Institute of Allergy and Infectious Diseases [NIAID], 2015). The sequence is then emitted into the cytoplasm of a cell, and begins a process of producing multiple times and quickly so that the virus spreads (NIAID, 2015). Once there is a large enough presence of infected cells, which can then be detected through HIV testing, the person infected will always be infected (Society, 2014). As HIV continues to attack the immune system, or the T-cells in our bodies, it can gradually overtake the immune system and progress to AIDS (i.e., acquired immunodeficiency syndrome).

Transmission

HIV is spread through contact with blood, semen, preseminal, rectal, vaginal fluids, and breast milk of people who are infected. There is evidence that HIV is not spread through casual contact through sweat, tears, saliva, feces, and urine (Centers for Disease Control and Prevention [CDC], 2015c). HIV is readily transmitted through unprotected sexual behavior and intravenous drug use with unsterilized needles and sharing of needles. It is less commonly transmitted via birth through an infected mother, receiving blood transfusions, being bitten by a person with HIV, needle sticks, deep open mouth kissing alone, or oral sex where there is no exchange of fluid (CDC, 2015c). The risk through these latter activities is still present, and is reduced further if there is no exchange of blood, if the infected person is on antiretroviral therapy (ART) and taking it as prescribed, and/or the person who is not infected is on pre-exposure prophylaxis (CDC, 2015c). Having another sexually transmitted disease, especially if untreated, and engaging in high-risk activities can also increase the risk of infecting another person. For healthcare workers, the CDC states the following:

> The risk of healthcare workers being exposed to HIV on the job (occupational exposure) is very low, especially if they use protective practices and personal protective equipment to prevent HIV and other blood-borne infections. For healthcare workers on the job, the main risk of HIV transmission is through accidental injuries from needles and other sharp instruments that may be contaminated with the virus; however, even this risk is small. Scientists estimate that the risk of HIV infection from being stuck with a needle used on an HIV-infected person is less than 1% (CDC, 2015c).

Needle sticks are not common in occupational therapy practice. However, it is vital that all occupational therapists (OTs) and occupational therapy assistants (OTAs) know the policies and procedures of their workplace for proper use of protective gear, such as gowns, masks, and gloves (CDC, 2007). These are used to not only protect one-self from being infected, but also to protect those who are already immunocompromised (e.g., the healthcare worker experiencing early onset of a cold could further immunologically compromise the client).

Course of HIV, Symptoms, and Related Conditions

There are three stages of HIV: (1) acute infection; (2) clinical latency (i.e., inactivity or dormancy); and (3) AIDS (CDC, 2015a). During the acute infection stage, within two to four weeks a flu-like symptom may appear called acute retroviral syndrome (U.S. Department of Health and Human Services, 2015). Symptoms can range from enlarged lymph nodes, to fever, headache, sore throat, rash, and fatigue. This natural response of the body indicates that the virus is replicating and attacking the immune system. People at this stage are at highest risk of transmitting the virus to others because there is a large percentage of virus in the blood (CDC, 2015a).

The amount of virus in the body at any one time is called viral load. In the clinical latency stage, often called the asymptomatic stage, people with HIV can still infect others, but the replication of the virus, particularly for those on ART, who can live for decades asymptomatically, is very low (U.S. Department of Health and Human Services, 2015). Once the viral load increases and CD4 or T-cell count declines, other symptoms of HIV may occur (CDC, 2015a). These include rapid weight loss, recurring fever or profuse night sweats, extreme and unexplained tiredness, prolonged swelling of the lymph glands in the armpits, groin, or neck, diarrhea that lasts for more than a week, sores of the mouth, anus, or genitals, pneumonia, red, brown, pink, or purplish blotches on or under the skin or inside the mouth, nose, or eyelids, and/or memory loss, depression, and other neurologic disorders (U.S. Department of Health and Human Services, 2015). If the CD4 count falls below 200, then the person is diagnosed with full-blown AIDS, the third stage (CDC, 2015a). At this stage, without medical interventions, the person may live for up to 3 years, but with an opportunistic infection, mortality is about 1 year. At this stage, viral load increases unless an individual receives medical care and cooperates with a routine medical regimen.

Common Diagnostic Tests

The blood test such as the enzyme-linked immunosorbent assay detects exposure to the virus. Home kits are readily available for self-testing. HIV is not readily detectable for at least 25 days postexposure. OTs and OTAs may work with people who cope with anxiety or other psychosocial concerns around the issue of HIV testing. It is important that OTs and OTAs continually update their knowledge of current tests available, and the confidentiality related to testing and test results in order to communicate effectively with clients. The Centers for Disease Control website is the most current and reliable source for such information (CDC, 2015b).

Universal Precautions

Table 24-1 provides information related to universal precaution recommendations from the CDC (2007). All OTs and OTAs should abide by such recommendations for the care of all clients in all healthcare settings, including community-based practice.

Table 24-1 Recommendations for Application of Standard Precautions for the Care of All Clients in All Healthcare Settings

Components	Recommendations
Hand hygiene	After touching blood, body fluids, secretions, excretions, contaminated items; immediately after removing gloves; between client contact
Gloves	For touching blood, body fluids, secretions, excretions, contaminated items; for touching mucous membranes and nonintact skin
Gown	During procedures and client-care activities when contact of clothing, exposed skin, blood/body fluids, secretions, and excretions are anticipated
Mask, eye protection (e.g., goggles), and face shield	During procedures and client-care activities likely to generate splashes or sprays of blood, body fluids, secretions, suctioning, and endotracheal intubation. During aerosol-generating procedures on clients with suspected or proven infections transmitted by respiratory aerosols (e.g., severe acute respiratory syndrome), wear a fit-tested N95 or higher respirator in addition to gloves, gown, and face/eye protection
Soiled client-care equipment	Handle in a manner that prevents the transfer of microorganisms to others and to the environment; wear gloves if visibly contaminated; perform hand hygiene
Environmental control	Develop procedures for routine care, cleaning, and disinfecting environmental surfaces, especially frequently touched surfaces in client-care areas
Textiles and laundry	Handle in a manner that prevents transfer of microorganisms to others and to the environment/wear gloves
Needles and other sharps	Do not recap, bend, break, or hand-manipulate used needles; if recapping is required, use a one-handed scoop technique only; use safety features when available; place used sharps in a puncture-resistant container
Client resuscitation	Use mouthpiece, resuscitation bag, and other ventilation devices to prevent contact with mouth and oral secretions
Client placement	Prioritize for single-client room if a client is at increased risk of transmission, is likely to contaminate the environment, does not maintain appropriate hygiene, or is at increased risk of acquiring infection or developing adverse outcome following infection
Respiratory hygiene/cough etiquette and source containment of infectious respiratory secretions in symptomatic clients, beginning at the initial point of encounter (e.g., triage and reception areas in emergency departments and physician offices)	Instruct symptomatic persons to cover mouth/nose when sneezing/coughing; use tissues and dispose in a no-touch receptacle; observe hand hygiene after soiling of hands with respiratory secretions; wear surgical mask if tolerated or maintain spatial separation >3 feet if possible

Reproduced from: CDC (2007).

Occupational Therapy and HIV/AIDS

OTs and OTAs can make a tremendous impact on the lives of people living with HIV/AIDS (PLWHA) on an individual to a population-based level. A public health prevention approach to assessment and intervention can be utilized (see Health Promotion and Wellness chapter).

Primary Prevention

At this stage, OTs want to prevent the transmission of HIV and reduce the incidence of infections in order to promote a healthy society and healthy communities. Building community awareness through educational programming can be implemented through HIV and health organizations in one's community. Another opportunity would be creating fact-filled occupation-based activities for high schools, such as creating a Jeopardy-type game and teams of high schoolers who would then be rewarded with gift cards or extra credit. This could be done in conjunction with the health classes.

Secondary Prevention

In secondary prevention, the intent is to target populations of people most at risk, such as people having unprotected sex or people who are sharing needles. Gay men and African Americans are among the populations most at risk. Programs such as harm reduction programs have been found to be effective (Coates, Richter, & Caceres, 2008; DiClemente et al., 2008). These programs can be educational and provide information through small groups of people who are at risk, with the OT or OTA using group dynamics, stress management, and life skills training to help people prevent further life choices that can put them more at risk for infection and for infecting others.

Tertiary Prevention

It is in tertiary prevention where occupational therapy services are most often utilized. People already infected are referred to occupational therapy for a variety of physical and psychosocial manifestations of the illness, which can include fatigue, sensory issues (e.g., neuropathies), and neurologic issues such as memory loss and dementia. It is important that OTs and OTAs understand occupational performance and help people participate fully in meaningful and self-satisfying occupations that promote quality of life as the ultimate goal of occupational therapy services.

Screening and Assessments

Evaluation focuses on clients' wants and needs and what they have done and currently do (American Occupational Therapy Association, 2014). The process of evaluation in occupational therapy relative to the HIV/AIDS population must include an occupational profile and an analysis of occupational performance. Client-centered assessments like the ones below yield additional information that helps to construct a more complete profile. Client-centered assessment and intervention demonstrates respect for and

understanding of a person's particular occupational life and lifestyle, without judgment or bias.

Pizzi Assessment of Productive Living for People with HIV/AIDS

The only occupation and client-centered assessment published and available in occupational therapy used with PLWHA is the Pizzi Assessment of Productive Living (Pizzi, 1993). The Pizzi Assessment of Productive Living is a semi-structured interview exploring physical, psychosocial, and environmental barriers and challenges that disrupt occupational performance (**Figure 24-1**).

Pizzi Occupational Loss Assessment

The Pizzi Occupational Loss Assessment is a criterion-referenced nonstandardized interview (Pizzi, 2010). It was developed to assess one's subjective sense of loss and its impact on daily life activity and occupational roles (**Figure 24-2**).

Other Assessments

There are other occupation-focused but not occupation-based assessments that address occupational performance in various areas. These assessments, which is not all inclusive list, include the Role Checklist, Worker Role Interview, School Function Assessment, Occupational Self-Assessment, and the SF-36 (Vaughn, 2014). Some client factor assessments include pain, strength and range of motion measures, visual perceptual measures, and fatigue scales. These can be administered to record one's current functional status as it impacts occupational participation in daily life occupations (**Table 24-2**).

Interventions

The ultimate goal of occupational therapy is to maximize one's occupational performance in self-selected occupations. All interventions must be client-centered. Each person responds to HIV/AIDS, physically and psychosocially, in different client-specific ways; thus it is crucial that OTs and OTAs treat each person and situation in a unique way. From a public health

Plzzi Assessment of Productive Living for Adults with HIV Infection and Aids

Demographics

Name _____ Age _____ Sex _____

Lives with (relationship) _____

Identified caregiver _____

Race _____ Culture _____ Religion _____ Practicing? _____

Primary occupational roles _____

Primary diagnosis _____

Secondary diagnosis _____

Stage of HIV _____

Past medical history _____

Medications _____

Activities of Daily Living (use ADL performance assessment)

Are you doing these now? _____

Do you perform homemaking tasks? _____

(For areas of difficulty) Would you like to be able to do these again like you did before? _____

　　　Which ones? _____

Work

Job _____ When last worked _____

Describe type of activity _____

Work environment _____

If not working, would you like to be able to? _____

Do you miss being productive? _____

Play/Leisure

Types of activities engaged in _____

_____

Are you doing these now? _____

If not, would you like to? _____ Which ones? _____

Is it important to be independent in daily living activities? _____

Physical Function

Active/passive range of motion _____

Strength _____

Sensation _____

Coordination (gross and fine motor/dexterity) _____

Visual-perceptual _____

Hearing _____

Balance (sit and stand) _____

Ambulation/transfers/mobility _____

Activity tolerance/endurance _____

Physical pain _____

　　Location _____

　　Does it interfere with doing important activities? _____

Cognition

Attention span, problem solving, memory, orientation, judgment, reasoning, decision making, safety awareness _____

Figure 24-1 Pizzi Assessment of Productive Living Form.

Plzzi Assessment of Productive Living for Adults with HIV Infection and Aids (continued)

Time Organization

Former daily routine (before diagnosis) _____

Has this changed since diagnosis? _____ If so, how? _____

Are there certain times of day that are better for you to carry out daily living tasks? _____

_____

Do you consider yourself regimented or flexible in organizing time and
activity? _____

_____

What would you change, if anything, in how your day is set up? _____

Body Image/Self-Image

In the last 6 months, has there been a recent change in your physical appearance? _____

How do you feel about this? _____

Social Environment

Describe support available and used by patient _____

_____

Physical Environment

Describe environments where patient performs daily tasks and level of support or impediment
for function _____

_____

Stressors

What are some things, people, or situations that are or were stressful? _____

_____

What are some ways you manage stress? _____

Situational Coping

How do you feel you are dealing with: _____

a) Your diagnosis _____

b) Changes in your ability to do things important to you _____

c) Other psychosocial observations _____

Occupational Questions

What do you consider co be important to you right now? _____

Do you feel you can do things important to you now? _____ In the future? _____

Do you deal well with change? _____

What are some of your hopes, dreams, and aspirations? _____

What are some of your goals? _____

Have these changed since you were diagnosed? _____

Do you feel in control of your life at this time? _____

What do you wish to accomplish with the rest of your life? _____

Plan _____

Short-term goals _____

Long-term goals _____

Frequency _____

Duration _____

Therapist _____

Figure 24-1 Pizzi Assessment of Productive Living Form. (*continued*)

Occupational Loss Assessment

Name: _____	Date: _____

Age: _____	Diagnosis: _____

Date of diagnosis: _____

Primary caregiver: _____

Key:	1.	No sense of loss
2.	Minor sense of loss
3.	Moderate sense of loss
4.	Major sense of loss

Please rate your sense of loss of not being able to do the following activities:

Taking care of myself	1	2	3	4
Work	1	2	3	4
Leisure/Recreation	1	2	3	4
Taking care of my home/apartment	1	2	3	4
Being with other people	1	2	3	4
Mobility/being able to get around	1	2	3	4
Other: _____	1	2	3	4
_____	1	2	3	4
_____	1	2	3	4

Things, people, situations or events I feel I must give up being involved with are:

_____
_____
_____

Things, people, situations, events I have already given up that I didn't want to give up are:

_____
_____
_____

Other Losses

Age	Loss	Rating	Pos/Neg
0-10	_____	_____	_____
11-20	_____	_____	_____
21-30	_____	_____	_____
31-40	_____	_____	_____
41-50	_____	_____	_____
51-60	_____	_____	_____
61-70	_____	_____	_____
70 plus	_____	_____	_____

Figure 24-2 Pizzi Occupational Loss Assessment Form.

Table 24-2 Occupation-Based Assessments

Assessment	Description	Type
Role Checklist	Elicits information about occupational roles	Semi-structured interview
Worker Role Interview	Assesses the ability for a person with a disability or injury to return to work with special attention to environmental and psychosocial factors	Standardized, semi-structured interview
School Function Assessment (SFA)	Used to evaluate student performance of school-related functional tasks	Standardized, criterion-referenced
Occupational Self-Assessment (OSA)	Assesses the value of occupations for each client based on perceptions of their own capabilities	Self-report standardized measure
SF-36	Assesses functional health and well-being from the client's point of view	Norm-referenced, self-report or professional administered interview

Data from: Coster, Deeney, Haltiwanger, and Haley (1998); Fenger and Kramer (2007); Oakley, Kielhofner, Barris, and Reichler (1986); Taylor, Lee, Kramer, Shirashi, and Kielhofner (2011); Ware and Sherbourne (1992).

perspective, especially in primary and secondary prevention, examples were cited above. In tertiary prevention, OTs and OTAs promote health and well-being and maximize occupational performance, engagement, and function for those with occupational challenges. Many of these occupational challenges can be addressed through relaxation techniques, structured routines, adaptive equipment, splinting, visual compensation, coping skills such as anxiety reduction techniques and stress management, and cognitive behavioral techniques. Environmental modification, energy conservation, work simplification, and health education, as well as caregiver training are also important aspects of intervention depending on the signs, symptoms, and stage of disease progression.

Expected Functional Outcomes

The following examples positively impact occupational performance:

- Help individuals adapt to a changed worker role or other important role by addressing the cause of disruption, and help them transition to occupations that incorporate components of that favored role;
- Adapt physical environments to minimize barriers to occupational performance and ensure safety;
- Educate in energy conservation and work simplification tasks;

- Train caregivers to help loved one in the end stage of AIDS to remain independent in self-care tasks;
- Develop new routines and time and activity management skills to include medication and medical visits;
- Help an individual develop assertiveness by setting boundaries with others;
- Recommend community resources and work with social workers to help individuals obtain and follow through with available and needed services;
- Activity of daily living (ADL) training with and without adaptive equipment;
- Develop self-advocacy and resilience skills to cope with stigma and discrimination;
- Working with caregivers to cope, as well as understand and help, with behavioral, cognitive, and neurologic changes that may occur.

Education and Training

Interventions can also include health and occupation-based educational sessions. Examples include education on safer sex and positioning when physically challenged, prevention information, harm reduction techniques (e.g., decreasing smoking but not quitting), and healthy eating to boost the immune system. Working in collaboration with other professionals, such as social workers, nutritionists, psychologists, physical therapists, and health educators, for example, is essential to educate PLWHA from multiple perspectives. Knowledge of other disciplines and their work with PLWHA can lead to appropriate professional referrals and interdisciplinary team intervention.

Reassessment

Function and health can be altered when clients change medications or become further immunocompromised. It is important that the OT reassess using the same evaluation tools used initially. This consistent approach helps determine if progress is being made or if there is a decline in function and occupational participation. Goals and plans can be altered accordingly.

Referrals and Discharge Considerations

After client-centered goals have been achieved, clients are discharged from occupational therapy. Recommendations to maintain or improve function and occupational participation are made relative to the clients' needs and discharge setting.

Settings and Contexts

Depending on the healthcare setting, therapists may be able to reassess an individual to determine occupational performance gains. In home care, for example, one can be seen several times to help ensure safety and functional abilities are intact prior to discharge from services. In a hospital acute care setting, a therapist may be able to implement an ADL program, recommend equipment, and then discharge the client. Irrespective of the setting, however, it is imperative that the person is treated with dignity and respect, and that they are afforded the same treatment as any other client. This helps to ensure that therapists uphold their standards of health care and remain ethical.

Management and Standards of Practice

Best practice in the delivery of occupational therapy services for PLWHA includes recognition of appropriate supervision, knowledge of the disease and remaining current about new developments, and providing ethical services.

Supervision

Appropriate supervision of an OTA varies from state to state. Both the OT and OTA must be knowledgeable regarding state regulations as this is crucial for best practice (American Occupational Therapy Association, 2009). The OT has an obligation to provide proper training and levels of supervision should the OTA have little or no experience with PLWHA. Likewise, it is obligatory for the OTA to become knowledgeable about PLWHA and the occupational challenges related to HIV/AIDS.

Current Knowledge

In just a few decades, HIV/AIDS progressed from a terminal illness to one managed as a chronic illness. Developments of new medications have dramatically changed the course of the illness. Social change and attitudes are slower, but continue to improve. Having knowledge of the most current information helps the practitioner provide best practice by being able to more effectively educate the client and provide options for living life fully.

Ethics

The American Occupational Therapy Association (2015) provides a framework for ethical best practice with PLWHA. Discrimination, bias, and prejudice continue to exist regarding this population of clients; however, occupational therapy professionals have an obligation to provide care that supports the ethical standards described in the Code of Ethics. These ethical standards, particularly those that support the core values of occupational therapy, such as justice, dignity, and equality, also support client-centeredness of the care delivered.

Other Considerations

This chapter concerns itself primarily with adults with HIV/AIDS. It must be recognized that children are also infected with HIV, but much less often today due to major medical breakthroughs that prevent perinatal infection. It is also critical for occupational therapy students to recognize and address the multiple occupational challenges and concerns of HIV/AIDS on unpaid caregivers, such as family members and the impact of HIV/AIDS on their occupational roles, routines, and lives.

Chapter 24 Self-Study Activities (Answers Are Provided at the End of the Chapter)

1. For each of the following signs and symptoms of HIV and AIDS that lead to occupational challenges, list one area of occupation that is potentially impacted and one potential occupational therapist intervention.

Signs, Symptoms, and Occupational Challenges	Area of Occupation	Intervention
Pain		
Altered cognition		
Poor endurance		
Visual impairment		
Stigma		
Depression		

2. **Case Study 1**

   Peter is a 45-year-old who is HIV positive and abuses intravenous drugs. He lives in a homeless shelter but receives occupational therapy in his personalized recovery-oriented service program. He hopes to find a job to become more independent and get his own apartment. What would be some occupational therapy services from which Peter can benefit?

3. **Case Study 2**

   Mary has full-blown AIDS and is on ARTs. She works full time as a teacher but is experiencing some beginning neurologic challenges including neuropathies in her hands and memory deficits. She is not adhering to her antiretroviral drug regimen. How could occupational therapy services assist Mary?

Chapter 24 Self-Study Answers

Signs, Symptoms, and Occupational Challenges	Area of Occupation	Intervention
Pain	Rest and sleep	Relaxation techniques, modalities, adapt sleep preparation routines
Altered cognition	IADL	Structure a routine, develop habits, and visual cues
Poor endurance	ADL	Adaptive equipment
Visual impairment	Education	Big print books, audiotaping lectures, and teacher education
Stigma	Social participation	Social anxiety reduction techniques and community education to diminish stigma
Depression	Work	Cognitive behavioral techniques, and motivational interviewing

IADL, instrumental activities of daily living; ADL, activities of daily living.

Case Study 1 Answer

Answer: Peter can benefit from life skills training, stress management, and vocational rehabilitation services that an OT can offer. These services are designed to help him develop the job skills necessary to interview well, obtain a viable job, and maintain employment.

Case Study 2 Answer

Answer: Mary could use some adaptive equipment for ADLs to compensate for the neuropathies. Splinting also could be efficacious, especially if the neuropathies become more severe. For her memory deficits, cognitive compensatory strategies could help, which would also assist with maintaining a drug regimen, as memory may be the reason she is not adhering to a routine.

References

American Occupational Therapy Association. (2009). Guidelines for supervision, roles, and responsibilities during the delivery of occupational therapy services. *American Journal of Occupational Therapy, 63*(6), 797–803. doi:10.5014/ajot.63.6.797

American Occupational Therapy Association. (2014). Occupational therapy practice framework: Domain and process (3rd ed.). *American Journal of Occupational Therapy, 68*(Suppl. 1), S1–S48. doi:10.5014/ajot.2014.682006

American Occupational Therapy Association. (2015). Occupational therapy code of ethics. *American Journal of Occupational Therapy, 69*(Suppl. 3), 6913410030p1–6913410030p8.

Centers for Disease Control and Prevention. (2007). *2007 guideline for isolation precautions: Preventing transmission of infectious agents in healthcare settings.* Retrieved from http://www.cdc.gov/hicpac/2007IP/2007ip_table4.html

Centers for Disease Control and Prevention. (2015a). *About HIV/AIDS.* Retrieved from http://www.cdc.gov/hiv/basics/whatishiv.html

Centers for Disease Control and Prevention. (2015b). *HIV basics.* Retrieved from http://www.cdc.gov/hiv/basics/

Centers for Disease Control and Prevention. (2015c). *HIV transmission.* Retrieved from http://www.cdc.gov/hiv/basics/transmission.html

Coates, T. J., Richter, L., & Caceres, C. (2008). Behavioural strategies to reduce HIV transmission: How to make them work better. *The Lancet, 372*(9639), 669–684. doi:10.1016/S0140-6736(08)60886-7

Coster, W., Deeney, T., Haltiwanger, J., & Haley, S. (1998). *School function assessment (SFA).* San Antonio, TX: Psychological Corporation.

DiClemente, R. J., Crittenden, C. P., Rose, E., Sales, J. M., Wingood, G. M., Crosby, R. A., & Salazar, L. F. (2008). Psychosocial predictors of HIV-associated sexual behaviors and the efficacy of prevention interventions in adolescents at-risk for HIV infection: What works and what doesn't work? *Psychosomatic Medicine, 70*(5), 598–605. doi:10.1097/PSY.0b013e3181775edb

Fenger, K., & Kramer, J. M. (2007). Worker role interview: Testing the psychometric properties of the Icelandic version. *Scandinavian Journal of Occupational Therapy, 14*(3), 160–172. doi:10.1080/11038120601040743

Greene, W. C. (2007). A history of AIDS: Looking back to see ahead. *European Journal of Immunology, 37*(Suppl. 1), S94–S102. doi:10.1002/eji.200737441

National Institute of Allergy and Infectious Diseases. (2015). *More on how HIV causes AIDS.* Retrieved from http://www.niaid.nih.gov/topics/hivaids/understanding/howhivcausesaids/pages/howhiv.aspx

Oakley, F., Kielhofner, G., Barris, R., & Reichler, R. K. (1986). The role checklist: Development and empirical assessment of reliability. *OTJR: Occupation, Participation and Health, 6*(3), 157–170. doi:10.1177/153944928600600303

Pizzi, M. (1993). HIV infection and AIDS. In H. S. Willard, C. S. Spackman, H. L. Hopkins, & H. D. Smith (Eds.), *Willard and Spackman's occupational therapy* (8th ed., pp. 716–729). Philadelphia, PA: Lippincott Williams & Wilkins.

Pizzi, M. (2010). Promoting wellness in end-of-life care. In M. E. Scaffa, S. M. Reitz, & M. Pizzi (Eds.), *Occupational therapy in the promotion of health and wellness* (pp. 493–511). Philadelphia, PA: F. A. Davis.

Sharp, P. M., & Hahn, B. H. (2011). Origins of HIV and the AIDS pandemic. *Cold Spring Harbor Perspectives in Medicine, 1*(1) a006841, 1–10. Retrieved from http://www.ncbi.nlm.nih.gov/pmc/articles/PMC3234451/pdf/cshperspectmed-HIV-a006841.pdf

Society, A. C. (2014). *HIV infection, AIDS, and cancer.* Retrieved from http://www.cancer.org/acs/groups/cid/documents/webcontent/002295-pdf.pdf

Taylor, R., Lee, S. W., Kramer, J., Shirashi, Y., & Kielhofner, G. (2011). Psychometric study of the occupational self-assessment with adolescents after infectious mononucleosis. *American Journal of Occupational Therapy, 65*(2), e20–e28. doi:10.5014/ajot.2011.000778

U.S. Department of Health and Human Services. (2015). *Symptoms of HIV.* Retrieved from https://www.aids.gov/hiv-aids-basics/hiv-aids-101/signs-and-symptoms/

Vaughn, P. (2014). Appendix 1: Common conditions, resources and evidence: HIV/AIDS. In M. E. Scaffa, B. A. B. Schell, G. Gillen, & E. S. Cohn (Eds.), *Willard & Spackman's occupational therapy* (12th ed., pp. 1148–1150). Philadelphia, PA: Wolters Kluwer Health/Lippincott Williams & Wilkins.

Ware, J. E., Jr., & Sherbourne, C. D. (1992). The MOS 36-item short-form health survey (SF-36). Part I: Conceptual framework and item selection. *Medical Care, 30*(6), 473–483. Retrieved from http://www.ncbi.nlm.nih.gov/entrez/query.fcgi?cmd=Retrieve&db=PubMed&dopt=Citation&list_uids=1593914

Lymphedema

Nicole R. Scheiman

Learning Objectives

- Identify the anatomic structures of the lymphatic system.
- Describe the physiologic structures and processes of the lymphatic system.
- Define lymphedema.
- Describe the signs and symptoms of lymphedema.
- Define and distinguish between primary and secondary lymphedema.
- Explain how lymphedema is diagnosed.
- Compare and contrast lymphedema and inflammation.
- Differentiate pathophysiologic changes and diseases of the lymphatic system.
- List potential precautions for individuals with lymphedema.
- Describe the basic principles of manual lymphatic drainage including indications and contraindications.
- Describe the basic principles of compression therapy (i.e., compression bandaging and compression garments) in the treatment of lymphedema including indications and contraindications.
- Explain skin care guidelines recommended for individuals with lymphedema.
- Describe basic components of an exercise plan for the treatment of lymphedema including indications and contraindications.
- Identify common surgical interventions for lymphedema.

Key Terms

- *Cellulitis*: A diffuse, acute infection of the subcutaneous connective tissue characterized typically by local heat, redness, pain, swelling, fever, and chills.
- *Comorbidity*: A disease or condition that can potentially exacerbate or aggravate the primary disease.
- *Congenital*: Present at birth.
- *Congestive heart failure (CHF)*: Abnormal condition or weakness of the heart that reflects impaired cardiac pumping leading to a buildup of fluids in the lungs and surrounding tissues. Caused by myocardial infarction, ischemic heart disease, or cardiomyopathy.
- *Deep venous thrombosis (DVT)*: A serious condition that results from a blood clot in one or more of the deep veins in the legs (i.e., most common), arms, pelvic, neck, or chest can be fatal.
- *Diuretic*: An agent (i.e., typically a medication) that promotes the production of urine output. Typically used to treat hypertension, CHF, and edema.
- *Filaria*: Nematode belonging to the superfamily Filarioidea. In humans, they may infect the lymphatic vessels and lymphatic organs, circulatory systems, connective tissues, subcutaneous tissues, and serous cavities.
- *Filariasis*: A chronic disease caused by the parasitic nematode worm *Wuchereria bancrofti* or *Brugia malayi*. This disease can result in elephantiasis.

- *Hereditary*: Relating to genetic characteristic transmission from parent to offspring; determined by genetic factors.
- *Lymph*: A thin, colorless, watery fluid originating in organs and tissues of the body that circulates through the lymphatic vessels and is filtered by the lymph nodes.
- *Lymphangiogram*: A radiograph of the lymphatic vessels and nodes.
- *Lymphangiography*: X-ray examination of lymph nodes and lymphatic vessels after an injection of a contrast medium.
- *Lymphatic system*: An immense, complex network of capillaries, vessels, valves, ducts, nodes, and organisms that help protect and maintain the internal fluid environment of the entire body by producing, filtering, and conveying lymph and by producing various blood cells. This system is a significant contributor to the body's immune system.
- *Lymphedema*: An abnormal accumulation of lymph fluid in the interstitial spaces, resulting in swelling.

The Lymphatic System

The lymphatic system (**Figure 25-1**) is part of a network of the structures listed above that work to move lymph from tissues to the bloodstream. The lymphatic system is essentially the body's waste filtration system as it works to remove impurities and comprises a large portion of the body's immune system. Lymph is a thin watery fluid that is produced in organs and body tissues. It circulates through lymphatic vessels and is filtered by lymph nodes. Lymph contains chyle, erythrocytes, and leukocytes (Thiadens, Steward, & Stout, 2010). Components of the lymphatic system include the following (Földi & Földi, 2006a; Zuther, 2005):

- Lymph vessels
- Lymph nodes
- Spleen
- Cisterna chyli
- Thymus gland
- Tonsils
- Lymphocytes
- Peyer's patches

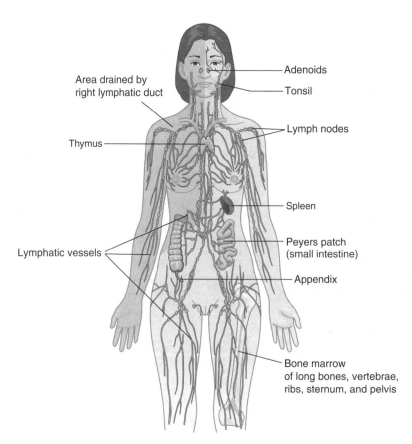

Figure 25-1 The lymphatic system.

Description

Lymphedema is a progressive condition that occurs when the transport capacity of the lymphatic system is unable to keep up with the lymphatic load. This condition results in an abnormal accumulation of water and proteins, which collect in the subcutaneous tissues (Zuther, 2005). If left untreated, lymphedema will gradually progress through its stages. Lymphedema may present in any part of the body including internal organs. In addition to lymphedema resulting in swelling, the affected area may feel tight and painful resulting in a potential disruption of the performance of daily activities (Burkhardt & Schultz-Krohn, 2013; Radomski, Anheluk, Grabe, Hopins, & Zola, 2014).

Lymphatic circulation can be impaired by lymph node dissection, irradiation of the lymphatics, or a tumor that has spread into the lymphatic vessels or nodes (Burkhardt & Schultz-Krohn, 2013). Lymphedema is a serious condition because of its long-term physical and psychosocial consequences. Currently, there is no cure for lymphedema; however, surgical advances are giving hope. Signs and symptoms of lymphedema include the following (Thiadens et al., 2010):

- Swelling in any part of the body
- Feeling of tightness or heaviness in the involved body part
- Decreased range of motion (ROM) due to the swelling limiting full joint movement
- Aching or discomfort in the involved body part
- Recurring infections
- Thickening or hardening of the skin known as fibrosis
- Skin texture and/or color changes in the involved body part

Because lymphedema is a complex condition, it is important for general occupational therapists (OTs) to be able to recognize the condition, understand the physiologic process, and be able to make the appropriate recommendations to specialists including the certified lymphedema therapists (CLT). Diagnosis of lymphedema is often made by the physician from the client's history and physical examination (Zuther, 2005).

Etiology and Pathology

The most common cause of lymphedema outside of the United States is from filariasis. Filariasis is a chronic disease caused by the parasitic nematode worm called *Wuchereria bancrofti* or *Brugia malayi*. In the United States, the highest incidence of lymphedema results from breast cancer treatments, primarily in individuals who receive radiation therapy following lymph node dissection (Zuther, 2005; Zuther & Norton, 2013).

Primary and Secondary Lymphedema

Lymphedema is categorized as primary or secondary lymphedema based on the etiology of the condition. Primary lymphedema can develop any time over the course of a lifetime. If diagnosed before an individual is 35 years old, it is called lymphedema praecox and if diagnosed after an individual is 35 years old, it is called lymphedema tarda. Secondary lymphedema can occur at any time with various conditions and disease states. Interestingly; however, the classification between primary and secondary has little influence on the treatment as the treatment is predominantly the same for both (Thiadens et al., 2010).

Primary Lymphedema

Primary lymphedema is a developmental abnormality (e.g., dysplasia) of the lymphatic system and may develop at any time over the individuals' lifetime. This abnormality can be either congenital or hereditary and can result from the following:

- *Aplasia*: The absence of lymph collectors, capillaries, or lymph nodes.
- *Hypoplasia*: The incomplete growth of lymph vessels. This is a decrease in the number of lymphatic vessels and the diameters of the vessels (i.e., the most common abnormality found).
- *Hyperplasia*: An increase in the diameter of the lymphatic vessels resulting in a malfunction of the valvular system, which leads to lymphatic reflux (Földi & Földi, 2006a).

Secondary Lymphedema

Secondary lymphedema results from a mechanical insufficiency of the lymphatic system and may be related to one or more of the following factors (Zuther, 2005; Zuther & Norton, 2013):

- *Dissection of lymph nodes*: results in fewer nodes available to process the lymphatic fluid.

- *Surgery*: can result in removal of lymph nodes/tissues.
- *Trauma*: such as burns and scar tissue formation can hinder the transport of lymphatic fluid.
- *Infection*: results in an inflammatory process that can cause fibrosis of the lymphatic tissues. Infection can result in an increase in the amount of lymphatic fluid paired with damage to the lymphatic tissues resulting in a combined insufficiency.
- *Malignancies*: malignant tumors can physically block lymphatic flow by compressing the lymphatic structures.
- *Chronic venous insufficiency*: lack of venous return, particularly in the lower extremities, results in an altered blood capillary pressure. The lymphatic system attempts to remediate this lack of homeostasis, which can result in a lymphatic insufficiency or lymphedema over time.
- *Immobility*: from disease or disability can result in a similar situation as venous insufficiency and may develop into lymphedema.
- *Self-induced*: typically caused from a tourniquet to an extremity, which creates a blockage of lymphatic function and results in lymphedema of the extremity distal to the tourniquet.
- *Radiation*: results in damage (e.g., fibrosis) to the lymphatic tissues and can result in subsequent lymphedema.

Secondary lymphedema precautions for lymphedema prevention in those with risk include the following factors (Swirsky & Sackett Nannery, 2008):

- Avoid injury to the skin
- Avoid heat
- Use precaution with exercise
- Do not have blood pressure measurements taken in an affected extremity
- Avoid compression of the affected extremity (e.g., from clothing and jewelry)
- Use caution with travel (e.g., airline travel and in tropical areas)
- Ensure best skin care practices
- Ensure proper nutrition and hydration

Common Diagnostic Tests for Lymphedema

In addition to the clients' subjective report and the physician history and physical examination, there are several diagnostic tests that can assist with the diagnosis of lymphedema. Two more common medical tests include magnetic resonance imaging (MRI) and computed tomography (CT). MRIs require the client to be placed into a magnetic field and uses radio waves to create images of organs and tissues. CTs provide physicians with a cross-sectional view of body segments, which reveals tissue density via x-rays. Lymphoscintigraphy testing uses a radioactive tracer to provide imaging of the lymph vessels and lymph nodes in addition to the speed and rate in which the lymph fluid flows through the vessels and nodes. This allows the physician to determine where dysfunction of the lymphatic system may be occurring. Indirect lymphology uses a water-soluble contrast medium which is injected intracutaneously to allow visualization of the superficial lymph vessels. Lastly, fluorescent microlymphangiography uses a fluorescent agent which is also injected intracutaneously to visualize cutaneous lymph vessels (Zuther, 2005; Zuther & Norton, 2013).

Stages of Lymphedema

Medical practitioners will often describe the client's lymphedema by "stage." Staging most frequently used is a four-stage model starting with Stage 0 through Stage 3 (**Table 25-1**).

Precautions and Contraindications

Precautions and contraindications for lymphedema treatment should be determined by the CLT and/or physician. Precautions may include the following (Zuther, 2005; Zuther & Norton, 2013):

- Rapid exacerbation of swelling may be a sign of a deep venous thrombosis (DVT) or blood clot
- Redness in the involved area may be a sign of infection
- History of cardiac disease, specifically congestive heart failure (CHF)
- Renal failure or insufficiency

General contraindications with lymphedema (Zuther, 2005; Zuther & Norton, 2013):

- Avoid heat in the involved extremity.
- No blood pressure measurements or intravenous needle sticks in the involved extremity.

Table 25-1 Stages of Lymphedema

Stage	Description
0	Stage 0 can also be called the prestage, subclinical, or latent stage of lymphedema. In Stage 0, there are no visible changes to the involved body part. The client may note a difference in sensation of the body part such as heaviness and tightness. Individuals often are in this stage months or years before more obvious signs of lymphedema are seen.
1	Stage 1 is also referred to as the mild stage. In this stage, the body part appears mildly swollen. When the skin is pressed it will temporarily dent or pit, which is commonly referred to as pitting edema. This stage is often considered reversible with proper treatment because the skin and tissues have not sustained long-lasting damage. Often elevation of an extremity in this stage will result in temporary edema resolution.
2	Stage 2 is also referred to as the moderate stage. In this stage, the affected body part continues to swell, elevation is no longer effective, and pitting of the skin no longer occurs. In this stage, changes to the tissues occur, including inflammation, thickening, and hardening of the tissues. Despite the fact that these changes cannot be reversed, with treatment the swelling can be managed.
3	Stage 3 is often referred to as the severe stage. This stage represents a significant increase in body part size, hardening of the skin, and various skin texture changes. Infections such as cellulitis, erysipelas, and lymphangitis are not uncommon.

Reproduced from Lymphology, 49 (2016), 170–184.

- No manual treatment with active infections (e.g., cellulitis), such as signs and symptoms of erythema, warmth, local edema, tenderness to touch, fever, and chills
- No exercise with pain present
- No ultrasound over the involved area for clients with a history of cancer
- Impaired arterial perfusion
- Malignant tumor

General contraindications may include (Zuther, 2005; Zuther & Norton, 2013):

- Cardiac edema
- Renal failure
- Acute infections
- Acute bronchitis
- Acute deep vein thrombosis
- Malignancies
- Bronchial asthma
- Hypertension

Local contraindications for the neck area may include (Zuther, 2005; Zuther & Norton, 2013):

- Carotid sinus syndrome
- Hyperthyroidism
- Clients' with advanced age may be at an increased risk of atherosclerosis in the arteries of the neck.

Local contraindications for the abdominal area may include (Zuther, 2005; Zuther & Norton, 2013):

- Pregnancy
- Dysmenorrhea
- Ileus
- Diverticulosis
- Aortic aneurysm
- Recent abdominal surgery
- Deep vein thrombosis
- Inflammatory conditions of the intestines (e.g., Crohn's disease, colitis, and diverticulitis)
- Radiation fibrosis and/or other skin complications as a result of radiation therapies
- Pain that is unexplained or with no root cause

Complications of Lymphedema

Inflammation is typically an acute condition that is temporary, whereas lymphedema is a chronic and progressive condition. Because lymphedema is a chronic and progressive condition, it is imperative that the practitioner addresses the client's edema needs promptly. This may mean referring the client to a certified lymphedema practitioner. It is important to address the edema needs of the client before addressing other goals as the edema can limit their ability to progress in other areas of occupation. Risks of not addressing edema needs include, but are not limited to, the progression of the condition, increased risk of infection, and increased risk of further disability/dysfunction (Zuther, 2005; Zuther & Norton, 2013).

Screening and Assessments

1. Standardized screenings and assessments
    A. *Lymphedema Quality of Life Assessment Tool (LYMQOL):* The LYMQOL is a condition-specific quality of life assessment tool for lymphedema of the limbs. This tool can be used both as a clinical assessment and as an outcome measure.
2. Semistandardized screenings and assessments for edema measurement:
    A. *Measuring tape:* Use of a measuring tape (inches/cm) to measure the circumferential girth at various predetermined points on the edematous limb. This allows the clinician to compare circumference before, during, and after therapeutic interventions to determine effectiveness of the treatment provided. Use of an anthropometric measuring tape is preferred, as it utilizes a weighted tape to ensure constant tension during measurements. There are various software systems available that will convert circumferential measurements to volumetric measurements for the practitioner.
    B. *Volumetric measurements:* Use of volumetric measuring devices to measure the amount of water displaced when the limb is submerged into the device enables the clinician to compare volume displacement before, during, and after therapeutic interventions (i.e., to determine the effectiveness of the treatment provided).
3. Nonstandardized screenings and assessments
    A. *Client evaluation/interview:* Determine functional limitations and indications for therapy, such as the Canadian Occupational Performance Measure. Living with lymphedema can significantly limit/prevent participation in occupations. Determining occupational deficits during the client evaluation and interview is important to guide your therapy plan.
    B. *ROM (AROM/PROM):* Determine joints with limited ROM due to joint structure/body habitus/edema. Edema can significantly limit joint motion. It is imperative to determine which motions are limited (i.e., passive and active limitation), as these limitations will directly affect participation in activities of daily living (ADLs)/instrumental activities of daily living (IADLs).

C. *Pain assessment:* Lymphedema is typically not painful; however, when tissues become very edematous, the fluid can compress the vessels, nerves, and soft tissues resulting in pain. The OT must complete a full pain assessment to determine the possible origins of pain and address them accordingly.
D. *Strength:* Chronic edema can result in decreased joint and soft tissue mobility, and decreased strength. OTs must determine the deficits and prescribe appropriate interventions. For clients who will be wearing compression garments, it is imperative that the OT address their upper body gross and fine motor strength in order to don and doff garments safely.
E. *Sensation:* Sensation can be altered with edema and must be assessed to determine if safety concerns are present. Further, if a client with lower extremity lymphedema has decreased sensation, they may not know if their bandages are applied with the correct tension and may inadvertently have them too tight/too loose.
F. *ADL observation:* Because lymphedema can significantly affect ADL abilities, OTs must observe clients' complete ADLs and make recommendations for environmental and/or adaptive equipment modifications.
G. *Postural assessment:* Unilateral edema in particular can result in alterations in posture and body mechanics. Accordingly, it is imperative for the OT to complete a postural assessment to determine the client's needs, such as ergonomic recommendations, environmental modifications, and home-exercise programs.

Interventions

Like other occupational therapy (OT) interventions, treatment for lymphedema is guided by theory, research, the experiences of the practitioners, and just as importantly, the clients' preferences, goals, and personal priorities (Gillen, 2014).

Interventions associated with lymphedema focus around edema management with the ultimate goal of achieving a higher level of independence with ADLs/IADLs and improvement of quality of life. Group intervention may also be very beneficial, especially to provide psychosocial support. Group interventions typically include exercise groups (e.g., aquatics) and social support groups (Swirsky & Sackett Nannery, 2008).

Expected Functional Outcomes

Functional outcomes expected as a result of receiving lymphedema treatment are specific to the individual and often include achieving independence with the daily tasks required to maintain improved lymphatic status (i.e., self-manual lymphatic drainage [MLD], bandaging, compression garments, skin care, and exercise). Treatments are designed to improve the quality of life of individuals with lymphedema; therefore, functional outcomes may also include return to occupations clients were previously unable to perform secondary to lymphedema status. For example, being able to stand for 30 minutes to safely cook a meal might be a functional outcome for someone with lower extremity lymphedema.

Impact on Occupational Performance

Occupation can be significantly limited by physical and mental changes precipitated by lymphedema; therefore, it is vital that the OT include occupation as part of their treatment plan. Therapeutic use of occupations and activities including group interventions should be incorporated when applicable.

Therapeutic Interventions

1. *Education and training*: Client education is quite extensive for the management of lymphedema and can include interventions from the following numbers 2 through 11 (Swirsky & Sackett Nannery, 2008; Zuther, 2005; Zuther & Norton, 2013).
2. *Deep breathing*: Deep breathing techniques can stimulate the abdominal lymphatics resulting in improved lymphatic flow in the trunk.
3. *MLD*: MLD is a type of gentle manual treatment designed to promote the natural drainage of lymph fluid, which carries waste products away from the tissues back toward the heart. When the client performs on him or herself, it is called "self-MLD."
4. *Decongestion exercises*: Exercises designed to increase muscle pumping action and promote lymphatic fluid movement are called decongestion exercises and are very beneficial to encourage lymphatic flow. Decongestive exercises depend on the abilities of the client and can range from gentle AROM to strengthening and aquatics.

5. *Lymphedema precautions for daily living*: It is imperative that the lymphedema therapists teach their clients how to reduce their risk of lymphedema (i.e., for those at-risk clients who currently do not have lymphedema), as well as teach their clients with lymphedema ways to decrease the risk of infection and edema progression.
6. *Protect the skin*: Protect the involved extremity from extremes such as overuse, excessive pressure, or extreme temperature changes (i.e., the skin is the largest organ of the body and is very important in preventing infections in those with lymphedema as the skin serves as a barrier to outside contaminants and prevents them from entering the body).
7. *Work with a lymphedema specialist*: An individualized exercise program will need to be established by a lymphedema specialist to achieve and/or maintain a healthy body weight. Excess adipose tissue can put strain on the lymphatic vessels and may increase one's risk of developing lymphedema. Clients must know the signs and symptoms of lymphedema and where to get help if needed.
8. *Multilayer compression bandaging*: Multilayer compression bandaging is a vital component of treatment for Stage 2 and Stage 3 lymphedema. It is important that the client understand the precautions of bandaging and be able to complete bandaging independently, or with caregiver assistance, and safely. There are special bandages (i.e., typically short-stretch and 100% cotton) used for lymphedema treatment. ACE bandages are never used for lymphedema wrapping. Bandages are used to achieve the smallest girth possible of the body area with lymphedema.

   Donning, doffing, wear, and care of various compression garments. Compression garments are typically fitted near the end of skilled lymphedema treatment, as they are designed to maintain girth reduction, not create girth reduction. Therefore, the lymphedema therapy practitioner will use multilayer compression bandaging to decrease girth during treatment and the client will be fitted for compression garments to maintain girth reduction achieved during treatment. The client must know how to safely and independently (i.e., or with a caregiver's assistance) don and doff the garments, know their wearing schedule, care of the garments, and garment replacement time frames.

Compression therapy includes multilayer medical compression bandaging, which is designed to reduce lymphedema and girth of the edematous body part. Compression garments are measured and ordered when the edematous body part is determined to be at its smallest girth. Absolute contraindications for compression therapy bandaging and garments may include:

- Cardiac edema
- Peripheral arterial diseases
- Reflex sympathetic dystrophy
- Acute infections

General contraindications and conditions for which compression must be used with caution may include:

- Hypertension
- Cardiac arrhythmia
- Decreased or absent sensation in the extremity
- Partial or complete paralysis
- Age
- Congestive heart failure
- Mild to moderate arterial disease
- Diabetes
- Malignant lymphedema

9. *Manual therapy/complete decongestive therapy*: Manual techniques are used to stimulate the lymphatic system and improve lymphatic flow. These techniques are incorporated with clients when there are no contraindications to increasing lymphatic fluid mobility.

10. *Home-exercise program*: Designed for lymphedema decongestion. Exercises are best completed while clients are in their compression for a "pumping" effect. Exercises can include general AROM, strengthening as tolerated; cardiovascular activity such as walking is particularly helpful for clients with lower extremity lymphedema. Aquatic exercises are very beneficial due to the external pressure from the water increasing the lymphatic pumping action.

11. *Surgical procedures*: While many advanced microsurgical techniques are being developed, some of the more common surgical procedures associated with lymphedema include debulking and liposuction. Debulking is completed to remove excess skin and subcutaneous tissue from the involved body part. This procedure does not fix the faulty lymphatic system and only serves to remove or debulk excess tissue after successful volume reduction in therapy. Liposuction involves surgically removing fatty tissues; however, this technique can destroy the lymphatic microcirculation and lymphedema can still occur after liposuction procedures. Surgeries that work to fix the lymphatic malfunction include lympholymphatic repair, lymphovenous repair, collector replacement, and enteromesenteric bridge (Ehrlich, 2007).

Medications Used in the Treatment of Lymphedema

Individuals with lymphedema may be prescribed diuretics. Diuretics work to remove the water portion in the lymph fluid and increase urine secretion. Diuretics may be a medical necessity for individuals with comorbidities such as hypertension and CHF; however, most experts agree that the use of diuretics for individuals with lymphedema is ineffective and can lead to further complications, as only water is removed and the proteins remain. Benzopyrenes are medication that include coumarin and flavonoids and have been shown to promote macrophage activity and the breakdown of proteins in the lymph fluid; however, they do not have the approval of the Food and Drug Administration in the United States. Antifungal medications are often prescribed for fungal infections, particularly in the finger and toenails. Antibiotics are often prescribed for individuals with lymphedema due to infections (Zuther, 2005; Zuther & Norton, 2013).

Reevaluation and Plan Modification

Reevaluation and plan modification or discontinuation occurs frequently in the treatment of those with lymphedema. Because there are many factors involved in the treatment of lymphedema and in achieving client independence with maintaining therapeutic gains, it is important that the plan of care be constantly updated as needed. Reevaluation is typically based on treatment facility practices and/or payer requirements. However, it is best to complete weekly measurements of the lymphedematous limb or body area in order to determine if the therapy is proving beneficial.

Plan modification is a crucial aspect for the lymphedema therapist. Because lymphedema can be a complex condition with various comorbidities, contraindications, and medical complications, the lymphedema therapist must be a highly trained and skilled practitioner and able to successfully modify the therapy plan for each treatment session.

Referrals and Discharge Considerations

Referrals made by the lymphedema therapist may include care providers or support services; common examples include:

- Compression garment fitter
- Dermatologist
- Diabetic shoe specialist
- Endocrinologist
- Exercise physiologist/fitness center
- Podiatry
- Psychologist
- Support groups
- Wound care center

Discontinuation of services is typically related to one or more of the following factors:

- Significant change in medical status warranting physician follow-up
- Independence achieved with the plan of care for self-lymphedema maintenance
- Noncompliance by the client

Management and Standards of Practice

It is important that OTs and occupational therapy assistants (OTAs) uphold standards and responsibilities and properly manage the direction of services to promote quality care. OTs and OTAs who participate in the evaluation and/or treatment of lymphedema should be trained extensively in the physiology and treatment of lymphedema. It is important for non-lymphedema–treating therapists to understand what lymphedema is and be versed in its identification, precautions, and indications and contraindications in order to make the appropriate referral to a CLT. Both

OTs and OTAs can become certified in lymphedema through various schools. Often the certification requires over 100 hours of coursework including hands on training. Currently, there is no regulation requiring therapists who treat individuals for lymphedema to have certification, but those in the lymphedema community strongly encourage it.

Chapter 25 Self-Study Activities (Answers Are Provided at the End of the Chapter)

1. Ms. Smith is being seen by OT status post a right total hip replacement (THR). You begin to educate her on how to properly get out of bed following her hip surgery precautions and she complains of pain in her right leg; while also stating that she feels feverish and has chills. You visualize redness in the surgical site area. You suspect the following:
   A. She is experiencing normal post-THR symptoms.
   B. She is having a reaction to her pain medications.
   C. She potentially has an infection.
   D. She is experiencing lymphedema.
2. You are working in a pediatric clinic with a newborn with oral motor limitations. It is your first treatment session and note that the baby's left leg is significantly larger than the right. You ask the mother and father about this anomaly and they state, "The doctor said it will go down as she grows." You ask if it has gotten better since her birth four weeks ago and they state "no." The baby appears to be in no pain or distress and the swollen leg is normal in color. You suspect that the baby could potentially have:
   A. Secondary lymphedema from the trauma of birth.
   B. Primary lymphedema in the edematous leg.
   C. Nothing, it is just a normal situation for this child.
   D. Diabetes.
3. You have received a referral for "OT to evaluate and treat for swelling." Upon further investigation, you learn that the client has secondary lymphedema in her right upper extremity and breast from breast cancer treatments. You are

not lymphedema trained or certified; therefore, you can do the following:

A. Treat her for the swelling because she is cancer-free at this time.

B. Refer her to a CLT.

C. Ask her to return in a week to wait for the edema to go down.

D. Fit her for a compression sleeve.

4. You are an OTA certified in lymphedema. You work in a skilled nursing facility and are eager to treat lymphedema; however, none of the OTs are trained or certified in lymphedema. You can:

A. Complete the evaluation yourself because you are the professional with the higher level of education for this diagnosis.

B. Complete the evaluation with the OT. You will do all the assessing and he/she will do the write-up of the evaluation.

C. Not treat this client because they need to be evaluated by an OT who is trained and/ or certified in lymphedema treatment. It is unfair and unethical for the evaluating OT to attempt an evaluation in an area in which they are not skilled/trained.

D. Skip the evaluation and begin treatment.

5. Match the term (left column) with the correct definition (right column).

Term	Definition
A. Cellulitis	**1.** ___Present at birth.
B. Comorbidity	**2.** ___An agent (e.g., medication) that increases urine output; typically used to treat hypertension, CHF, and edema.
C. Congenital	**3.** ___Nematode belonging to the superfamily Filarioidea; may infect the lymphatic vessels and organs in humans.
D. CHF	**4.** ___A chronic disease caused by the parasitic nematode worm *Wuchereria bancrofti* or *Brugia malayi*.
E. DVT	**5.** ___A condition that reflects impaired cardiac function, (e.g., myocardial infarction and ischemic heart disease).

F. Diuretic	**6.** ___A thin watery fluid originating in organs and tissues of the body that circulates through the lymphatic vessels.
G. Filaria	**7.** ___X-ray examination of the lymph nodes and the lymphatic vessels after an injection of contrast medium.
H. Filariasis	**8.** ___A disease or condition that can potentially exacerbate or aggravate the primary disease.
I. Hereditary	**9.** ___Relating to genetic characteristic transmission from parent to offspring.
J. Lymph	**10.** ___A diffuse, acute infection of the skin and subcutaneous tissue (e.g., local heat, redness, pain, swelling, and fever).
K. Lymphangiogram	**11.** ___Protects and maintains the internal fluid environment of the body by producing, filtering, and conveying lymph.
L. Lymphangiography	**12.** ___An abnormal accumulation of tissue fluid in the interstitial space.
M. Lymphatic system	**13.** ___A blood clot in one or more of the deep veins in the legs, arms, pelvic, neck, or chest; can be fatal.
N. Lymphedema	**14.** ___A radiograph of the lymphatic vessels and nodes.

Chapter 25 Self-Study Answers

Question I

A. She is experiencing normal post-THR symptoms: those symptoms are not normal post-THR.

B. She is having a reaction to her pain medications: this is not a normal reaction to pain medications.

C. She potentially has an infection: correct—these are common symptoms for infection, especially since it is near a surgical site.

D. She is experiencing lymphedema: incorrect, these are not typical symptoms for lymphedema.

Question 2

A. Secondary lymphedema from the trauma of birth: there was no mention of a traumatic birth, only oral motor limitations.

B. Primary lymphedema in the edematous leg: because the edema is not going down and there was no indication of trauma, infection, or injury, one might suspect primary lymphedema and further examination by a physician is warranted.

C. It is just a normal situation for this child: edema is not normal.

D. That the baby must have diabetes: diabetes does not typically cause unilateral edema.

Question 3

A. Treat her for the swelling because she is cancer-free at this time: you are not trained to treat lymphedema.

B. Refer her to a CLT: correct so that her needs are adequately met.

C. Ask her to return in a week to wait for the edema to go down: incorrect, she has been diagnosed with lymphedema, it is a chronic progressive condition; therefore, it will not go down on its own.

D. Fit her for a compression sleeve: false, you are not trained to do this nor is it appropriate at this time; compression sleeves are fitted after the involved body part has been reduced through lymphedema treatment.

Question 4

A. Complete the evaluation yourself because you are the professional with the higher level of education for this diagnosis: false, as an OTA you cannot perform evaluations.

B. Complete the evaluation with the OT. You will do all the assessing and he/she will do the write-up of the evaluation: false, as an OTA you cannot complete the evaluation.

C. Not treat this client because they need to be evaluated by an OT that is trained and/or certified in lymphedema treatment. It is unfair and unethical for the evaluating OT to attempt an evaluation in an area in which they are not skilled/trained: correct, the client must be evaluated by a trained/certified lymphedema therapist.

D. Skip the evaluation and begin treatment: clients must be evaluated in order for treatment to be initiated.

Question 5

1. C
2. F
3. G
4. H
5. D
6. J
7. L
8. B
9. I
10. A
11. M
12. N
13. E
14. K

References

BreastCancer.Org. (2014, March 25). *Stages of lymphedema*. Retrieved from http://www.breastcancer.org/treatment/lymphedema/how/stages

Burkhardt, A., & Schultz-Krohn, W. (2013). Oncology. In L. W. Pedretti, H. M. Pendleton, & W. Schultz-Krohn (Eds.), *Pedretti's occupational therapy: Practice skills for physical dysfunction* (7th ed., pp. 1215–1227). St. Louis, MO: Elsevier Mosby.

Ehrlich, A. B. (2007). *Voices of lymphedema: Stories, advice, and inspiration from patients and therapists*. San Francisco, CA: Lymph Notes.

Földi, M., & Földi, E. (2006a). Lymphostatic diseases. In M. Foldi & E. Foldi (Eds.), *Foldi's textbook of lymphology for physicians and lymphedema therapists* (pp. 223–319, 2nd ed.). San Francisco, CA: Mosby Elsevier.

Földi, M., Földi, E. (2006b). Lymphostatic diseases. In M. Foldi & E. Foldi (Eds.), *Foldi's textbook of lymphology* (223–319). Munich, Germany: Elsevier. With contributions by L. Clodius and H. Neu.

Gillen, G. (2014). Occupational therapy interventions for individuals. In B. A. B. Schell, G. Gillen, & E. S. Cohn (Eds.), *Willard & Spackman's occupational therapy* (12th ed., pp. 322–341). Philadelphia, PA: Wolters Kluwer Health/Lippincott Williams & Wilkins.

Kubik, S., Kretz, O. (2006). Anatomy of the lymphatic system. In M. Földi & E. Földi (Eds.), *Földi's textbook of lymphology* (1–149). Munich, Germany: Elsevier. With contributions by M. Manestar and G. Molz.

Radomski, M. V., Anheluk, M., Grabe, K., Hopins, S. E., & Zola, J. (2014). Cancer. In M. V. Radomski & C. A. T. Latham (Eds.), *Occupational therapy for physical dysfunction* (7th ed., pp. 1368–1387). Philadelphia, PA: Wolters Kluwer Health/Lippincott Williams & Wilkins.

Swirsky, J., & Sackett Nannery, D. (2008). *Coping with lymphedema*. New York, NY: Avery Publishing Group.

Thiadens, S., Steward, P. J., & Stout, N. L. (2010). *100 questions & answers about lymphedema*. Sudbury, MA: Jones and Bartlett Publishers.

Zuther, J. E. (2005). *Lymphedema management: The comprehensive guide for practitioners*. New York, NY: Thieme.

Zuther, J. E., & Norton, S. (2013). *Lymphedema management: The comprehensive guide for practitioners* (3rd ed.). New York, NY: Thieme.

Dysphagia

Shari Bernard

Learning Objectives

- Describe the common symptoms of dysphagia.
- Compare and contrast the five types of dysphagia.
- Describe the anatomic structures involved with dysphagia.
- Describe appropriate interventions for clients with dysphagia based on assessment findings.
- Describe appropriate referral and discharge considerations for clients with dysphagia.

Key Terms

- *Aspiration*: When secretions, fluids, food, or other foreign substances enter the lungs below the vocal cords.
- *Fluoroscopy*: A type of radiographic imaging that produces continuous x-ray images that can be viewed on a monitor.
- *Videofluoroscopic swallowing study (VFSS)*: An examination using fluoroscopy with barium added to food to capture images of a swallow with foods of varied textures and consistencies.

Description

Groher and Crary (2009) define dysphagia as a swallowing disorder that can involve any of the stages of swallowing, including oral, pharyngeal, and esophageal. However, dysphagia is not a primary diagnosis, but rather a symptom of an underlying disease; therefore, dysphagia is associated with various diagnoses. For example, dysphagia may be associated with Parkinson's disease, multiple sclerosis, amyotrophic lateral sclerosis, cerebral palsy, muscular dystrophy, and myasthenia gravis. Additionally, other causes may include cerebrovascular accident, traumatic brain injury, spinal cord injury, brain tumors, head/neck and esophageal cancers, generalized weakness, and the normal aging process (Groher & Crary, 2009). Anatomy of the head and neck is depicted and described in **Figure 26-1**.

Types of dysphagia to consider are as follows:

1. *Paralytic*: Results from lower motor neuron involvement, observed by weakness or sensory impairment (e.g., myotonic dystrophy, Guillain–Barré syndrome, and neuromuscular diseases).
2. *Pseudobulbar*: Results from upper motor neuron involvement, observed by varying tone of oral and pharyngeal structures or decreased coordination: multiple sclerosis, cerebrovascular accident, and head injury.
3. *Mechanical*: Caused by a loss of oral, pharyngeal, or esophageal structures possibly from trauma or surgery (e.g., edema, lesion, or foreign body).
4. *Acute dysphagia*: Some improvement is to be expected following intubation/extubation.
5. *Chronic dysphagia*: Function will plateau and deficits will remain (e.g., dementia, effects from radiation, and age-related changes).

Anatomy plays an important role in dysphagia management. The following provides a description of the relevant anatomy:

- *Pharynx*: The passage way for food or liquid from the base of the tongue leading into the esophagus.
- *Epiglottis*: A cartilaginous structure at the base of the tongue that covers the trachea during swallowing.
- *Esophagus*: A muscular tube with a mucous membrane lining that extends from the pharynx to the stomach (i.e., a passageway).

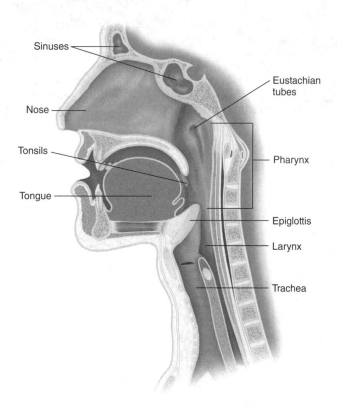

Figure 26-1 Anatomy of the head and neck.

- *Larynx*: The airflow passage way that houses the vocal cords.
- *Trachea*: Commonly referred to as the "windpipe," the trachea is a membrane reinforced by cartilaginous rings that extends from the larynx to the bronchial tubes (i.e., a passageway to and from the lungs).

Etiology and Pathology

The presence of dysphagia implies that there is a dysfunction with the anatomy (e.g., mechanical obstruction) or the motor function (i.e., functional obstruction) of the oral cavity, the pharynx, or the esophagus. Lieberman et al. (1980) report that about half of the populations with Parkinson's disease have dysphagia and Calcagno, Ruoppolo, Grasso, De Vincentiis, and Paolucci (2002) report that 34% of clients with multiple sclerosis have dysphagia. Similarly, Singh and Hamdy (2006) report that 23–50% of clients experience challenges with swallowing after a stroke. Aspiration in stroke occurs in 29–81% of clients with silent aspiration (i.e., no physical

signs of difficulty with swallowing) present in half of those individuals with acute stroke (Altman, Yu, & Schaefer, 2010).

The swallowing process is commonly affected by the normal aging process, impacting a growing number of individuals older than 60 years (National Foundation of Swallowing Disorders, 2013). It is estimated that 40–50% of older individuals residing in long-term care facilities have swallowing disorders (Easterling & Robbins, 2008) and 15–33% of nursing home clients report having trouble swallowing medication (Morris, 2005). Conversely, 33% of elderly people who are non-institutionalized reported that they have a swallowing disorder and 38% reported that they have a history of dysphagia (Roy, Stemple, Merrill, & Thomas, 2007). Clinical presentation and common diagnostic tests for dysphagia are described in **Table 26-1**.

Clinical Presentation

The clinical presentation for dysphagia varies widely. Signs and symptoms associated with dysphagia may include being unable to swallow or pain while swallowing, feeling food stuck in the throat, chest, or behind the breastbone, drooling, speaking in a hoarse voice, experiencing regurgitation or frequent heartburn, unexpected weight loss, and coughing and/or gagging with swallowing, as well as requiring food cut into smaller pieces or avoiding certain foods all together (Mayo Clinic, 2015).

Table 26-1 Common Diagnostic Tests

Diagnostic Tests and Specialist	Possible Finding(s)
Clinical dysphagia evaluation (OT or speech pathologist)	Visible signs of aspiration such as coughing/choking or oral motor difficulties
Video fluoroscopic swallow study (OT or speech pathologist)	Rule out aspiration, and observe for obstruction, and residue
Fiberoptic endoscopic swallowing evaluation (speech pathologist)	Visualize structures for damage or dysfunction (e.g., vocal cords), and rule out aspiration

Data from Groher & Crary 2016.

Screening and Assessments

Multidisciplinary dysphagia teams are necessary for optimal care (Crary & Groher, 2003). Providers may include a dietician, physician, radiologist, occupational therapist (OT), occupational therapy assistant (OTA), nurse, and speech and language pathologist. Examples of dysphagia screening tools include the Gugging Swallowing Screen (Trapl et al., 2007) and the Self-Report Symptom Inventory (Wallace, Middleton, & Cook, 2000). Team members may begin with screening for dysphagia as mentioned above and if signs and/or symptoms of dysphagia are identified, a referral to occupational therapy can be made for further evaluation. Correspondingly, dysphagia screening and early intervention have been shown to save both client and hospital costs (Martino, Pron, & Diamant, 2000).

Clinical Dysphagia Evaluation

There are five phases of normal swallowing that need to be evaluated. The stages are as follows:

1. *Preoral*: Evaluates how food and drink are brought to the mouth (e.g., independence in feeding).
2. *Oral preparatory*: Evaluates how food is chewed and manipulated by the lips, cheeks, and tongue (e.g., no spillage or drooling from the mouth).
3. *Oral*: Evaluates how the bolus of food is propelled to the pharynx (e.g., is food well chewed and is oral cavity cleared adequately).
4. *Pharyngeal*: Evaluates how the swallow response is initiated (e.g., is swallow efficient and is coughing or choking observed).
5. *Esophageal*: Evaluates how food and drink travel through the esophagus and into the stomach (e.g., complaints of food getting caught in throat or reflux symptoms).

Key components that may comprise a complete dysphagia evaluation include:

- Chart review and client interview
- Assess level of cognition and alertness
- Evaluation of oral motor function
- Strength of volitional cough
- Evaluation of respiratory status

- Change in voice quality
- Assess ability to perform oral cares
- Optimal positioning
- Ability to self-feed
- Trials of oral intake with various consistencies
- Eating assessment tools
- Quality of life concerns
- Special circumstances (e.g., tracheostomy)

In addition, during mealtime, an OT can complete a feeding evaluation/mealtime observation to establish a baseline for the client's eating habits, as well as the caregivers' habits or routines during meals (American Occupational Therapy Association, 2014).

Standardized Assessment Tools

The following include examples of common assessments used in dysphagia care. They are as follows:

1. *Functional Oral Intake Scale*: The Functional Oral Intake Scale may be used to document the functional level of oral intake of food and liquid for persons with dysphagia (Crary, Mann, & Groher, 2005).

   Tube Dependent (levels 1–3)

   Level 1—No oral intake

   Level 2—Tube dependent with minimal/inconsistent oral intake

   Level 3—Tube supplements with consistent oral intake

   Total Oral Intake (levels 4–7)

   Level 4—Total oral intake of a single consistency

   Level 5—Total oral intake of multiple consistencies requiring special preparation

   Level 6—Total oral intake with no special preparation, but must avoid specific foods or liquid items

   Level 7—Total oral intake with no restrictions

2. *Eating Assessment Tool (EAT-10;* **Figure 26-2***)*: The purpose of administering the EAT-10 is to assess if a client has challenges swallowing efficiently and safely. It is important to discuss findings from this assessment with a physician if the total score is 3 or higher (i.e., the total possible score is 40 points).

Eating Assessment Tool (Eat-10)

Date: _____

Name: _____ MR#: _____

Height: _____ Weight: _____

Please briefly describe your swallowing problem.

_____

_____

Please list any swallowing tests you have had, including where, when, and the results.

_____

_____

To what extent are the following scenarios problematic for you?

Circle the appropriate response	0 = No problem 4 = Severe problem				
1. My swallowing problem has caused me to lose weight.	0	1	2	3	4
2. My swallowing problem interferes with my ability to go out for meals.	0	1	2	3	4
3. Swallowing liquids takes extra effort.	0	1	2	3	4
4. Swallowing solids takes extra effort.	0	1	2	3	4
5. Swallowing pills takes extra effort.	0	1	2	3	4
6. Swallowing is painful.	0	1	2	3	4
7. The pleasure of eating is affected by my swallowing.	0	1	2	3	4
8. When I swallow food sticks in my throat.	0	1	2	3	4
9. I cough when I eat.	0	1	2	3	4
10. Swallowing is stressful.	0	1	2	3	4
	Total EAT-10:				

Figure 26-2 Eating Assessment Tool (EAT-10) standardized tool.

Reproduced with permission from Belafsky, P. C., Mouadeb, D. A., Rees, C. J., Pryor, J. C., Postma, G. N., Allen, J., & Leonard, R. J. (2008). Eating Assessment Tool, EAT-10.

Additional Assessment Tools

1. *Fiberoptic Endoscopic Evaluation of Swallow (FEES)*: The FEES is an examination used for the observation of swallow abnormalities and is usually completed with a speech and language pathologist.

2. *Videofluoroscopic swallowing study (VFSS)*: The VFSS is an examination used for observation of swallowing abnormalities.
   - It is the most commonly used instrumental tool (i.e., the gold standard).
   - Uses fluoroscopy to capture images of a swallow when a variety of foods and textures are being taken orally.

- Barium contrast in varied consistencies is added to the food, so it can be seen on the video fluoroscopic swallow study.
- The VFSS is performed in a radiology suite with a radiologist present along with the OT.

Frazier Free Water Protocol

The Frazier Water Protocol is an option available as part of dysphagia rehabilitation. It is designed to allow clients with dysphagia who are on diet restrictions that include thickened liquids to also have regular water as part of their diet (Panther, 2005). The clients follow specific guidelines to decrease their risk of developing aspiration pneumonia while continuing oral intake of water, even with diet restrictions that call for use of thickened liquids.

Interventions

Based on evaluation findings, the OT practitioner must consider the following key points:

- Safe diet recommendations
- Proper positioning
- Instruction in aspiration precautions and signs of aspiration
- Instruction on good oral care habits
- Compensatory techniques
- Exercises
- Alternative method for feeding
- Further evaluation with instrumental assessment

Expected Functional Outcomes

Occupational therapy outcomes are commonly focused on reengaging clients back into meaningful, purposeful, and productive lives. The following demonstrates specific occupational therapy outcomes related to dysphagia care (American Occupational Therapy Association, 2014):

- *Occupational performance and participation*: The act of swallowing/eating/feeding; keeping and manipulating food or fluid in the mouth and swallowing it. Setting up, arranging, and bringing food or fluid from the plate or cup to the mouth.

Ensuring occupational performance including access to participation in meaningful and enriching occupations by using compensatory strategies to ensure engagement is also a desired outcome of treatment.

- *Prevention*: Education on use of appropriate positioning and seating during oral intake.
- *Health and wellness*: Resources for everyday life that could include participation of a person in an oral care improvement group at a long-term facility.
- *Quality of life*: The client's life satisfaction that may include use of quality of life tools and surveys to report client satisfaction with current oral intake levels.
- *Participation*: Engagement in desired occupations like a client recovering from a stroke and using techniques to learn to swallow or self-feed again.
- *Role competence*: The ability to effectively meet the demands of roles in which the client engages. The client is able to demonstrate proper use of a thickening agent to thicken liquids to a nectar thick level.
- *Well-being*: The ability to feel contentment with one's health. A client may be a member of a stroke support group where they are able to discuss feeding issues that cause embarrassment and provide encouragement to one another.

Impact on Occupational Performance

Feeding and eating are major areas of focus in occupational therapy practice and are classified as activities of daily living that typically occur three times/day. The following types of interventions provide an overview of the types of interventions that may help improve the occupational performance of those experiencing dysphagia:

- *Restorative intervention*: Exercises and eating activities.
- *Modified intervention*: Compensatory techniques to help client through acute illness.
- *Direct intervention*: Interventions that address client factors and swallowing performance skills within the context of eating.
- *Indirect intervention*: Interventions that address strengthening, client factors, and swallowing performance skills outside the context of eating.

An important safety consideration with dysphagia intervention includes educational instruction on general aspiration precautions. These precautions include the following:

- Sit upright for all oral intake
- Remain upright for 20–30 minutes after oral intake to allow pooling to clear
- Take small bites and sips
- Chew food completely
- Empty the mouth before adding more
- Avoid oral intake when overly fatigued
- Avoid using a straw
- Avoid talking during meal time
- Eat smaller meals more frequently
- Be aware of signs of aspiration

Additional dysphagia interventions include education and training in areas such as diet, positioning, exercise, compensatory training, aspiration management, and oral care. The following points discuss these areas in further detail:

1. *Diet modifications*: Consider use of thickened liquids and/or easy to eat soft foods. Observe during a mealtime to confirm diet modifications are being tolerated with no signs of aspiration.
2. *Positioning*: Head and trunk positioning are important considerations for seating. Head turning or tilting is a common technique to help direct the bolus in the proper route down the esophagus.
3. *Exercises*: Tongue and lip strengthening can be used to assist with bolus formation and propulsion.
4. *Compensatory techniques*: Dry or second swallow, chin tuck, and effortful swallow are techniques used to clear residue following a single swallow, and to direct a bolus in the proper route decreasing risk of aspiration.
5. *Consequences of aspiration*: Dysphagia can cause aspiration pneumonia if food or secretions are aspirated as the result of an abnormal swallow mechanism (Loeb, McGeer, McArthur, Walter, & Simor, 1999).
6. *Importance of oral care*: Effective oral care relating to clients with dysphagia can decrease the risk of developing aspiration pneumonia (Franceschini, 2007). Good oral hygiene requires brushing all areas of the mouth to make sure the bacterial colonies are disrupted and cleaned away. Aspiration of oropharyngeal pathogens is the main cause of nursing home-acquired pneumonia (Shay, 2002). In addition, poor oral health is strongly correlated with an increased risk of aspiration pneumonia.

Types of Occupational Therapy Interventions

There are five main areas of occupational therapy interventions in dysphagia care. They are as follows (American Occupational Therapy Association, 2014):

1. *Occupations and activities*: A client can purchase groceries and prepare a meal with meal modifications that are required for decreasing the risk of aspiration.
2. *Preparatory methods and tasks*: A client works on hand to mouth active range of motion in preparation for self-feeding.
3. *Education and training*: A client is instructed in aspiration precautions and ways to be aware of aspiration if it occurs.
4. *Advocacy*: An OT can advocate for improvement in oral care procedures in a long-term care facility.
5. *Group interventions*: Participation in a group that helps to support the use of adaptive equipment needed during mealtime.

National Dysphagia Diet

Finally, OT can incorporate the National Dysphagia Diet (NDD) into a client's plan of care, which was published in 2002 by the American Dietetic Association (National Dysphagia Diet Task Force, 2002). The NDD is a classification of foods and liquids that can assist in standardizing terminology and defining food and liquid textures. The OT should clarify with their practice setting to see if the NDD is being used and any protocols that may be in place.

Quality of Life and Ethical Considerations

Quality of life is an area of concern for all clients. It is important to address important factors that contribute to quality of life and, in many cases, result in ethical dilemmas or considerations. These considerations are as follows:

- The changes that occur in the swallowing mechanism as we age
- End-of-life wishes
- Dysphagia in geriatrics in terms of preserving quality of life for elderly clients
- Compensatory techniques
- Dietary modifications
- Positional strategies
- Rehabilitation protocols based on dysfunction
- Discuss medication administration strategies with clients and/or caregivers
- Inform clients and/or caregivers of alternative options and resources
- Discuss the consequences of choice with clients and/or caregivers
- Increase eating satisfaction
- Promote positive feeding interactions
- Know your client's wishes, values, and beliefs

Referrals and Discharge Considerations

Groher and McKaig (1995) revealed residents in a nursing home were on a lower level diet than what they could actually tolerate. Keeping this in mind, it is very important to reevaluate a client's status with regard to tolerance of their current diet on a regular basis. Based on the goals of the client's diet levels, as the client plateaus in progress or meets their goals, they can then be dismissed from skilled occupational therapy. A screening process can be used to assess a client who requires further evaluation or a diet modification. Within the screening process, an OT can observe if a client is having signs or symptoms of aspiration and compare the client's level of performance with different diet consistencies.

Management and Standards of Practice

Dysphagia is an excellent specialty area for the OT and the OTA to work collaboratively. As it is a specialty area in feeding, eating, and swallowing, it will be best served by an experienced OT and OTA who have training specifically for dysphagia evaluation and treatment.

As in all settings, the OT directs the evaluation process, determines the need for services, and develops the intervention plan. The OT delegates aspects of the therapy intervention to the OTA to perform the interventions with the appropriate level of supervision. The OT is responsible for determining the continuation, modification or discontinuation of services, as well as completing and interpreting client outcomes. The OTA must be familiar with the evaluation results and goals. They can work collaboratively with the OT in assisting with the development of a plan of care. The OTA is responsible for knowing the results of measurable outcomes and to work collaboratively to exchange information that assists the OT in the development of the intervention plan.

Chapter 26 Self-Study Activities

Answer the following case study multiple-choice questions.

Mr. B is an 80-year-old male who was hospitalized for aspiration pneumonia. He presented with a fever, coughing, and decreased appetite, and he has a history of Parkinson's disease. Mr. B's daughter reports he was eating supper the night before last and started to cough and choke when swallowing water. Mr. B has no history of dysphagia and was tolerating a general texture food diet prior to being hospitalized. He does not participate in oral care regularly. Mr. B was referred to occupational therapy for a dysphagia evaluation to rule out aspiration. Upon initial bedside assessment, Mr. B was alert and able to demonstrate normal oral motor skills and he said, "I just swallowed the wrong way." With oral intake during evaluation, Mr. B tolerated pudding and a cracker with no coughing or choking. When he was given sips of water, immediate coughing was observed. Further evaluation was completed with a VFSS, which revealed Mr. B was aspirating on thin liquids. A chin tuck maneuver was completed during the VFSS, which eliminated aspiration with thin liquids. Recommendations included education of aspiration precautions and signs of aspiration, education of a good oral care routine, and instruction in the use of a chin tuck maneuver during swallowing of thin liquids.

1. All of these can be seen as clinical presentation of dysphagia except:
   A. Drooling
   B. Pain with swallowing

    C. Fainting

    D. Coughing

2. Recommendations for decreasing the risk of developing aspiration pneumonia can include:

    A. Swishing/spitting with a mouth rinse

    B. Brushing teeth

    C. Flossing teeth

    D. All of the above

Match the following terms with their appropriate definitions:

1. Dysphagia	**A.** Passageway for food or liquid from the base of the tongue leading into the esophagus
2. Pharynx	**B.** Airflow passageway that houses the vocal cords
3. Epiglottis	**C.** Passageway for food to pass through and into the stomach
4. Larynx	**D.** Food or liquid passes the vocal cords
5. Trachea	**E.** Chin tuck
6. Esophagus	**F.** Fluoroscopic examination showing images of a swallow using a variety of food consistencies with barium added
7. Mechanical dysphagia	**G.** A swallowing disorder that can involve any of the stages of swallowing including oral, pharyngeal, and esophageal
8. Aspiration	**H.** Loss of swallow mechanism structures from possible trauma, surgery, or lesion
9. Videofluoroscopy	**I.** A cartilage structure assisting in the safe swallow mechanism
10. Compensatory technique	**J.** Windpipe

Chapter 26 Self-Study Answers

Case study multiple-choice question answers:

1. C

2. D

Matching answers:

1. G

2. A

3. I

4. B

5. J

6. C

7. H

8. D

9. F

10. E

References

Altman, K. W., Yu, G. P., & Schaefer, S. D. (2010). Consequence of dysphagia in the hospitalized patient: Impact on prognosis and hospital resources. *Archives of Otolaryngology—Head & Neck Surgery, 136*(8), 784–789. doi:10.1001/archoto.2010.129

American Occupational Therapy Association. (2014). Occupational therapy practice framework: Domain and process (3rd ed.). *American Journal of Occupational Therapy, 68*(Suppl. 1), S1–S48. doi:10.5014/ajot.2014.682006

Belafsky, P. C., Mouadeb, D. A., Rees, C. J., Pryor, J. C., Postma, G. N., Allen, J., & Leonard, R. J. (2008). Validity and reliability of the Eating Assessment Tool (EAT-10). *Annals of Otology, Rhinology & Laryngology, 117*(12), 919–924.

Calcagno, P., Ruoppolo, G., Grasso, M. G., De Vincentiis, M., & Paolucci, S. (2002). Dysphagia in multiple sclerosis—prevalence and prognostic factors. *Acta Neurologica Scandinavica, 105*(1), 40–43.

Crary, M. A., & Groher, M. E. (2003). *Introduction to adult swallowing disorders.* St. Louis, MS: Butterworth-Heinemann.

Crary, M. A., Mann, G. D., & Groher, M. E. (2005). Initial psychometric assessment of a functional oral intake scale for dysphagia in stroke patients. *Archives of Physical Medicine and Rehabilitation, 86*(8), 1516–1520. doi:10.1016/j.apmr.2004.11.049

Easterling, C. S., & Robbins, E. (2008). Dementia and dysphagia. *Geriatric Nursing, 29*(4), 275–285. doi:10.1016/j.gerinurse.2007.10.015

Franceschini, T. (2007, October 27–28). *Lecture: Dysphagia practice: Taking services to the next level of evidence based practice.* Rochester, MN: Mayo Clinic.

Groher, M. E., & Crary, M. A. (2009). *Dysphagia: Clinical management in adults and children.* St. Louis, MO: Elsevier Health Sciences.

Groher, M. E., & Crary, M. A. (2016). *Dysphagia: Clinical management in adults and children* (2nd ed.). St. Louis, MO: Elsevier.

Groher, M. E., & McKaig, T. N. (1995). Dysphagia and dietary levels in skilled nursing facilities. *Journal of the American Geriatrics Society, 43*(5), 528–532. Retrieved from http://www.ncbi.nlm.nih.gov/pubmed/7730535

Lieberman, A. N., Horowitz, L., Redmond, P., Pachter, L., Lieberman, I., & Leibowitz, M. (1980). Dysphagia in Parkinson's disease. *American Journal of Gastroenterology, 74*(2), 157–160.

Loeb, M., McGeer, A., McArthur, M., Walter, S., & Simor, A. E. (1999). Risk factors for pneumonia and other lower respiratory tract infections in elderly residents of long-term care facilities. *Archives of Internal Medicine, 159*(17), 2058–2064. doi:10.1001/archinte.159.17.2058

Martino, R., Pron, G., & Diamant, N. (2000). Screening for oropharyngeal dysphagia in stroke: Insufficient evidence for guidelines. *Dysphagia, 15*(1), 19–30.

Mayo Clinic. (2015). *Diseases and conditions: Dysphagia.* Retrieved from http://www.mayoclinic.org/diseases-conditions/dysphagia/basics/symptoms/con-20033444

Morris, H. (2005). *Dysphagia in the elderly, Country Doctor.* Retrieved from www.ask.com

National Dysphagia Diet Task Force. (2002). *National Dysphagia Diet: Standardization for optimal care.* Chicago, IL: American Dietetic Association.

National Foundation of Swallowing Disorders. (2013). *How aging affects our swallowing ability.* Retrieved from http://swallowingdisorderfoundation.com/how-aging-affects-our-swallowing-ability/

Panther, K. (2005). The Frazier Free Water Protocol. *SIG 13 Perspectives on Swallowing and Swallowing Disorders (Dysphagia), 14*(1), 4–9. doi:10.1044/sasd14.1.4

Roy, N., Stemple, J., Merrill, R. M., & Thomas, L. (2007). Dysphagia in the elderly: Preliminary evidence of prevalence, risk factors, and socioemotional effects. *Annals of Otology, Rhinology & Laryngology, 116*(11), 858–865.

Shay, K. (2002). Infectious complications of dental and periodontal diseases in the elderly population. *Clinical Infectious Diseases, 34*(9), 1215–1223. doi:10.1086/339865

Singh, S., & Hamdy, S. (2006). Dysphagia in stroke patients. *Postgraduate Medical Journal, 82*(968), 383–391. Retrieved from http://www.ncbi.nlm.nih.gov/pmc/articles/PMC2563739/

Trapl, M., Enderle, P., Nowotny, M., Teuschl, Y., Matz, K., Dachenhausen, A., & Brainin, M. (2007). Dysphagia bedside screening for acute-stroke patients: The Gugging Swallowing Screen. *Stroke, 38*(11), 2948–2952. doi:10.1161/strokeaha.107.483933

Wallace, K. L., Middleton, S., & Cook, I. J. (2000). Development and validation of a self-report symptom inventory to assess the severity of oral-pharyngeal dysphagia. *Gastroenterology, 118*(4), 678–687.

Occupational Functioning: Mental Health Days 18–19

Mental Health Conditions

Sophia Kimmons and Regina Parnell

Learning Objectives

- Describe criteria and symptoms of mental health conditions covered in this chapter.
- Describe the core concepts and assumptions of occupational practice models relevant to mental health practice.
- Describe the core concepts and assumptions of the psychosocial occupational therapy interventions in various practice settings.
- Differentiate the roles of the occupational therapist (OT) and occupational therapy assistant (OTA) in the management of occupational therapy services in mental health settings.
- Apply knowledge of occupational therapy interventions to practical and clinical case scenarios.

Key Terms

- *Adaptive behavior*: A type of behavior that can be adjusted based on other behaviors or situations, thereby allowing the individual to function in a practical and socially appropriate manner.
- *Occupational adaptation*: The ability to achieve occupational performance, which is often times facilitated by the OT by implementing strategies to overcome difficulties with functioning.
- *Service competency*: The observed and documented achievement of clinical reasoning and judgment related to specific assessment and intervention processes for occupational performance.
- *Social skills*: Interaction with others using verbal and nonverbal communication skills, along with the ability to modify communication based on verbal and nonverbal cues from others.

Introduction

This chapter will cover psychosocial occupational therapy, which will include an overview of the primary mental health diagnoses commonly seen in mental health settings and corresponding assessments and interventions typically used with these populations. The chapter will provide the description, pathology, clinical presentations, screening and assessment tools, impact on occupational performance, and interventions for each of the identified conditions, as well as referrals and discharge considerations, safety precautions, and risk factors for each diagnostic category. When applicable, general information on medication class, purpose, common side effects, and occupational therapy involvement in managing medications will be discussed. Lastly, the mental health conditions covered in this chapter are organized to match the *Fifth Edition of Diagnostic and Statistical Manual of Mental Disorders (DSM-5)*, which is the standard classification of mental disorders used by health professionals in the United States (American Psychiatric Association, 2013a). The seven categories include: neurodevelopmental, disruptive, impulse control and conductive disorders, bipolar and depressive disorders, schizophrenia spectrum and psychotic personality disorders, substance-related and addictive disorders, and trauma stress–related disorders.

People diagnosed with mental health conditions range in age from infancy through older adulthood. Diagnoses were categorized according to the *Diagnostic and Statistical Manual of Mental Disorders (DSM-IV)* multiaxial guidelines until the introduction of the *DSM-5* (Sadock, Sadock, & Ruiz, 2015). The *DSM-5* is used to determine the range and severity of a condition based on the client's symptoms. Axis I is the top level of the *DSM* classification scheme, defines clinical disorders, and includes the most commonly recognized diagnoses (e.g., depression and schizophrenia). Axis II defines the presence of any personality disorder. Axis III refers to general medical conditions. Axis IV includes information about the psychosocial and environmental challenges. Axis V provides a determination about the client's global assessment of functioning (Bruce, Borg, & Bruce, 2002; Early, 2009).

Evaluation and Intervention Processes

The client evaluation process incorporates the development of an occupational profile, as well as an assessment of the client's occupational performance. In addition to gathering key client data such as demographics, medical history, current diagnoses, and reason for admission, information regarding the client's occupational history, routines, values, and interest is also explored. Relevant assessments are then used to determine the client's occupational performance strengths and challenges.

Assessments refer to the measurement of more specific or narrow aspects of client factors, client occupational performance, and contexts. Some tools are appropriate for use across the life span, while others were designed with specific age groups in mind. The purpose of assessments is to provide valuable information about the individual as follows: (1) identify deficits and strengths, (2) identify skills and habits, (3) identify goals and objectives, (4) identify functional abilities, (5) identify values and interests, and (6) identify contextual environments (Early, 2009).

Standardized and Nonstandardized Assessments

Standardized assessments are used to establish a baseline, to evaluate the efficacy of interventions and to compare a client's assessment results against normative data for a specific population. Procedures for administering standardized assessments must be strictly followed (Early, 2009). Nonstandardized assessments include specific tasks and/or questionnaires but lack consistent procedures for administering the assessments and cannot (i.e., typically) be compared against normative data for a specific population. Nonstandardized assessments may be tailored to the individual and situation (Early, 2009). Psychosocial assessments throughout the life span are categorized and described in **Table 27-1**.

Interventions

The intervention process, planning, implementation, and review targets outcomes intended to promote health and well-being. The occupational therapist (OT) and client collaborate on the intervention plan and the selection of objective goals based on best available evidence. Table 8 in the Occupational Therapy Practice Framework III (OTPF III) specifies five basic intervention approaches: (1) create, (2) establish, (3) maintain, (4) modify, and (5) prevent (American Occupational Therapy Association, 2014). Client responses are monitored and modified when appropriate to support client progress and success. The OTPF III also identifies 10 potential outcomes to consider during intervention and discharge planning (American Occupational Therapy Association, 2014). Each of these intervention strategies requires knowledge of human development, specific disease processes, and an appreciation for human resilience and potential. The following provides a guide based on the five intervention approaches that are suggested by the American Occupational Therapy Association (2014):

- *Create and promote*: When the goal of the intervention is to generate and encourage skills, the underlying assumption is that a skill set has failed to develop. For example, a developmental delay occurs and as a result, the client has minimal ability in communication and social participation.
- *Establish and restore*: This is appropriate when the loss of function has occurred. In such instances, the client has some previous experience with a skill set and needs assistance with the restoration of function.
- *Maintain*: This approach is appropriate when a client has the potential to experience a loss of function if certain behaviors, practices, or disease processes continue.
- *Modify*: Appropriate when some functional ability has been permanently lost or diminished.
- *Prevention*: This intervention approach is often used to prevent acquired health conditions. This is an appropriate intervention strategy when an individual has an identified risk factor for injury, illness, or disease. This approach also encourages individuals to modify their environments and behaviors to minimize the risk of injury, acquiring a particular health condition, or both treatment approaches.

Table 27-1 Psychosocial Assessments Throughout the Life Span

Age	Assessment Name	Purpose
Life span	Allen Cognitive Level (ACL) Screen	A quick screen (i.e., part of a body of the Allen Battery of assessment tools) used to provide an initial estimate of cognitive function, which must be validated by further observations.
	Allen Diagnostic Module (ADM)	A set of craft projects used to determine a client's cognitive level and functional limitations.
	Assessment of Communication and Interaction Skills (ACIS)	A MOHO is a formal observation tool used to determine skill levels during performance of occupations.
	Holmes–Rahe Life Change Inventory	An assessment used to help measure a client's stress load.
	Kohlman Evaluation of Living Skills (KELS)	An interview and set of observations used to assess a client's ability to perform basic living skills.
	Leisure Diagnostic Battery (LDB)	A set of instruments designed to assess a client's leisure functioning.
	Life Skills Profile (LSP)	A measure of aspects of functioning, which affects how successfully clients with schizophrenia lived in a community or hospital.
	Mini-Mental State Examination (MMSE)	A questionnaire used to screen and measure cognitive impairment.
	Occupational Case Analysis and Interview Rating Scales (OCAIRS)	An instrument used to measure a client's occupational adaptation.
	Modified Interest Checklist	A checklist on leisure interests that influence a client's activity choices.
	Occupational Performance History Interview II (OPHI II)	A semistructured interview used to obtain information on a client's life history in areas of work, play, and self-care performance.
	Role Checklist	A checklist used to obtain information on a client's perceptions of their participation in occupational roles.
	Social Functioning Scale	An instrument used to evaluate areas crucial to community living for clients with schizophrenia (e.g., social engagement and withdrawal).
Adolescence	Adolescent Coping Scale (ACS)	A self-report inventory designed to assess utilization of coping strategies across differing specific and non-specific situations.
	Adolescent Role Assessment (ARA)	A semistructured interview used to evaluate a client's involvement in occupational roles (i.e., occupational choices) over time.
	Adolescent Leisure Interest Profile (ALIP)	A self-report interview used to explore a client's leisure interest and participation, as well as their feelings about leisure.
	Coping Inventory	A self-report form used to provide a profile of coping styles and behaviors, which may help or interfere with constructive coping strategies.
	Family Stress and Coping Interview (FSCI)	A questionnaire designed to examine the experiences of parents of children with developmental disabilities.
Adulthood	Activity Card Diagnostic (Activity Card Sort)	An interview used to assess and develop a client's participation in instrumental, leisure, and social activities.
	ACL Screen	A quick screen (i.e., part of the ACL Battery of assessment tools) used to provide an initial estimate of cognitive function, which must be validated by further observations.
	Barth Time Construction (BTC)	A client- or group-constructed color-coded chart used to assess time, usage, roles, and underlying skills and habits.
	Community Integration Questionnaire (QIC)	A questionnaire used to measure participation in home, social, and productive activities after traumatic brain injury.

(continues)

Table 27-1 Psychosocial Assessments Throughout the Life Span (*continued*)

Age	Assessment Name	Purpose
	Comprehensive Occupational Therapy Evaluation (COTE)	A behavior rating scale used in mental health settings to help identify client behaviors that impact occupational performance.
	Milwaukee Evaluation of Daily Living Skills (MEDLS)	Measures the ability to perform basic and complex ADL for lower functioning clients with long-term psychiatric challenges.
	Model of Human Occupation Screening Tool (MOHOST)	An assessment designed to address a majority of MOHO concepts in order to gain an overview of a client's occupational functioning.
	The Canadian Occupational Performance Measure (COPM)	An individualized outcome measure used to detect change in a client's self-perception of occupational performance over time.

Data from Asher, 2014; Brown, Stoffel, and Munoz, 2011; Early, 2009.

Treatment Settings

Individuals with mental health disorders may receive treatment in a variety of psychosocial healthcare settings. These settings are broadly divided into two categories: traditional and community. Traditional settings are typically based on the medical model where the individual is defined as the client. They include inpatient and outpatient models and often are affiliated with a hospital. Community settings are also called nontraditional sites.

Early (2009) outlines the following venues in which occupational therapy practitioners can view individuals as clients or consumers:

- *Traditional inpatient setting*: A full medical team, including a psychiatrist, internist, psychologist, nurse, OT, social worker, and various support personnel are available to support client needs.
    - *Acute care*: Short-term care, ranging from a few days to a few weeks.
    - *Long-term care*: Inpatient care for extended periods of time (e.g., months to years).
- *Community outpatient settings*: Large agencies that provide a wide range of services offer transitional housing, day treatment, and supportive skills training.
    - *Day treatment*: Facilities that provide day treatment offer services during daytime working hours.
    - *Consumer-run facilities (e.g., clubhouses)*: These facilities are run and sometimes owned and operated by individuals with histories of mental illness.

- *Community residential settings*:
    - *Halfway house*: Help individuals who are recovering from various addictions and facilitate their ongoing recovery.
    - *Adult foster care*: Housing for adults who require some assistance with activities of daily living (ADLs) and supervision.
    - *Semi-independent living*: Assistance for adolescents who are unfit for independent living.
    - *Home health care*: Intervention in the natural environment that involves the family and the client in a collaborative relationship.
- *Supportive employment settings*
    - Transitional Employment Program (TEP): Is a program in which staff members work with community businesses to employ individuals in the TEP for six-month intervals.
    - *Prevocational and vocational rehabilitation program*: Helps individuals develop skills that are necessary for jobs and job-like situations.

Client-Centered Clinical Reasoning

People diagnosed with mental health disorders maintain their unique personhood despite any health condition label. Core personality traits often remain intact and manifest in treatment as individual strengths, challenges, personal likes, and dislikes. Individuals make the greatest and most meaningful gains when treatment approaches are based on their unique characteristics and not solely on the symptoms of the disorder; it is important to keep this in mind (Brown, Stoffel, & Munoz, 2011).

Commonly used interventions may include the following (Brown et al., 2011; Early, 2009):

- Social skills
- Physical motor
- Communication
- Leisure
- Relaxation
- Self-awareness
- ADLs
- Instrumental ADLs (IADLs)
- Emotional regulations
- Self-expression
- Cognition
- Social participation
- Role play
- Low impact aerobic
- Assertiveness training
- Woodworking
- Progressive muscle relaxation
- Journaling
- Cooking
- Budgeting
- Anger management
- Writing
- Board games
- Support group

Common Diagnostic Tests

To assist with diagnosing the various disorders, especially with a new onset, the physician may order various tests. Some of the more common tests are used to aid in diagnosis as described in **Table 27-2**.

Medications

Medications are often categorized in association with the disorders and are used to manage the symptoms and behaviors associated with the disorder. The client receiving mental health services may be prescribed various types of medications, as outlined under each diagnosis below.

Table 27-2 Common Diagnostic Tests

Diagnostic Tests	Possible Finding(s)
Blood and urine tests	Used to evaluate overall health and to detect and assess a wide range of disorders, such as infection, kidney disease, diabetes, anemia, thyroid disease, leukemia, and abnormal hormone levels.
Magnetic resonance imaging, computerized tomography, and positron emissions tomography	Used to evaluate and assess a wide range of structural changes and abnormalities in different organs and organ systems, such as tumors, cancer, blood flow to and from organs, and brain and spinal cord disorders (e.g., intracranial bleeding and hydrocephalus), and infection.
X-ray	Used to evaluate overall health and to detect and assess a wide range of disorders, such as bone fractures and other abnormalities of bone, joint abnormalities, ingested items, the size and shape of the heart, changes in the density of certain soft tissues, and specific types of fluid collection.
Electroencephalogram	Used to evaluate and assess electrical activity of the brain and specific types of brain disorders, such as epilepsy, sleep disorders, brain tumors, and coma.

Data from Sadock, Sadock, and Ruiz, 2015.

Occupational Therapy Theories and Frames of Reference in Mental Health

OTs use theory-based principles to inform and guide their treatment approaches. Theories refer to statements or principles that conceptualize and interpret aspects of human occupation and behavior. Theories assist OTs with determining when, how, and why a particular human phenomenon exists.

The term "frame of reference" refers to a specific formulation of concepts, which includes four basic components: (1) the theoretical base or explanation of the concept, (2) the criteria for determining function and dysfunction as it relates to the concept, (3) statements regarding evaluation and assessment tools, and (4) statements regarding intervention methods (Bruce et al., 2002).

Claudia Allen's Cognitive Disabilities Frame of Reference

Allen is an OT who believes cognition affects a person's ability to perform. This frame of reference defines functional ability as the capacity to use mental energy to guide motor and speech performance (Cole, 2012). There are 6 levels and 52 modes (Cole, 2012). Level 1 is the lowest and indicates severe impairment and Level 6 is the highest and indicates little to no impairment. The identification of a level serves as a predictor to current and future functioning. Allen further believes a person is motivated by biological factors such as "can do" (i.e., realistic ability), psychological factors "will do" (i.e., relevance), and social factors "may do" (i.e., possibility) (Cole, 2012). A person will be further impacted by the environment, emotions, activity complexity, and familiarity.

Gary Kielhofner: Model of Human Occupation (MOHO) Frame of Reference

Kielhofner was an OT who hypothesized that humans have the innate drive to explore and master their environment. Doing, exploring, and taking actions help organize and maintain us. Occupational behavior is the outcome of an interaction among the person, the occupational task, and the environment. The process of exploring, creating, and controlling the environment is human occupation. Order occurs when there is exploration, competence, and achievement and disorder occurs when there is helplessness, incompetence, and inefficacy (Cole, 2012).

Lorna Jean King: Sensory Integration

King was an OT who believed that the human brain is innately organized to program a person to seek out stimulation that is organized and beneficial and input from the sensory system can facilitate or inhibit the state of the entire organism. Input from each system influences every other system and the whole organism (Dirette, 2015).

Psychodynamic: Object Relations Frame of Reference

This approach draws from Freud, Jung, and other noted theorists, which describes that a person's psychological construct or their mental state has an effect on occupational and social behaviors (Brown et al., 2011). The approach provides a means of understanding and supporting inner life (e.g., feelings, thoughts, and emotions). This theory provides explanations for conscious and unconscious mental processes, perceptions, thoughts, and feelings, and the relationship with the human and nonhuman environment (Bruce et al., 2002).

Ecological Models

Ecological Models include Person–Environment–Occupation (PEO), Person–Environment–Occupation–Performance (PEOP), and Ecology of Human Performance (EHP). PEO is a conceptual framework developed by a group of Canadian OTs, which focuses on the person, environment, and occupation (Strong et al., 1999). These models view the individual holistically, recognizing the influence that environments have on a client's ability to satisfactorily engage in meaningful tasks. OTs working with mental health populations can utilize these theories to support client-centered interventions, which consider performance in clinical, community, and home environments (Brown et al., 2011).

Client-centered and occupation-based therapies are essential components of all frames of reference, and therefore assessment and intervention. They are delineated as follows:

Client-Centered Treatment Planning

- Human beings possess the ability to direct their growth and development.
- People are likely to act in a confused manner if there is conflict in what they want and what others want.
- If the OT practitioner is nondirective, the client will become more directive.
- People will become more knowledgeable and aware of thoughts and feelings by experiencing them (Early, 2009).

Occupation-Based Treatment Planning

- Achieve maximal engagement in occupations.
- Plan and goals focus on situations and interventions that are important to occupations.
- The OT practitioner uses the actual occupation, occupational task, or activity (Early, 2009).

Evaluation

In order to facilitate a client-centered approach, obtain information regarding the individual's skills, abilities, wants, and needs. Early (2009) provides the following steps for the OT to follow when obtaining and assessing data, and implementing a treatment plan:

- *Data gathering*: Key data include basic demographic information and a medical history, including current diagnosis, values, and interest. Methods include observations, interview, past history, and assessment.
- *Assessment*: Determines client's strengths and challenges or weaknesses based on a specific set of assessments utilized in the evaluation process. Assessments may focus on client factors

and their occupational performance, as well as environmental or contextual factors.

- *Treatment planning*: Develop a plan that includes consideration of past history, deficits, and assets regarding occupations, skills, and other areas of occupational therapy practice including the framework, goals, and plans to meet goals. The plan will also include safety considerations.
- *Precautions and contraindications*: Safety precautions and risk factors are determined by examining a combination of factors. Some diagnoses have inherent deficits associated with the progression of the disorder (e.g., Alzheimer's disease). Sometimes precautions are based on the setting in which treatment is provided (e.g., an inpatient setting versus a community setting).
- *Implement plan*: Present the plan to the client as indicated in the treatment plan.

Psychosocial Disorders

Neurodevelopmental Disorders

Disorders that occur during childhood as a result of environmental conditions, and care during gestation may affect development and/or behaviors that occur before the age of 18. The *DSM-5* lists seven categories of neurodevelopmental disorders. This chapter will present information on the three types most commonly treated in clinical or community settings where mental health is the primary focus: autism spectrum disorders (ASD), attention deficit/hyperactivity disorder (AD/HD), and intellectual disabilities (IDs) (American Psychiatric Association, 2013b). Neurodevelopmental disorders addressed in settings where the focus is primarily on education or physical dysfunction are covered in the pediatric chapter content.

Autism Spectrum Disorder

Description: ASD presents with persistent difficulties in social communications and social interaction (American Psychiatric Association, 2013a). Clinical presentation and diagnostic criteria are described in **Table 27-3**.

Pathology

- *Genetic*: ASD is an inherited disorder through the genes (Brown et al., 2011).

Table 27-3 ASD Clinical Presentation/Diagnostic Criteria

Signs/Symptoms	Description
Symptoms	Absence or failure of back and forth conversation and the ability to initiate or respond to social interactions.
Nonverbal communication	Deficit in understanding body language and lack of eye contact, facial expressions, and nonverbal communication.
Relationships	Deficits in developing, maintaining, and understanding relation, and absence of interest in others.
At least two of the following	
Movement	Stereotypical or repetitive motions (e.g., lining up toys, repeating the same phrase, echolalia, and idiosyncratic phrases).
Repetition	Insistence on sameness, ritualistic patterns, and extreme distress with changes.
Fixation	Highly restricted, fixated interest, strong attachment, or fixation on unusual objects.
Sensory	Hyper or hyporeactive to sensory stimuli or unusual interest in sensory aspects of the environment. Adverse reaction to different sounds and textures, and fascination with lights and movement.
Occurrence	Symptoms occur during early development. Symptoms significantly impair social and occupational performances. Disturbances are not better explained by other conditions.

Data from American Psychiatric Association, 2013a.

- *Neuroanatomical*: Brain volume and hemispheres of the brain show an increase in volume (Brown et al., 2011).
- *Immunizations*: Measles, mumps, and rubella vaccine have been associated with ASD, yet no scientific evidence supports the connection (American Psychiatric Association, 2013b).
- *Prenatal and perinatal care*: Prenatal care and/or abnormalities that occur during birth (American Psychiatric Association, 2013a).

Screening and Assessments

- *Adolescent Sensory Profile*: Used to determine client's sensory processing patterns and effects on functional performance (Vaughn, 2014).
- *Bayley Scales of Infant Development*: Measures fine and gross motor skills, cognition, behavior, and social emotional development (Stultz, 2014).
- *Child Occupational Self-Assessment*: Evaluates how children describe their own perceptions about occupational competency and values (Brown et al., 2011).
- *Occupational Performance History Interview*: Evaluates life history in the areas of work, play, and self-care performance (Brown et al., 2011).
- *Scales of Independent Behavior—Revised*: Assesses adaptive and maladaptive behavior (Stultz, 2014).
- *School Function Assessment*: Evaluates functional task performance in schools (Stultz, 2014).
- *Sensory Processing Measure*: Measures sensory functioning in home, school, and community (Stultz, 2014).

Interventions and Impact on Occupational Performance

Children with this disorder typically have difficulties in areas of occupation, performance skills, and client factors. Particularity in performing basic ADLs, interacting or socializing with others, interpreting environmental stimuli, communicating with others, and ritualistic behaviors that significantly impact school performance (Brown et al., 2011). Interventions for autism are described in **Table 27-4**.

Attention Deficit/Hyperactivity Disorders

- *Description*: AD/HD presents with persistent inattention or hyperactivity with impulsive behaviors (American Psychiatric Association, 2013b).
- *Pathology*: Although the etiology of AD/HD is not certain, common causes thought to contribute to the development of this condition include genetics, neurotransmitter abnormalities, prenatal exposure to maternal toxins, and low birth weight (American Psychiatric Association, 2013b).
- *Clinical presentation/diagnostic criteria*: AD/HD is classified by six or more symptoms, persisting for at least six months, with negative effects on social,

Table 27-4 Autism Interventions: Therapeutic Use of Self, Occupations, and Activities

Psychosocial interventions	Social skills training: Approaches to facilitate development of social skills through practice, role play, modeling, and coaching.
	Managing communication: Activities to improve communication skills through education, social groups, and the use of technology.
	Manage sensory processing and integration: Ayres Sensory Integration approaches to organize and regulate sensory input.
	Perceptual motor skills: Facilitate development of perceptual motor skills by incorporating tasks that require fine motor, visual motor, visual perception, and bilateral coordination.
	Managing self-care: Help establish daily routines around performance of self-care tasks.
	Managed supportive employment: Individualize career planning to match client preferences and to accommodate the client's social, cognitive, and performance skills.
Preparatory methods and tasks	Age-related activities.
	Supportive, structured, and least distracting environment.
	Brief 1:1 play and art therapy.
	Match shapes or colors.
	Shred/rip paper.
	Use soft cloth to make circles on a table.

Data from Early, 2009.

occupational, and academic activities, and 5 or more for teens 17 or older (American Psychiatric Association, 2013b). See **Table 27-5** for signs and symptoms.

Screening and Assessments

- *Emotional Problems Scale*: Assesses emotional and behavioral challenges in individuals with mild intellectual impairment (Integrated Assessment LLC, 2015).
- *Functional Independence Measure (FIM)*: Measures independent performance in ADLs, mobility, and communication (Asher, 2014).
- *Matson Evaluation of Social Skills in Individuals with Severe Mental Retardation (MESSIER)*: Measures social skills of people with severe developmental delays (Asher, 2014).

Table 27-5 AD/HD Signs and Symptoms

Signs/Symptoms	Description
Inattention	Overlooks or misses details
	Difficulty remaining focused
	Mind seems elsewhere
	Starts task and loses focus
	Messy and disorganized work does not meet deadlines
	Avoids and dislikes tasks requiring mental effort
	Loses items needed for a task
	Distracted by extraneous stimuli
	Forgets daily activities
Hyperactivity/ impulsivity	Fidgets and taps hands or feet
	Leaves place when he/she should be seated
	Runs or climbs or feels inner restlessness
	Unable to play quietly
	Uncomfortable being still for extended periods of time
	Talks excessively
	Blurts out answers before completion of a question
	Difficulty waiting for his/her turn
	Interrupts or intrudes on others

Data from American Psychiatric Association, 2013a.

Interventions and Impact on Occupational Performance

Children with this disorder may demonstrate extreme difficulty with socialization, academics, emotional regulations, and performance patterns, habits, and routines (Early, 2009); interventions are described in **Table 27-6**.

Intellectual Disabilities

- *Description*: Intellectual and adaptive functioning deficits in conceptual, social, and practical domains occur during development, resulting in the need for lifelong assistance and support (American Psychiatric Association, 2013b).
- *Pathology*: Limitations in intellectual and adaptive function is evident in childhood. Pre- and perinatal

Table 27-6 AD/HD Interventions: Therapeutic Use of Self, Occupations, and Activities

Therapeutic use of self	Obtain the client's attention (e.g., say his/her name loudly)
	Touch gently, yet firmly on the arm or the shoulder; with caution
	Pay attention to nonverbal cues
	Speak positively in a matter-of-fact and calming tone
Psychosocial interventions	Social skills and assertiveness training
	Managing self-care and occupational roles
	Managing attention
	Supportive employment
	Perceptual motor skills
	Coping and stress management skills
	Training in safety and emergency responses
Preparatory methods and task	Simple familiar age-related activities
	Structured tasks with sequencing steps
	Creative and repetitive activities or tasks
	Incorporating classical music or the client's favorite tune

Data from Early, 2009.

factors have been linked to severe and profound deficits in intellectual development. People with this diagnosis often have comorbid developmental or medical disorders (American Psychiatric Association, 2013b).

- *Clinical presentation*: The individual must meet all three criteria as outlined in **Table 27-7** for clinical presentation and **Table 27-8** for severity levels.

Medications for IDs: Mood stabilizers, stimulants, and antipsychotics may be prescribed; however, caution is exercised when prescribing antipsychotics for children. The purpose of commonly prescribed medications is as follows (Krumbach, 2014):

- *Risperdal*: An antipsychotic commonly used to treat aggression.
- *Ritalin*: A stimulant commonly used to treat inattention.
- *Amphetamines*: A stimulant commonly used to treat AD/HD (e.g., Adderall©).

Complications and side effects: Amphetamines may result in withdrawal reactions, especially if used regularly for a long period of time or in high doses. In such cases,

Table 27-7 ID Clinical Presentation/Diagnostic Criteria

Signs/Symptoms	Description
Intellectual	Deficits in reasoning, problem-solving, planning, abstract thinking, judgment, and academics, as well as experiences with learning are confirmed by both clinical assessment and individualized standardized intelligence testing.
Adaptive functioning	Deficits in adaptive functioning that result in a failure to meet developmental and sociocultural standards for personal independence and responsibility, and interfere with one or more daily life activity.
Occurrence	Onset of the deficit during a developmental period.

Data from American Psychiatric Association, 2013a.

withdrawal symptoms (e.g., severe tiredness, sleep challenges, and mood changes) may occur if medication use stops suddenly. Abnormal drug-seeking behavior (i.e., addiction) increases the risk if there is a history of alcohol or drug use (Sadock et al., 2015).

Childhood neurodevelopmental precautions: Children with IDs may have challenges with ambulation, seizures, and other chronic physical conditions, which need to be considered during the clinical assessment and intervention planning process (Rogers, 2010).

Screening and Assessments

- *Emotional Problems Scale*: Assesses emotional and behavioral challenges in individuals with mild intellectual impairment (Integrated Assessment LLC, 2015).
- *Family Stress and Coping Interview*: A specific interview tool to obtain information about coping and family dynamics (Brown et al., 2011).
- *FIM*: Measures independent performance in ADLs, mobility, and communication (Asher, 2014).
- *MESSIER*: Measures social skills of people with severe developmental delays (Asher, 2014).
- *Dynamic occupational therapy cognitive assessment for children (DOTCA-Ch)*: Assesses a child's learning potential (Asher, 2014).

Interventions and Impact on Occupational Performance

Children with this disorder may have mild to profound involvement. Children classified as having a more mild spectrum demonstrate difficulty in areas of occupation

Table 27-8 ID Specifiers and Severity Levels

	Specifiers/Severity Level		
Severity	Conceptual Deficits	Social Deficit	Practical Deficits
Mild	May develop reading and math skills with limited comprehension.	Difficulty in accurately reading social cues and assessing risk.	Difficulty assessing well-being and performing advanced ADLs.
Moderate	Language and learning develops slowly, and typically does not advance past elementary level.	Limited social judgment and decision making.	Requires extensive training for extended periods to perform and may demonstrate maladaptive disruptive behaviors.
Severe	Diminished or absent understanding of written language or concepts of time, numbers, or money.	Spoken language vocabulary and grammar are greatly limited.	Cannot make responsible decisions and requires supervision at all times for ADLs. At risk for self-injury.
Profound	May have sensory and motor deficits and may perform simple tasks using objects in a goal-directed manner.	Little to no understanding of symbolic speech or gestures. Engages in mostly nonverbal communication. Enjoys relationships with known family or caregivers.	Totally dependent on caregivers with some isolated functions (i.e., with great assistance). Typically enjoys music, movies, and physical activity. Maladaptive behaviors may be present.

Data from American Psychiatric Association, 2013a.

such as education, work, and social participation, performance skills, cognition, communication, and social skills. Children classified as having symptoms more in line with the more severe end of the spectrum will have more profound involvement. The child with profound intellectual delay will likely also show difficulty in toileting, motor control, and walking, which may affect health with associated and secondary conditions (Brown et al., 2011). See **Table 27-9** for interventions.

Childhood Neurodevelopmental Referrals and Discharge Considerations

OTs may pay close attention to changes in mental status. For example, mental health concerns such as conduct and anxiety disorders are prevalent with individuals diagnosed with ID and must be considered during the discharge process (Brown et al., 2011). Additional consideration should be directed on adultlike roles and work (Brown et al., 2011). OTs are uniquely skilled to assess, implement services, and/or make recommendations to address mental health issues and vocational strategies.

Disruptive, Impulse Control, and Conduct Disorders

Conduct (Behavior) Disorders

- *Description*: A repetitive and persistent pattern of behavior in which basic rights of others, societal norms or rules are violated prior to age 10 (*DSM-5*, 2013).
- *Pathology*: Exposure to secondhand smoke has been linked to this condition. Abnormalities in brain function have been detected with a decreased dopamine response and disruptions in frontal lobe activity. Genetic factors are shown to contribute to the development of this disorder (American Psychiatric Association, 2013b).
- *Clinical presentation/diagnostic criteria*: Individuals must meet at least three criteria in the past 12 months as outlined in **Table 27-10**.

Table 27-9 ID Interventions: Therapeutic Use of Self, Occupations, and Activities

Therapeutic use of self	Obtain the client's attention
	Touch gently, yet firmly on the arm or the shoulder; with caution
	Pay attention to nonverbal cues
	Speak slowly and positively in a matter-of-fact and calming tone
Psychosocial interventions	Social skills training
	Managing self-care
	Managed supportive employment
	Perceptual motor skills
Preparatory methods and task	Modify the environment to minimize stimuli
	Use like environments when performing skills
	Sensory stimulating activities

Data from Early, 2009.

Table 27-10 Conduct (Behavior) Disorder Clinical Signs and Symptoms

Signs/Symptoms	Description
Aggression	Bullies, threatens, or intimidates others
	Initiates physical fights
	Has used a weapon
	Physically cruel to people
	Physically cruel to animals
	Steals
	Forces others into sexual acts
Destructive	Deliberately sets fires
	Deliberately destroys others' items without the use of fire
Deceitfulness or theft	Breaks into someone else's house
	Lies to obtain favors or avoid obligations
	Steals items without confrontation
Serious violations	Stays out all night before the age of 13 despite parental limits
	Has run away from home overnight at least twice, or once for a longer period of time
	Truant from school before the age of 13

Data from American Psychiatric Association, 2013a.

Screening and Assessments

- *Bay Area Functional Performance Evaluation*: Assesses how clients may function in task-oriented and social settings (Asher, 2014).
- *Adolescence Role Assessment*: Semistructured interview to evaluate the client's involvement in occupational roles over time (Asher, 2014).
- *Children's Assessment of Participation and Enjoyment & Preferences for Activities of Children (CAPE & PAC)*: Measures participation and engagement in activities (Asher, 2014).

Interventions and Impact on Occupational Performance

A client presenting with a conduct disorder will display antisocial behaviors that may include criminal activity, and therapy will affect all domains and aspects of occupational functioning. Clients may find it difficult to follow protocols for classroom work and adjust to new settings (Brown et al., 2011). See **Table 27-11** for interventions.

Oppositional Defiant Disorder (ODD)

- *Description*: Pattern of angry, negativistic, and defiant behavior lasting six months.

Table 27-11 Conduct (Behavior) Disorder Interventions: Therapeutic Use of Self, Occupations, and Activities

Therapeutic use of self	Calm, firm, and nonjudgmental explanation of behaviors
	Remove from a session if unwanted behaviors do not cease
	Firm and matter-of-fact communication
Psychosocial interventions	Social skills training
	Managing self-care
	Personal behavior and self-regulation
	Anger management and conflict resolution
	Assertiveness training
Preparatory methods and task	Avoid physical contact
	Clarify relationships and expectations
	Use vigorous gross motor exercises (e.g., kneading clay)

Data from Early, 2009.

- *Pathology*: Deficits and injuries to the parts of the brain may contribute to patterns of behavior. Pre and perinatal factors, as well as familial and environmental triggers have been correlated with this disorder (American Psychiatric Association, 2013a).
- *Clinical presentation/diagnostic criteria*: Must meet at least four symptoms for six months as outlined in **Table 27-12**.

Disruptive, impulse control, and *conduct disorder precautions*: When a person is diagnosed with disruptive behavior disorders, a sense of control is threatened that may present with increased aggression, which may be triggered by change (e.g., environment and expectations) (Brown et al., 2011).

Screening and Assessments

- *Parent–Child Relationship Inventory*: Measures attitudes and quality of the parent–child relationship (Asher, 2014).
- *Child Behavior Checklist*: A reported record of a child's competencies and challenges (ASEBA, 2015).
- *CAPE & PAC*: Measures participation and engagement in activities (Asher, 2014).
- *Coping Inventory*: Measures adaptive and maladaptive coping skills (Asher, 2014).

Interventions and Impact on Occupational Performance

A client presenting with ODD typically displays hostile defiant behaviors, which affect social, academic, and

Table 27-12 ODD Clinical Signs and Symptoms

Signs/Symptoms	Description
Angry/irritable mood	Loses temper
	Touchy and/or easily annoyed
	Angry and/or disrespectful
Argumentative/ defiant	Argues with authority figures and/or adults
	Defies and/or refuses to comply with requests and/or rules from authority figures
	Deliberately annoys others
	Blames others
Vindictiveness	Spiteful on at least two occasions

Data from American Psychiatric Association, 2013a.

Table 27-13 ODD Intervention: Therapeutic Use of Self, Occupations, and Activities

Therapeutic use of self	Calm, firm, and nonjudgmental explanation of behaviors
	Remove from a session if unwanted behaviors will not cease
	Avoid power struggles
Psychosocial interventions	Social skills training
	Managing self-care
	Personal behavior and self-regulation
	Anger management and conflict resolution
	Reward-based interventions
Preparatory methods and task	Minimize environmental distractions
	Clarify relationships and expectations
	Relaxation techniques
	Incorporate the child's interests

Data from Early, 2009.

occupational functioning when their sense of control is threatened (Brown et al., 2011). See **Table 27-13** for interventions.

Disruptive, Impulse Control, and Conduct Disorders: Referrals and Discharge Considerations

Children diagnosed with disruptive behavior disorders are often challenged and left with decreased self-esteem. Remain mindful that skill deficits are more pronounced in times of stress and may not accurately reflect the child's abilities. As the child progresses in age and skill level, the child may be assessed for work function (Brown et al., 2011) and may benefit from a referral to vocational rehabilitation.

Bipolar and Depressive Disorders

This group of clinical conditions is characterized by a loss of control and sense of great distress. The *DSM-5* has two broad categories: bipolar and related disorders (i.e., seven types) and depressive disorders (i.e., eight types) (American Psychiatric Association, 2013a). This section will focus on the three major types of mood disorders

primarily seen in occupational therapy practice. They are as follows:

- *Bipolar I (raging)*: Characterized by manic and major depressive episodes (American Psychiatric Association, 2013b).
- *Bipolar II*: Characterized by past or current episodes of hypomania and depression (American Psychiatric Association, 2013b).
- *Major depression*: Characterized by marked diminished pleasure in all or most ADLs (Sadock et al., 2015).
- *Pathology*: The pathophysiology of bipolar and major depression has not been determined but a significant genetic component, as well as biochemical, psychodynamic, and environmental factors have been identified (American Psychiatric Association, 2013b). See **Table 27-14** for clinical presentation.

Bipolar medication management: Medications are used to reduce manic symptoms and stabilize mood in individuals with bipolar disorders. Sadock et al. (2015) report common bipolar medications and side effects as follows:

- *Lithium*: A mood stabilizer primarily used to treat episodes of manic depression. Common side effects include weight gain, nausea, slow cognitive function, polyuria (i.e., excessive urine output), polydipsia (i.e., abnormally great thirst), tremors, or taste of metal.
- *Depakote*: An anticonvulsant used as a mood stabilizer to treat bipolar disorder.
- *Risperdal*: An antipsychotic medicine used to treat schizophrenia and symptoms of bipolar disorder.
- *Anticonvulsants*: Anticonvulsant drugs used as mood stabilizers to treat or prevent bipolar disorder.

Depression medication management: Antidepressants elevate and stabilize mood. Sadock et al. (2015) provide a list of commonly prescribed medications for depression below:

- Monoamine oxidase inhibitors and tricyclic antidepressants may be effective in the treatment of depression; however, dangerous side effects typically preclude their use.
- Serotonin–norepinephrine reuptake inhibitors (SNRIs) are antidepressants used to relieve symptoms of depression.
- Cymbalta is an SNRI used to treat depression, as well as pain-associated peripheral nerve pain and fibromyalgia.

Table 27-14 Bipolar and Depressive Disorder Clinical Presentations/Diagnostic Criteria

Episode	Description
Mania	A distinct period of abnormally persistent elated, expansive or irritable mood, or goal direct activity or action lasting one week, that requires hospitalization
	Presence of three or more signs, or four if only an irritable mood is present
	Inflated self-esteem or grandiosity
	Decreased need for sleep
	More talkative than usual and pressure to talk
	Flight of ideas
	Distractibility
	Psychomotor agitation—increases activity
	Excessive involvement in activities with high potential for harm (e.g., sexual)
Hypomanic	A distinct period of abnormally persistent, elated, expansive or irritable mood, or goal-directed activity or action lasting four consecutive days
	Presence of three or more signs, or four if only an irritable mood is present
	The disorder is not severe enough to cause disturbance in social or occupational functioning
	May not require hospitalization
Depression	Decrease in mood, feelings of sadness or emptiness for the majority of the day; nearly every day
	Presence of five or more of the following signs/symptoms: <ul><li>Crying episodes</li><li>Decreased interest or pleasure in almost all activity</li><li>Weight loss</li><li>Daily insomnia or hypersomnia</li><li>Psychomotor agitation or retardation</li><li>Fatigue or loss of energy</li><li>Feelings of worthlessness or excessive guilt</li><li>Diminished ability to think or concentrate or indecisiveness</li><li>Recurrent thoughts of death</li></ul>

Data from American Psychiatric Association, 2013a.

- Wellbutrin, Lexapro, Paxil, and Zoloft are selective serotonin reuptake inhibitors (SSRIs) used to treat depression.

SNRIs and SSRIs may cause insomnia, drowsiness, and nausea, which typically subside after four to six weeks;

however, changes in sex drive (i.e., decreased sex drive, lack of orgasm, and delayed ejaculation) may occur and last longer and significantly impact medication compliance (Sadock et al., 2015).

Bipolar and depressive disorder precautions: Clients may be at a higher risk for suicide and alcohol use, and caregivers may be equally stricken with the stigma of mental illness, as their loved one has been diagnosed with a mental health disorder (Brown et al., 2011).

Screening and Assessments

- *MOHOST*: Addresses client's engagement in occupation (Asher, 2014).
- *ACL test*: Quick assessment of the client's learning and problem-solving skills (Asher, 2014).
- *Bay Area Functional Performance Evaluation*: Assesses how clients may function in task-oriented and social settings (Asher, 2014).

Interventions and Impact on Occupational Performance

A client diagnosed with a mood disorder may have significant challenges in the areas of occupation and performance skills in school, work, home, and the community. People with mood disorders may also see interference in co-occupational roles such as caring for and developing a bond with a child (Brown et al., 2011). See **Table 27-15** for interventions.

Bipolar and Depressive Disorder Referrals and Discharge Considerations

Referrals and recommendations may be appropriate for a peer support person. If the client has the required skill set, encourage clients to engage in supportive social activities and or supportive work (Bonjuklian, 2014).

Schizophrenia Spectrum Disorders

- *Description*: Schizophrenia spectrum disorders include a group of clinical conditions characterized by delusions, hallucinations, disorganized speech, and behavior, as well as social and occupational dysfunctions. The *DSM-5* lists eight types of

Table 27-15 Bipolar and Depressive Disorder Interventions: Therapeutic Use of Self, Occupations, and Activities

Bipolar and Depressive Symptoms	Intervention Approaches
Depression	Initially may require one-to-one care
	Match the client's tempo
	Accept the client's feelings
Mania	Be aware of flattery and grandiosity
	Focus on behaviors and minimize praise
	Use a calm and matter-of-fact style of communication
	Establish and enforce limits
Psychosocial interventions	Social skills training
	Medication management
	Managing self-care, habits, routines, and roles
	Managed and supportive employment
	Executive functioning and perceptual skills
	Emotional regulation
	Values clarification
	Time, stress, and money management
	Reestablish regular habits and routines
	Help the client assess self-worth positively
	Help the client understand the disease process
Preparatory methods and task	Gross motor exercises
	Client-centered activities from limited choices (e.g., a tedious task)
Depression	Help the client assess self-worth positively
	Structured, short-term, simple, successful, and familiar activities
	Use predictable materials
	Reestablish regular habits and routines
	Allow verbal expression
	Crafts (e.g., mosaics, leatherwork, and woodworking)
Mania	Minimize environmental distractions
	Semistructured, short-term, simple, successful, and familiar activities
	Crafts (e.g., copper tooling, beading, and leatherwork)

Data from Early, 2009.

schizophrenia (American Psychiatric Association, 2013b). This section will focus on the two types most commonly seen in occupational therapy (i.e., schizophrenia and schizoaffective disorder).

- *Pathology*: No single cause has been identified but vulnerability to these conditions has been linked to genetic mutations and a positive family history for the disorder. Current research focuses on the role of brain chemistry and physiology on psychotic disorders (American Psychiatric Association, 2013b).

Schizophrenia

A severe brain disorder characterized by delusions, hallucinations or disorganized speech, and behavior and/or social/emotional withdrawal (American Psychiatric Association, 2013b; Sadock et al., 2015). Continuously diminished functioning and cognitive changes are noted within a six-month time frame. **Table 27-16** outlines the clinical presentation for schizophrenia.

Schizoaffective

- *Description*: Onset typically presents with uninterrupted periods of illness where there is a major episode of depression or mania associated

Table 27-16 Schizophrenia Clinical Presentation/ Diagnostic Criteria

Signs/Symptoms	Description
Cognitive/perceptual	Two or more of the following for a 1-month period of time: • Delusions (i.e., a false belief despite evidence to the contrary) • Hallucinations (i.e., the perception of something not present) • Disorganized-incoherent speech • Disorganized behaviors and catatonia • Diminished emotional expression (i.e., negative symptoms)
Occupational functioning	Decline in normal performance in one or more of the following areas: • Work • Interpersonal • Self-care

Data from American Psychiatric Association, 2013a.

with schizophrenia. Delusions or hallucinations are present for two or more weeks, and major mood episodes are present in the majority of clients (American Psychiatric Association, 2013b). Continuously diminished functioning and cognitive changes are noted within a six-month time frame. **Table 27-17** outlines the clinical presentation for a schizoaffective disorder.

Medications for schizophrenia *spectrum disorders*: Antipsychotic medications are designed to eliminate distorted thoughts; the first- and second-generation medications are presented below (Sadock et al., 2015).

Typical first-generation medications include the following:

- *Haldol*: Used to reduce hallucinations, aggression, and negative thoughts (e.g., harming others)
- *Prolixin*: Used to reduce hallucinations, delusions, and inappropriate behaviors

Table 27-17 Schizoaffective Clinical Presentation/ Diagnostic Criteria

Signs/Symptoms	Description
Cognitive/perceptual	Two or more of the following for a 1-month time period: • Delusions • Hallucinations • Disorganized-incoherent speech • Disorganized behavior(s) and catatonia • Diminished emotional expression (i.e., negative symptoms)
Functioning	Decline in normal performance in one or more of the following areas: • Work • Interpersonal • Self-care
Bipolar type	The presence of both manic and depressive symptoms
	A distinct period of abnormally persistent elated, expansive or irritable mood, or absence of goal-directed activity
Major depression type	The presence of depressive symptoms
	Decrease in mood, feelings of sadness or emptiness for most of the day; nearly every day

Data from American Psychiatric Association, 2013a.

Atypical antipsychotic second-generation medications include the following:

- *Zyprexa*: Used to reduce hallucinations and improve cognition
- *Risperdal*: Used to reduce hallucinations and improve cognition
- *Seroquel*: Used to reduce hallucinations and improve concentration
- *Abilify*: Used to reduce hallucinations and improve concentration

Common side effects may include the following:

- *Typical*: Sedation, sun sensitivity, dry mouth, constipation, and orthostatic hypotension. Movement disorders: akathisia, dystonia (i.e., sustained muscle contraction) and tardive dyskinesia.
- *Atypical*: Weight gain, diabetes, movement disorders, sedation, cardiac effects, dry mouth, constipation, and blurred vision.
- *Schizophrenia spectrum disorder precautions*: Requires maximal supervision due to risk of a client harming self or others when actively delusional or hallucinating. A client may require close supervision to safely complete tasks due to poor attention span, memory skills, and inability to make appropriate decisions based on information in the environment (Sadock et al., 2015).

Screening and Assessments

Various assessments can be used to gather information on clients with schizophrenia spectrum disorder. These assessments are as follows (Asher, 2014):

- *Draw-A-Person Test*: Psycho projective personality test to screen for emotional or behavior disorders.
- *ACL test*: Quick assessment of client's learning and problem-solving skills.
- *Bay Area Functional Performance Evaluation*: Assesses how clients may function in task-oriented and social settings.

Interventions and Impact on Occupational Performance

A client diagnosed with a psychotic disorder such as schizophrenia may show a progressive decline in areas of occupation, particularly basic ADLs, work, and leisure, as well as an alteration in sensory perception and all

Table 27-18 Schizophrenia Spectrum Disorder Intervention: Therapeutic Use of Self, Occupations, and Activities

Therapeutic use of self	Redirect attention to a neutral topic
	Reality-based success activities
	Do not make quick movements or gestures or stand behind the client
	Calm, firm, and supportive tone
	Frequent concrete feedback
Psychosocial interventions	Social skills training and interaction
	Develop habits and routines
	Manage self-care
	Manage supportive employment
	Cognitive and perceptual motor skills
	Work and productivity
Preparatory methods and tasks	Structured, simple, and suited to intellectual ability
	Success-oriented with use of predictable materials
	Gross motor exercises
	Controlled and stable environment that facilitate interaction with others in real-life activities
	Avoid activities that may reinforce non-reality thinking or increase frustrations and fears
	Activities with music or dance, television, eating, and crafts using wood, leather, or metal

Data from Early, 2009.

other performance skills, due to changes in cognitive impairment. In addition, there may be noted changes in client factors, performance patterns, and activity demands (Brown et al., 2011). See **Table 27-18** for interventions.

Schizophrenia Spectrum Disorder Referrals and Discharge Considerations

People diagnosed with psychotic or mood disorders are likely to require community supports to minimize repeated hospitalizations such as Assertive Community Treatment, partial day hospitalization, and/or psychosocial rehabilitation clubhouses in addition to community mental health services and family psycho education. Furthermore, people may require assistive living such as adult foster care or assisted living residential care (Brown et al., 2011), or a social support program, (i.e., peer support specialist and supportive employment) (Bonjuklian, 2014).

Personality Disorders

- *Description*: Personality disorders are an enduring pattern of inner experiences and behaviors that deviates from what is expected in society and may include areas of cognition, emotional regulations, interpersonal relations, and controlling one's behavior (American Psychiatric Association, 2013a).
- *Pathology*: Various factors contribute to the pathology of personality disorders; these factors are as follows (Brown et al., 2011):
  - *Genetics*: A family member likely has the same or a different personality disorder.
  - *Biological*: May be related to hormonal changes and/or overactive or physiological abnormalities in the amygdala.
  - *Environmental factors*: High reactivity to stimuli has been shown to be a risk factor. Childhood trauma, verbal abuse, and impaired social relationships may contribute to the development of this disorder.
  - *Personality disorder precautions*: The client will act out by demonstrating extreme quick unpredictable behaviors that often disrupt or cause attention to be focused on them in an effort to self-soothe. The client is also at a greater risk for self-harming (i.e., cutting, biting, burning, picking, and self-medicating behaviors). The client may discontinue sessions abruptly and disturb the effectiveness of group sessions (Brown et al., 2011).

Cluster A personality disorders: Includes paranoid, schizoid, and schizotypal diagnoses and is characterized as odd and eccentric behaviors with discomfort in interpersonal relations (American Psychiatric Association, 2013a). See **Table 27-19** for clinical presentation.

Cluster B personality disorders: Includes antisocial, borderline, narcissistic, and histrionic diagnoses and are characterized as dramatic, emotional, and erratic (American Psychiatric Association, 2013a). See **Table 27-20** for clinical presentation.

Table 27-19 Cluster A Personality Disorders Clinical Presentation/Diagnostic Criteria

Types	Description
Paranoid	Pervasive distrust and suspiciousness of others beginning in early adulthood
	The behaviors are present in a variety of contexts as indicated by four or more of the following: • Preoccupied with unjust doubts about others • Reluctant to confide in others due to fear • Reads hidden meanings into remarks • Persistently bears grudges and/or is unforgiving • Perceives attacks on his or her character • Has recurrent suspicions without sufficient basis or justification
Schizoid	A pervasive pattern of detachment from social relations and restricted range of emotions
	Indicated by four or more of the following: • Neither desires nor enjoys close relationships • Almost always chooses solitary activities • Has little or no interest in having sexual experiences • Takes pleasure in few, if any, activities • Lacks close friends or confidants • Appears indifferent to praise or criticism • Shows emotional coldness or detachment

Data from American Psychiatric Association, 2013a.

Cluster C personality disorders: Includes avoidant and dependent, and obsessive–compulsive diagnoses described as anxious and fearful (American Psychiatric Association, 2013a). See **Table 27-21** for clinical presentation.

Screening and Assessments

- *COPM*: Designed to measure a client's perception of their occupational performance over time (Asher, 2014).
- *COTE*: For use in mental health settings to help identify client behaviors that impact occupational performance (Schell, Gillen, & Scaffa, 2014).
- *Bay Area Functional Performance Evaluation*: Assesses how clients may function in task-oriented and social settings (Asher, 2014).

Interventions and Impact on Occupational Performance

A client presenting with any of the identified personality disorders will likely have difficulty with occupational

Table 27-20 Cluster B Personality Disorders Clinical Presentation/Diagnostic Criteria

Types	Description
Antisocial	A pervasive pattern of disregard for and violation of the rights of others. The individual is at least 18 years old with evidence of conduct disorder before age 15
	Displays three or more of the following behaviors: • Failure to conform to social norms • Repeated lying • Impulsivity • Irritability and aggression • Reckless disregard for safety of self or others • Consistent irresponsibility • Lack of remorse or rationalize hurting others
Borderline	A pervasive pattern of instability in interpersonal relationships and self-image beginning during early adulthood
	Presents in a variety of contexts in five or more of the following: • Frantic effort to avoid real or imagined abandonment • Extreme idealizing or devaluing of relations • Markedly and persistent unstable self-image • Impulsivity that has potential for self-harm • Recurrent suicidal gestures, threats, or mutilation • Intense moods • Chronic feeling of emptiness • Intense anger or inability to control anger • Transient stress-related paranoia or disassociation

Data from American Psychiatric Association, 2013a.

performance including I/ADLs, work, social participation, communication, and leisure. Interventions will most likely focus on emotional regulations and coping, as well as beliefs and values (Brown et al., 2011). See **Table 27-22** for interventions.

Personality Disorder Referrals and Discharge Considerations

Mindfulness is a significant intervention when working with people diagnosed with borderline personality disorder. Supportive employment may also be

Table 27-21 Cluster C Personality Disorders Clinical Presentation/Diagnostic Criteria

Types	Description
Avoidant	A pervasive pattern of social inhibition, feelings of inadequacy, and hypersensitivity to negativity
	Indicated by four or more of the following:
	• Avoids occupational activities that involve significant interactions
	• Is unwilling to get involved with others unless certain he or she will be liked
	• Shows restraint within intimate relationships for fear of being shamed
	• Preoccupied with being criticized or rejected
	• Is inhibited in new interpersonal situations
	• Views self as socially inept, unappealing, or inferior
	• Reluctant to take personal risk
Dependent	A pervasive and excessive need to be taken care of that leads to submissive and clinging behaviors
	Indicated by five or more of the following:
	• Has difficulty making everyday decision without excessive advice
	• Needs others to assume responsibility for most areas of his or her life
	• Has difficulty expressing disagreement with others
	• Goes to extreme lengths to obtain support
	• Feels uncomfortable or helpless when alone
	• Urgently seeks another relationship when a close relationship ends
	• Unrealistically preoccupied with fears of being left to take care of self

Data from American Psychiatric Association, 2013a.

helpful in assisting with and maintaining employment (Brown et al., 2011).

Anxiety and Stress-Related Disorders

- *Description*: Anxiety and stress-related disorders are typically due to a response to an external traumatic event that interferes with a variety of

Table 27-22 Personality Disorder Interventions: Therapeutic Use of Self, Occupations, and Activities

Therapeutic use of self	Build rapport through trust, respect, and empathy
	Establish firm limits and consistent expectations
	Provide realistic appraisal and feedback
Psychosocial interventions	Social and interpersonal skills training
	Symptom reduction
	Manage fear(s)
	Emotional regulation
	Relaxation exercise (e.g., yoga)
	Assertive communication
Preparatory methods and task	Safe and comfortable environments
	Success-oriented activities
	Role playing

Data from Early, 2009.

social and work functions (American Psychiatric Association, 2013a).

- *Pathology*: Studies show genetic, structural and functional neuroanatomical, neurotransmitter, hormonal, cognitive, psychological, and environmental factors may contribute to the development of anxiety and stress-related disorders. Results of the stress response and underlying factors are additionally activated by a perceived threat (Brown et al., 2011).

Anxiety Disorders

Generalized Anxiety

Characterized by excessive fear, anxiety, and/or worry about a number of events or activities for a time period of six months or more, in which the client may be exposed to scrutiny (American Psychiatric Association, 2013b). See **Table 27-23** for clinical presentation.

Social Anxiety

- *Description*: Marked fear or anxiety about one or more social situations for six months or more, in which the client may be exposed to scrutiny (American Psychiatric Association, 2013a). See **Table 27-24** for clinical presentation.

Table 27-23 Generalized Anxiety Clinical Presentation/Diagnostic Criteria

Signs/Symptoms	Description
Thinking/physical	Has difficulty controlling anxiety with three or more of the following: • Restlessness or feeling excited, anxious, or on edge • Easily fatigued • Difficulty concentrating • Irritability • Muscle tension • Sleep disturbance (e.g., difficulty falling or staying asleep or unsatisfied sleep)
Functioning	Impaired social and occupational functioning

Data from American Psychiatric Association, 2013a.

Table 27-24 Social Anxiety Clinical Presentation/Diagnostic Criteria

Signs/Symptoms	Description
Fear beliefs	Beliefs will be negatively evaluated or act in a way that will not be accepted by others
	Fear is out of proportion of an actual threat or situation
	Avoids situations or endures them with extreme anxiety or fear
Functioning	Impaired social, occupational, or other functioning

Data from American Psychiatric Association, 2013a.

Panic Disorder

- *Description*: Commonly seen as an abrupt surge of intense fear or intense discomfort that peaks within minutes (American Psychiatric Association, 2013b). See **Table 27-25** for clinical presentation.

Obsessive-Compulsive Disorder (OCD)

- *Description*: The presence of obsession, compulsions, or both that consume thoughts and actions and last more than one hour while posing an interruption to daily functioning. See **Table 27-26** for clinical presentation.

Table 27-25 Panic Disorder Clinical Presentation/Diagnostic Criteria

Signs/Symptoms	Description
Fear attack	Four or more of the following are present during feelings of fear: • Heart palpitations • Sweating • Trembling • Shortness of breath • Feelings of choking • Chest pains • Abdominal distress or nausea • Dizzy, unsteady, and light headed • Chills and heat sensations • Numbness and tingling • Derealization or depersonalization • Fear of losing control • Fear of dying
Functioning	The following symptoms may be present for 1 month: • Persistent concern or anxiety about additional attacks or their consequences • Significant maladaptive change in behavior (e.g., behaviors designed to avoid attacks)

Data from American Psychiatric Association, 2013a.

Table 27-26 OCD Clinical Presentation/Diagnostic Criteria

Signs/Symptoms	Description
Obsessions	Repeated thoughts in a person's head
	Recurrent and persistent thoughts, urges, or images that are experienced as intrusive and unwanted
	Attempts to ignore or suppress symptoms by excessive acts
Compulsions	Repeated behaviors as a result of excessive thoughts
	Repetitive thoughts (e.g., counting or repeating words)
	Repetitive physical acts (e.g., hand washing or checking rituals)

Data from American Psychiatric Association, 2013a.

Hoarding

- *Description*: A persistent difficulty discarding or parting with possessions regardless of their values. See **Table 27-27** for clinical presentation.

Posttraumatic Stress Disorder (PTSD)

Description: The emotional, mental, and physical response to an extremely stressful events or threat of death after the age of six; for the duration of one month. See **Table 27-28** for clinical presentation.

Medications for PTSD: Medications are used to control or alleviate symptoms of anxiety; however, they do not

Table 27-27 Hoarding Clinical Presentation/ Diagnostic Criteria

Signs/ Symptoms	Description
Thoughts	Perceived need to save items and distress occurs with the idea of discarding the items
	Results in an accumulation of possessions that congest and clutter living areas, and compromises intended use
	Interferes with the ability to maintain safe environments

Data from American Psychiatric Association, 2013a.

Table 27-28 PTSD Clinical Presentation/Diagnostic Criteria

Signs/ Symptoms	Description
Thoughts	Exposure to actual or threatened death, serious injury, or sexual violence in one or more of the following: • Directly experiences trauma • Directly witnesses an event or events as they occurred to others • Experiences repeated or extreme exposure to aversion details of traumatic events (e.g., first responders)
Intrusive thoughts	One or more of the following are associated with a traumatic event: • Recurrent involuntary and intrusive distressing memories • Recurrent distressing dreams about trauma • Flashbacks (i.e., reliving the traumatic event) • Intense prolonged psychological distress with external cues that resembles any aspect of the root trauma • Marked physical reactions to internal symbolic cues
Behaviors	• Persistent avoidance of stimuli associated with trauma • Avoid or put forth extreme effort to avoid memories associated with trauma • Avoid or put forth extreme effort to avoid external reminders (e.g., people, places, conversations, and objects) associated with trauma
Mood	• Negative alteration in cognition and mood • Inability to remember important aspects of the trauma (e.g., amnesia, head injury, or deliberate use of alcohol or drugs) • Persistent negative beliefs or expectations about one's self (e.g., "I am bad" and "No one can be trusted") • Persistent distorted thoughts about cause or consequences of the trauma that leads to self-blame • Persistent diminished interest or participation in significant activities • Feelings of detachment from others • Persistent inability to experience positive emotions (e.g., does not feel happiness or satisfaction)
Alertness	Marked alteration in arousal and reactivity associated with the trauma as evidenced by two or more of the following: • Irritable behavior and angry outbursts (e.g., with little or no provocation) toward objects or others • Reckless or self-destructive behaviors • Hypervigilance • Exaggerated startle response • Difficulty with concentration • Sleep disturbances

Data from American Psychiatric Association, 2013a.

cure it (Vaughn, 2014). Sadock et al. (2015) classify these medications as follows:

- *Benzodiazepine*: A class of antianxiety drugs primarily used to produce calming effects:
  - Alprazolam (Xanax)
  - Lorazepam (Ativan)
- *Antidepressants*: A class of drugs that reduce symptoms of depressive disorders; medication of choice for anxiety include:
  - Celexa
  - Paxil
  - Zoloft

Benzodiazepines may cause a client to become physiologically and psychologically dependent. Abrupt withdrawal results in insomnia, diarrhea, and sun sensitivity.

Common medications for personality disorders include:

- *Lithium*: Mood stabilizer
- *Paxil*: Antidepressant (i.e., improves/elevates mood)
- *Risperdal*: Antipsychotic (i.e., improves clarity of thought)
- *Valium*: Produces a calming effect and relaxes muscles

Anxiety- and stress-related disorder precautions: A client with an anxiety-related disorder is at risk of developing other conditions such as depression, substance abuse, and eating disorders, as well as other major mental health conditions. Working with and caring for a client with this disorder is emotionally and physically consuming. In addition, physical injuries may occur with people experiencing PTSD (Vaughn, 2014).

Screening and Assessments

- *Assessment of Motor and Process Skills*: Assesses the quality and context of ADL performance (Vaughn, 2014).
- *Bay Area Functional Performance Evaluation*: Assesses how clients may function in task-oriented and social settings (Asher, 2014).
- *Beck Anxiety Inventory*: Self-report inventory on feelings of anxiety (Vaughn, 2014).
- *COTE*: Used in mental health settings to identify client behaviors that impact occupational performance (Schell et al., 2014).

- *Milwaukee Evaluation of Daily Living Skills*: Measures the client's ability to perform basic and complex ADLs (Schell et al., 2014).
- *Occupational Circumstances Assessment Interview and Rating Scale (OCAIRS)*: Based on MOHO, documents an individual's participation in occupations (Asher, 2014).
- *Occupational Self-Assessment*: Self-report establishing priorities for change (Vaughn, 2014).

Interventions and Impact on Occupational Performance

Anxiety disorders can be extremely debilitating and interfere greatly with all areas of occupation, activity demands and performance patterns, particularly with social participation and learning. These disorders can create situations where burden on the occupational performance of the client's family and society may be present (e.g., may miss family, work, and spousal events). People with PTSD are at a significantly high risk for diminished well-being and quality of life (Brown et al., 2011). See **Table 27-29** for interventions.

Table 27-29 Anxiety- and Stress-Related Disorder Interventions: Therapeutic Use of Self, Occupations, and Activities

Therapeutic use of self	Identify and recognize triggers
	Reality testing: do not engage in physical issues and causes
	Supportive self-appraisal through supported expressions
	Calm redirection
Psychosocial interventions	Social skills training
	Medication management
	Visual or social expressions
	Sensory processing–related techniques
	Stress management and relaxation exercise
	Coping skills and problem-solving
Preparatory methods and task	Short-term and familiar activities
	Safe and subdued environments
	Guided choices
	Repetitious acts and gross motor activities
	Journal writing
	Simple cooking
	Crafts and small woodworking projects

Data from Early, 2009.

Anxiety and Stress-Related Disorder Referrals and Discharge Considerations

Cognitive behavioral therapy is a significant intervention with known efficacy in successfully managing anxieties by reducing the catastrophe associated with the event by challenging the distorted thoughts related to the fear (Brown et al., 2011). Occupational therapy practitioners may recommend support groups and family therapy for caregivers (Vaughn, 2014).

Feeding and Eating Disorders

- *Description*: Eating disorders are considered disorders of the mind and body, and are characterized by an intense fear of being fat and quest for thinness. The disorder is derived from the struggle to feel accepted and competent within cultural family, or social environments. Adolescents are particularly at risk with a greater prevalence in females (Brown et al., 2011).
- *Pathology*: The cause is multifaceted and can be associated with personality, genetics, family function, social, and cultural factors. Personality traits may include people who have low self-esteem and are fragile or anxious, along with a tension between the need to belong and a desire to be independent. Genetics and family structure may also contribute to the pathology, including alcohol or drug abuse, overvaluing appearance and thinness, and/or excessive or absent parental control. Precipitating factors include perceptions and thoughts about self, their appearance, or the future that is caused by vulnerability particularly as one moves from one milestone to another. Perpetuating factors include complimenting a client on his or her appearance after losing weight (Brown et al., 2011).

Anorexia Nervosa

- *Description*: An intense fear of becoming fat accompanied by behaviors that prevent weight gain, even though he or she may have a low weight with a persistent lack of recognition that his or her weight is low.

- *Clinical presentation*: A low body weight, intense fear of gaining weight, and a disturbance in the perception of his or her weight and/or their body shape. See **Table 27-30** for clinical presentation.

Bulimia Nervosa

- *Description*: Recurring episodes of binge eating and compensatory behaviors to prevent weight gain.
- *Clinical presentation/diagnostic criteria*: Behaviors occur at least once a week for three months. See **Table 27-31** for a list of clinical presentations.

Medications for anxiety *and stress-related disorders*: Medication cannot cure this disorder; however, it can help control binging and purging. Antidepressant and antianxiety medications may be prescribed for depression and anxiety disorders (Griffin, 2014).

Feeding and eating disorder precautions: Monitor clients for signs of relapse in dysfunctional eating behaviors and/or other maladaptive behaviors such as excesses, obsessions, or extreme neglect (Brown et al., 2011).

Table 27-30 Anorexia Nervosa Clinical Presentation

Signs/Symptoms	Description
Binge-eating/purging	Any occurrence throughout the last 3 months
	Recurrent episodes of binging or purging
	Purging (e.g., self-induced vomiting, misuse of laxatives, or enemas)
Restricting	No episodes of binging or purging throughout the last three months
	Maintains weight with diet, exercise, or fasting

Data from American Psychiatric Association, 2013a.

Table 27-31 Bulimia Nervosa Clinical Presentation

Signs/Symptoms	Description
Binge	Eats large portions of food within a two-hour period
	Inability to stop eating
Purge	Self-induced vomiting, misuse of laxatives or enemas, fasting or excessive exercise

Data from American Psychiatric Association, 2013a.

Screening and Assessments

- *Adolescent Role Assessment*: Semistructured interview to evaluate client's involvement in occupational roles over time (Asher, 2014).
- *Eating Disorders Inventory*: Self-report measures symptoms of eating disorders (Griffin, 2014).
- *Leisure Interest Measure*: Measures level of interest in leisure activities (Asher, 2014).
- *KELS*: Interview and observations to assess client's ability to perform basic living skills (Asher, 2014).
- *Occupational self-assessment*: Self-report establishing priorities for change (Griffin, 2014).

Interventions and Impact on Occupational Performance

Chronic long-term effects of binging and purging will greatly affect body structures and functions which could be life-threatening. Common occupational concerns include maladaptive eating and lifestyle habits, meal planning, and impaired independent living skills. Clients are also found to have impaired communication and assertion skills and difficulty with stress management, as well as being resistant to change (Brown et al., 2011). See **Table 27-32** for interventions.

Feeding and Eating Disorder Referrals and Discharge Considerations

Family therapy may be indicated to observe and educate family dynamics and effects on recovery. Strategies should be implemented to help family members cope and assist in the client's recovery. Community follow-up is important to monitor the weight of a client with an eating disorder and to support and effectively respond to stressors. A resource such as the National Association of Anorexia and Associated Disorders can be given to clients and/or caregivers (Griffin, 2014).

Substance-Related Disorders

- *Description*: Substance disorder primarily includes individuals involved in the use and abuse of alcohol and illicit drugs (Brown et al., 2011).

Table 27-32 Feeding and Eating Disorder Interventions: Therapeutic Use of Self, Occupations, and Activities

Therapeutic Use of Self	Unconditional Acceptance
	Expectation of change
	Allow opportunity for positive control
	Calm, firm, and supportive tone
Psychosocial interventions	Social skills training
	Adult role meal planning and preparation
	Realistic exercise routine
	Assertiveness and communication skills
	Stress management and relaxation strategies
	Body image improvement
	Lifestyle redesign and independent living skills
	Relapse prevention
Preparatory methods and task	Explore occupational interests and role play
	Relevant activities related to current trends, fashions, and technology
	Meal planning
	Group discussions
	Visual and social expression
	Projective and dramatic arts
	Crafts
	Journaling

Data from Brown et al., 2011; Early, 2009.

- *Pathology*: Genetics, temperament, sociocultural influences, environmental factors, and/or the presence of a mental illness may contribute to the chronic use of illicit substances (Brown et al., 2011).
- *Clinical presentation*: See **Table 27-33** for clinical presentation.

The following medications are commonly used for substance abuse and use disorders (Brown et al., 2011):

- *Antianxiety*: Produce a calming effect and may relax muscles
- *SSRI antidepressants*: Elevates mood (i.e., used when depression accompanies a disorder)
- *Acamprosate and Disulfiram* (i.e., *Antabuse*): Used to treat alcohol dependency (i.e., in combination with counseling)
- *Methadone*: Used to reduce drug cravings (e.g., heroin)

Table 27-33 Substance-Related Disorders Clinical Presentation/Diagnostic Criteria

Types	Description
Substance use disorders	The mild to severe form of the chronically relapsing, and compulsive use of alcohol, cannabis, opium, or prescription drugs
Alcohol	Often taken in large amounts
Cannabis	Persistent desire and unsuccessful effort to stop or cut down on use
Hallucinogen	Great deal of time is spent in obtaining the substance
Inhalants	There is often a craving or strong desire for the substance
Opioid	Recurrent use interferes with work, school, or home
Stimulant	Continued use despite interferences
	Gives up or reduces all activities
	Recurrent use in situations that are hazardous
	Continues despite physical challenges related to substance
	Develops an increased tolerance for the substance
Substance-induced disorders	The mental disorder that is caused by the use of substances that may include the following: • Mood such as depression • Psychosis or cognition such as paranoia • Mental thinking and processing, such as memory • Physical weight loss or weakness

Data from American Psychiatric Association, 2013a.

There are various methods that can be used to adhere to prescribed medications. Brown et al. (2011) provide suggestions for medication management techniques as follows:

- Reminder system
- System for tracking medication use
- Design a supportive environment
- Self-monitoring tasks
- Reinforcement
- Maintain caregiver quality of care
- Medication education
- Destigmatize disorder as a mental illness

Substance-related disorder precautions: Monitor clients for signs of withdrawal including, but not limited to, rapid heart rate, anxiety, hyperactivity, and convulsions. Long-term illicit drug use may lead to other complications such as heart, liver, and/or pancreatic diseases, as well as cognitive and social issues (Carifio, 2014).

Screening and Assessments

Screenings and assessments are used to determine the presence of the disorder and the effects on day-to-day performances using the following tools:

- *Addiction Severity Index (ASI)*: Ratings indicate interviewer's estimate of the client's need for additional treatment in several key challenging areas (Carifio, 2014).
- *Coping Behaviors Inventory*: Assesses behaviors and thoughts used to control heavy drinking (Carifio, 2014).
- *MOHOST*: Addresses client's engagement in occupation (Asher, 2014).
- *OCAIRS*: Based on MOHO, documents an individual's participation in occupations (Asher, 2014).
- *Role Checklist*: Used to gather information about a client's occupational roles (Asher, 2014).
- *Routine Task Inventory*: Assesses cognitive ability in the context of routine daily activities (Asher, 2014).
- *University of Rhode Island Change Assessment*: Evaluates motivation for change (Brown et al., 2011).

Interventions and Impact on Occupational Performance

Substance-related disorders typically have a negative impact on all occupational roles, including the inability to make healthy and safe choices and maintaining quality of life (Brown et al., 2011). See **Table 27-34** for affected systems and resultant symptoms, and **Table 27-35** for interventions.

Substance-Related Disorder Referrals and Discharge Considerations

A 12-step spiritual support program such as Alcoholics Anonymous (i.e., AA) or Narcotics Anonymous

Table 27-34 Substance-Related Disorders Systems and Symptoms

Systems	Symptoms
Cognition	Memory loss, inattention, and aphasia
Psychosocial	Sadness and difficulty concentrating
Psychological	Hallucinations and delusions
Neurological	Restlessness and panic attacks

Data from Brown et al., 2011.

Table 27-35 Substance-Related Disorder Interventions: Therapeutic Use of Self, Occupations, and Activities

Therapeutic use of self	Monitor relapse behaviors
	Monitor and minimize use of defense projection and rationalizing
	Manage transference and counter transference
	Provide matter-of-fact communication
Psychosocial interventions	Use of time leisure as a major focus
	Educate the client and family on codependency and enabling
	Relapse prevention and condition education
	Cognitive and perceptual beliefs
	ADLs, IADLs, and nutritional support
	Social skills, interaction, and communication skills
	Work-related skills
	Stress management, coping, and relaxation
	Acquisitions and development of roles and skills
Preparatory methods and task	Structured, controlled, and stable environments (e.g., lighting)
	Paper and pen activities
	Daily life task and leisure exploration
	Craft woodworking, leather crafting, and cooking tasks as appropriate

Data from Brown et al., 2011; Early, 2009.

(i.e., NA), and family education and support groups such as Al-Anon have shown to be successful intervention programs for clients with substance-related disorders (Brown et al., 2011).

Summary of Referrals and Discharge Considerations in Mental Health Settings

Evaluations refer to the comprehensive appraisal of a client's condition, environmental circumstance, deficits, potential for success, and recommendations for discharge setting and resources. An evaluation utilizes one or more individual assessment tools to make these determinations (Schell et al., 2014). The reevaluation of skill levels in the psychiatric setting occurs 30 days after the initial evaluation or with a doctor's order.

Table 27-36 OT Versus OTA Roles in Mental Health Settings

OT roles	Assessment, evaluation, intervention planning, and intervention plan implementation
	Initiates, manages, guides, and documents the evaluation
	Selects theoretically and culturally relevant approaches for evaluation
	Has the final responsibility for obtaining and interpreting the information needed for intervention planning
	Formulates an intervention plan, which can be implemented directly by the OTA under the supervision of an OT
OTA roles	Assessment, intervention planning, and intervention plan implementation
	Collects information and administers assessments with service competency
	Records observations and results
	Contributes to the evaluation and ongoing assessment under the supervision of the OT
	Implements the intervention plan under the supervision of the OT

Data from Early, 2009.

Management and Standards of Practice

OTs in mental health settings will follow professional association guidelines in line with governing bodies (e.g., American Occupational Therapy Association, Public Health, and The Joint Commission) to provide evaluation and reevaluation standards.

Roles of the OT and occupational therapy assistant (OTA) are delineated throughout occupational therapy practice. **Table 27-36** provides a more specific breakdown regarding the OT and OTA relationship for practice in mental health settings.

Chapter 27 Self-Study Activities

1. Please read the case study and then respond to the questions provided.

   Jack, age 14, was admitted to an acute care facility for teens. Jack had not attended school for seven days, and during an impulse episode, he broke into the school science lab and destroyed several of his peer's lab experiments. The medical record review revealed that his father drinks alcohol daily. During the initial interview with the OTA, Jack reported remaining in bed for long periods of time, avoiding classmates and family, and feeling tired and like it was a waste of time to go to school.

A. Jack has verbalized many risk factors that may result in long-term substance use. What intervention is BEST used to help prevent Jack from developing that disorder?

B. Jack described symptoms related to a mood disorder. What assessment tools can the OT use to determine Jack's mood and his occupational behaviors?

C. What environmental considerations MUST the OT remain mindful of while presenting group interventions?

2. Psychosocial Theories and Frames of References Learning Activity

Please write in the author of a theory or frame of reference commonly used in psychosocial practice and the corresponding key beliefs. Use the psychosocial theories and frames of references learning worksheet provided below or a method of your choosing.

Theory	Author	Key Beliefs

Chapter 27 Self-Study Answers

Question I Answers

A. Psycho education about the alcohol condition, stress management, coping, and relaxation skills activities (Early, 2009).

B. *Bay Area Functional Performance Evaluation*: Assesses how clients may function in task-oriented and social settings (Asher, 2014). *Adolescence Role Assessment*: Semistructured interview to evaluate client's involvement in occupational roles over time (Asher, 2014). *Emotional Problems Scale*: Assesses emotional and behavioral challenges (Integrated Assessment LLC, 2015). *Draw-A-Person Test*: Psycho projective personality test to screen for emotional or behavioral disorders (Asher, 2014).

Child Behavior Checklist: Provides a record of the child's competencies and challenges (ASEBA, 2015)
CAPE & PAC: Measures participation and engagement in activities (Asher, 2014, p. 338).
Coping Inventory: Measures adaptive and maladaptive coping skills (Asher, 2014).

C. Minimize environmental distractions
Clarify relationships and expectations
Incorporate the child's interests
Help to assess positive self-worth
Use predictable materials
Reestablish regular habits and routines
Allow verbal expression
Provide a safe and comfortable environment
Incorporate success-oriented activities

Question 2 Answers (Psychosocial Theories and Frames of References Learning Worksheet)

Theory	Author	Key Beliefs
Cognitive Disability	Claudia Allen	Believes cognition affects a client's ability to engage in occupational performance. Defines functional ability as the capacity to use mental energy to guide motor and speech performance. There are six levels and 52 modes. Level 1 is the lowest and indicates severe impairment and Level 6 is the highest where there is little to no impairment. The identification of a level serves as a predictor to current and future functioning. This frame believes a person is motivated by biological factors such as "can do" (i.e., realistic ability), psychological factors "will do" (i.e., relevance), and social factors "may do" (i.e., possibility). A client will be further impacted by the environment, emotions, activity complexity, and familiarity (Cole, 2012).
MOHO	Gary Kielhofner	Humans have the innate drive to explore and master their environment. Doing, exploring, and taking actions help organize and maintain us. Occupational behavior is the outcome of an interaction among the client, the occupational task, and the environment. The process of exploring, creating, and controlling the environment is human occupation. Order occurs when there is exploration, competence, and achievement. Disorder occurs when there is helplessness, incompetence, and inefficacy (Cole, 2012). MOHO describes the relationship between three dynamic systems and how they work toward motivation (Brown et al., 2011).
Psychodynamic	Sigmund Freud, Carl Jung	The client's psychological construct or their mental state has an effect on occupational and social behaviors. This approach provides a means of understanding and supporting inner life—feelings, thoughts, and emotions. This theory provides explanations for conscious and unconscious mental processes, perceptions, thoughts and feelings, and the relationship between the human and nonhuman environment (Bruce et al., 2002).
Sensory Integration	Lorna Jean King	The human brain is innately organized to program a person to seek out stimulation that is organized. Input from the sensory system can facilitate or inhibit the state of the entire organism. Input from each system influences every other system and thereby the organism as a whole (Dirette, 2015).
Ecological frames of reference • PEO • PEOP • EHP	Christiansen and Baum (1997), Dunn, Brown, and McGuigan (1994), Law et al. (1996)	Focus on the client, environment, and occupation. These models view the individual holistically, recognizing the influence that environments have on a client's ability to satisfactorily engage in meaningful tasks. OTs working with mental health populations can utilize these theories to support client-centered interventions, which consider performance in clinical, community, and home environments (Brown et al., 2011).

References

American Occupational Therapy Association. (2014). Occupational therapy practice framework: Domain and process (3rd ed.). *American Journal of Occupational Therapy, 68*(Suppl. 1), S1–S48. doi:10.5014/ajot.2014.682006

American Psychiatric Association. (2013a). *Desk reference to the diagnostic criteria from DSM-5.* Washington, DC: American Psychiatric Publishing.

American Psychiatric Association. (2013b). *Diagnostic and statistical manual of mental disorders: DSM-5* (5th ed.). Washington, DC: Author.

ASEBA. (2015). *Childhood behavior checklist.* Retrieved from http://www.aseba.org/forms/schoolagecbcl.pdf

Asher, I. E. (2014). *Asher's occupational therapy assessment tools: An annotated index* (4th ed.). Bethesda, MD: American Occupational Therapy Association, Inc.

Bonjuklian, A. (2014). Appendix I: Common conditions, resources, and evidence: Schizophrena and schizoaffective disorder. In B. A. B. Schell, G. Gillen, & M. E. Scaffa (Eds.), *Willard & Spackman's occupational therapy* (12th ed., pp. 1173–1176). Philadelphia, PA: Wolters Kluwer Health/Lippincott Williams & Wilkins.

Brown, C., Stoffel, V., & Munoz, J. P. (2011). *Occupational therapy in mental health: A vision for participation.* Philadelphia, PA: F.A. Davis Co.

Bruce, M. A., Borg, B., & Bruce, M. A. (2002). *Psychosocial frames of reference: Core for occupation-based practice* (3rd ed.). Thorofare, NJ: SLACK Incorporated.

Carifio, C. M. (2014). Appendix I: Common conditions, resources, and evidence: Substance abuse disorders. In B. A. B. Schell, G. Gillen, & M. E. Scaffa (Eds.), *Willard & Spackman's occupational therapy* (12th ed., pp. 1182–1184). Philadelphia, PA: Wolters Kluwer Health/Lippincott Williams & Wilkins.

Christiansen, C., & Baum, C. M. (1997). *Occupational therapy: Enabling function and well-being* (2nd ed.). Thorofare, NJ: SLACK Incorporated.

Cole, M. B. (2012). *Group dynamics in occupational therapy: The theoretical basis and practice application of group intervention* (4th ed.). Thorofare, NJ: SLACK Incorporated.

Dirette, D. K. (2015). Theory that guides practice: Our map. In K. Sladyk & S. E. Ryan (Eds.), *Ryan's occupational therapy assistant: Principles, practice issues, and techniques* (5th ed., pp. 72–91). Thorofare, NJ: SLACK Incorporated.

Dunn, W., Brown, C., & McGuigan, A. (1994). The ecology of human performance: A framework for considering the effect of context. *American Journal of Occupational Therapy, 48*(7), 595–607. Retrieved from http://www.ncbi.nlm.nih.gov/pubmed/7943149

Early, M. B. (2009). *Mental health concepts and techniques for the occupational therapy assistant* (4th ed.). Philadelphia, PA: Wolters Kluwer Health/Lippincott Williams & Wilkins.

Griffin, T. (2014). Appendix I: Common conditions, resources, and evidence: Eating disorders. In B. A. B. Schell, G. Gillen, & M. E. Scaffa (Eds.), *Willard & Spackman's occupational therapy* (12th ed., pp. 1144–1145). Philadelphia, PA: Wolters Kluwer Health/Lippincott Williams & Wilkins.

Integrated Assessment LLC. (2015). *Effective assessment for persons with mild intellectual disabilities, mental retardation, and borderline intelligence.* Retrieved from http://integrated-assessment.com/

Krumbach, A. P. (2014). Appendix I: Common conditions, resources, and evidence: Attention deficit/hyperactivity disorder. In B. A. B. Schell, G. Gillen, & M. E. Scaffa (Eds.), *Willard & Spackman's occupational therapy* (12th ed., pp. 1112–1117). Philadelphia, PA: Wolters Kluwer Health/Lippincott Williams & Wilkins.

Law, M., Cooper, B., Strong, S., Stewart, D., Rigby, P., & Letts, L. (1996). The Person–Environment–Occupation model: A transactive approach to occupational performance. *Canadian Journal of Occupational Therapy, 63*(1), 9–23.

Rogers, S. L. (2010). Common conditions that influence children's participation. In J. Case-Smith (Ed.), *Occupational therapy for children* (6th ed., pp. 146–192). St. Louis, MO: Mosby.

Sadock, B. J., Sadock, V. A., & Ruiz, P. (2015). *Kaplan & Sadock's synopsis of psychiatry: Behavioral sciences/clinical psychiatry* (11th ed.). Philadelphia, PA: Wolters Kluwer.

Schell, B. A. B., Gillen, G., & Scaffa, M. E. (2014). *Willard & Spackman's occupational therapy* (12th ed.). Philadelphia, PA: Wolters Kluwer Health/Lippincott Williams & Wilkins.

Strong, S., Rigby, P., Stewart, D., Law, M., Letts, L., & Cooper, B. (1999). Application of the Person–Environment–Occupation model: A practical tool. *Canadian Journal of Occupational Therapy, 66*(3), 122–133. Retrieved from http://www.ncbi.nlm.nih.gov/pubmed/10462885

Stultz, S. (2014). Appendix I: Common conditions, resources, and evidence: Autism spectrum disorders. In B. A. B. Schell, G. Gillen, & M. E. Scaffa (Eds.), *Willard & Spackman's occupational therapy* (12th ed., pp. 1114–1117). Philadelphia, PA: Wolters Kluwer Health/Lippincott Williams & Wilkins.

Vaughn, P. (2014). Appendix I: Common conditions, resources, and evidence: Anxiety disorders. In B. A. B. Schell, G. Gillen, & M. E. Scaffa (Eds.), *Willard & Spackman's occupational therapy* (12th ed., pp. 1106–1109). Philadelphia, PA: Wolters Kluwer Health/Lippincott Williams & Wilkins.

Group Dynamics

Doreen Head and Sophia Kimmons

Learning Objectives

- Describe the scope and limits of group activities and skills through the lenses of theory and evidence-based practice.
- Identify group leadership guidelines by drawing from occupational therapy (OT) frames of reference and the Occupational Therapy Practice Framework III (OTPF III).
- Demonstrate knowledge of key principles, roles, and functions of the OT professional in program planning and intervention in accordance with the American Occupational Therapy Association's (AOTA) standards of practice.
- Apply knowledge of OT assessments and interventions for therapeutic groups that maximize health and wellness of the group and its members.

Key Terms

- *Activity analysis*: The breaking down and review of the demands, performance skills, and cultural aspects of an activity.
- *Client centered*: The focus of any aspect of service with emphasis on the client.
- *Group dynamics*: The interactions between each of the parts of a group including activity, people, culture, and the environment.
- *Group roles*: The various roles each group member plays that either help manage or maintain group processes or that may serve to disrupt the group process.
- *Occupations*: Meaningful and purposeful activities that people engage in to occupy their time.
- *Therapeutic use of self*: The OT practitioner deliberate use of emotions and skills as a therapeutic tool.

Introduction

Therapeutic groups are used for many purposes including practicality and cost-effectiveness, to learn to develop relationships and trust others through self-disclosure, and for the value gained from feedback and support each member gives to one another. Group dynamics is the interaction between the group members and the activity process and performance within an environment. This chapter will address group dynamics including group development, group interpersonal relations, and group performance as a method for guiding occupational therapy (OT) practice.

Group Development

Consideration of the group as a mode of intervention will also include the use of OT frames of reference, varying group models, and the OTPF III (American Occupational Therapy Association, 2014). Each of these concepts provides guidance, definitions, and validation toward evidence-based OT practice.

Frames of Reference

There are various frames of reference that are commonly used in psychosocial OT (Bruce, Borg, & Bruce, 2002), which are outlined below:

1. *Canadian Occupational Performance Model (COPM)*: The COPM was developed to guide service delivery to a diverse group of clients and healthcare settings; it is also referred to as an open-system model (McColl et al., 2005).

2. *Model of Human Occupation (MOHO)*: This model asserts that human beings possess an innate drive to explore and master their environments (Kielhofner, 2008).

3. *Sensory Integration (SI)*: SI theory asserts that the human brain seeks out stimulation that is organized and beneficial for individuals' sensory systems (Ayres, 1977).

4. *Cognitive Disabilities*: This model postulates that a person's ability to use mental energy to guide motor and speech performances will help to predict his or her functioning environments (Toglia, Golisz, & Goverover, 2014).

Group Models

Different group models are used to accomplish specific goals. Each group has a purpose and is structured and designed to focus on specific skill development. Four common group models are outlined below:

1. *Task-oriented group*: The purpose of the task-oriented group is to provide members a shared working experience (e.g., publishing an electronic newsletter) (Scaffa, 2014). Collaboration results in an environment where productive and nonproductive behaviors can be observed and addressed. Through shared experiences, group members begin to recognize the relationship between thinking, feeling, and behavior. Shared experiences also reinforce the notion that one's behavior often has an effect on others, as well as the accomplishment of group tasks and goals. Alternatives to nonproductive behaviors can be identified, tested, and reinforced. This process strengthens members' egos and leads to improved functioning of the group and its members (Cole, 2012).

2. *Developmental group*: This group hypothesizes that OT treatment should be a "recapitulation of ontogenesis" (Scaffa, 2014). In other words, group processes can repeat the normal course of development, allow opportunities for the individual to return to the earliest developmental lag, and progress until the person reaches the expected developmental level. The model further indicates that successful participation in group interaction skill

building is related to successful community living (Cole, 2012).

3. *Directive group*: This group is designed to provide consistent and structured experiences for individuals who are minimally functioning and acutely mentally ill. Group levels include the following: exploration, competence, and achievement (Kaplan, 1988).

4. *Integrative group*: This group features a five-stage format that is designed to stimulate the senses, encourage movement, and facilitate adequate social interaction, competency, and preferred occupational behaviors (Cole, 2012).

Occupational Therapy Practice Framework

This framework presents a group of domains and aspects designed to guide OT practice in all settings while serving any given population. **Table 28-1** provides a summary of the OTPF III (AOTA, 2014).

Group Interpersonal Relations

Interpersonal relations include the interactions of each group member including the OT practitioner and the roles of each participant. The following is true of member roles: roles are interchangeable, and healthy individuals will assume many roles, which can enhance group functioning by supporting role formation and modeling adaptive and functional behaviors. The role that each member assumes is based on his/her past experiences and social skills that are consistent with the adaptive–maladaptive continuum. This area will cover leaders' roles, adaptive and maladaptive group roles, and maladaptive behaviors often displayed in group settings.

Leader Roles

The leader's role is to facilitate the group so that individuals and the group will work toward the final stage of maturity where the members of the group can express behavior that is both negative and positive. To

Table 28-1 Occupational Therapy Practice Framework Domains and Process

Occupations
- Activities of daily living (ADLs)
- Instrumental activities of daily living (IADLs)
- Rest and sleep
- Education
- Work
- Play
- Leisure
- Social participation

Client factors
- Values
- Beliefs
- Spirituality
- Body functions
- Body structures

Performance skills
- Motor skills
- Process skills
- Social interaction skills

Performance patterns
- Habits
- Routines
- Roles
- Rituals

Context
- Cultural
- Personal
- Temporal
- Visual

Environments
- Physical
- Social

Modified from AOTA, 2014.

Table 28-2 Types of Leadership Styles

Autocratic	Democratic	Laissez-faire
• The leader has complete control and facilitates vis-à-vis aggression. • *Authoritative*: Dictatorial and commanding of obedience. • *Authoritarian*: Leader makes independent decisions and is not responsive to the group members. • Used with members functioning at a lower level and require increased structure.	• Input or feedback and the freedom of choice help facilitate group cohesiveness. • Used with members functioning at higher cognitive levels and most effective in conjunction with client-centered approaches (e.g., MOHO, psychodynamic, and cognitive-behavioral).	• Leader deliberately refrains from interfering in the process and does not direct behavior or rules. The group members develop guidance or structure. • Used most effectively with humanistic and psychodynamic concepts (e.g., MOHO).

Data from Richards, 2014.

Occupational Therapist's Role and Leadership Style

The goals of the group, the characteristics of the group members, and the leader's therapeutic use of self determine one's leadership style (Cole, 2012). See **Table 28-2**

accomplish this, the leader will need to develop roles and an appropriate leadership style (Cole, 2012; Scaffa, 2014).

for types of leadership styles. Cole (2012) cites five key characteristics OT practitioners should exude:

- Maintain client-centered group goals and activities that are safe, meaningful, and age appropriate.
- Maintain an awareness of his or her strengths and weaknesses and model acceptable and desired behaviors.
- Provide a nonjudgmental and unconditional positive regard for every person in the group.
- Guide the client through the group experience and encourage members to reflect and learn about the process by directing and/or participating in the group.
- Act as a gatekeeper and control the direction of the group to match the clients' needs and type of group selected.

Occupational therapist roles on reaching group maturity include the following:

1. *Plan*: Guide the group toward a predetermined focus.
2. *Attentive to feeling*: Explore and express personal issues and emotions.

3. *Actively participate*: Take an active role; engage in the activity and process.
4. *Give feedback*: Provide an honest assessment, both negative and positive, being careful not to single out or belittle.
5. *Be open to feedback*: Manage one's emotions and be mindful of such defenses as rationalizing, withdrawing, denying, and/or internalizing the comment(s).
6. *Take responsibility*: Accurately assess situation(s) and take steps to improve the group as needed (Cole, 2012).

Cole (2012) identifies advantages of co-leadership groups led by two or more practitioners as follows:

1. *Mutual support*: Provides greater opportunities to complete tasks, meet the needs of group members and/or the group leaders.
2. *Increased objectivity*: Allows for the comparison of observations and feedback for greater understanding, which can lead to successful goal attainment.
3. *Collective knowledge*: Provides more knowledge and experience for the task, group facilitation, and participants.
4. *Modeling*: Leans toward the demonstration and development of different co-leadership styles.
5. *Different roles*: The OT practitioner's ability to play different roles helps to strengthen group processes during facilitation and management of group activities.

In addition, there are various group member roles exhibited in different types of groups. The three main types of groups include adaptive, maintenance, and mal-adaptive (Cole, 2012). See **Table 28-3** for delineation of roles depending on group assignment.

There are also various challenging behaviors present in groups. These behaviors may include the following:

- *Monopolist*: The person who takes over and dominates the group.
- *Silent member*: The person who sits quietly and does not actively engage or participate in the group process.
- *Attention-getter*: The person who will use any means to divert attention from others and onto themselves (e.g., self-deprecating, help rejecting, or self-love).
- *Psychosis*: The person who is out of touch with reality (American Psychiatric Association, 2013; Cole, 2012).

Activity Group Process: Group Protocol

Group protocols provide an extensive and detailed plan that includes the identification of populations, selection of a frame of reference, selection of an intervention focus, writing a group intervention plan outline, and planning goal-directed sessions. The group goals provide the foundation and purpose for which the group is meeting. It also provides direction and reason for the group being together, and without it, groups may fall apart. Group protocols also provide a task or activity to work toward a goal to accomplish, as well as to establish a commonality between group members. The protocol is a method used for group design and provides the format used for each group session. Although many designs are available, this section will discuss the group interaction styles, and Cole's seven-step, holistic, client-centered model for the OT group (Cole, 2012).

In general, there are five group interaction skills. Mosey (1973) indicates that to effectively facilitate the progression and development of the person's skill levels, people are placed one level above their performance. **Table 28-4** provides a description of the various group skills and corresponding definitions. In terms of group leadership, **Table 28-5** provides a summary of the seven-step model for group leadership as identified by Cole (2012).

Group Performance

When considering group performance, it is necessary to consider not only the formation of the group, but also the ongoing assessment of functioning and safety. According to Yalom and Leszcz (2005), there are three stages of group development:

1. *Orientation*: Hesitance with regard to participation stems from an individual's need to see how the group can assist him or her in achieving a set of predetermined goals. During this stage, members "size each other up in order to determine whether or not they belong as they search for acceptance and approval" (p. 36).
2. *Conflict*: As members acclimate to the group and compete for power and control, they begin to feel comfortable with contributing personal comments and criticism. Dominance, rebellion, differences,

Table 28-3 Task Roles for Adaptive, Maintenance, and Maladaptive Groups

Group	Task Roles
Adaptive group	• *Initiator–contributor*: Individual suggests new ideas. • *Information seeker*: Individual asks for facts. • *Opinion seeker*: Individual asks for feelings about issues. • *Information giver*: Individual provides facts. • *Opinion giver*: Individual expresses feelings not necessarily based on facts. • *Elaborator*: Individual spells out suggestions and gives examples. • *Coordinator*: Individual pulls ideas together. • *Orienter*: Individual focuses on goals. • *Energizer*: Individual prods or arouses. • *Procedural technician*: Individual performs tasks. • *Recorder*: Individual writes down key points.
Maintenance group	• *Encourager*: Individual praises and accepts others. • *Harmonizer*: Individual settles differences. • *Compromiser*: Individual gives in to disputes. • *Gatekeeper*: Individual keeps communication going. • *Standard setter*: Individual expresses norms. • *Observer*: Individual records and offers record to group for feedback. • *Follower*: Individual goes along with the mood and decisions of the group.
Maladaptive group	• *Antigroup*: Individual is self-centered (i.e., egocentric). • *Aggressor*: Individual belittles or attacks others. • *Blocker*: Individual prevents progression. • *Recognition seeker*: Individual calls attention to him or herself. • *Self-confessor*: Individual expresses personal challenges. • *Playboy*: Individual is disruptive and disinterested. • *Dominator*: Individual controls, manipulates, or interrupts others. • *Help seeker*: Individual tries to get sympathy and views him or herself as being victimized. • *Special-interest pleader*: Individual pretends to speak on behalf of others to express his or her own biases.

Data from Cole, 2012.

Table 28-4 Group Skill Definitions

Group Skills	Description
Parallel	Individual's work or play in the presence of others.
Project	Members are involved in short-term tasks cooperatively or competitively.
Egocentric–cooperative	Members jointly decide on a long-term activity and carry it throughout completion.
Cooperative	Individuals have common interests, concerns, and values, and activity is of little importance.
Mature	Individuals of different backgrounds, ages, interests, and ideas take on roles for task development and group member satisfaction.

Data from Bryant et al., 2014; Cole, 2012; Early, 2009; Scaffa, 2014.

Table 28-5 Seven-Step Model for Group Leadership

Seven Steps	Description
Introduction	• Occupational therapist introduction (e.g., name, title, and group topic). • Members greet group by saying their name (e.g., acknowledge members and help members learn each other's names). • Friendly "hello" when members are late entering the group. • Set the mood (e.g., environment, facial expressions, body language, media used, lighting, reduce clutter, and have equipment ready).
Activity	• Consider many factors (e.g., knowledge of clients' health conditions, corresponding dysfunctions, and assessments). • Intervention planning, activity analysis, and synthesis. • Clinical reasoning (i.e., therapeutic goals, apply knowledge of their abilities and disabilities, knowledge and skill of the leader, and adaptation of the activity). • Timing of the group (e.g., keep it fairly short and simple, and the activity should be no longer than one-third of the total session). • Group norms (e.g., rules of behavior, attitudes, and expectations of the group). • Be aware of the behaviors of group members, such as wandering or being preoccupied. • Meet the needs of most of the group members.
Sharing	• After completing an activity, each member is asked to share the experience with the group, which varies with each experience. • Make sure each of the members' contributions are verbally or nonverbally acknowledged. • Be supportive, provide encouragement and reassurance, and role model the sharing process.
Processing	• This step reveals important and relevant information about the client and encourages members to express their feelings. • Feelings are easy to express if they reflect positive experiences. • Feelings are difficult to express if they reflect negative experiences.
Generalizing	• Address the cognitive learning aspects of the group. • Sum up the group members' responses into a few general principles. • Look at patterns, opinions, commonalities, disagreements, and conflicts among group members. • Make the activity exciting and interesting.
Application	• Help the group understand how the principles learned during the group session can be applied to everyday life.
Summary	• Verbally emphasize the most important aspects of the group so that the members will be understood and remembered. • Points to emphasize should come from the group. • Review the goals, the content, and the process of the group.

Data from Bryant et al., 2014; Cole, 2012; Scaffa, 2014.

and conflicts arise within the group during this phase of the group's development.

3. *Cohesiveness*: Group solidarity results from members resolving initial conflicts and is punctuated by a shared sense of closeness, trust, and support.

Occupational therapists must be aware of the different stages of group development, which include many aspects and stages of group cohesiveness and maturity. The next phase includes an understanding of group norms. See **Table 28-6**.

The OT and occupational therapy assistant (OTA) must also consider the context in which groups are carried out and how they impact client performance individually and in a group setting. The AOTA and the American Psychological Association discuss the following analysis and adaptation of the environment, which may include the following:

• Physical environment includes the physical setting and the objects within the environment.
• Social environment includes environmental demands, such as people, culture, and rules of behavior.

Table 28-6 Established Group Norms	
Norms	**Criteria**
Explicit	Consistent rules: • *Social*: Confidentiality, waiting turns, and discussions remain in the group, supportive, and nonjudgmental. • *Punctuality*: Begin and end the group on time and arrive and leave at designated times. • *Work related*: Carry out task as directed or instructed. • *Group organization*: Behavior management, follow rules, and address disruptive behaviors (e.g., ask the person to leave after three disruptions).
Implicit	Indirectly implied evolving rules based on observations of nonverbal behavioral observations: • Give permission to behave emotionally with acceptance and offering support. • Imitate acts through social reinforcement. • Adapt behaviors based on nonverbal acts (i.e., extinction of negative behaviors and acknowledgment of positive behaviors).
Positive	Acts that create cohesiveness and trust: • Negotiate. • Compromise.
Negative	Acts that create dissension: • Interrupting or disrupting a group in process. • Subgrouping. • Avoiding topics or becoming directly involved. • Criticizing or blaming others.

Data from Bryant et al., 2014; Cole, 2012.

- Observations of the physical and social environments and the process of altering these environments to meet the needs of the individual and the group (AOTA, 2014; American Psychiatric Association, 2013).

Finally, it is critical to understand safety implications and considerations. First and foremost, OT providers must maintain universal precautions by observing infection control protocols with all clients at all times. Cole (2012) provides a list of suggestions for attempts at controlling the surrounding environment:

1. Keep track of keys and sharps, such as scissors, pens, and pencils.

2. Ensure restricted items are not taken from a treatment area to the ward or hospital floor. For example, items that can be used as weapons or to deface property.
3. Prepare the treatment area before the client enters the room.
4. Do not leave a client unattended.
5. Be selective about who is in the surrounding environment during the time of the group.
6. Alert the client to potential dangers related to planned activities.
7. Follow safety precautions for hazards and toxins.
8. Do not substitute or recycle containers; use original containers with labels.
9. Have knowledge of and use proper safety equipment.
10. Provide structure and manage the group to maintain emotional and physical safety.
11. Attend to and take all threats, medical complaints, and emergencies seriously.

Referrals and Discharge Considerations

As an OT prepares for client discharge to a medical, home, or community setting, collaboration with appropriate professionals within the treatment setting (e.g., physician, psychiatrist, occupational therapist, and social worker) and caregivers must be established. The client and/or their advocate must be included in the discharge and/or referral planning process. Goals and objectives for further treatment should be established and clearly communicated with the appropriate individuals.

Management and Standards of Practice

All intervention plans that are implemented should be carried out as documented in the client's treatment plan by either the OT or OTA. Any changes should be discussed with the OT and follow facility protocols. All information regarding the client must be confidential and not discussed in open, public places such as staff rooms or elevators. Nothing should be photocopied, taken home, or captured by any form of social media.

Chapter 28 Self-Study Activities

Case Scenario 1

Amanda is a 25-year-old single woman with an 11th grade education. She lives with her parents and two young children (ages 4 and 5 years old) fathered by two different men. The relationships between her and her children's fathers are strained causing her to be very angry. Amanda was recently discharged from the hospital with a diagnosis of depression. Prior to treatment, Amanda presented with symptoms of mood swings, crying spells, angry outbursts, and poor sleeping patterns. She is financially unable to move out on her own and relies on her parents for shelter and childcare; however, she becomes frustrated and argumentative with her parents when they remind her of house rules and evening curfews. Amanda typically leaves her parents' home nearly every evening to hang out with her friends to drink alcohol and smoke marijuana. She returns home late at night and has a hard time getting up to get the children ready for school. She is noncompliant with her antidepressant medicine and plans to ask her doctor for a medical marijuana prescription. She has a personal goal of passing a General Education Development (GED) test and securing stable employment to financially care for her children.

Case Scenario 1 Questions

1. What are Amanda's challenges and strengths?
2. What are appropriate long-term goals?
3. What are appropriate short-term goals that would address her long-term goals?
4. How should the OT prioritize Amanda's goals?
5. What types of activities should be suggested for her to engage in to reach her goals?
6. What frame of reference/theory supports the intervention choices?

Case Scenario 2

A recent OT graduate begins her first job at an acute, inpatient, locked, psychiatric unit in a general hospital. The clients are diagnosed with a wide variety of acute psychiatric disorders. The present OT is planning on retiring soon after 20 years of employment and typically leads the same type of discussion groups each day with little variety. The new OT would like to revise the current unit activity schedule to implement techniques learned in her OT education program.

Case Scenario 2 Questions

1. How should the OT propose her new ideas to her supervisor?
2. What type of activity groups should she plan to conduct?

Case Scenario 3

Matthew has been married for 10 years to Sharon, his high school sweetheart. They have three children with another expected in six months. Sharon enjoys being a homemaker while Matthew works 10 hours a day in their family-owned hardware store. Matthew's father, a widower, recently experienced a stroke and it was decided, due to Matthew's personal values, that he move into their home while he recovers. Sharon loves her father-in-law; however, she is finding it overwhelming to care for her father-in-law's special needs, take care of the children, prepare meals, and manage the household. She has a routine now but is concerned that something will need to change when the new baby arrives.

Case Scenario 3 Questions

1. What community support groups should the OT recommend?
2. What types of activities are appropriate for Sharon to engage in to address her issues?
3. What frame of reference/approach is appropriate to support the OT's treatment interventions?

Case Scenario 4

Jerry is a 64-year-old man who has lived in various homeless shelters for the last three years after falling on hard times when his factory job closed. His wife passed away 10 years ago and he has no children or family members in the state where he lives. He has tried to find employment; however, he feels his age and limited skill set are keeping him from getting a job. He was admitted to the hospital for symptoms of depression and is preparing for discharge.

Case Scenario 4 Questions

1. What should the OT focus on first in preparation for discharge?
2. Who should the OT work with on the healthcare discharge team?
3. What type of community resources should the OT recommend?

Chapter 28 Self-Study Answers

Case Scenario 1

1. *Strengths*: 25-year old; lives with her parents; recently discharged; personal goal of earning a GED; and securing stable employment to financially care for her children.
   Challenges: Single woman with an 11th grade education; two young children (ages 4 and 5 years old) fathered by two different men; relationships between her and her children's fathers are strained; financially unable to move out on her own and relies on her parents for shelter and childcare; drinks alcohol and smokes marijuana; noncompliant with her antidepressant medication; medical marijuana prescription.
2. Earn a GED and skilled trade; independent housing, medication compliance; drug- and alcohol-free lifestyle. Improve relationships with the fathers of her children and parents.
3. Medication compliance, abstinence from alcohol and marijuana, prepare for/seek out GED courses, look for employment, and anger management.
4. Address medication compliance and drug/alcohol use, enhance self-esteem, and strengthen relationship with supportive parents.
5. Explore job interests and skills, worksheets to prepare for GED and job applications, coping skills, relaxation, and parenting.
6. MOHO and/or developmental.

Case Scenario 2

1. If appropriate for the setting, request to schedule a meeting with her supervisor to discuss her ideas. If approved by her supervisor, include the outgoing OT in the planning sessions for her valuable experience.
2. *Variety of diagnosis*: Depression, manic behavior, schizophrenia, personality disorders, obsessive thoughts, and compulsive behaviors.
   Variety of activities: ADLs, task groups, stress management, community resource, employment groups, money management, anger management, assertiveness training, time management, problem solving, goal setting, meal preparation, home maintenance, interpersonal and social skills, gross motor skills, life skills, and self-esteem.

Case Scenario 3

1. Explore home services provided by the insurance provider. A support group for new mothers offered at a hospital.
2. Stress reduction, exercise, time management, home organization. Consult with therapist(s) on interventions and home modifications for her father-in-law.
3. MOHO for Matthew and Sharon, a sensory motor approach and Allen's cognitive disabilities for the father-in-law.

Case Scenario 4

1. Work with the discharge planner to make sure Jerry has housing. Provide information on community resources that provide employment and skill building.
2. Social work and nursing.
3. Support groups and return to work programs.

References

American Occupational Therapy Association. (2014). Occupational therapy practice framework: Domain and process (3rd ed.). *American Journal of Occupational Therapy, 68*(Suppl. 1), S1–S48. doi:10.5014/ajot.2014.682006

American Psychiatric Association. (2013). *Diagnostic and statistical manual of mental disorders: DSM-5* (5th ed.). Washington, DC: Author.

Ayres, A. J. (1977). Cluster analyses of measures of sensory integration. *American Journal of Occupational Therapy, 31*(6), 362–366. Retrieved from http://www.ncbi.nlm.nih.gov/pubmed/879252

Bruce, M. A., Borg, B., & Bruce, M. A. (2002). *Psychosocial frames of reference: Core for occupation-based practice* (3rd ed.). Thorofare, NJ: SLACK Incorporated.

Bryant, W., Fieldhouse, J., Bannigan, K., Creek, J., & Lougher, L. (2014). *Creek's occupational therapy and mental health* (5th ed.). Edinburgh, UK: Churchill Livingstone/Elsevier.

Cole, M. B. (2012). *Group dynamics in occupational therapy: The theoretical basis and practice application of group intervention* (4th ed.). Thorofare, NJ: SLACK Incorporated.

Early, M. B. (2009). *Mental health concepts and techniques for the occupational therapy assistant* (4th ed.).

Philadelphia, PA: Wolters Kluwer Health/Lippincott Williams & Wilkins.

Kaplan, K. (1988). *Directive group therapy: Innovative mental health treatment*. Thorofare, NJ: SLACK Incorporated.

Kielhofner, G. (2008). *Model of human occupation: Theory and application* (4th ed.). Baltimore, MD: Lippincott Williams & Wilkins.

McColl, M. A., Law, M., Baptiste, S., Pollock, N., Carswell, A., & Polatajko, H. J. (2005). Targeted applications of the Canadian Occupational Performance Measure. *Canadian Journal of Occupational Therapy, 72*(5), 298–300. Retrieved from http://www.ncbi.nlm.nih .gov/pubmed/16435590

Mosey, A. C. (1973). *Activities therapy*. New York, NY: Raven Press.

Richards, G. (2014). Management and leadership. In W. Bryant, J. Fieldhouse, K. Bannigan, J. Creek, & L. Lougher (Eds.), *Creek's occupational therapy and mental health* (5th ed., pp. 120–131). Edinburgh, UK: Churchill Livingstone/Elsevier.

Scaffa, M. E. (2014). Group process and group intervention. In B. A. B. Schell, G. Gillen, & M. E. Scaffa (Eds.), *Willard & Spackman's occupational therapy* (12th ed., pp. 437–451). Philadelphia, PA: Wolters Kluwer Health/Lippincott Williams & Wilkins.

Toglia, J. P., Golisz, K. M., & Goverover, Y. (2014). Cognition, perception, and occupational performance. In B. A. B. Schell, G. Gillen, & M. E. Scaffa (Eds.), *Willard & Spackman's occupational therapy* (12th ed., pp. 779–815). Philadelphia, PA: Wolters Kluwer Health/Lippincott Williams & Wilkins.

Yalom, I. D., & Leszcz, M. (2005). *The theory and practice of group psychotherapy* (5th ed.). New York, NY: Basic Books.

Pediatric Occupational Functioning Days 20-21

Pediatric Assessments

Robin Mercer and Beth Angst

Learning Objectives

- Describe core concepts of pediatric assessments, including the purpose and appropriate methods.
- Compare and contrast the standardized evaluation tools and skilled observation methods.
- Describe the developmental sequence for gross and fine motor skills, feeding, sensory processing, and visual motor control.
- Apply knowledge of assessments to the provided chapter learning activities.

Key Terms

- *Chronological age*: Age in years, months, and days since the person's birth.
- *Criterion referenced*: The measurement of performance based on a description of expected outcomes.
- *Developmental age*: Estimated age based on physical and mental maturation.
- *Norm-referenced*: The measurement of performance against a predefined population based on the same performance criteria.
- *Standardized test*: The same protocol used for administration and scoring of an assessment.

Introduction

This chapter reviews the important aspects of evaluations in pediatrics. The underlying theory is the same as with the adult population in that the purpose of a pediatric evaluation is to obtain a sense of challenges, strengths, weaknesses, and functional goals. The evaluation of children requires an occupational therapist (OT) to have a strong understanding of typical development, as well as knowledge of the different assessments available. It also relies more on an ability to use other means of gathering information, such as interviewing the parents or caregivers and using skilled observations because children are not always willing or able to cooperate with standardized testing.

Screening and Assessments

The purpose of a pediatric evaluation is to assess what the child wants and needs to do, what strengths support and what weaknesses or challenges interfere with childhood occupations. Childhood occupations include play, school activities, and self-help skills (American Occupational Therapy Association, 2014; Case-Smith, 2010; Mulligan, 2014; Rogers, 2010).

Factors to Consider for Specific Pediatric Conditions

When performing assessments in the pediatric population, the whole child needs to be taken into account. The age and developmental level of the child often dictate the important areas to assess more than the specific diagnosis. All children should be assessed for strength, tone, developmental level, and implications for activities of daily living (ADLs). A basic familiarity with the condition is required to understand the long-term implications such as if it is a static or progressive disorder and if the condition affects cognition to a level that will alter expected outcomes. **Table 29-1** provides a list of conditions with brief suggestions of areas that are likely to be of concern.

Table 29-1 Pediatric Conditions and Evaluation Areas

Diagnosis	Most Likely Areas to Evaluate
Autism spectrum disorders	Sensory processing and ADLs
Burns	ROM and the need for splinting
Cardiac conditions	Strength, endurance, and feeding in infants
Congenital anomalies	ROM and the need for assistive devices to complete ADLs
Cystic fibrosis	Endurance and ADLs
Developmental coordination disorders	Sensory processing, gross and fine motor skills, and ADLs
Developmental disabilities	Tone, overall developmental level of gross and fine motor skills
Juvenile rheumatoid arthritis	ROM, stamina, and the need for assistive devices for ADLs
Muscular dystrophy	Strength, tone, ADLs, and the need for assistive devices
Musculoskeletal (e.g., limb deficiencies)	ROM, ADLs, play skills, and the need for assistive devices
Neural tube defects (e.g., spina bifida or myelomeningocele)	Tone, strength, developmental level, and the need for assistive devices
Neuromuscular disorders (e.g., cerebral palsy, including ataxia, spastic, and athetoid types)	Tone, strength, developmental level, feeding, and the need for adaptive equipment
Peripheral nerve injuries (e.g., brachial plexus injuries)	Active range, strength, and the need for splinting
Prematurity	Feeding, positioning, and environmental stimulation, or sensory input
Traumatic brain injury	Tone, ROM, and ADLs including feeding

Data from Rogers, 2010.

Evaluation Process

A comprehensive evaluation is completed to determine eligibility, assist with diagnosis, plan intervention, and reevaluate, as well as contribute to clinical research. The evaluation may be conducted in one of a variety of settings depending on the initial concerns and the reason for the assessment. These typically include educational, outpatient (e.g., mental health facilities) and inpatient settings, as well as assessment participation, and the inclusion of parents or caregivers as described below.

- *Assessment participation*: Follow a client-centered practice model. For children, this will involve play and observation in the environment where the child is having difficulty. If possible, this may include the home, classroom, or playground, but observation may also have to be completed in a hospital setting with a simulation of typical activities.
- *Include parents or caregivers*: They may give the OT pertinent information about the child's history, as well as information on their perception of the child's difficulties and how these challenges impact family life. Parents may assist in getting the child to participate in the evaluation process to help determine if the performance is typical.

Assessment Methods

Standardized Assessments

The choice of which test to give is based on a number of issues, including the reason for the referral, availability of tests, and the occupational therapy practitioner's level of competence in conducting a given assessment. Standardized tests (see **Table 29-2**) must be administered according to the test protocol; using the standardized test materials for the scores to be valid. Calculate chronological age and adjust for prematurity. Norm-referenced assessments compare the child's score to that of a sample group that was assessed when the test was developed. Common pediatric assessments that are norm-referenced include, but are not limited to, the following.

Criterion-Referenced Measures

Criterion-referenced assessments measure group skills into functional or developmental areas, by age level. Common pediatric assessments that are criterion-referenced include, but are not limited to, the assessments outlined in **Table 29-3**.

Table 29-2 Standardized Assessments

Test Name	Author(s)	Age Ranges	What It Tests
Battelle Developmental Inventory	Newborg (2005)	Birth–8 years	Personal social skills, adaptive behavior (e.g., self-help), psychomotor, communication, and cognition
Bayley Scales of Infant Development	Bayley (2005)	1–42 months	Cognitive and motor development
Beery–Buktenica Developmental Test of Visual-Motor Integration (VMI)	Beery, Buktenica, and Beery (2010)	2–65+ years	Visual-motor integration deficits
Bruininks–Oseretsky Tests of Motor Skills, second edition	Bruininks and Bruininks (2005)	4.5–14.5 years	Gross motor, upper limb, and fine motor proficiency
DeGangi–Berk Test of Sensory Integration	Berk and DeGangi (1983)	3–5 years	Sensory processing difficulties
Developmental Test of Visual Perception (DTVP-2)	Hammill, Pearson, and Voress (1988)	4–10 years	Visual perceptual and visual motor integration
Miller Assessment for Preschoolers (MAP)	Miller (1988)	2 years 9 months–5 years 8 months	Sensory motor foundations, motor coordination, verbal and nonverbal skills, and performance on complex tasks
Motor-Free Visual Perception Test (MVPT-3)	Colarussi and Hammill (2002)	4–70 years	Visual perceptual abilities that do not require motor involvement
Peabody Developmental Motor Scales, second edition (PDMS-2)	Folio and Fewell (2000)	Birth–5 years	Gross and fine motor skills
Sensory Integration and Praxis Test	Ayres (2004)	4–9 years	Sensory integration processes
Test of Visual Motor Skills–Revised	Gardner (1995)	3–13 years	Eye–hand coordination skills needed to copy geometric designs
Test of Visual Perceptual Skills non motor (TVPS-3)	Martin (2006)	4–18 years	Visual perceptual skills

Data from Mulligan, 2014; O'Brien and Williams, 2010; Richardson, 2010; Stewart, 2010.

Table 29-3 Criterion-Referenced Assessments

Test Name	Ages	What It Tests
Hawaii Early Learning Profile (Furuno et al., 2004)	Infants, toddlers, and young children	Developmental needs, intervention goals, and tracks progress
School Function Assessment (Coster, Deeney, Haltiwanger, & Haley, 1998)	Kindergarten through grade 6	Student's level of participation, supports needed, and activity performance on specific school tasks
Evaluation Tool of Children's Handwriting (ETCH) (Amundson, 1995)	Grades 1–6	Manuscript and cursive handwriting skills
Gross Motor Function Measure revised (GMFM) (Russell, Rosenbaum, Avery, & Lane, 2002)	Children whose motor skills are at or below a 5-year-old level	Gross motor function in children with cerebral palsy and Down syndrome

Data from Mulligan, 2014; Stewart, 2010.

Observation Assessments

Some assessments are set up as observational tools and include, but are not limited to, the following:

- *Childhood Autism Rating Scale* (CARS 2) (Schopler, Reichler, & Renner, 2002): Age 2 years and older; distinguishes children with autism from children with other cognitive delays, and helps determine severity of autistic symptoms.
- *Erhardt Developmental Prehension Assessment* (Revised) (Erhardt, 1994): Looks at components of arm and hand development in children with cerebral palsy or other neurologic impairments.
- *Knox Preschool Play Scale* (Revised) (Parham & Fazio, 1997): Birth to six years; assesses play behaviors.
- *WeeFIM* (Hamilton & Granger, 1991): 6 months to 6 years; looks at self-care, mobility, and cognitive skills to determine the amount of caregiver assistance required.

Skilled observation is essential to the pediatric OT. Children do not always comply with standardized testing, often making the scores invalid. Children act differently in different environments and with different people. Important information can be gathered through skilled observation that is not covered on a standardized developmental assessment. Skilled observation of neuromotor status includes tone, strength, posture, interviews with the child and the referral source (e.g., physician, school teacher or psychologist, clinic staff) if appropriate, and with the parents or caregivers. This gives background information and validation of information gathered through more formal assessments. Assessments that are set up as questionnaires will assist with the interview process. They include, but are not limited to, the following:

- *Sensory Profile 2* (Dunn, 2014): Birth to 14 years 11 months and caregiver questionnaire. There is also an adolescent/adult sensory profile for ages 11 and older (Brown & Dunn, 2002).
- *Ages and Stages Questionnaire* (Bricker & Squires, 1999): Birth to 5 years, including communication, gross motor, fine motor, problem-solving, and personal-social.
- *Canadian Occupational Performance Measure* (COPM) (Law et al., 2005): Helps identify family priorities for children with special needs.
- *Pediatric Evaluation of Disability Inventory* (PEDI) (Haley, Coster, Ludlow, Haltiwanger, &

Andrellos, 1992): 6 months to 7.5 years. Measures capabilities and performance in self-care, mobility, and social function.

Specific Assessment Areas

Arena assessments are conducted with a team of professionals and use a transdisciplinary approach. Generally one discipline takes the lead with the child while the other professionals observe. **Tables 29-4** and **29-5** contain reflexes and reactions that are not typically covered in standardized tests.

Muscle Tone

The evaluation of tone is a skilled observation that involves handling the child and observing his or her functional movement patterns.

- Hypotonia is noted when there is a decreased amount of resistance when a muscle is moved through available range of motion (ROM). A soft feeling to the muscle, hypermobile joints, a slouched posture, and facial drooping may also be noted.
- Hypertonia is noted when there is increased resistance or tension when a muscle is moved through available ROM. Decreased joint mobility, fisted hands, scissoring of the extremities, arching, and retraction or tightness of facial muscles may also be noted.

Strength and ROM

Not different in theory from adults but may require skilled observation because the child cannot always follow specific instructions for a manual muscle test.

- Observe functional strength and range by noting the ability to complete an activity and also monitoring endurance. Can he or she reach against gravity to get a toy? Can the motion be repeated several times? Is it a smoother motion when they are in sidelying, reaching with gravity eliminated, or are they able to reach over their head in sitting?
- Specific ROM measurements are valuable, in particular, for children with cerebral palsy or other disorders that result in increased tone, as well as with children with burn injuries. The treatment will be designed to maintain or increase the ROM, so specific measurements will assist with monitoring progress.

Table 29-4 Reflexes, Righting, Equilibrium, and Protective Reactions

Reflex	How to Test	Age Reflex Emerges	Age Reflex Fades
Rooting	Stroke the side of mouth and observe the head turning toward the stimulus	28 weeks gestation	3–7 months (i.e., longer in babies who are nursed)
Sucking	Place a finger on the roof of the infants mouth and observe sucking ability	28 weeks gestation	3–7 months
Palmar grasp	Press a finger into the palm and observe the fingers flexing in a tight grip	30 weeks gestation	3–4 months
Asymmetrical tonic neck	In supine, turn the head to one side and note extension of the arm and the leg on the face side and flexion of the limbs on the skull side	1 month	4 months
Symmetrical tonic neck	Prone over lap, flex the neck, and observe the arms flex and the legs extend; extend the neck and observe the arms extend and the legs flex	4 months	10 months
Moro	Support in a semi-reclined position and momentarily release support to observe for abduction, extension and external rotation of the arms, followed by flexion and adduction	28 weeks gestation	4 months

Data from Bazyk and Case-Smith, 2010; Mulligan, 2014; O'Brien and Williams, 2010; Stewart, 2010.

Table 29-5 Development of Automatic Reactions

Reaction	How to Observe	Age Response Emerges
Protective responses	In sitting, gently push the child off balance to the front, each side, and back, and observe for arm extension and placement to prevent falling	Front: 6–7 months Side: 7–10 months Back: 9–12 months
Head righting	In sitting or held suspended, tilt the child gently from side to side and from front to back and observe the child moving the head in the opposite direction to maintain head alignment with their body	3–4 months
Neck on body righting	In supine, rotate the child's head to one side; note if body rotation and the child rolling to prone occurs as a unit or segmentally	Segmental rolling emerges at 4–5 months
Body on body righting	In supine, rotate the child's hips to one side; observe the child rotate the upper body and roll over to align the body	Segmental rolling emerges at 4–5 months
Equilibrium reactions	Test in prone, supine, four point, and standing. Tilt the supporting surface to one side and then the other. When tilted to the left, observe for lateral flexion of the right side of the trunk with rotation; when tilted to the right, observe for lateral flexion of the left side of the trunk with rotation; all with head righting	Prone: 5–6 months Supine: 7–8 months Sitting: 7–10 months Quadruped: 9–12 months Standing: 12–20 months

Data from Mulligan, 2014.

Gross Motor Development

The developmental sequence is based on developing mobility, stability, or both in weight-bearing, and then mobility and stability in nonweight-bearing for increased skill level. It is developed not only through improving strength and balance, but also as a response to processing of sensory input including vestibular, proprioceptive, and visual (Exner, 2010; Mulligan, 2014; O'Brien & Williams, 2010). See **Table 29-6**.

Sensory Processing

A clear understanding of the many aspects of sensory processing is necessary to evaluate sensory challenges properly. This includes an understanding of

Table 29-6 Gross Motor Development

Age in Months	Prone and Supine Skills	Sitting and Four Point Skills	Standing and Walking
2–4 months	In prone, the shoulder girdle begins to protract, and weight-bearing occurs through the lower body. The child is able to lift the head and maintain posture. In supine, the child is able to maintain the head in neutral and can achieve some neck flexion in pull to sit. The child visually tracks and can get his or her hands to the mouth	Unable to sit unsupported; rounded back in supported sit	Stepping reflexes when held in standing
4–6 months	In prone with hand propping and extended elbows. The child is able to roll from prone to supine. In supine, with midline play and the arms over the chest, the child is able to play with his or her feet. The child can roll to sidelying	Can sit with hand support to the front or sides. Can momentarily free a hand. Can weight bear in quadruped position. Pivots in prone or may scoot backward	Partial weight-bearing in supported standing
6–9 months	The child can assume a quadruped position and begin to rock and may crawl. The child rolls from prone to supine and from supine to prone with rotation	Moves in and out of sitting, sits well, and begins to creep	Stands supported and can bear full weight through the legs
9–18 months		Crawls well	Cruises along furniture or walks with hands held. Walks independently at 12–18 months

Data from J. Case-Smith, 2010; Mulligan, 2014.

Table 29-7 Sensory Integration Terms

Response	Description
Adaptive response	A successful response to an environmental challenge
Body scheme	The brain's map of body parts and how they interrelate
Perception	The organization of sensory data into meaningful units
Praxis	The ability to conceptualize, organize, and execute nonhabitual motor tasks
Ideation	The ability to conceptualize a new action to be performed in a given situation
Sensory defensiveness	Characterized by over responsivity in one or more sensory systems
Sensory integration	Organization of sensation for use
Sensory modulation	Ability to generate a response that is appropriately proportionate to the incoming sensory stimuli
Sensory registration	Process by which the central nervous system attends to stimuli
Sensory processing	Referring to the handling of sensory information by neural systems
Vestibular	Pertaining to receptors and organs that detect head position, movement, and gravity
Somatosensory	Pertaining to the tactile and proprioceptive systems.

Data from Parham and Mailoux, 2010.

modulation, registration, defensiveness, discrimination, and proprioception, as well as motor planning or praxis (see **Tables 29-7** and **29-8**) (Mulligan, 2014; Parham & Mailoux, 2010). Methods to obtain this information include the following formal assessments, including interviews and questionnaires and informal observations, including clinical observations.

Table 29-8 Sensory Integration Responses	
Response	**Description**
Gravitational insecurity	The child reacts negatively to movement, especially when the head is moving backward
Hyper-responsivity	The child reacts defensively to ordinary sensory input and frequently demonstrates activation of the sympathetic nervous system
Hypo-responsivity	The child tends to ignore sensory stimuli that would produce a response in most individuals
Sensory seeking	The child searches out specific sensory input at a higher frequency and/or intensity
Tactile defensiveness	The child tends to react negatively to clothing, dislikes having shoes off, and has a tendency to weight bear on the fingertips rather than the palms
Over responsiveness	Disorder used interchangeably with hyper-responsivity
Under responsiveness	Disorder used interchangeably with hypo-responsivity

Data from Parham and Mailoux, 2010.

Fine Motor Development

In regard to fine motor, it is generally accepted that motor skill development occurs from proximal to distal; however, new theories such as the systems theory of motor development have presented an alternative viewpoint. Irrespective of this ongoing debate, evaluation of fine motor skills should incorporate an evaluation of overall postural control; for example, head control, balance, tone, and strength. Fine motor skills may also be impaired due to sensory impairments such as tactile, proprioceptive, and visual deficits (Exner, 2010).

Development of Grasp

Grasp (see **Table 29-9**) is the attainment of an object with the hand, release is intentional letting go at a specific time and place, and reach is the extension and movement of the arm for grasping or placing (Exner, 2010). Grasp develops from a reflexive pattern with no voluntary control, to a voluntary palmar grasp. At about six months, a radial palmar grasp develops. By six to nine months, grasp patterns with active thumb use develops and by 9–12 months, a neat pincer grasp develops (Exner, 2010).

In-Hand Manipulation

Development of in-hand manipulation requires movement and stability in various degrees of supination, wrist stability, opposed grasp, isolated thumb and finger movements, control of the transverse metacarpal arch,

disassociation of the radial and ulnar sides of the hand, and control of fingertip force (see **Table 29-10**).

- Bilateral hand use involves the coordination of both hands. Hands are used either together, such as throwing a large ball, or one for stability and the other for movement, such as holding a piece of paper to cut with scissors.
- Tool use includes the purposeful use of an object to manipulate another object; for example, silverware, writing instruments, and scissors.

Handwriting Evaluation Considerations

Handwriting evaluation includes domains, legibility, speed, and ergonomic factors described as follows (Case-Smith, 2010):

- *Domains*: Letter formation, copying, both near and far point, writing dictated words, and writing from original thought.
- *Legibility*: Size, formation, alignment, and spacing.
- *Speed*: Measured in relation to peer and classroom expectations.
- *Ergonomic factors*: Posture, pencil grip, stability, and mobility of the upper extremities.

Visual Motor/Visual Perception

Visual acuity, visual fields, and oculomotor control may require an evaluation by an optometrist or ophthalmologist; however, the OT can perform a functional

Table 29-9 Types of Refined Grasp

Type	Age	Description	Example
Pincer (i.e., two-point or pad to pad)	10 months	Opposition of the thumb to index finger pad	Picking up a piece of cereal
Lateral pinch	3 years	Partial thumb adduction, MCP flexion and a slight IP flexion with the pad of the thumb against the radial side of the index finger	Using a key in a lock
Power grasp	5 years	Used to control tools or objects stabilizing with the ulnar side of the hand and controlling the position and use with the radial side	Scooping ice cream
Three jaw chuck (i.e., three-point pinch)	3–5 years with increased strength	Opposition of the thumb simultaneously to the index and middle finger pads	Tripod grasp on a pencil
Spherical grasp	18 months–3 years	Wrist extension, finger abduction, and some degree of IP and MCP flexion	Holding a ball
Cylindrical grasp	18 months–3 years	Palmar arch is flattened and the fingers are only slightly abducted with IP and MCP flexion graded to fit the object's size and weight	Holding a glass
Hook grasp	18 months–3 years	Fingers adducted with flexion at the IP joints and flexion or extension of the MCP joints	Carrying a pail
Disk grasp	18 months–3 years	Finger abduction graded according to the size of the object, hyperextension of the MCP joints, and flexion of the IP joints	Unscrewing the lid of a jar

IP, interphalangeal joint; MCP, metacarpophalangeal joint.
Data from Exner, 2010.

Table 29-10 Types of In-Hand Manipulation

Skill	Description	Example
Finger to palm translation	Grasping an object with the pads of the fingers and thumb and moving it into the palm of the hand	Picking up coins to hold in a hand
Palm to finger translation	Isolated control of the thumb and finger flexion moving toward finger extension	Taking coins from the palm of the hand and putting them in a vending machine
Shift	Linear movement of an object on a finger's surface to allow for repositioning	Separating two pieces of paper
Simple rotation	Fingers act as a unit with the thumb in an opposed position while turning an object 90° or less	Unscrewing a small cap
Complex rotation	Rotation of an object 180° to 360° as the fingers move independently and alternate with the thumb	Turning a pencil to use the eraser

Data from Exner, 2010; Mulligan, 2014.

assessment to determine if a referral for further testing is appropriate. Review the standardized tests that assess visual spatial and visual motor functioning (Mulligan, 2014; Schneck, 2010).

- *Visual acuity*: This needs to be formally assessed by an optometrist or ophthalmologist, and assessed for the ability to track, localize, and focus on objects.

- *Visual tracking/oculomotor control*: Look for the ability to separate eye movement from head movement, the ability to smoothly follow across midline, and the ability of the eyes to work together.
- *Functional vision*: Can the child complete puzzles, find objects on a page or with a variety of other objects, copy from near or far points, sort objects, and move around obstacles?

- *Sensitivity to visual stimuli*: Visual reactivity to stimuli such as bright lights.
- *Form perception*: Constancy, closure, and figure ground recognition.
- *Spatial perception*: Position in space, depth perception, and topographic orientation.
- *Visual motor integration*: How the eyes and hands work together; generally assessed through tracing or copying designs.

Feeding/Oral Motor

Information on feeding requires input from family members, in addition to the information gathered from an evaluation of the child. The time it takes to complete a meal, the diet appropriate for nutrition, the diet appropriate for the child's culture, and the stress involved in getting the child to participate are all important aspects that are not directly found by conducting an oral motor assessment. When conducting an oral motor evaluation, overall development, as well as positioning for feeding is evaluated. The sensory responses to smell, taste, and texture are also part of the evaluation (also see **Table 29-11** for developmental sequences of eating) (Schuberth, Amirault, & Case-Smith, 2010).

Activities of Daily Living

ADLs need to take into account the context of the task and where the task is being carried out (e.g., home, school, and community), the developmental level of the child, and the social environment, including cultural differences in expectations (Case-Smith, 2010; Schuberth et al., 2010; Shepherd, 2010) (see **Tables 29-12** and **29-13** for self-feeding and dressing developmental time frames).

Toileting

The approximate age for toilet training is 2.5–3 years; by 3–3.5 years they should be independent with the exception of wiping or managing fasteners on clothing. Complete independence in toileting is 4–5 years, including washing hands and managing clothing.

Referrals and Discharge Considerations

Pediatric evaluations differ from adult evaluations in that every diagnosis needs to be considered in the context

Table 29-11 Developmental Sequence of Eating

Age	Types of Food	Sucking/Drinking	Biting/Chewing
0–3 months	Liquids only	Suckling pattern	None
4–6 months	Liquids or pureed	Suckling pattern is more mature	Primitive phasic bite with a munching pattern
9 months	Soft foods and mashed table foods	Can begin cup drinking	Voluntary biting and munching with a diagonal pattern
12–18 months	Coarsely chopped foods	Primarily from a cup	Begin rotary chewing and controlled sustained bite on harder objects

Data from Mulligan, 2014; Schuberth et al., 2010.

Table 29-12 Self-Feeding Skills

Age in Months	Self-Feeding Skills Observed
5–7	Takes pureed food from a spoon
6–9	Attempts to hold a bottle, holds a cracker or cookie and attempts to eat it, and may grab a spoon but sucks on either end
9–13	Finger feeds self a portion of the meal and is more proficient with cup drinking
12–14	Dips a spoon into food but not yet skilled enough to be independent
15–18	Scoops food with a spoon and brings the spoon to the mouth
24–30	Interested in using a fork, proficient in using a spoon with mixed consistency foods, and can drink from a straw

Data from Mulligan, 2014; Schuberth et al., 2010.

Table 29-13 Dressing

Age (years)	Dressing Skills
1	Cooperates in dressing and pulls off shoes and socks
2	Removes unfastened front opening garments and helps pull down pants
2.5	Removes elastic waist pants, puts on front opening coat/shirt, and unbuttons large buttons
3	Puts on pullover shirt, puts on shoes without fasteners, puts on socks, pulls pants down independently, zips and unzips if already engaged, and buttons large buttons
3.5	Snaps or hooks in front, unzips separating zipper, buttons series of three to four buttons, can dress with supervision for correct orientation of front and back of garments
4	Removes pullover garment, zips, buckles, puts on shoes, laces but cannot yet tie, and consistent with front and back of garments
5	Ties and unties knots and dresses unsupervised
6	Closes back zipper, ties bows, buttons back buttons, and snaps back snaps

Data from Mulligan, 2014.

of the child's age and overall development. In adulthood, the expectation of performance at various ages is relatively stable. During childhood, however, there are vast changes in expectations of performance as the child grows and develops. Knowledge of a general developmental sequence in gross motor, fine motor, oral motor, and self-care is invaluable in determining areas of evaluation and the need for treatment. Referrals to various healthcare professionals may occur if the OT obtains evidence of challenges that are outside of the scope of practice for occupational therapy. This may occur through observation, screening, or child and/or parent report. A discharge plan is proposed when the child has achieved their proposed goals and is successfully participating in their occupations, which usually takes place through a gradual decrease in occupational therapy services.

Management and Standards of Practice

While there are a variety of standardized tests available, they are limited in the chronological ages, developmental ages, and cognitive levels that can be tested. Much of the information needed for a comprehensive evaluation and the development of a treatment plan comes from skilled observation and the interview with the caregiver and the child when appropriate. Regardless of the specific diagnosis, tone, strength, and overall ability to participate in ADLs, school, and play are important evaluation considerations. OTs and occupational therapy assistants work together to provide the most appropriate care possible for each individual child.

Chapter 29 Self-Study Activities (Answers Are Provided at the End of the Chapter)

Case Study 1

A 7-year-old female comes for an occupational therapy evaluation to a hospital-based outpatient facility. The prescription from the physician states, "left hemiplegia, evaluate and treat." You are provided with her developmental history and learn she was born three months premature, was on a ventilator, and was tube fed until she was six months old. She is currently in a general education setting with some resource room support. She does not get occupational therapy services at school. Her mother reports the child has had therapy in the past, but not in the last 12 months. The child is ambulatory without assistive devices, but does wear an ankle foot orthosis on her left foot. She walks with her left arm in a slight flexor synergy pattern.

1. After meeting the child and her mother, what should the occupational therapy practitioner do first?
   A. Give her a standardized fine motor assessment, adjust for prematurity, and decide on eligibility for treatment based on those results.
   B. Interview the child, as well as the parent about what has been done in the past, what

the current limitations are, and what they are hoping to improve.

    C. Inform the mother that because her daughter is school aged, all treatment will have to be provided in school.

    D. Provide a splint for her left hand.

2. When assessing the need for a splint, the following should be considered:

    A. Range of motion, both active and passive

    B. Past trials of splints and outcomes of use

    C. The amount of tone present

    D. All of the above

    E. B and C

3. Her mother reports that the child is having difficulty with buttoning and zipping. The OT would assess this by:

    A. Asking her to show you how she zips and buttons

    B. Giving her a visual motor standardized assessment since she may not be able to see the buttonholes or where the zipper engages

    C. Watching how she manages with two-handed activities like lacing cards or stringing beads

    D. Giving her assistive devices such as a button hook or a loop on the end of her zipper

    E. A and C

    F. A and B

4. It is necessary to do a standardized assessment to formulate goals.

    A. True

    B. False

Case Study 2

You are a school OT called in to evaluate a 3-year-old child with autism. He is currently in a special education preschool classroom. He is able to follow simple one-step directions but is having frequent meltdowns, crying, covering his ears, and running around the room. He communicates by pointing or using one word.

1. The main areas for the OT to assess in his school setting include:

    A. Fine motor and oral motor skills

    B. Sensory processing and handwriting

    C. Sensory processing and self-help skills

    D. Oral motor and self-feeding

2. Assessing his sensory processing can be completed by:

    A. Using a questionnaire to be completed by a staff member or parent, such as the Sensory Profile

    B. Observing his reaction to stimuli in the environment

    C. Asking him what bothers him

    D. All of the above

    E. A and B

Pediatric ADL Skill Development Activity

Answer "yes" or "no" to the following questions, assuming the children are developing typically.

1. Can an 18-month-old sit on a potty chair for short periods?

2. Can a 13-month-old remove his socks?

3. Can a 30-month-old zip her jacket?

4. Can a 3-year-old tell someone he needs to go to the bathroom?

5. Would you expect an 18-month-old to be toilet trained?

6. Can a 2.5-year-old unbutton large buttons?

7. Can a 4-year-old lace shoes?

8. Can a 3-year-old dress unsupervised?

9. Can a 2-year-old remove a pullover shirt?

10. Can a 14-month-old cooperate with dressing by pushing his or her arms through sleeves?

11. Would you expect a 3-year-old to be mostly toilet trained during the day?

12. Can a 4-year-old button a series of three to four buttons?

13. Can a 42-month-old snap in the front?

14. Should you expect complete toilet training (i.e., bowel and bladder) between 4 and 5 years of age?

15. Would you expect a 36-month-old to engage a separating zipper?

Postural Control Worksheet

Match the stimulus with the reflex or automatic righting, equilibrium, or protective reaction that you would expect to observe.

Stimulus	Answer	Options
1. In sitting, displace the child forward so he or she could possibly fall.		A. Body on body righting B. Moro reflex C. Symmetrical tonic neck
2. Place your finger into a newborn's palm.		D. Rooting E. Asymmetrical tonic neck
3. In supine, rotate the infant's head and observe either log rolling or segmental rolling.		F. Palmar grasp

Stimulus	Answer	Options
4. The child is in a supported position sitting on a ball. Displace the child gently and watch the trunk and head.		G. Protective reaction H. Neck on body righting I. Equilibrium reactions J. Head righting
5. A 5-month-old is in a prone position over your lap. Flex or extend the head and observe the extremities.		
6. Stroke the side of a 2-month-old's cheek. Observe the head turning toward the stimulus.		
7. Tilt a 7-month-old while in a supported sitting position and observe the head movement in the opposite direction to maintain alignment with the body.		
8. In the supine position, turn the head of a 2-month-old to one side. Observe the extension of the arm on the face side and flexion of the arm on the skull side.		
9. Support a full-term newborn in a semi-reclined position and release the head; support momentarily. Observe the arm movements.		
10. In the supine position, rotate an infant's hips to one side. Observe the upper body rotating or segmental rolling.		

Chapter 29 Self-Study Answers

Case Study 1

1. The correct answer is B. Standardized tests would not give an OT the appropriate and needed information. The school is not able to provide treatment beyond what is educationally relevant and the OT does not know if the child would benefit from a splint.

2. The correct answer is D. If the child has full active ROM, a splint would not be necessary, and if she has too much tone, it may not be possible to fit one effectively. Conversely, it would not be necessary to provide a splint if the child has one but has never worn it (e.g., noncompliance).

3. The correct answer is E. Using alternate activities will allow an OT to assess hand function and see if it is a motor difficulty or just difficulty with the concept of buttoning or zipping, which would not necessarily be only watching her zip or button. Providing assistive devices is a treatment possibility, but not used to assess initially.

4. The correct answer is false. Many standardized assessments are not normed on children with disabilities. A child may score as age appropriate on a standardized assessment if they can complete the activities with their dominant hand only, but that does not take overall function into account.

Case Study 2

1. The correct answer is C. While a child with autism may have deficits in all of the above areas, his reaction to sensory stimuli is impacting his abilities in the classroom. He is too young to look at handwriting, and his oral motor skills are not the area that is interfering with his ability to fully access the curriculum.

2. The correct answer is E. He is unable to communicate effectively enough to be able to answer what is bothering him.

Answer Key for Worksheet 1: Pediatric ADL Skill Development

Answer yes or no to the following questions, assuming the children are developing typically.

1. Can an 18-month-old sit on a potty chair for short periods? **Yes**
2. Can a 13-month-old remove his socks? **Yes**
3. Can a 30-month-old zip her jacket? **No**
4. Can a 3-year-old tell someone he needs to go to the bathroom? **Yes**
5. Would you expect an 18-month-old to be toilet trained? **No**
6. Can a 2.5-year-old unbutton large buttons? **Yes**
7. Can a 4-year-old lace shoes? **Yes**
8. Can a 3-year-old dress unsupervised? **No**
9. Can a 2-year-old remove a pullover shirt? **No**
10. Can a 14-month-old cooperate with dressing by pushing his or her arms through sleeves? **Yes**
11. Would you expect a 3-year-old to be mostly toilet trained during the day? **Yes**
12. Can a 4-year-old button a series of three to four buttons? **Yes**
13. Can a 42-month-old snap in the front? **Yes**
14. Should you expect complete toilet training (i.e., bowel and bladder) between 4 and 5 years of age? **Yes**
15. Would you expect a 36-month-old to engage a separating zipper? **No**

Postural Control Worksheet Answers

1.	G
2.	F
3.	H
4.	J
5.	C
6.	D
7.	I
8.	E
9.	B
10.	A

References

American Occupational Therapy Association. (2014). Occupational therapy practice framework: Domain and process (3rd Edition). *American Journal of Occupational Therapy, 68*(Suppl. 1), S1–S48. doi:10.5014/ajot.2014.682006

Amundson, S. J. (1995). *Evaluation tool of children's handwriting (ETCH)*. Homer, AK: OT Kids.

Ayres, A. J. (2004). *Sensory integration and praxis tests manual*. Los Angeles, CA: Western Psychological Services.

Bayley, N. (2005). *Bayley scales of infant development* (3rd ed.). San Antonio, TX: PsychCorp.

Bazyk, S., & Case-Smith, J. (2010). School-based occupational therapy. In J. Case-Smith & J. C. O'Brien (Eds.), *Occupational therapy for children* (6th ed., pp. 713–743). Maryland Heights, MO: Mosby/Elsevier.

Beery, K., Buktenica, N., & Beery, N. (2010). *Beery-Buktenica developmental test of visual-motor integration (VMI)* (6th ed.). San Antonio, TX: Pearson, PsychCorp.

Berk, R., & DeGangi, G. (1983). *DeGangi-Berk test of sensory integration*. Los Angeles, CA: Western Psychological Services.

Bricker, D., & Squires, J. (1999). *Ages and stages questionnaires: A parent-completed, child-monitoring system* (2nd ed.). Baltimore, MD: Brookes.

Brown, C., & Dunn, W. (2002). *Adolescent/adult sensory profile: User's manual*. San Antonio, TX: Psychological Corporation.

Bruininks, R. H., & Bruininks, B. D. (2005). *Bruininks-Oseretsky test of motor proficiency* (2nd ed.). Circle Pines, MN: American Guidance Service.

Case-Smith, J. (2010). Development of childhood occupations. In J. Case-Smith & J. C. O'Brien (Eds.), *Occupational therapy for children* (6th ed., pp. 56–83). Maryland Heights, MO: Mosby/Elsevier.

Colarussi, R., & Hammill, D. (2002). *The motor-free visual perception test* (3rd ed.). Ann Arbor, MI: Academic Therapy Publications.

Coster, W., Deeney, T., Haltiwanger, J., & Haley, S. (1998). *School function assessment (SFA)*. San Antonio, TX: Psychological Corporation.

Dunn, W. (2014). *Sensory profile: User's manual*. San Antonio, TX: Psychological Corporation.

Erhardt, R. P. (1994). *Erhardt developmental prehension assessment* (Revised). San Antonio, TX: Psychological Corporation.

Exner, C. (2010). Evaluation and intervention to develop hand skills. In J. Case-Smith & J. C. O'Brien (Eds.), *Occupational therapy for children* (6th ed., pp. 275–324). Maryland Heights, MO: Mosby/Elsevier.

Folio, M. R., & Fewell, R. R. (2000). *The Peabody Developmental Motor Scales* (2nd ed.). Austin, TX: Pro-ED.

Furuno, S., O'Reilly, K., Hosaka, C. M., Inatsuka, T. T., Allman, T. L., & Zeisloft, B. (2004). *The Hawaii early learning profile.* Palo Alto, CA: VORT.

Gardner, M. (1995). *Test of visual-motor skills—Revised* (2nd ed.). Hydesville, CA: Psychological and Educational Publications.

Haley, S. M., Coster, W. J., Ludlow, L. H., Haltiwanger, M. A., & Andrellos, P. J. (1992). *Pediatric evaluation of disability inventory* (2nd ed.). San Antonio, TX: Psychological Corporation.

Hamilton, B. B., & Granger, C. U. (1991). *Functional independence measure for children (WeeFIM)* (2nd ed.). Buffalo, NY: Research Foundation of the State University of New York.

Hammill, D., Pearson, N. A., & Voress, J. K. (1988). *Developmental test of visual perception (DVPT-2)* (2nd ed.). Austin, TX: Pro-ED.

Law, M., Baptiste, S., Carswell, A., McColl, M. A., Polatajko, H., & Pollock, N. (2005). *Canadian occupational performance measure* (4th ed.). Toronto, ON: Canadian Association of Occupational Therapy Publications.

Martin, N. (2006). *Test of visual-motor skills* (3rd ed.). Ann Arbor, MI: Academic Therapy Publications.

Miller, L. J. (1988). *Miller assessment for preschoolers.* San Antonio, TX: Psychological Corporation.

Mulligan, S. (2014). *Occupational therapy evaluation for children: A pocket guide* (2nd ed.). Philadelphia, PA: Lippincott Williams & Wilkins.

Newborg, J. (2005). *Battelle developmental inventory* (2nd ed.). Itasca, IL: Riverside.

O'Brien, J., & Williams, H. (2010). Application of motor control/motor learning to practice. In J. Case-Smith & J. C. O'Brien (Eds.), *Occupational therapy for children* (6th ed., pp. 245–274). Maryland Heights, MO: Mosby/Elsevier.

Parham, L., & Mailoux, Z. (2010). Sensory integration. In J. Case-Smith & J. C. O'Brien (Eds.), *Occupational therapy for children* (6th ed., pp. 325–372). Maryland Heights, MO: Mosby/Elsevier.

Parham, L. D., & Fazio, L. S. (1997). *Play in occupational therapy for children* (2nd ed.). St. Louis, MO: Mosby.

Richardson, P. K. (2010). Use of standardized tests in pediatric practice. In J. Case-Smith & J. C. O'Brien (Eds.), *Occupational therapy for children* (6th ed., pp. 216–244). Maryland Heights, MO: Mosby/Elsevier.

Rogers, S. L. (2010). Common conditions that influence children's participation. In J. Case-Smith & J. C. O'Brien (Eds.), *Occupational therapy for children* (6th ed., pp. 146–192). Maryland Heights, MO: Mosby/Elsevier.

Russell, D. J., Rosenbaum, P. L., Avery, L., & Lane, M. (2002). *Gross motor function measure: User's manual.* Malden, MA: Blackwell Publishing.

Schneck, C. M. (2010). Visual perception. In J. Case-Smith & J. C. O'Brien (Eds.), *Occupational therapy for children* (6th ed., pp. 373–403). Maryland Heights, MO: Mosby/Elsevier.

Schopler, E., Reichler, R. J., & Renner, B. R. (2002). *Childhood autism rating scale* (2nd ed.). Los Angeles, CA: Western Psychological Services.

Schuberth, L. M., Amirault, L. M., & Case-Smith, J. (2010). Feeding interventions. In J. Case-Smith & J. C. O'Brien (Eds.), *Occupational therapy for children* (6th ed., pp. 446–473). Maryland Heights, MO: Mosby/Elsevier.

Shepherd, J. (2010). Activities of daily living. In J. Case-Smith & J. C. O'Brien (Eds.), *Occupational therapy for children* (6th ed., pp. 474–517). Maryland Heights, MO: Mosby/Elsevier.

Stewart, K. B. (2010). Purposes, processes, and methods of evaluation. In J. Case-Smith & J. C. O'Brien (Eds.), *Occupational therapy for children* (6th ed., pp. 193–215). Maryland Heights, MO: Mosby/Elsevier.

Specialized Pediatric Interventions

Beth Angst and Robin Mercer

Learning Objectives

- Describe the core concepts and assumptions of intervention strategies and approaches used in pediatric populations.
- Describe clinical reasoning skills used by occupational therapy practitioners in providing interventions to pediatric populations.
- Describe principles for providing intervention services for pediatric populations in clinical settings.
- Compare and contrast early intervention, school-based, hospital-based, and outpatient-based services available for pediatric populations.
- Compare and contrast intervention strategies and approaches used in the treatment of pediatric populations.
- Apply knowledge of intervention strategies and approaches to provided pediatric clinical case scenarios.

Key Terms

- *Dyspraxia*: Apraxia that results in difficulty with motor planning necessary to perform tasks.
- *Equilibrium*: The ability to maintain balance and posture.
- *Individualized Education Program (IEP)*: A plan developed by an educational institution typically in elementary and secondary programs that ensures teaching and learning modifications for children with disabilities.
- *Individuals with Disabilities Education Act (IDEA)*: A law that ensures free and appropriate public education for students with disabilities.

- *Sensory processing*: A complex organization of neurologic processes regarding the sensation of a person and their environment.

Description

Treatment in the pediatric population is often more based on an assessment of the individual child's particular needs, rather than being diagnoses driven. In fact, sometimes occupational therapists (OTs) and occupational therapy assistants (OTAs) treat children who do not yet have a definitive diagnosis. The OTs should identify a child's individual strengths and challenges and develop a treatment plan to address these abilities and limitations. It is important during treatment to discuss with the caregivers and medical team any precautions (e.g., not lifting a baby up under their arms for approximately six weeks after cardiac surgery). It is also important to be aware of the child's level of cognitive functioning to provide appropriate directions and instructions during treatment and to base treatment on that child's level of understanding. Treatment may need to be based more on developmental age rather than on chronological age. The OT provider should always strive to make treatment as fun and engaging as possible.

Treatment Settings

OTs provide treatment to children in a variety of settings. Although treatment interventions can be utilized in different treatment environments, each environment requires a unique treatment approach. Each setting has its own specific rules and regulations, influenced by such things as federal policies and insurance guidelines that govern the type of treatment the occupational therapy team may provide.

Early Intervention Services

Early intervention provides services for children from birth to 3 years of age. These children have been identified as having an established developmental delay or are determined to be at either a biologic and/or an environmental risk of developing a delay in function. The emphasis of early intervention is on how the child functions within the family unit and uses a family-centered approach. Accordingly, the goal of early intervention is to "prevent or minimize the physical, cognitive, emotional, and resource limitations of young children disadvantaged by biologic or environmental risk factors" (Myers, Stephens, & Tauber, 2010, p. 681).

Part C of the Individuals with Disabilities Education Act (IDEA 2004) establishes the policies and procedures that each state must follow for early intervention services. It establishes occupational therapy as a primary service within the early intervention setting. Occupational therapy can be provided in addition to other services, but due to its assignment as a primary service, occupational therapy can also be the only service the child receives through early intervention. Correspondingly, the individualized family service plan (IFSP) is a map of the services that will be provided to the family. It outlines the services that will be received, who will provide them, and where they will be provided.

School-Based Services

The primary role of the OT in a school-based setting is to support the child's academic challenges inclusive of their surrounding environment (Wright-Ott, 2010). OTs providing school-based services must have an understanding of the school context and the federal laws and regulations that guide them and they need to apply their understanding of the occupational therapy domain within these boundaries.

For example, the IDEA (2004) requires "free appropriate education in the least restrictive environment for students with disabilities attending public schools." It also "stipulates that individually designed special education and related services must be provided to students 3 to 21 years of age, if the student needs such services to benefit from her or his education" (Bazyk & Case-Smith, 2010, p. 714).

OTs in school-based settings must provide services that are "educationally relevant, by contributing to the development, or improvement of the child's academic and functional school performance" (Bazyk & Case-Smith, 2010, p. 717). Services may be provided directly to the child, provided on behalf of the child, or provided to teachers and other staff working with the child. An IEP is developed for all children receiving school-based services. The IEP is the resulting legal document that is completed by the IEP team, including parents, during the formal planning process. The IEP establishes what services and programs the child will need in order to participate in school and receive their "appropriate education."

Two essential aspects of the IEP include goal writing and establishing short-term goals. Goals are written for the IEP based on what the child is expected to obtain within 1 year; short-term goals are not necessarily completed in the school setting. Occupational therapy practitioners must relate their goals and activities to the general education curriculum and extracurricular activities. Deficits that do not impact the child's participation in the education curriculum or extracurricular activities will not be addressed in a school-based program. A plan for addressing progress must be provided at least as often as the progress reports are received for students without disabilities.

Consulting in a School-Based System

The school-based OT provides support within the school environment to make both the child's and the teacher's jobs easier. They provide a valuable role not just in direct client care but also in consulting with the teachers and staff. Their unique medical background and knowledge base can help enhance the multidisciplinary team's decision-making process. Along with effective communication and interaction skills, the occupational therapy practitioner will need a full understanding of the challenge(s), an awareness of appropriate interventions, and an understanding of the educational system in order to fulfill their role as a consultant and advocate. Intervention strategies when consulting typically include the following:

- Reframe the teacher's perspective (e.g., educate the teacher on the student's particular diagnosis and sensory processing disorder)
- Improve student skills

- Adapt tasks
- Adapt the environment
- Adapt routines

School-Based Mental Health Services

Mental health services have traditionally been provided in hospitals subscribing to the medical model or in community mental health centers. There is currently a growing movement to address these issues in the school system where more children can be reached. "Approximately one in five children ages 9 to 17 have a diagnosable emotional or behavioral disorder, with the most common being anxiety, depression, conduct disorders, and attention deficit/hyperactivity disorder (ADHD)" (Bazyk & Case-Smith, 2010, p. 737). OTs need to integrate mental health strategies into the school environment, including the school curriculum, routines, and classroom settings; some examples include the following:

- Informally observe all children for behaviors that might suggest mental health concerns or limitations in social–emotional development; bring concerns to the educational team.
- Provide tips for promoting successful functioning throughout the school day, including transitioning to classes, organizing work spaces, handling stress, and developing strategies for time management.
- Consult with teachers to modify learning demands and academic routines to support a student's development of specific social–emotional skills.
- Develop and run programs to foster social participation for students struggling with peer interaction.
- Identify ways to modify or enhance school routines to reduce stress and the likelihood of behavioral outbursts (Bazyk & Case-Smith, 2010).

Hospital-Based Services

Most hospital-based care focuses on the acute-onset challenges and provision of services for diagnoses that are of low occurrence but of high complexity. Services may be provided in an acute inpatient setting, acute rehabilitation setting, and/or an outpatient setting. Services may also be provided in a dedicated children's hospital or as part of a generalized hospital setting that services both adult and pediatric populations.

Hospital-based services support a family-centered care approach. Treatment is provided with the child and the caregivers as integral parts of the medical decision-making team. The OT shares their evaluation findings with the family in terms that are meaningful to them and involves the caregiver and child in the process of establishing treatment goals.

Treatment in a hospital-based setting is guided by accrediting and regulatory agencies. OTs working in the hospital setting must have knowledge of the guidelines from the Centers for Medicare and Medicaid Services, and accreditation boards such as The Joint Commission and the Commission on Accreditation of Rehabilitation Facilities. They also must have an understanding of the guidelines from the various third-party payers their clients may possess.

Goal Setting

Goals in medically based treatment must be "explicitly stated, measurable, and functionally relevant" (Dudgeon & Crooks, 2010, p. 791). The goals must have a clear target for the child's functional outcomes. Long-term goals are established based on the outcomes expected at the end of the child's length of stay. Short-term goals are established as interim steps to reach that goal.

Characteristics of Intervention

Evaluation and treatment must be streamlined, prioritized, and efficient to address the child's needs in a relatively brief period of time. Due to this limited time period, discharge plans generally begin at the time of onset of treatment.

The OT must have knowledge of a broad range of diagnoses, assessments, interventions, and modalities to address the wide variety of needs of this population. Within this setting, the OT functions as an integral part of an interdisciplinary care team.

Focus of Interventions

- Preventing secondary disability and restoring performance skills.
- Addressing neuromuscular and musculoskeletal complications.
- Addressing skin care: pressure sore prevention.
- Addressing perceptual, cognitive, and behavior impairments.

- Resuming and restoring occupational performance.
- Adaptations for activities of daily living (ADLs) and associated skills.

Outpatient Services

Interdisciplinary outpatient clinics provide monitoring and intervention for children with chronic health risks and disabilities either as follow-up for hospitalizations or for treatment of medical needs that do not require direct hospitalization. Treatment must be medically oriented and focused on the child's current health status and level of development. The emphasis must be on functional improvements and the child's ability to participate in their home and community activities.

Neonatal Intensive Care Unit

The neonatal intensive care unit (NICU) is a specialized setting within the acute care hospital system. Traditionally, occupational therapy in the NICU has focused on rehabilitation, developmental stimulation, and therapy-targeted specific challenges (e.g., low tone, feeding issues). Currently, treatment in this setting is moving toward involving the OT from the time the child is admitted to the NICU rather than waiting for children to be medically stable enough to tolerate hands-on treatment. Protective and preventive care is becoming the focal point of treatment. The OT focuses on managing the infant's environments to support proper overall development. Where previously the emphasis was on direct contact or "hands-on" approach, the more current emphasis is on "protecting the fragile newborn from excessive or inappropriate sensory input" (Hunter, 2010, p. 652).

Intervention Strategies

The field of occupational therapy has always held as one of its central tenets the importance of looking at the whole being and involving the person in functional and meaningful activities or occupations. Some traditional intervention strategies only focus on improving specific deficits in motor dysfunction. When used in isolation, these intervention strategies are usually not successful in improving the functional skills of children. They lack an overall examination of the whole being and how multiple systems need to interact to produce purposeful movement. Pediatric OTs need to identify the areas impacting function and address these areas within the context of the whole task. OTs must remember that skills are only functional when the task can be completed throughout various environments. Intervention strategies should hold a dynamical systems theory approach. "Movement is dependent upon task characteristics and an interaction among cognitive, neuromusculoskeletal, sensory, perceptual, socioemotional, and environmental systems. The interaction among systems is essential to predictive and adaptive control of movement" (O'Brien & Williams, 2010, p. 247). The intervention strategies listed below should be used to address the client's deficits in the context of whole task activities and how these tasks are completed in various ways and throughout variable environments.

Developmental Positioning

Neonatal Positioning Issues

Due to a lack of available rooms, full-term infants typically have a flexed posture in the womb with midline positioning of their head and extremities. They typically sustain a flexor bias (i.e., physiological flexion) during their newborn months. Temporary tightness of the hips, knees, and elbows provides feedback to return to this flexed resting position as the baby begins to experiment with extensor movements of the trunk and extremities. This allows for the development of hand-to-mouth activities, self-regulating behaviors, and antigravity control.

Preterm infants are generally hypotonic at birth. They have not had the boundaries of the womb to promote flexor posturing and to limit extension behaviors. Their resting positioning is generally very flat, with extension and abduction of the arms and legs and asymmetrical positioning of the head to one side. They do not start in a flexed position and their movements into extension are not met with any feedback to encourage a more flexed position. Left unchecked, extension and arching becomes the movement pattern for infants who are premature and greatly limits their functional development.

Positioning devices should be used with infants born prematurely and any infants with low tone, to provide appropriate boundaries that promote flexion posturing. Families should be instructed on handling and carrying techniques to support these appropriate postures and encourage equilibrium.

Principles for General Pediatric Populations

Working in various developmental positions is very important in the pediatric population. Weight-bearing provided through developmental positions works to improve strength in the shoulder girdle and the upper extremities (UEs). Facilitation of weight shifting in various developmental positions increases the development of proximal stability and postural control. Static weight-bearing in developmental positions can provide an inhibitory effect on tone, and dynamic weight shifts over a stable base can provide a facilitatory effect on tone. Back to sleep programs and frequent positioning in car seats and carriers result in many of today's infants spending much of their time in the supine position. Care should be taken to encourage a "back to sleep, tummy to play" approach with tummy time (i.e., prone positioning) being encouraged during the waking (e.g., play) hours of the day. Caregivers of newborns, especially when special needs are of concern, should be instructed on the benefit of tummy time and of age-appropriate activities to encourage multiple developmental positions throughout the day (see **Table 30-1**).

Proximal Stability/Postural Control

Appropriate proximal stability and postural control help to provide a basis from which functional gross motor and fine motor skills develop, which includes the ability to isolate oral movements required during eating. If proximal stability and postural control are inadequate, the child will develop compensatory strategies and inefficient movement patterns. Their movement patterns will lack the adjustable stability that is a key component of normal movement. This will greatly affect the child's ability to progress through developmentally appropriate areas of occupation. Early facilitation of appropriate postural control and proximal stability through therapeutic handling and positioning are imperative to allow the child to progress through all areas of development with the most efficient patterns possible. Working on unstable surfaces, providing activities to promote movement through developmental positions, and reaching outside of the child's base of support and/or above the child's center of gravity can be effective ways to address

proximal stability and postural control. Handling techniques should be provided to allow the child to work through the activity experiencing the best movement patterns possible.

A child who lacks proximal stability and/or postural control will often seek stability from other areas of the body or may look for opportunities to seek outside stability. They might demonstrate a nice open hand in supine but when brought up to sitting they will demonstrate bilateral fisting. They may brace themselves on their UEs during sitting or standing. Movement patterns such as these will impact their ability to develop and complete fine motor activities and ADLs. They might also demonstrate shoulder elevation, cervical extension, and/or clenching of their jaw, impacting their ability to isolate oral movements and control a bolus during eating. Though handling during therapy sessions is a great way to help develop stability and control, the occupational therapy practitioner cannot be with the child 100% of the time. Care should be taken to provide appropriate positioning during daily activities (e.g., school activities, feeding sessions, ADLs, and play activities).

This does not always mean expensive positioning devices are required. It can simply involve a parent bundling their infant during bottle-feeding, providing towel rolls to offer lateral support to a child in their high chair, having the child support their feet on a box during desk activities at school, or using towel rolls to assist with chest support when a child is playing in prone. Instructing parents, teachers, and all caregivers on proper handling and positioning techniques is imperative to helping the child develop or gain stability and postural control.

Strengthening

Just as in the adult population, a child with decreased strength in areas such as the trunk, UEs, and/or facial musculature can experience a significant loss in functional skills. Unlike the adult population, a young child cannot be expected to complete a rote exercise program with any amount of success. Individual rote exercise programs also do not support a dynamical systems theory approach. Addressing decreased strength in the pediatric group, especially those less than approximately 6 years of age, can test the OT's ability to embed therapeutic activities into occupations. Strengthening activities for young children must be incorporated into occupational tasks, such as lifting a weighted ball up onto a slide for it to roll

Table 30-1 Developmental Positions

Position	Benefits	Disadvantages	Play/Treatment Ideas
Supine	1. *Encourages*: • Hands to reach and engage • Midline activities • Eye contact 2. *Develops*: • Stomach muscles (i.e., body flexion) • Movement control of the legs and flexibility 3. Enables the hands to reach and touch the leg 4. Recommended position to reduce sudden infant death syndrome (SIDS)	1. Can encourage extensor tone 2. May not challenge the child enough (i.e., provides too much support) 3. Can encourage external rotation deformities of the arms and legs (i.e., may need outside positioning to decrease these deformities) with children who have weakness and low tone	1. Hold toys at midline to encourage reaching 2. Involve feet in play and encourage reaching to the feet (e.g., place rattles on the feet) 3. Place towel rolls along the child's side and shoulder to support the arms and encourage activities in midline
Prone	1. *Develops*: • Head control • Muscles in the shoulders and the arms • Muscles in the back • Hip muscles 2. Initiates posterior weight shift 3. Facilitates development of flexor tone in premature infants 4. Improves oxygenation and ventilation in premature infants 5. Reduces reflux, especially if the head of surface is elevated 30° 6. Can help reduce hip flexion contractures	1. Associated with increased risk of SIDS in infants 2. If not properly positioned, can cause flattened, frog leg positioning 3. Infants with weak and/or low tone may not have enough strength to clear airway 4. Makes visual exploration more difficult 5. Less face-to-face contact with caregivers	1. Place age-appropriate toys in front of the child 2. Lay in front of the child and talk to the child 3. Use towel rolls under the chest with the arms over a roll to assist with head extension
Prone on elbows	1. *Develops*: • Head control • Muscles in the shoulders and the arms • Muscles in the back • Cocontraction 2. Ability to weight shift posteriorly to the hips 3. Ability to weight shift side to side when reaching	1. Infants with weak and/or low tone may not be able to obtain or sustain this position 2. Can result in decreased visual exploration if difficulty sustaining cervical extension and controlling rotational movements are present 3. Can result in a frog leg positioning	1. Place toys on higher surfaces to encourage head up positions 2. Use a roll at the level of the chest to provide support as needed 3. Support the shoulders or the elbows as needed 4. Provide pressure downward or toward the hips to encourage posterior weight shifting
Prone on extended elbows	1. *Develops*: • Head control • Muscles in the shoulders and the arms • Muscles in the back • Cocontraction • Ability to weight shift when reaching 2. Elongates the hip and stomach muscles	1. Infants with weak and/or low tone may not have enough strength to obtain or sustain this position 2. Can result in frog leg positioning	1. Use higher surfaces to support toys 2. Place the child off the edge of a wedge or use a Boppy pillow for support as needed 3. Provide support at the shoulders as needed 4. Use an air splint to assist with elbow extension

Table 30-1 Developmental Positions (*continued*)

Position	Benefits	Disadvantages	Play/Treatment Ideas
Side-lying	1. Develops the rib cage 2. Encourages rolling when reaching for toys 3. Encourages midline orientation of the head and the extremities 4. Keeps hands together and makes it easier to touch or hold a toy 5. Allows for shoulder movement in a gravity-eliminated plane 6. Facilitates hand to mouth 7. Helps to decrease extensor patterning when positioned appropriately (i.e., requires less effort to move) 8. Right side-lying can improve gastric emptying 9. Left side-lying can assist with decreasing reflux	1. May be difficult to maintain position of a child with increased extensor patterning 2. Left side-lying can decrease gastric emptying 3. Right side-lying can increase reflux symptoms	1. Place a toy next to the child's hand to encourage exploration 2. Brush a toy against the back of the hand to encourage reaching 3. Facilitate hips forward to encourage rolling to prone, and hips back to encourage rolling to supine 4. Use a roll behind the child to assist with sustaining position 5. Place a toy at eye level to encourage eye contact and reaching of the hands up to the toy 6. Place a toy at levels between the shoulder and the hip to encourage downward eye gaze

Side sitting	1. *Encourages*:
	  • Cocontraction
	  • Weight shift
	  • Unilateral reaching
	  • Rotational components of movement
		1. May be difficult to sustain this position with children who have low tone, athetosis, or spasticity
		2. Need to ensure proper shoulder alignment on the weight-bearing side to prevent injury
			1. Use to initiate weight-bearing on the hemi side to decrease tone
			2. Provide proprioceptive input to increase activity in the shoulder, elbow, and wrist joints
			3. Side sit to the more functional side to encourage use of the hemi side
			4. Use a splint or cast to support elbow extension
			5. Place toys to the weight-bearing side to increase weight shift in that direction
			6. Place toys at higher levels to encourage movement out of the base of support

Sitting	1. Facilitates balance 2. Good alerting posture 3. Good visual exploration 4. Encourages social interaction	1. Can cause increased fixation patterns if the child is not strong enough to stay up against gravity 2. Children with low tone and weakness will likely have difficulty raising their hands against gravity. May weight bear on their hands for support 3. Children with low tone and weakness may show a forward flexed position that can impact respiratory effort (e.g., may see pushing into extension) 4. Children with increased tone may be unable to sustain this position and frequently push into extension	1. Place activities on a table surface to encourage more upright positions. Increase the height of the table for more upright positioning and to facilitate reaching 2. Perform activities on the floor in front of the child to encourage chin tuck, downward eye gaze, and forward flexion 3. Move the support and facilitation provided by the OT from the shoulders down to the rib cage, and down to the hips as the child's strength and stability increases

(*continues*)

Table 30-1 Developmental Positions (*continued*)

Position	Benefits	Disadvantages	Play/Treatment Ideas
Four-point	*Develops*: • Muscle control and strength in the shoulders, arms, hips, legs, and back • Cocontraction • Balance with weight shifting • Trunk stability	1. Can be difficult to keep in proper positioning 2. If too difficult, the child will assume a locked, static position that decreases function and contributes to deformities	1. Place a roll under abdomen for support as needed 2. Use a splint to support elbow extension 3. Place a toy to the side to encourage reaching and weight shifting to that side 4. Support the shoulder and the opposite hip to facilitate weight shift
Standing	1. Frees UE for prehension and manipulation 2. Facilitates higher level neurologic integrations	1. Requires the child to have a good stability to be successful 2. May be hard to move the arms against gravity and the child may seek fixation	1. Complete ADL activities at a sink or counter 2. Improve dynamic balance (e.g., shoot baskets) 3. Use table top board games with a focus on keeping the UEs off of the table surface

Data from Case-Smith, 2010.

down and knock over bowling pins, pushing a toy grocery cart with weights inside, completing activities with wrist weights on, and finding items that have been buried in Theraputty. Care needs to be taken to instruct families and caregivers on carryover of strengthening activities into the home environment. Children can help with such things as carrying groceries in from the car, putting groceries away, picking up and carrying items during toy cleanup, and pulling wet clothing from the washer to place in the dryer. Home play activities can be developed to encourage activities like crawling, reaching overhead, transitioning from sitting to kneeling, and four-point, and/or standing.

Muscle Tone

Abnormal muscle tone needs to be addressed as soon as possible in the pediatric population. Abnormal tone leads to the development of abnormal movement patterns resulting in high energy and inefficient patterns that impact all areas of function. Normal movement patterns are based on flexible synergy patterns. These patterns have consistent characteristics in their sequence of movements and the ratios of joint movement, but are

flexible in nature in order to allow for completion of the specific task at hand. Children with abnormal muscle tone, such as children with cerebral palsy, muscular dystrophy, stroke, or traumatic brain injuries, develop synergistic movement patterns that are fixed and repetitive. These patterns prevent the completion of functional tasks as they lack gradation and flexibility. It is important to use therapeutic techniques to help the child normalize tone so that he or she develops movement patterns that are as normal, fluid, and efficient as possible.

Spasticity Management

Management of spasticity is usually under the decision making of the physician. The OT contributes to this decision-making process by providing input to the physician on how the client's tone relates to their ability to complete functional tasks. Often, a child's increased tone makes it difficult for them to complete a task. However, some children may use their tone to assist them in the completion of a task and reducing or changing the tone may result in the child becoming less functional. The OT needs to be able to recognize this in order to aid the physician in the decision-making process. The physician may decide to use oral medications that impact tone on a more global basis or they may decide on a baclofen pump or the use of neural blocks, such as Botox, that can target a more specific area. Some children may also receive surgical interventions such as tendon lengthening or dorsal rhizotomies. The OT needs to be aware of the medical management techniques available to be able to suggest what might best help their client's functional status. They also need to be aware of what techniques were used in order to assess and address the changes noted. For example, a child who receives Botox to their wrist flexors will have a decrease in tone to that area. This then presents an opportunity for the OT to work on improving the biomechanical alignment and functional use of the wrist and fingers through casting and/or splinting, strengthening the weakened and overstretched extensor muscles, and incorporating a large gamut of activities to involve the affected hand in functional tasks.

Improving Postural Tone and Control

In order to obtain desired movement and engage in activities, children with decreased proximal tone and control will develop fixation positions and increase their distal tone to gain more proximal control. Working on activities to improve proximal stability can decrease the need for this compensation.

Inhibition

Activities such as static weight-bearing on the extremity, pressure to the thenar eminence, prolonged stretch, and neutral warmth can provide an inhibitory impact on tone. Slow sustained traction with deep massage can help reduce muscle tone to an area that allows for increased range and movement.

Serial Casting

Serial casting is an excellent technique to provide neutral warmth and prolonged stretch to an area to help decrease tone. However, serial casting alone will generally not provide a prolonged effect. It must be combined with activities to facilitate functional movement patterns of the joints proximal and distal to the area being casted. The cast inhibits movement of the area into synergistic or compensatory patterns during functional movement of the extremity. Along with understanding the care and precautions of the cast, the OT must take great care to be sure that the caregivers have a home exercise program of activities that incorporate movement of the joints proximal and distal to the area being casted.

Splinting

Splinting children, especially a child with increased tone, is one of the challenges of working in pediatric occupational therapy. The smaller size of the UEs, especially the hands, means that you have a smaller lever arm to work with, making it more difficult to properly secure the joints, especially when tone is pulling in the opposite direction. This can be further complicated by the fact that children have more hypermobility to their joints than what is generally seen in the adult population. In the child with increased tone this may mean that their hypertonic joints are pulled into quite severe deformities or that the laxity in joints proximal or distal to the hypertonic area can make it more difficult to maintain proper positioning. Some splints used in children with increased tone are noted below:

- *Air splint*: Come in a variety of sizes and can be used to position a tonal area and provide neutral warmth and pressure to help inhibit tone. To promote functional improvement, the splint must be combined with activities to encourage more functional involvement of the joints proximal and distal to the tonal area.
- *Antispasticity*: Best used to help alignment and prevent deformity prior to the development of spasticity. These splints can be difficult to apply and can be difficult to keep on depending on the amount of tone and the size of the hand.
- *Neoprene*: Provides neutral warmth and pressure. May require the use of stays to keep the client with higher levels of tone from pushing back into tonal positioning.
- *Weight-bearing*: Splints used to position the hand and wrist in a more extended position allows for improved positioning during weight-bearing activities.

Managing Low Tone

Hypotonia is often an issue in premature infants, children with muscular dystrophy, children with Down syndrome, some children with autism, and some forms of cerebral palsy. The child's nutritional status and state of arousal can have a significant impact on them appearing hypotonic. Children with chronic, poor nutritional intake can be hypotonic partially because they lack the protein needed to allow for muscle development. A child can also show more increased tone when they are alert and interacting, but this same child will appear more hypotonic when tired or sleeping.

Facilitation

Infants and children with low tone often lack the ability to work against gravity. Working in gravity-eliminated planes such as side-lying and/or elevated on a wedge can facilitate increased movement in low tone areas. Working with good support on unstable surfaces, using faster movements, and increasing proprioceptive input to the area can help facilitate tone. Incorporating vestibular input into treatment, especially when combined with proprioceptive input, is an excellent way to improve overall tone. Use of cold stimulation is another way to help increase tone. This is especially useful when working with low oral and facial tone. The use of cold drinks, cold pacifiers, cold oral probes, and cold washcloths, for example, can help increase tone and elicit a response in the oral cavity.

Splints

Splints and orthotics are generally thought of for use in children with increased tone. However, children with low tone can also benefit greatly from splints or orthotics. Specialized trunk and extremity supports that provide deep pressure, assist with proprioception, and result in improved support and stability can be very beneficial for children with low tone. Pediatric medical garments, such as Benik vests (www.benik.com) and TheraTogs (www.theratogs.com), may be used in therapy, at home, and in school environments. Dynamic shoulder splints designed to prevent subluxation of the hypotonic shoulder may also be useful. Therapeutic taping, such as Kinesio taping, can be a good alternative to splinting for providing increased stability and facilitation in hypotonic areas including joint, trunk, and facial musculature.

Constraint-Induced Therapy

Constraint-induced therapy involves casting or splinting for the noninvolved or less involved extremity to facilitate use of the more involved extremity. A bivalve cast, permanent cast, or splint is fabricated for the uninvolved extremity. This makes it more difficult for the child to use the casted extremity in activities, and encourages the child to recruit the use of their involved or weaker extremity in order to be able to complete the desired activity. Components of successful constraint-induced therapy include the following:

- Often used with children with diagnoses such as brachial plexus injuries and hemiplegia.
- Must sustain the use of a cast or splint on the noninvolved side for extended periods during the day.
- Activities need to be provided to engage the involved extremity in repetitive motions for extended periods.
- More successful in cases of neglect where the involved extremity has reached a point of function that will allow the client to use the extremity in activities without excessive frustration.

Sensory Integration (SI)

Not all pediatric occupational therapy practitioners have the opportunity to work in a facility that is set up for the sole purpose of sensory integrative treatment. These facilities differ significantly from the multipurpose treatment environments in which many pediatric OTs provide their services. However, this does not mean that pediatric OTs who do not have access to specific sensory integrative gyms will not use sensory integrative techniques in their treatment sessions. In fact, all pediatric occupational therapy providers should have knowledge of these techniques because they can help to address many treatment needs of the pediatric population and can be adapted for use in most treatment environments. An understanding of sensory processing needs of the child and acknowledging and addressing these needs appropriately in the treatment session can often increase the success of the treatment plan when standard treatment approaches alone may not achieve the desired result.

SI Defined

The term SI refers to how the body takes in and processes sensory information for function. When sensory information is taken in and appropriate integration of that information occurs, the person makes appropriate, adaptive responses to the environmental stimuli. SI is also used to refer to a treatment approach for treating those who have difficulty in sensory processing. When viewing a treatment session with a skilled OT using a sensory integrative approach, it may seem that the OT is doing little more than encouraging a child to play; however, the OT is carrying out a well thought out and flexible treatment plan. The goal of this plan is to help clients obtain an appropriate sensory basis with just the right amount of challenge to their system. This will help them learn to take in sensory information and allow that information to be appropriately processed and integrated. Occupational therapy providers who treat children with an SI approach require advanced training and extended hands-on experience under the guidance of well-experienced mentors. The understanding of the field is constantly growing and changing and the OT must work to stay up to date on the newest approaches and theories.

Basis of Treatment for SI

The basis of sensory integrative treatment is providing the child with opportunities to make adaptive responses. The child is able to take in appropriately selected sensory input and organize that information to accomplish a given goal. The child's adaptive response comes from within and cannot be forced upon the child. The OT sets up an environment to help elicit the adaptive response but the child must be an active participant in order to integrate the information appropriately and develop a "successful, goal-directed action" in response to the input (Parham & Mailloux, 2010).

Classic SI Treatment/Ayres Sensory Integration

Ayres Sensory Integration (ASI®) treatment is used when the child requires assistance in integrating sensory information to improve their performance in a specific sensory area. It is an individually based treatment that is geared to the specific needs of a specific child. The occupational therapy provider is skilled at providing balance between a structured treatment session while allowing the child freedom to explore and experience sensory stimuli in a safe, nonthreatening environment. They may take the child to an area that is rich in the type of sensory input the child needs. Within that environment, the child will have the opportunity to experience sensory input in varying degrees and combinations. The OT is constantly assessing and adjusting treatment on a

moment-by-moment basis as they judge the child's adaptive response to the input. The OT is constantly trying to adjust the environment to provide the child with an effortful challenge that is not so challenging it overwhelms the child. In order for this intervention approach to be effective, the child must be an active participant in treatment. Simply imposing the stimulation on the child in some passive way will not generate adaptive responses. The inner drive of the child must be challenged and developed so the child becomes actively engaged in the activity.

Treatment environments for ASI sessions are composed with a wide variety of items to provide input to all of the sensory systems. OTs need to have a clear understanding of the various properties of all the activities and which sensory system or systems will be challenged during that activity. They must have an understanding of how to grade activities to encourage more or less input based on the child's responses during treatment. The OT must have a clear understanding of the child's needs and be able to help structure the treatment session to provide that "just right challenge" to allow the child to continue to make adaptive responses within the environment. Treatment sessions focus primarily on the integration of tactile, proprioceptive, and vestibular input. These three systems provide the basis of organization for sensory input. The visual and auditory systems are considered distal systems and need integration of the proprioceptive, tactile, and vestibular systems for proper function. When many people think of ASI treatment, they visualize the various pieces of suspended equipment and feel that all children need vestibular treatment. Great care needs to be taken in regard to vestibular input. It should never be imposed on a child or provided through passive means. Vestibular input is very powerful and greatly impacts arousal levels and autonomic nervous system responses. It can take several hours to process, so reactions due to overstimulation may not actually occur until several hours posttreatment. For this reason, treatment using vestibular input should only be provided under the direction of well-trained professionals. Vestibular input does not simply mean the use of a swing. Up and down movement such as jumping jacks, going up and down stairs, and sitting on inflated surfaces can also provide vestibular input. Vestibular input can also be provided through movement in a horizontal path such as that provided when riding a scooter board, bike, or wagon. More specific treatment ideas can be viewed in **Tables 30-2** to **30-4**.

Table 30-2 Tactile System

Type of Dysfunction	Purpose of Treatment/ Expected Outcome	Treatment Strategies
Modulation disorders tactile defensiveness	• Maintain an optimal state of arousal in the presence of tactile input • Decrease overreaction to tactile input • Improve social–emotional skills • Improve organizational skills • Improve fine motor skills	• Combine tactile, proprioceptive, and vestibular input • Respect the child's personal space (i.e., do not impose) • Use deep pressure and firm touch input • Reduce sensory overload in the environment, use natural light, and work in small spaces to reduce the threat of uncontrolled tactile input • Use a Benik vest or air splint to provide deep pressure • Use activities in various textures (e.g., beans, rice, and a ball pit) • Provide tools for use in various textures (e.g., sand, beans, and rice) • Cover equipment with textured materials • Allow the child control over tactile input • Use wide paint brushes and textured mitts for "painting" skin
Hyporesponsiveness to touch/tactile discrimination disorders	• Improve body scheme • Gradually improve localization, two-point discrimination, and stereognosis • Improve hand skills and the ability to manipulate objects • Improve motor planning (e.g., secondary to dyspraxia) • Improve peer interaction	• Encourage movement in pressure (i.e., body socks and in a pool) • Use items such as shaving cream, finger paints, or lotions (e.g., have the child dip their finger and write on the body to identify letters) • Place stickers of various sizes on the arms and/or the legs and have the child find them with their eyes open and eyes closed • Use an obstacle course with different textured equipment • Arts and crafts • Beans, rice, and sand activities

Data from Bundy, Lane, Murray, and Fisher, 2002; Comprehensive Program in Sensory Integration, 2003; Dunn, 1999.

Table 30-3 Proprioceptive System

Type of Dysfunction	Purpose of Treatment/ Expected Outcome	Treatment Strategies
Hyporesponsiveness/ poor proprioceptive discrimination	• Improve ability to discriminate force • Improve body scheme	• Activities that include jarring, jerking, or sudden stopping/starting • Activities that provide resistance during movement, compression, or stretching • Use of weights (e.g., cuff weights, weighted balls, or a weighted vest) • Have the child help push and pull equipment (e.g., set up or clean up the session) • Wheelbarrow walking, prone on elbows, bear crawling, and crab walking activities • Tug of war, push, and pull activities • Looking for items in play-dough or Theraputty • Carrying groceries • Blow toys, straw games, and resistive chewing activities

Data from Bundy et al., 2002; Comprehensive Program in Sensory Integration, 2003; Dunn, 1999.

Table 30-4 Vestibular System

Type of Dysfunction	Purpose of Treatment/ Expected Outcome	Treatment Strategies
Gravitational insecurity	• Improve tolerance of movement activities • Improve organization of behavior • Improve body scheme	• Respect fear behaviors and do not force movement • Work to gain trust • Work with the child near the ground to start • Give the child control over the movement • Keep swings low, so the child can stop the swing with their feet • Use swings attached from two suspension points • Provide activities that require proprioception • Provide linear vertical movement such as jumping on a trampoline
Poor bilateral integration	• Improve rhythm of movements • Improve sequencing of movements • Improve organization of behavior	• Activities that require symmetrical patterns (e.g., catching a ball, rowing, and pulling up on a trapeze bar with both hands) • Activities that require alternating patterns (e.g., hand over hand pulling on a rope, tug of war, and wheelbarrow walking) • Use rhythmic songs and clapping games
Poor postural–ocular control	• Improve overall balance and postural control • Improve ocular motor skills • Improve organization of behavior • Improve tonic extension, tonic flexion, lateral flexion, and rotation	• Use NDT principles to facilitate appropriate postural responses • Prone on extended arms over a bolster with weight shifting • Supine on a scooter board and pulling self along • Activities that require a stable visual field while moving (e.g., throwing at a target while swinging) • Sit on a ball during fine motor activities • Work on an easel or vertical surface • Weight shift while prone on elbows
Intolerance to movement	• Improve tolerance of movement activities • Improve organization of behavior • Improve body scheme	• Minimize vestibular input • Start with slow head turning and progress to linear movements against gravity • Provide opportunities for increased proprioception during movement • Provide linear vestibular input with resistance to movement (e.g., sitting on scooter board and pulling hand over hand on a rope to move on a carpeted surface)

Data from Bundy et al., 2002; Comprehensive Program in Sensory Integration, 2003; Dunn, 1999.

Consultation

Children with SI challenges are often misunderstood and are frequently thought to have behavioral, psychological, and/or emotional challenges. It is important for the OT involved with children with SI challenges to provide education to all who are involved in their care. The results of individual ASI treatment are most often not instantaneous. People involved with the child's care (e.g., families, caregivers, and teachers) often require assistance with strategies to allow the child a more immediate adaptive response in order to function within their current environments. Providing activities such as the use of a weighted pencil to increase proprioceptive feedback during writing, replacing their chair with a therapy ball to increase their ability to keep calm, alerting their state by obtaining periodic proprioceptive and vestibular input, or providing a brushing and joint compression program prior to bedtime or a possible stressful event are typically useful strategies.

Fine Motor

Efficient and refined fine motor skills are required for proper engagement in many occupations found within the pediatric population. For example, children need fine motor skills to participate in writing tasks at school, to complete grooming tasks, to complete dressing tasks, for play activities, and for feeding skills. Unlike the adult population that likely has full development of their fine motor skills and may be working to regain those skills, children might be trying to develop these skills amid many impacting factors. The development of fine motor skills is much more difficult if you are obligated to develop them with an underlying basis of high tone, limited range of motion, decreased strength, decreased visual skills, and/or decreased sensory processing skills. Children require repetition and extended practice to develop fine motor skills. If repetition and practice occurs in an environment of tonal impairment, strength deficits and/or sensory processing deficits, then compensatory strategies tend to develop and inefficient fine motor skills often result. The OT is challenged to analyze the child's level of fine motor function, to prioritize all factors impacting the development of fine motor skills, and complete a treatment plan that will successfully progress the child through fine motor development.

Type of Treatment

The type of treatment the child may receive to address deficits in their fine motor skills is dependent upon the setting in which the child is receiving treatment. Fine motor skills play a large role in the child's ability to participate within the classroom setting and meet their educational needs. Treatment in the school setting will more likely address the use of adaptive techniques, equipment, and technology to allow the child to increase their function within the school environment. Treatment in outpatient settings may focus more on the underlying issues that result in the child's fine motor deficits and may address the balance, stability, strength, or tonal issues impacting the quality and efficiency of the child's fine motor movements.

Challenges That Affect Hand Skills

Many factors can impact the development and refinement of fine motor skills such as the control of postural functions, amount of available range of motion, quality of tone, amount of strength, quality of visual–perceptual skills, ability to process tactile and proprioceptive input, socioeconomic status, and gender and role expectations. Since hand skill development is a result of two motor systems, one that impacts postural control and stability and the other that allows for isolated finger movement, an understanding of the deficits impacting the child's fine motor skills can greatly help to guide the OT in treatment decisions.

General Treatment Strategies

Treatment for fine motor skills rarely focuses solely on the fine motor skill itself. A treatment session will often start in a more gross motor way to address sensory processing, improve tone and strength, provide proprioceptive input to increase awareness in the arms and hands, and address proximal control and stability. It will then refine down to focusing on specific fine motor control. A session may start with a child working through an obstacle course, progress to pulling themselves along a rope while on a scooter board, move to stacking large blocks, then completing a pattern with large pegs in a resistive board, and finally finish with working on picking up pennies to put in a penny bank. Throughout the process of treatment planning and during treatment intervention, the OT has many issues to consider and address in order to facilitate development and progression of a child's fine motor skills.

Positioning of the Child

A child may be able to demonstrate the best fine motor control in one position but the actual task they need this fine motor skill for must be completed in another position. The occupational therapy practitioner will need to work with the child to continue to progress the refinement of their fine motor skills, as well as progressing their ability to complete fine motor skills in a variety of positions. To help further refine the level of skill, the occupational therapy practitioner will work with the child in the position they can best complete the fine motor skill in at the present time. The occupational therapy provider will then continue to work on improving proximal stability, strength, and/or tonal abnormalities that may be impacting the child's ability to progress this skill to other positions. The OT may need to look at providing outside support to allow the child to complete their fine motor skills in a more functional position while simultaneously addressing stability and tone deficits. For example, the child may tip to the right side while sitting in their high chair, causing them to weight bear on their right UE, and preventing them from using their right hand during finger feeding. The OT might place towel rolls along either side of the child's trunk to support them in a more upright posture, thus allowing them to practice using their hands and fingers to refine their pinch skills and participate in finger feeding.

Postural Tone and Control

Poor postural tone and control can impact the development of fine motor skills as children will tighten and fixate their UEs to gain proximal control. This decreases their ability to isolate their arm movements for proper hand placement and to isolate their finger movements for proper manipulation skills. Children with low tone throughout the trunk and poor trunk stability have difficulty participating in fine motor skills due to the need to weight bear on their UEs. Providing appropriate positional support during the activity can increase fine motor control. Providing activities such as vestibular and proprioceptive input on a therapy ball prior to engaging in a fine motor activity can increase postural tone and control and improve the basis for refinement of fine motor skills. Children with increased tone have poor postural control and a tendency to push into extensor positioning. Providing appropriate hip flexion to help break up tone and providing activities to encourage slow rotational movements, external rotation at the shoulder, and supination at the forearm can help break up tonal patterns. Activities in weight-bearing also help to inhibit tone and provide ease of movement for isolation of hand skills.

Muscle Strength

Children with decreased strength seek positions of stability. Their fine motor skills are characterized by decreased dexterity and coordination. Providing exercises with clay or Theraputty to work the fingers against resistance will help to address underlying muscle weakness in the hands. Other activities to address underlying muscle weakness may include completing a peg design on a resistive board, opening lids on various size containers, pinching clothespins to hang items on a clothesline, or mixing cookie dough with hands. Children with decreased muscle strength will benefit from working on a surface such as a table or wheelchair tray where they can support their forearms on the surface and allow for increased isolation of wrist and finger movements. Mobile arm supports can also be beneficial for children with very low muscle strength to allow more gravity-eliminated movement and improve reach.

Isolation of Arm and Hand Movements

In order for fine motor skills to develop in an efficient and coordinated manner, the child must be able to isolate their arm and hand movements from each other and from total body movement patterns. Isolating arm and hand movements can be encouraged through games and songs like pat a cake, and "itsy bitsy" spider. The movements of elbow flexion and extension, wrist flexion and extension, and forearm supination and pronation need to be completed in an integrated and coordinated manner to effectively and efficiently complete reach, grasp, and release activities. These movements must also be performed in isolation. For example, the child will not be able to effectively grasp the object if elbow extension is accompanied by pronation and wrist flexion. This results in poor placement of the hand to the object and causes the child to develop compensatory movements such as lateral trunk flexion to raise the fingers to the level of the object. Appropriate observation and analysis of where the isolation and coordination breaks down will determine the treatment approach. For example, supination is best facilitated with the elbow in full flexion and then slowly worked into being integrated with more elbow extension and shoulder flexion. With the forearm supported on a surface, supination can be elicited by presenting objects in a more vertical orientation. Care must be taken to attend to trunk stability and overall positioning so that isolation of arm and hand movements can occur with the least amount of compensation possible.

Reach

Compensatory strategies for reaching develop when children are faced with abnormalities in areas such as tone, strength, or stability. They learn to reach with the use of compensatory movements like shoulder elevation, adduction, internal rotation, and/or lateral trunk flexion. They may have difficulty directing the hand to the object and cannot coordinate hand opening to grasp the object. When they attempt to reach, they may be unable to sustain an upright body position and fall into the direction of the reach. To address these deficits, the occupational therapy practitioner should provide proper positioning so that the child has the best possible postural control and visual attention to the task at hand. OTs can position themselves to provide shoulder support and handling techniques as needed for the arm, wrist, and fingers to facilitate elbow extension, supination, and wrist and finger extension in preparation for grasp. The occupational therapy practitioner will place objects to encourage reaching, being cognizant of such things as the distance of the object from the child, the height it is above or below the child's center of gravity, whether the child will require reaching across midline, whether the object is placed vertically to encourage supination or horizontally to encourage pronation, and/or whether the object is placed behind the body to encourage rotation with reaching.

Grasp

Children with grasp challenges may demonstrate fisting, thumb adduction and flexion, wrist flexion, and/or excessive forearm pronation. They often lack thumb opposition and cannot grade the grasp response. Treatment to promote grasping skills should begin with a focus on preparing the hand for proper grasp. Activities that manage tone, such as facilitating wrist extension, and promoting an open hand position with decreased cortical thumbing should be addressed as needed prior to focusing on grasp. Activities that provide proprioceptive and tactile input can increase awareness of the hand. Object selection is very important when addressing grasp. The size and the shape of the object will determine the type of grasp that should be elicited. A larger, firm, smooth object is generally a good place to start to address a grosser grasp. A smaller object with well-defined edges is a good place to start for refining finger and thumb control. The smaller the object presented, the more precision will be required to manage the object in grasp. If too small of an object is presented, the effort to grasp it will be too great and precision of grasp will be lost. When addressing control and precision of grasp, it is best to work on grasp alone and remove reaching from the equation. Grasp develops from a point of stability. Start to work on grasp with the arm well supported. The object being presented should be held by the occupational therapy practitioner and presented to the volar surface of the child's fingers

for grasp. Running an object from proximal to distal along the dorsal surface of the hand can encourage hand opening or relaxation to allow for grasp. Release of the object by the OT occurs after the child has sustained the grasp. Once mastered at this level, the occupational therapy practitioner can progress to presenting the object in the OT's hand where slight movement of the hand can adjust the object for grasp. When this is mastered, the object can be placed on a surface for the child to obtain. Objects should initially be presented in line with the shoulder and as grasp progresses the object can be moved further away and then finally toward midline. When practicing grasp, a variety of objects varying in size, weight, and shape should be presented as treatment progresses. The occupational therapy provider should be prepared with a large variety of objects in the treatment area to encourage many attempts at grasp. Involving the child in imaginary play and working them through a play scheme will provide a variety of objects to explore and will encourage multiple transitions between grasp patterns.

Carry

Sustaining a grasp to move an object from one place to another is very important in the functionality of fine motor skills. Carrying an object generally requires sustained wrist extension and finger flexion. Sustaining this positioning can be encouraged by holding an object and using it to manipulate another object, such as batting at a suspended ball with a cylindrical object like a therapy cone or dowel rod. Children with increased tone may have difficulty sustaining proper positioning while manipulating smaller objects. Initiating therapy with a larger, cylindrical-shaped object may provide more pressure to the thenar eminence (i.e., the place of tonal control of the UE) and improved relaxation of the hand. Smaller objects actually accentuate the pull into a tonal pattern as they encourage more movement into flexion.

Anticipatory Control

A fine motor task actually begins with the first visual attention to the object. Before the arm moves for reach or the hand moves for grasp, there is already a plan developed of how to move the arm, how to shape the hand, and how much force to use to begin manipulation of that object. This is developed through repetition of being able to grasp and explore various objects. To develop this among the many things that can impact a child's fine motor skills, the child must be presented with a large variety of objects that differ in shape, weight, and size. Initially, the child should have multiple repetitions of objects that are of the same size, shape, and weight to develop the motor plan for such objects. As this becomes integrated, the occupational therapy provider can begin grading the activities and adjusting the size, shape, and weight of objects being presented. Verbal cueing of the movements required can assist with developing anticipatory control. The occupational therapy practitioner should use statements such as "big, open hand, it's going to be heavy" or "small, light fingers" to help the child prepare for appropriate grasp. This can progress to asking the child what is needed before starting the movement required for the activity.

Voluntary Release

Voluntary, controlled release must accompany grasp and manipulation skills for activities to be fully functional in nature. Voluntary release relies on the child's ability to open the hand, demonstrate appropriate stability for arm placement, and be able to accurately judge placement of the object. Treatment for release may begin with weight-bearing techniques to increase proprioception and help normalize tone. It can then progress to providing handling techniques to guide the extremity to the location of reach and/or providing thenar eminence pressure to assist with release of the object. Working on release generally begins with working further away from the body. Working at midline facilitates pronation and flexion and makes release more difficult, especially in kids with higher tone. Reaching out to the side, or to the side and down toward the floor, encourages release of the object. Initial treatment will focus on just letting go of the object with no specific target of release. A larger object can be used to allow the occupational therapy practitioner to grasp a portion of the object when the placement for release has been obtained. The object stabilized in the therapy provider's grasp allows the child to initiate release. This stabilization is decreased as treatment progresses. The child moves on to being able to release once their hand is stabilized on a surface and then to release into space. Treatment can progress to the child releasing an object into a wide-open container and then into smaller openings as skill of voluntary release improves.

In-Hand Manipulation

Children having difficulty with in-hand manipulation skills often become frustrated with tasks because they frequently drop objects and are slow in execution of tasks. The child will often seek supportive surfaces so that they can change the position of the object in their hand by placing the object on the surface and then re-grasping the object in a different position. They may have limited finger isolation and lack controlled finger movements; lack palmar arch control so they cannot cup the hand to sustain grasp of an object within the palm; have great difficulty or are unable to sustain more than one object in the hand at the same time; and may tend to move the object to their fingertips by holding their hand down, so that the object falls from the palm into the fingertips. Treatment to address decreased hand manipulation skills should focus on increasing proprioceptive and sensory awareness within the hand, addressing any tonal abnormalities, and improving arch formation and control. Dynamic weight-bearing on the hands will help to address arch formation in the hand. Having the child place their hand on a mound of Theraputty or clay during weight-bearing can assist with providing pressure into the hand and help to shape the arches. Placing objects in the clay and having the child work to pull them out can be used to encourage weight-bearing activities. Isolation of the ulnar side of the hand from the radial side of the hand is also needed for in-hand manipulation skills. The child can be encouraged to hold items in the palm of their hand using their ring and little finger while picking up objects with their index finger, middle finger, and thumb. If this is too difficult, self-adhesive tape can be used to hold the little and ring fingers in place or the occupational therapy practitioner can hold Thera-Band® over the fingers and hand to help stabilize them during movement of the index, middle fingers, and thumb. Palm to finger movement of the object can be addressed by initially placing the object more distally in the fingers with the hand supported on a surface. The occupational therapy practitioner can gradually change initial placement of the object more proximally along the palmar surface as a means of grading the activity.

Bilateral Hand Use

Many fine motor tasks require coordination of the use of both hands. At times, one hand serves as more of a stabilizer while the other hand is the primary manipulator.

Other bilateral hand activities require both hands to be completing simultaneous or reciprocal manipulation of the object or objects. Children who have difficulty with keeping both UEs at midline will have greater difficulty with bilateral hand skills. Further difficulties can arise when children also have difficulty visually attending to two objects. Activities to facilitate bilateral hand skills generally begin with more gross activities such as pushing a child-size grocery cart with two hands or carrying a large ball. Activities like wheelbarrow walking can increase reciprocal movement of the UEs while providing proprioceptive input and strengthening to assist with bilateral hand coordination. Construction toys come in a variety of shapes and sizes and are an excellent means of encouraging bilateral hand use. ADL activities like buttoning and zipping are prime bilateral hand activities and can be graded from large sizes completed on dressing boards or dressing dolls to smaller sizes completed on clothing worn by the child. Children with diagnoses such as hemiplegia or brachial plexus injuries will have difficulty integrating bilateral hand tasks and generally require increased encouragement to use the affected hand in activities. When used in an activity, the affected hand is most often used as the stabilizer.

Handwriting

Just as in fine motor skills, development of handwriting skills can be difficult for a child if they are trying to develop these skills amid issues like increased tone, poor proximal stability, decreased muscle strength, decreased processing of proprioceptive input, and decreased visual motor skills. Handwriting is noted to have a strong connection to eye–hand coordination but is less dependent on dexterity skills. When children begin to develop handwriting skills, they rely heavily on vision to guide their movements. However, as handwriting skills develop, proprioceptive and kinesthetic inputs become more dominant in guiding movements. As was the case with treatment for fine motor skills, handwriting treatment is different depending on the setting in which the child receives the treatment. Handwriting can greatly impact the child's ability to participate in their educational plan, and is therefore generally a part of treatment provided within the school system. Compensatory strategies, accommodations, and adaptations will be used to allow the child to improve their function in the school environment in a more immediate manner. Remedial approaches

to improve function in an area impacting handwriting are often addressed simultaneously with compensatory strategies, accommodations, and adaptations. Insurance companies will often categorize work on handwriting skills under the jurisdiction of the school environment and not approve work on handwriting in outpatient settings. Therefore, outpatient settings will often focus on handwriting skills through addressing such things as UE strength, proprioception, tone management, trunk stability, and shoulder girdle stability. Several treatment approaches are used in addressing a child's difficulty with handwriting skills. Often the best treatment for children who are challenged by issues with handwriting is found in the fastidious combination of various approaches.

Neurodevelopmental Treatment Approach

The neurodevelopmental treatment (NDT) approach focuses on addressing deficits in a child's postural support and movement patterns. This approach will focus on such things as modulating tone, improving proximal stability, and improving hand function in order to prepare the hands and the body for handwriting. An NDT approach might include activities like working prone on elbows to improve cocontraction through the neck, shoulder girdle, elbows, and wrists, as well as jumping activities to increase tone. This approach may also include having a child complete chair push-ups to provide input to their arms and hands prior to completing a writing task.

Acquisitional Treatment Approach

The acquisitional approach has four prime areas. These areas are practice, repetition, feedback, and reinforcement. This is the approach where handwriting interventions fall. There is a focus on spacing, size, and alignment during writing. This approach may use special paper with color-coded lines to help the child orient each part of the letter appropriately.

Sensorimotor Treatment Approach

The sensorimotor approach focuses on multisensory writing activities. In this approach, the occupational therapy practitioner may place the child's paper on an easel for more vertical orientation and increased wrist extension during writing. An occupational therapy provider may have the student work in the schoolyard with sidewalk chalk or may have the student write with crayons on sandpaper to increase sensory feedback during writing. The child may work with finger paints while drawing letters with their fingers on paper plates. A student may use Popsicle® sticks to draw letters in the frosting of their cupcakes or cake.

Biomechanical Treatment Approach

The biomechanical approach focuses on changes to the student context. In this approach, the occupational therapy practitioner may work to improve a child's sitting posture by lowering their chair so that they can have their feet well supported on the ground. They may increase the height of their table surface to encourage a more upright sitting posture. The occupational therapy practitioner may utilize pencil grips if the child demonstrates too much tension during pencil grasp. This increased tension typically results in a very static pencil grasp and early fatigue during writing. The occupational therapy practitioner can also explore changing the type of writing tool used by the student.

Psychosocial Treatment Approach

In the psychosocial approach, OTs may decide to place students in a writing group. For example, they may decide to have the student write Valentine cards to pass out to class members.

Selection and Positioning of the Activity

Pediatric OTs frequently use a variety of toys as tools to both engage children and facilitate a desired result. Especially in the infant or a very young child, it is not possible for the OT to simply give a list of directions and have that child complete the activity with the movement patterns that the OT desires. Therefore, pediatric OTs must become skilled at choosing a specific toy/activity and place the toy/activity so that it facilitates the child to practice the desired movement pattern or skill. If the occupational therapy practitioner wants the child to hold a position, then an activity should be chosen that requires more time to complete. If more dynamic movements are required, then the activity should be less static and more dynamic as well. For instance, to provide more sustained

weight-bearing in side sitting, an occupational therapy provider would have the child place pegs into a resistive pegboard or complete a shape in the form of a puzzle. These activities require greater focus on placement. If an occupational therapy practitioner wants the child to work on weight shifting, but they are not yet strong enough to hold that position for any prolonged period, then the occupational therapy practitioner might have the child pick up a block placed at midline and drop it into a wide mouth bucket placed to the desired side of weight shift. This activity requires less refinement and less focus on placement making it more dynamic in nature. If the activity is not bringing about the desired result, then the occupational therapy provider should consider changing the type of activity and/or the specific placement of the activity. The occupational therapy practitioner may want to change the height of the surface at which the child is completing the activity. Children who tend to pull into extension may benefit from a lower surface that will bring their eyesight down to the activity and cause an increase in flexion of the trunk and neck. With some children, sitting on the floor and trying to engage in an activity that is resting on the floor may result in too much forward flexion and negatively impact their breathing. This may cause them to resist fine motor practice or to only engage in the fine motor activity for short periods of time. Placing the activity on a small table or bench in front of the child will allow them to more actively engage in the activity through promoting trunk extension. Careful consideration to choice and positioning of the task is often what transforms the activity from being a simple play activity to one of therapeutic value.

Feeding/Nippling

Whether treating children with difficulty in nippling, drinking from a cup, or taking solid foods, the OT needs to develop a treatment plan that is holistic in nature. Focusing simply on the oral cavity and the amount of food that is gone from the plate or the amount of liquid gone from the bottle/cup will result in missing some key components that may be impacting the child's feeding skills. For instance, the child may be able to take in all of the food on their plate but may do so with such a high-energy process that they are actually burning all the calories they might have gained from the food. They may show appropriate oral strength and oral movement, but may be breathing so hard that they cannot coordinate the swallow with their respiratory effort. The OT needs to be able to develop a treatment plan to address the child's ability to regulate their state of alertness, provide the most appropriate respiratory support, have support for their tone and stability needs, provide them with the proper equipment to maximize their feeding skills, and ensure safety during the feeding process. The OT will work closely in coordination with the family, physician, and nutritionist to provide the best possible treatment plan.

Nippling

Nutritive versus nonnutritive sucking. See **Table 30-5**.

Nippling Interventions

Managing Environments

When working on nippling, especially in the premature infant, care should be taken to control the stimulation within the environment. Dimming the lights and providing minimal auditory input or controlled, consistent

Table 30-5 Nippling		
	Nonnutritive Sucking	**Nutritive Sucking**
Developmental progression	Present at 27 weeks gestation. Well integrated by 34 weeks.	Present at 32 weeks. Well integrated by 37 weeks.
Rate	Two sucks per swallow.	One suck per swallow.
Pattern	4–13 sucks per burst alternating with 3–10-second rest breaks.	10–30 sucks per burst initially. See variability in bursts and rest periods getting longer as feeding progresses.
Stimulus	Dry stimulus like finger or pacifier. Or just mouthing movements without stimulus.	Liquid from nipple/breast.
Suck/swallow/breathe ratio	6–8 sucks per swallow/breathe.	One suck per swallow/breathe.
Benefits	Helps regulate state control. Reduces stress. Assists with initiation of nutritive sucking pattern.	Obtains nutrition.

Data from Hunter, 2010; Schuberth, Amirault, and Case-Smith, 2010.

sound like rhythmic music can help with regulation during feeding.

Infant Level of Arousal

Most NICUs are moving from scheduled feeding times to cue-based, infant-driven feeding schedules. An individualized program is developed for the infant based on their medical status, ability to obtain a stable, alert status, and feeding readiness cues like awakening for feeds, rooting, and nonnutritive sucking behaviors. An infant needs to demonstrate a stable, alert status throughout the feeding. The infant may show signs of being overstressed, like arm and hand extension (i.e., stop sign), finger splaying, and hiccupping and/or increased fussing. They may also show a decreased state of arousal, like being difficult to arouse and/or being difficult to keep awake once initially alert. Managing the environment as noted above, bundling the infant to help control extraneous movements and inputs, or unbundling the infant to help increase arousal are techniques that can be used to help an infant manage their level of arousal so they are ready for nippling.

Postural Stability

Providing the infant with proper support through bundling and secure positioning can help improve postural stability for nippling. Working with the infants in prone positioning during playtimes also helps increase postural stability. Care should be taken during feeding to ensure the infant's head is kept in a neutral position with a proper chin tuck.

Positioning

Careful consideration needs to be given to positioning during nippling. Infants are often fed in a more reclined position. This may be more difficult for some infants as gravity pulls the formula back too quickly causing poor coordination of the swallow. It can also pull the tongue into a more retracted position interfering with the infant's ability to properly grasp the nipple and initiate negative pressure. An upright position can allow greater control of formula flow and improve tongue positioning. An infant who has difficulty keeping an alert state during nippling may also benefit from a more upright position. Breastfeeding is typically completed in side-lying as the infant is oriented toward the breast. This side-lying position can also be used with bottle-feeding. If an infant has better tongue, lip, and cheek control to one side, then putting that side down in the side-lying position will allow the formula to fall to the side with more functional movement and allow the infant better control. An infant may also have better breathing patterns in side-lying where gravity is not directly acting on the diaphragm (i.e., gravity-reduced positioning). Prone positions with prone feeding bottles can also be used to help a child with severe tongue retraction.

Preparation for Oral Stimulation

Controlled oral stimulation prior to feeding might help organize the infant's oral movements in preparation for nutritive sucking. Stroking the infant by the side of the mouth to elicit a rooting response can open the infant's mouth and prepare them for a sucking response. Stroking the tongue with a finger or pacifier and allowing the infant to organize their sucking on a pacifier first can help prepare the infant. Stimulation to the hard palate will encourage tongue elevation and can help initiate a swallow.

Jaw/Tongue Support

Infants will at times have difficulty with controlling and organizing their oral movements for a nutritive sucking pattern. Providing jaw support can provide the stability the infant needs to coordinate their tongue, lips, cheeks, and jaw movements for a nutritive pattern. Using a single finger support under the jaw for tongue stability may be all the child needs to help organize oral movements. Other infants will require support under the jaw and along both cheeks to organize a nutritive sucking pattern. This three-point support pattern is generally completed with the feeder placing their middle finger under the chin, their index finger on one cheek, and thumb on the other cheek. The thumb and index finger are generally placed along the lower jawbone on either side with a gentle pressure in and forward to provide the stability the infant needs. Support is slowly decreased as the infant's skills improve.

Flow Rate

If the child is having difficulty coordinating their swallow in a timely manner, coughing, gagging, and a loss of formula from the oral cavity may be observed. Slowing down the rate at which the formula moves through the oral cavity can allow the infant the time needed to coordinate the trigger for swallowing. Flow rate can be managed by changing the position of the infant as noted above. It can also be changed by thickening the formula with cereal or by changing the nipple to one designed with a slower flow rate.

Respiratory Concerns

During the swallowing process, the infant must interrupt their respirations for a fraction of a second to allow for the swallow. Infants who have respiratory challenges will have difficulty coordinating their sucking and swallowing with their breathing. The infant's respiratory status will greatly impact their ability to nipple. The OT should try different feeding positions to assess their impact on the infant's respiratory status. As discussed above, the OT should also assess if controlling the formula's rate of flow will help the child coordinate their swallow with their breathing.

Nipple Styles

Several different nipple styles of various sizes, shapes, and flow rates are available on the market. The OT should assess the infant's feeding skills and match the properties of the nipple used to the baby's current skill level. Larger diameter nipples can help provide stability for the tongue. Some nipples are softer and have faster flow rates. These can be used for babies with decreased strength of suck. Other nipples have slower flow rates and can be useful for babies who have difficulty coordinating their suck/swallow/breathe patterns.

Feeding Interventions

Environmental Adaptations

Children need to be able to eat and drink in a variety of environments; however, trying to develop new skills in a variety of different environments will often be too challenging for the child. Oftentimes, treatment will begin in a stable environment where outside stimulation is well controlled. Regularly scheduled meals are typically the best way to help a child develop appropriate feeding skills. Care should also be given to the overall length of the mealtime. Children who have difficulty controlling boluses can often take an extended time at meals. Here again, children may actually end up burning more calories in the process of eating than they are gaining from the food. Treatment may include: limiting meal time, providing foods that are easier to manipulate, providing supplemental feedings, and providing exercises to improve the strength and coordination of oral movements. Arranging the order of foods at mealtimes is another type of environmental adaptation that can be provided in feeding treatment. Providing the challenging foods first and in a limited amount can allow the child to consume these before they are too fatigued. Children who have difficulty fully clearing the oral cavity upon swallow may benefit from alternating bites of food with sips of liquid.

Positioning Adaptations

During meals, children should be supported so that they can stabilize their trunk, head, and neck in midline with symmetrical alignment. This can provide the stability needed to better isolate their oral motor skills. Keeping the chin tucked and preventing hyperextension of the neck helps to decrease the risk of aspiration by allowing improved protection of the airway. It also prevents over-lengthening of the swallowing musculature which makes swallowing more difficult. Proper positioning might be completed by a specialized wheelchair, feeder seat, or by simply using towel rolls with the child's standard high chair to provide lateral support, and/or under their legs to provide increased hip flexion. Positioning of the caregiver also needs to be taken into consideration. Caregivers who stand above the child's level lead to head, neck, and trunk extension causing decreased control during the swallow and opening of the airway, both increasing the risk of aspiration.

Sensory Processing Interventions

Children with decreased oral motor skills will have difficulty tolerating various sensory inputs due to their inability to manage these textures in the oral cavity. Some of these children will have had medical complications that limit oral exploration and/or depress some of their oral reflexes. Treatment for these children should include opportunities to explore various sensory inputs through play and positive exploration experiences. Activities should be under the child's control as much as possible. With infants who are too weak to even bring their hands to their mouth, passively bringing their hand to their mouth or positioning them in side-lying to allow easier hand-to-mouth movement is a good place to begin oral exploration. See **Tables 30-6** and **30-7** for additional activity ideas for sensory interventions.

Neuromuscular Interventions

Children with neuromuscular disorders often have tone and strength challenges that dominate their oral movements and interfere with feeding skills. They often have

Table 30-6 Activities for Children with Oral Sensory Challenges
• Provide various textured objects safe for oral exploration such as textured teethers, chewy tubes, and pacifiers
• Provide vibrating items like toothbrushes, vibrating toys, and vibrating teethers
• Provide linear rocking and deep pressure to the body prior to oral treatment/feeding
• Wear a Benik vest for calming pressure during feeding
• Provide perioral tactile input with a washcloth. Begin with static deep pressure and progress to light moving pressure. Try different textures of washcloths/fabrics
• Gradually introduce new textures
• Gradually introduce new flavors

Data from Schuberth et al., 2010.

Table 30-7 Activities for Children with Low Registration Challenges/Decreased Oral Awareness
• Provide strong flavors like pickle juice, BBQ sauce, or sour sprays
• Provide chewing activities with Thera-Band tubing, teethers, or chewy tubes
• Provide increased input with resistive chewing on things like sour gummy worms or licorice
• Provide vibratory input through vibrating toothbrushes, vibrating toys, or vibrating teethers
• Provide cold input through placing pacifiers in a freezer, dipping objects in ice water, chewing ice, or eating ice cream
• Try firmer boluses like meat dipped in steak sauce for increased flavor as well

Data from Schuberth et al., 2010.

difficulty isolating their oral movements from total body tonal patterns and cannot manipulate a bolus within the oral cavity, often losing the bolus from the oral cavity. Children with medical issues may have required intubation and/or sedation and often have experienced periods of being NPO (i.e., receiving nothing by mouth). The fast twitch muscle fibers that are seen in many of the muscles involved in feeding are quicker to demonstrate atrophy during disuse. This results in weakness in the oral motor musculature and impacts oral intake skills. See **Table 30-8** for suggested interventions for common neuromuscular issues.

Table 30-8 Common Neuromuscular Issues and Possible Interventions

Low tone: Open mouth position, drooling, and drooping cheeks	• Cold stimulation to the face and oral cavity • Utilize sour flavors • Use a Nuk® brush dipped in sour flavors to stretch the cheeks in an arc from the upper jaw to the lower jaw • Provide proprioceptive input through resistive blowing toys • Provide proprioceptive input through resistive chewing
Jaw weakness: Clenched jaw or open mouth position, drooling, and food loss	• Repetitive chewing against resistive input (e.g., licorice, raw fruit, or raw vegetables); can be placed in a meshed bag or gauze if the child cannot control the pieces obtained from biting • Repetitive chewing on Thera-Band tubing or chewy tube teethers • Sustaining bite on Thera-Band tubing and trying to "pull" tubing from the mouth
Tonic bite reflex	• If this reflex occurs when bringing a utensil to the mouth, keep the utensil still in front of the mouth but not touching, and wait. Stimulus for the reflex may be the movement of the spoon toward the mouth, when movement is gone, the reflex may be released and the child may be able to open his or her mouth and accept the utensil • Feed in a quiet, calm environment. Overstimulation increases tonic bite reflex • Provide forward flexion with rounded shoulders and chin in a tucked position • Keep the body well supported with the feet on a surface and the trunk slightly forward flexed • If tonic bite occurs on a spoon, do not pull on the spoon as this will result in increased biting. Provide as minimal input to the spoon as possible and wait for a release • Provide sustained pressure to the temporomandibular joint to help release • Use a rubber-coated, metal spoon for feeding to reduce the chance of biting through a plastic spoon and/or damaging the teeth
Tongue thrust	• Usually accompanied by jaw and trunk extension. Provide forward trunk flexion and chin tuck • Exercises to increase lip closure and provide a boundary for the tongue • Encourage tongue lateralization; place the bolus to the side of the mouth or tastes onto the inner cheek • Stimulate the posterior portion of the hard palate to encourage proper placement of the midblade portion of the tongue (i.e., contact with inner surface of the upper, posterior gums) • Facilitate jaw strength and control • If tongue thrust occurs just during swallow, practice holding a very small amount of fluid in the mouth and keep the jaw closed during swallowing
Tight retracted lips and cheeks	• Passive stretching and massage exercises for perioral and intraoral areas • Practice using just lips to clear food items like yogurt, pudding, or thickened liquids from a flat bowled spoon • Encourage blowing bubbles and/or activating blow toys

Data from Schuberth et al., 2010.

Adaptive Equipment

Numerous types of adaptive devices to assist with feeding issues are currently readily available on the market, especially through Internet sites. Adaptive equipment is available that can assist with allowing a child to be more independent with self-feeding skills, and with allowing more controlled presentation of the food by the child or the feeder to increase safety during feeding.

See **Table 30-9** for examples of using adaptive equipment for feeding.

Food Modifications

Successful feeding therapy relies on a good knowledge of the properties of various food consistencies and textures and the ability to match these to the child's oral motor skills. An understanding of how to manipulate

Table 30-9 Examples of Adaptive Equipment for Feeding

Scoop plates, scoop bowls, and plate guards	• Helps the child fill his or her spoon or fork by providing an edge that traps food and allows it to be pushed onto a spoon or fork
Dycem, suction cups on bowls, and plates	• Stabilizes the bowl or plate to make it easier for the child to obtain food onto the utensil
Curved handled utensils	• Brings the bowl of the spoon or tongs of fork into alignment with the mouth when range of motion is more limited at the elbow and/or wrist
Spoon with shallow bowl	• Requires less lip control to clear a bolus from the spoon
Spoon with bumps or ridges	• Provides increased sensory input and improves awareness of food placement
Cold utensil	• Increases awareness of food placement
Wide handled utensil	• Requires less refined grasp and control
Weighted utensils	• Can help dampen ataxic movements and improve control of hand-to-mouth movement
Shorter straw	• Easier to obtain liquid; the longer the straw, the more sustained, negative pressure is required
Straw with smaller diameter	• Easier to obtain liquid; the wider the straw, the more sustained, negative pressure is required
Cut out cup	• Allows the cup to be tipped up more without the child having to extend their head and neck. Can provide increased control during drinking

Data from Schuberth et al., 2010.

food textures and consistencies to progress the child to a more age-appropriate diet is also required. The property of liquids is that they move freely and are hard to contain. Children who have limited oral motor strength, range, and/or coordination will have difficulty managing the speed at which thin liquids can move. Thickening the liquid to a nectar or honey consistency can provide the child with more time to coordinate the movements they need as the thicker the liquid the slower the flow rate. Thicker liquids also provide more sensory input through increased density. This can improve coordination of movement by providing increased awareness of the liquid within the oral cavity. Providing cold, thickened liquid can further increase this awareness and also increases the triggering of a swallow. Thickening the liquid is also a way to help control the movement of the liquid when the child is learning to transition to drinking from an open cup. Foods with cohesive and smooth consistencies are easier to manage when the child has limited oral motor skills. They do not require as much coordination of lip, cheek, and tongue movements and are more easily managed with more primitive skills. Crunchier, denser foods, or foods that are sticky or tacky require greater intrinsic control of the tongue and coordination of tongue, cheek, lip, and jaw movements. Foods with mixed consistencies, containing a liquid and a solid component (e.g., soups, some stage three infant foods, and stews) are harder to control. These require

the ability to hold the solid portion in the mouth while swallowing the liquid portion and then going back to manipulate the solid. OTs working with children who have feeding difficulties will need to become familiar with food chaining techniques that can help the child gradually progress from their current food preferences to more challenging and age-appropriate foods. Food chaining techniques include such things as working on biting and chewing skills by starting with a crunchy solid that is easily dissolved, then moving up a level to something that requires a little more manipulation but softens and mashes, then working up to a crunchy solid that requires full biting and chewing. For example, the therapist may begin by presenting the child with veggie-straws, progress to graham crackers, and then work up to apple slices.

Self-Feeding

Self-feeding skills are often limited in children who have limited range of motion, decreased strength, tonal impairments, decreased hand skills, cognitive impairments, and/or sensory processing deficits. As these deficits are addressed in therapy, self-feeding skills will slowly improve. Therapy should also address techniques to improve self-feeding skills in the face of existing motor/sensory impairments. The child may benefit from a raised table or tray to provide arm support and assist with hand-to-mouth control. The occupational therapy practitioner may use a hand over hand technique to assist with hand-to-mouth control. As skills progress, the occupational therapy provider can decrease support at the forearm or elbow. A large variety of adaptive equipment, as noted above, can also be obtained to help the child improve their self-feeding skills. Chaining techniques, where the OT does most of the task and the child completes either the first step or the last step and works to gain more and more of the steps, can also be used.

Behavioral Interventions

Children with feeding difficulties often have at least some component of behavioral issues intertwined with their feeding challenges. Though medical issues and/or oral motor skill deficits are usually the underlying causes of feeding difficulties, parents often feel that their inability to feed their child is a reflection on their parenting skills. They will try anything to get their child to eat. By the time they reach an OT for assistance, the child may have received so many different inputs and changes that they often respond with refusals in an attempt to gain control. Oftentimes refusing what enters their mouth is the only point of control that the child may be able to obtain. The OT is then faced with the need to address not only such things as the various range of motion, strength, and tonal impairments that might impact oral feeding skills, but must also address the behavioral components that have developed around feeding. The OT must work with all caregivers to learn how to set clear limits and expectations that are at the appropriate level for the child's current feeding skills. They need to work to decrease the stress that surrounds the feeding process. Treatment often focuses on a combination of providing positive reinforcement when the child's behavior reflects actual fulfillment of the expected outcome and ignoring behaviors that do not meet the outcome. It often takes effort to help the families understand the need to say less during feedings. It is often the first response to correct all negative behaviors with verbal cues. However, it needs to be understood, that even negative reinforcement is a form of reinforcement and attention that will often hinder the feeding process for the child (i.e., achieving the child's desired goal of not eating). The OT may desire to seek the help of a behavior management specialist to assist with developing a plan for addressing behavioral issues around feeding.

Activities of Daily Living

General Treatment Interventions

ADL treatment needs to be addressed based on what is meaningful and useful to the child and the family. Treatment should be based on family preferences, what is age appropriate for the child, and what is realistic based on the child's level of functioning and expected progress. The OT will need to take the time to identify cultural issues that are important to the family and how these issues will impact the child's ADL skills. Treatment approaches should incorporate the idea that ADL skills must be completed in a variety of different environments (e.g., home, school, and public restrooms and so on).

Treatment to Restore or Maintain Performance

This treatment approach addresses the underlying body structure and function that can be impacting the completion of ADL tasks. It identifies the underlying issues with in-hand manipulation such as UE range of motion, strength, grip strength, eye–hand coordination skills, and stability.

Compensatory Treatment Approach

This approach uses a different physical technique, a different position, or substitutes a different movement pattern to complete ADLs. Children may complete dressing in bed, long sitting on the floor with their back against a corner of the room, or taught an adaptive method of putting their coat on (e.g., placing it on the floor with the collar facing them, putting both arms in their jacket and flipping it over their head). The child may use some type of assisted technology to help them complete the task. Technology should be able to assist without being too cumbersome or make it inconvenient to use. The technology should allow the child to complete the task more efficiently than they could without the device. Adaptations to the environment include controlling sensory input, and making architectural changes (e.g., roll in showers, lower closet rods, and lower countertops).

Preventative Treatment Approach

In many cases, planning ahead can help with managing ADL tasks. Looking at the day's activities and planning appropriate clothing can assist with a child's independence in ADLs. Dressing in yoga or sweat pants instead of pants that have buttons and/or zippers may make it easier for a child to manage their clothing during toileting. Packing a Ziploc bag with supplies the child needs for a catheterization session and then packing their school bag with one bag for each catheterization session that will occur while they are at school can help the child remember the steps of catheterization and increase independence. Packing the child's curved spoon, and scoop bowl in their lunch box or being sure they have a duplicate set at school will help increase their independence during lunch or snack time. Providing a picture board in the coatroom at the school to help sequence the activities of putting coats and boots on and off will also encourage more independence.

Coaching and Education

Treatment for ADLs may focus on discussion, education, and problem-solving sessions with the child and family. Discussions can focus on safety in ADL completion for both the child and the caregiver, coping strategies for ADL skills in various environments, and specific techniques to use in the completion of ADLs. Education can be completed to instruct the parent(s) on how to best position themselves and the child during completion of ADL tasks when the child is more dependent on caregivers.

Specific Treatment Interventions

Improving Toileting Independence

Improving toileting independence is often a challenging task. Pediatric OTs must have knowledge of treatment techniques that encompass assisting parents with improving the ease of diapering to help children with neurogenic bowel and bladders learn timed evacuation, catheterization techniques to, and ultimately independence with, standard toileting. Children must also be able to complete the task in various environments with different bathroom configurations throughout any given day. In many situations, occupational therapy practitioners work to improve toileting tasks by improving fine motor and dexterity skills, sequencing and memory skills, and addressing tone, strength, range of motion, and balance skills. Children with hypersensitivity to tactile, olfactory, and/or auditory input can have difficulty with toileting tasks due to the many sensory aspects involved in the task and contained within the environment. Helping the family to manage the environmental stimuli can improve toileting independence.

Catheterization and Colostomy Management

OTs are most often involved in catheterization and colostomy management by addressing issues of sequencing, hand skills, sensory awareness, balance, positioning, and adaptive equipment. Treatment to help improve catheterization skills may have a child work on organizing sequencing cards to identify and remember the steps of the task, using tactile input to find a hole in which to place a peg in a pegboard, sitting on a therapy ball while playing catch with a beach ball to improve balance while using both hands in an activity, and assessing the need for a long-handled mirror. Therapy should also include assessment and planning for the best location in which the child can complete these tasks for appropriate privacy.

Diapering

Children with increased tone may at times demonstrate tonal patterns that result in trunk and hip extension, with adduction of the legs. This tonal position can make diapering and toileting hygiene very difficult to complete. Teaching parents to place a towel roll under the child's hips to increase hip/trunk flexion and teaching them to gently move the child slowly through hip flexion a few times prior to trying to abduct and externally rotate the legs can assist with breaking up tone to make diapering easier. Working on positioning, tonal management, and range of motion can assist with improving ease of diapering and hygiene.

Adaptations for Toileting

Multiple types of toileting aids are available on the market. Children with poor dexterity skills may benefit from a universal cuff to hold a catheter or a toilet tissue aide to hold and position toilet tissue. Children with decreased balance may benefit from a toilet reducing ring or toilet seat with arms. Children with decreased mobility may improve their independence with toileting by using a bedside commode in their bedroom, so they have room to transfer from their wheelchair.

Improving Independence in Dressing

As with many tasks in the pediatric population, the child must learn dressing tasks in the context of their range of motion, tonal, cognitive, and sensory challenges. Independence can be further complicated by the fact that parents often protect their children with developmental, sensory, and/or motor limitations for longer periods. The expectations for independence in tasks like dressing are often suppressed until later age ranges than what is typically seen in children without such challenges. It is the OT's job to help these families develop realistic, age-appropriate expectations for their children.

Limitations in Cognitive Skills and Sensory Perception

Sequencing and memory tasks related to dressing need to be practiced with children who have cognitive and sensory perception deficits. Using color-coded tags can help children match clothing to enhance dressing skills. A chart can be constructed that shows the sequence of dressing with each section color coded to match a bin containing that piece of clothing. Backward chaining techniques can be useful in teaching dressing tasks when cognitive skills are limited. Here, the parent might place the shirt over the child's head, place each arm in the proper sleeve, and then have the child pull the shirt down around their trunk. After this is mastered, the parent may expect the child to place the second arm in the sleeve and pull the garment down. They would slowly continue to add the previous step until all portions of the task are mastered.

Physical or Motor Limitations

Children with limitations in dexterity skills may benefit from adaptations such as the use of button hooks, attaching loops to their pants to slide their hands through to help with pulling pants up, or applying rings to zippers to allow them to pull the zipper up by hooking a finger through the loop. They may benefit from shoes that slip on or have hook and loop closures or elastic laces. Children with balance deficits may do better with getting dressed sitting on their bed with their back supported in a corner or being taught to dress in the side-lying position. Children with severe motor limitations can be a challenge for their caregivers to dress, and the occupational therapy providers will need to work with their parents to develop strategies to assist with dressing. Many caregivers will place their child supine on a surface to try and dress them. This can cause an increase in extensor tone and extensor posturing that will actually make it more difficult for the child to be dressed. If the child is small enough, it may be beneficial to dress the child lying prone across the caregiver's lap. Children

with poor trunk and head control can benefit from being placed in sitting on their caregiver's lap with their back supported against the caregiver's chest. Children with physical or motor limitations will generally require increased, graded practice to learn dressing skills. Therapy activities can be provided to help a child practice the components of dressing. For instance, any activity that practices placing an item in a slot can be addressed to work on buttoning skills. It may begin with placing coins in a bank and then progress to a more bilateral hand activity (e.g., having the child hold a piece of cardboard with a slot in it and place a large button through the slot). A child can work on learning to place their legs into clothing by practicing sitting on a therapy ball with their feet supported and then raising one leg up to place a hoop around their foot.

Improving Independence with Bathing or Showering

Safety is a major concern for children during bathing and showering and this should be a primary focus of the occupational therapy treatment when addressing independence in this area.

Establishing or Restoring Performance

Addressing the child's tone, range of motion, balance, and cognitive, sensory, and/or motor issues will improve their skills in bathing or showering. Treatment might also include activities to improve body awareness such as songs like "head, shoulders, knees, and toes" or games like "Simon Says." Using body paints or shower gels to encourage the child to wash an area can also heighten focus on areas to bathe.

Adapting the Task or Environment

Children with hypersensitivity issues may dislike the bathing experience. Preparing the child for bathing by providing deep pressure before starting the bath and using deep pressure when washing may be helpful. Care should be taken that all children are well supported during the bathing process. If the child is noted to startle easily, they may push into extension and are at risk of being hurt while in the tub. Many seating devices are available that can provide the child with appropriate support during bathing. Focus should also be on the position of the caregiver and their ability to be safe during the bathing process.

Prevention/Education for Bathing Safety

Using nonslip mats in and outside of the tub/shower, using covers for the faucets to prevent the child from hitting their head, and applying grab bars to assist the child with getting in and out of the tub should be considered. Careful monitoring of water temperature and checking temperature before getting in to the tub should be taught; especially with children who may have decreased sensation. Care should also be given to instruct caregivers on proper body mechanics and safety in lifting a child who will be wet from the bath.

Home Programs

A large part of success in pediatric intervention is dependent on the family's ability to help carry over treatment techniques and functional gains into life outside of the therapy room. A child may be positioned to complete an appropriate movement pattern for the 30–90 minutes a week he or she is in therapy, but if this is not reinforced at times in the home environment, that leaves 9,990 to 10,050 minutes a week for the child to work on developing inappropriate movement patterns. OTs, however, need to be prudent in establishing realistic expectations for home programs. Strict home programs that add another task to the already stressful day of the family of a child with an injury or disability may not be successful. Home program activities need to be embedded in and around the normal daily activities of the family. Appropriate involvement of the families in therapy goals, good communication with caregivers on a regular basis, and clear, concise, verbal, written, and/or illustrated instructions on ways to help the family integrate therapeutic techniques into everyday activities are all paramount to successful intervention.

Establishing a Partnership

- Recognize the child and family (e.g., parents, siblings, and grandparents) as part of the therapy team.
- Recognize and listen to the parents' insights into how their child functions outside the therapy setting.
- Establish goals for treatment in collaboration with the family and what is important in their family unit.

- Facilitate parent empowerment.
- Gain an understanding of the many factors that can impact a family's ability to complete a home program (e.g., work schedule, activities of other siblings, and cognitive levels).

Recognizing Diversity

- Do not assume everyone does things exactly like you and your family.
- Therapy providers need to gain an understanding of each family's particular makeup (e.g., ethnic background and religious beliefs) in order to make any home program successful for that family. For example, establishing a feeding therapy program with foods that are not part of the child's cultural dietary practices may address your goal but will not increase the child's function within their environment.

Communication Strategies

- Communication needs to match the child/family's level of understanding.
- *Formal meetings*: Such as an IEP to establish goals and plan of care for the child.
- *Informal meetings*: Before therapy to establish changes/follow-through since the last treatment and after therapy to summarize session and home activities.
- *Written communication*: Establish a journal that the OT writes in to communicate with the family (e.g., home program handouts).
- Emails and electronic communications.
- Phone calls.

Home Program Considerations

- *Realistic*: Do not give a long list of exercise to do. If exercises need to be completed, prioritize the exercises and introduce a few of the most important ones for the home program. Remember that many children may not be able to afford specialized equipment for the home. Be creative at adapting household items to meet their home program needs.
- *Understandable*: Written and illustrated handouts at the family/child's level should be provided if possible. Demonstrate the home program to the family and

have them teach it back to you. Use interpreters to translate for the family/child if needed.

- *Value to family*: Take time to find out the family/child's goals and use these to develop home activities. Take time to discuss with the family/child how this program relates to their goals.
- *Easy to complete in daily routine*: Home programs should not be an additional burden on the family/child. Be creative at adapting activities that are already a part of their daily routine so that the activities overtly help to address their goals (e.g., a baby who needs to work on shoulder girdle and trunk strength could be required to pull to sit after each diaper change rather than just being picked up).

Managing Behavior in Therapeutic Situations

When encountering behavior difficulties with a child in the pediatric population, especially in a very young child, the OT should be asking, what is this child trying to tell me? Children may demonstrate behavioral difficulties for several reasons, including being requested to do an activity that is too difficult, perceiving the activity to be too easy, and/or having a sensory processing disorder that interferes with their ability to function in the given situation. Identifying the stimulus that resulted in the given behavior will provide the key to managing the behavior during the treatment session. Do not automatically assume that the child is simply a behavioral challenge. Try to figure out why the behavior is being elicited.

Referrals and Discharge Considerations

Pediatric interventions are most often completed using a team-oriented approach. The OT will often facilitate a referral to another discipline to maximize treatment outcomes by seeking ways to address the child's and the family's goals that may fall outside of the occupational therapy scope of practice. Through referral and collaboration with other healthcare professionals such as professionals from the educational setting, the OT can augment the child's participation in occupations by facilitating carryover of activities between disciplines. The discharge plan should be formulated from the beginning of the therapeutic

interventions, along with goals for functional outcomes. Consideration for discharge should be given when the child has achieved all their functional goals and successfully participates in their occupations. Consideration for discharge should also be given when, despite the OT's best treatment practices, the child is showing a change from progress to plateau in the performance of their occupations.

Management and Standards of Practice

There are times when the OT may feel like they are implementing an endless array of treatment interventions. The occupational therapy practitioner must give close consideration for the appropriateness of the intervention given the child's chronological and developmental age, and cognitive and medical status. The occupational therapy provider must also ensure that their own skills are up to date with current intervention theories and strategies. They should work in collaboration with OTAs and members of other disciplines to ensure the best functional outcome for each individual child.

Chapter 30 Self-Study Activities (Answers Are Provided at the End of the Chapter)

Worksheet I: Settings

Define which specialized pediatric setting would be most appropriate for intervention services for children in the following case scenarios. Choose from the following possible intervention settings:

- **A.** Early intervention
- **B.** School based
- **C.** Hospital-based acute
- **D.** Hospital-based outpatient

Case One: Alonzo is a child with Down syndrome who has an active IFSP. Where would Alonzo most likely receive services? _____

Case Two: Jennifer is a 3-year-old girl with spastic diplegia whose family is concerned about her development. Her UE tone and strength are within normal limits. Who would be most appropriate to provide consultative services? _____

Case Three: Jonathan is an 8-year-old boy who is demonstrating handwriting difficulties and fine motor delays that are interfering with his ability to produce written work at a pace equal to his peers. He may benefit from assistive technology. Where would he most likely be referred for an evaluation for occupational therapy services? _____

Case Four: Tyrone is a 10-year-old boy status postfracture to his radius and is having difficulty with writing postsurgery. Where would he most likely be referred for evaluation for occupational therapy services? _____

Case Five: Julie is a 6-year-old female with left hemiparesis due to a stroke. She demonstrates significant range and strength limitations and increased tone in her left hand. She is able to self-ambulate around the school environment. She uses classroom tools appropriately. Where would she most likely receive therapy services? _____

Case Six: Natasha is a 5-year-old girl with a history of a brain tumor whose parents are concerned about her IEP. She has endurance and coordination issues. She frequently drops objects and has difficulty with her dressing and feeding skills. Which setting would help the parents address these issues? _____

Case Seven: Michael is a 13-year-old male who was involved in a motor vehicle accident in which he sustained a concussion and a fractured femur. Michael and his parents are concerned about him being able to perform lower extremity dressing and carry his books at school due to his external fixator. Where would Michael most likely be referred to help his family address their concerns? _____

Worksheet 2: Developmental Positions

Developmental positions are frequently used in interventions with the pediatric population to help develop desired strength, proximal stability, and skill. Match the developmental position with the skill it helps to facilitate.

A. Supine	_____ Facilitates the development of head control, muscles of the trunk, back and hips, and balance.
B. Prone	_____ Encourages hands to reach and engage, and encourages midline activities. Facilitates development of stomach muscles through body flexion in older infants. Facilitates extension in premature infants. Easy visual attention.

C. *Side-lying*	_____ Develops muscles of the trunk, back, and hips. Strengthens muscles of the arm. Allows the child to accept body weight to one side.
D. Prone on elbows	_____ Facilitates head control and helps develop muscles of the shoulders, arms, back, and hips. Facilitates hand-to-mouth activities. Facilitates development of flexor tone in premature infants.
E. Side sitting	_____ Facilitates hands together and makes it easier to touch or hold a toy. Facilitates hand and head at midline. Relaxes the child and requires less effort to move the body. Encourages extremity flexion and adduction. Develops the rib cage. Encourages rolling when reaching for toys.
F. Ring sitting	_____ Helps develop muscle control and strength in the shoulders, arms, hips, legs, and back. Helps to facilitate balance with weight shifting.
G. Four-point, quadruped	_____ Facilitates the development of muscles of the shoulders, arms, and back, head control, and the ability to weight shift when reaching.

Worksheet 3: Tone Questions

1. Pick the statement that best describes normal postural tone.
    A. It must be high enough to withstand gravity.
    B. It provides the background on which movement is based.
    C. Easy movement is only available if postural tone is low enough to allow it to happen.
    D. All of the above
2. Which statement is not true about muscle tone?
    A. Tone is highly influenced by gravity.
    B. Your emotional state can influence your muscle tone.
    C. Muscle tone allows movement against an outside source.
    D. Tone allows smooth, coordinated movements.

3. If the child you are treating has increased tone in the flexor muscles of the arm resulting in severe elbow flexion, you would expect that:
   A. The extensor muscles are also tight.
   B. The extensor muscles are overstretched and weak.
   C. The extensor muscles have not been affected because they are innervated differently.
   D. All of the above.

4. You are working with a 4-year-old male who has increased tone in his right biceps muscle. This tone is noted to increase with participation in all functional activities. Which technique is the best option to help decrease tone?
   A. Tap the muscle belly to inhibit or deactivate the muscle.
   B. Use quick stroking movements along the muscle with the muscle on stretch.
   C. Cast the arm for stretch and neutral warmth.
   D. Provide slow, firm massage strokes with stretch.

5. Evan is a 3-year-old male with a history of cerebral palsy. He has significantly increased tone in his right UE. He is holding his right UE in elbow and wrist flexion. You know that his increased tone is interfering with his ability to participate in occupations. What is the best option for the OTA to perform during treatment?
   A. Place the child in supported sitting and slowly stretch and move his right UE through full range.
   B. During home program instruction, encourage the parents to hand him things to his left UE.
   C. Position him in right side sitting with support at his elbow and have him shoot baskets with his left hand.
   D. Provide vibration to the right UE.

6. You are working with the family of a 5-year-old child with cerebral palsy who has increased extensor tone. The family has difficulty getting the child from supine to sitting after changing his diaper. Which of the following statements best describes how you would teach the parents to bring their child from a supine to a sitting position?
   A. Tell them to place their hand behind his head and slowly push him up into a sitting position because hip flexion helps to break up tone.
   B. Tell them it would be easiest to hold him by his hands and slowly pull him into a sitting position.

C. Tell them to hold his upper arms and gently lift and turn the shoulders to rotate the trunk slightly and then come up.
D. Tell them to flex his legs and knees so they face up in the air and use your body to hold his legs in this position; then, holding his upper arms near the shoulders, gently lift his shoulders up and toward you as you use your body to push his legs back so that he ends up in a sitting position.

7. Alex is a 4-year-old male with a history of hypotonia. He sits with a forward posture with his ribs resting on his hipbones. He can use his UEs in activities within his base of support and below his center of gravity, but without crossing midline. The best activity to improve overall tone and help increase his trunk stability to free his UEs for improved use includes which of the following?
   A. Position him in sitting on a platform swing and have him throw beanbags into a basket while slowly swinging in wide, full circles.
   B. Position him in sitting on a therapy ball and support him on the lateral sides of his trunk to facilitate appropriate trunk alignment and provide firm, quick pressure into the ball; then have him shoot beanbags into a basket that is above his head and off to the left.
   C. Position him in sitting on a therapy ball and support him on the lateral sides of his trunk to facilitate appropriate trunk alignment and provide firm, quick pressure into the ball; then have him place beanbags into a basket that is at his shoulder height and in front of him.
   D. Have him shoot baskets at shoulder level while he is sitting stable on the ground in tailor sitting and you are providing slow stroking to his extensor and abdominal muscles to increase his trunk stability.

Worksheet 4: Facilitating In-Hand Manipulation

Interventions for enhancing a child's in-hand manipulation skills need to be embedded into everyday play activities. Match the treatment activity with the type of in-hand manipulation skill it would help facilitate. After identifying the skill, place an "S" next to the options that would be completed with stabilization.

In-hand manipulation skills:

A. Shift
B. Translation (fingers to palm)
C. Translation (palm to fingers)
D. Rotation (may be simple or complex depending on the object's orientation)

Treatment activity:

_____ 1. You are playing a basketball game where you have the child crumple up sheets of paper and then throw them in a container.

_____ 2. You are playing a game of Uno and have the child pick up and deal the cards one at a time from the deck sitting on the table.

_____ 3. You are completing a puzzle that is made of colored blocks. The blocks have different colors on each of their sides. You are placing the blocks into the palm of the child's hand, and the child needs to turn them until he or she finds the right side to put them in.

_____ 4. During a coloring activity, what in-hand manipulation skill is used when removing a crayon from the box and preparing to color with it?

_____ 5. The child is holding fabric in one hand while trying to button with the other.

_____ 6. You have the child hold pennies in one hand and move them one at a time to place them in a bank.

_____ 7. In preparation for placing the pennies into a bank, you have the child pick five pennies up from the palm of your hand, one at a time.

_____ 8. You have the child string beads.

_____ 9. You are working on a cutting task. To move the paper in the nonpreferred hand during cutting, what type of in-hand manipulation skill is used?

_____ 10. You are placing a fish cracker into the palm of the child's hand and allow the child to eat the cracker.

Worksheet 5: Feeding Scenario

1. Jacob is a 4-week-old infant born at 34 weeks gestational age. He has a diagnosis of broncho-pulmonary dysplasia and is currently on oxygen via a nasal cannula. He was referred to occupational therapy for assistance with his nippling skills. The nurses report that he initiates sucking on the nipple but then quickly stops. He loses a lot of the formula from the oral cavity. What intervention strategies should be considered for Jacob?

2. Jennifer is an 8-week-old infant born at 24 weeks gestational age. She has a cardiac abnormality and demonstrates hypotonia throughout her body. She spends much of her day sleeping in a side-lying position. When supported in an upright position she tends to demonstrate an open mouth position. When presented with the bottle she demonstrates weak mouth closure and initiates a suck but does not seem to obtain much from the bottle. After about five minutes of working on the bottle, she tends to become drowsy and wants to fall back to sleep. What intervention strategies should you consider when working with Jennifer?

3. Antoine is a 6-year-old male with a history of cerebral palsy who has been referred to you for treatment based on his feeding difficulties. You observe his parents feeding him and note that they hold him in their lap during feedings. Antoine is noted to push into extensor patterns with his trunk, and his arms go into a high guard position (i.e., arms abducted to about 90° with elbows flexed) and his neck goes into extension. He almost lies in his parent's lap during feeding. You worry about aspiration in this position due to the neck extension. How would you instruct his parents to position him?

4. Jessica is a 2-month-old female who is on gastric tube (i.e., g-tube) feedings due to aspiration noted on her modified barium swallow. Her parents hope to be able to feed her orally in the future. You are working on a program with the family to help Jessica be able to progress from tube feedings to oral feedings. What might you recommend to the family to help Jessica maintain a suck pattern in preparation for later oral feedings?

5. Angelica is a 4-year-old female with low tone of an unknown etiology. She demonstrates low tone throughout her trunk, extremities, and facial area. During feeding she tends to demonstrate an open mouth posture and often loses the bolus from the oral cavity. What interventions might you do in treatment to help decrease her open mouth posture during spoon feedings?

6. John is a 3-year-old male who is having challenges transitioning to drinking from a regular cup. When he attempts to drink from the cup, the liquid spills between the cup and his lips. The liquid that enters the oral cavity makes him cough and sputter. What can you do to help John learn how to transition to a regular cup?

7. Elijah is a 5-year-old male who demonstrates poor motor control. With UE reaching activities he often demonstrates over or underreaching of his target. He frequently uses too much force in activities. His parents report that their major concern

for him at this time is his inability to scoop food off of his plate. What could you do to help Elijah improve his ability to complete this task?

8. Tiffany is a 4-year-old female who demonstrates a weak gross grasp and poor grip reflex. She attempts to self-feed with a spoon but often ends up dropping the spoon when attempting to scoop the food onto the spoon, bringing the spoon to her mouth, or both. She is becoming very frustrated with the task overall and often refuses to eat unless her parents feed her. What can you do to help Tiffany complete this task more independently?

Worksheet 6: ADL

1. You are working with a child and have him place pennies into a penny bank. What ADL skill could you be addressing with this activity?
   A. Tying shoes
   B. Donning shirt
   C. Buttoning
   D. Zipping

2. You are working with a child and are completing an activity where the child is sitting on a bench and you have placed five hoops around the child's waist. You have the child take the hoop from around his or her waist, up over the head, and then try to throw the hoop onto a post a few feet in front of him or her. What ADL skill are you most likely addressing with this activity?
   A. Zipping
   B. Donning a shirt
   C. Doffing a shirt
   D. Buttoning

3. You are working with a child and have the child play tug of war with you to help strengthen his or her grasp. What ADL skill are you most likely addressing with this activity?
   A. Buttoning
   B. Pulling up pants
   C. Zipping
   D. Brushing hair

4. You are having a child grasp a beanbag animal, then put his or her arm through a tube (e.g., an empty oatmeal container with both ends cut off), and then drop the animal into a basket. What ADL skill are you most likely addressing with this activity?
   A. Buttoning
   B. Donning a shirt

   C. Zipping
   D. Pulling up pants

5. You are working with a child in treatment and begin by having the child pinch and pull Thera-putty. You then use a pair of plastic, child-size tweezers to pick up small plastic animals placed at arm's length and then sustain the grasp to place them in a small container near the child's body. What ADL skill are you most likely addressing with this activity?
   A. Zipping
   B. Donning pants
   C. Buttoning
   D. Tying

6. You are working with Tony, a 7-year-old boy. In treatment, you have him play Connect Four, a game where you place checkers in slots and see who is the first to get four in a row of a particular color. What ADL skill are you most likely addressing with this activity?
   A. Feeding skills
   B. Gross grasp skills
   C. Buttoning skills
   D. Bathing skills

7. You are working with a child with an intellectual disability (ID), and his parents are concerned because he is not yet toilet trained at 4 years of age. What do you tell his parents?
   A. There are larger diapers available and they should call their durable medical equipment company to get some because it is not likely that he will be toilet trained.
   B. Many children with ID just take longer to potty-train and you can help them with some strategies to progress him along.
   C. They should begin to remodel their bathroom because it is likely that he will not be independent with toileting.
   D. Children with ID have difficulty with sequencing activities, and because toileting requires the appropriate sequencing of several tasks, it is unlikely that the child will be able to be toilet trained.

8. The child you are trying to dress continues to go into an asymmetric tonic neck reflex (ATNR) pattern. What would be the best thing to tell the parents to do to help make dressing the child easier?
   A. Gently roll the baby toward you so that the baby's head comes into midline and his or her arms relax, making dressing easier.

   B. It will be easier to get the shirt on if you dress the extended arm first and then the flexed arm.

   C. It will be easier if you dress the flexed arm first and then the extended arm because the flexed arm is closer to the head and easier to get in.

   D. It would be best to dress the child in a sitting position because this is how a child at that age would be dressing.

9. A 5-year-old, Luke, has decreased UE strength and decreased hand strength. He is having difficulty with pulling up his pants after they are put on. Your goal is for him to be independent in donning his pants. What would be the best activity to use during treatment?

   A. Placing his leg through a ring

   B. Placing rings over his feet

   C. Playing tug of war

   D. Stepping into a box

10. Jennifer is an 8-year-old female with a history of developmental delay. She has difficulty with putting her clothes on in the appropriate order. Which activity would be most appropriate to incorporate into treatment?

   A. Play games or sing songs that help to identify body parts

   B. Use a set of sequencing cards that depict a child completing the different stages of dressing

   C. Change Jennifer's positioning during dressing, and have her sit supported in the corner to dress

   D. Provide wrist loops to make it easier for Jennifer to pull up her clothing

Worksheet 7: Case Scenarios

1. A 7-year-old child presents with difficulty with handwriting skills. During writing tasks, the student rests with at least one arm on the desk and after a short period will have their chest resting against the front of the desk. During writing, their letters are of different sizes, and have poor spacing. Their writing is at times very faint. Their hands fatigue quickly. They have difficulty sustaining grasp on their pencil and will either drop the pencil or frequently end up holding it in more of a gross grasp pattern.

   1. What would be the best SI activity to complete with this child?

     a. Swinging on a tire swing

     b. Completing an obstacle course that involves crawling under objects and pushing objects

     c. Searching for objects in a container of rice

     d. Finger painting

   2. What would be the best activity to complete with this child?

     a. Completing a puzzle on the floor in prone on elbows

     b. Completing a puzzle in side sitting to their dominant side

     c. Straddling a bolster using both hands to lift rings and place them on a post at chest level

     d. Sitting on a ball and completing a table top game

Chapter 30 Self-Study Answers

Worksheet 1: Settings

Case One: A. An IFSP or individualized family service plan is a result of the evaluation completed on an at-risk child that has been referred to early intervention. It is an outline of the family's services and who is providing them.

Case Two: A. Jennifer is age 3 years or younger and at risk of developmental delay. She does not currently demonstrate significant tonal involvement that is greatly impacting her function. She would be best served in the least restrictive environment of early intervention services provided in the home or consultative group setting.

Case Three: B. He is school aged, and his delay has a direct impact on his educational performance.

Case Four: D. Although his difficulty is with writing and may impact his educational performance, it is due to a temporary impairment. School-based therapy services are not provided when a student has a temporary impairment. Rehabilitation is more appropriately addressed in the outpatient therapy setting.

Case Five: D. Although she demonstrates significant impairment with her left UE, she is independent in her educational setting and would not qualify for school services.

Case Six: B. The parent's issue is with the IEP. An IEP is an individualized education plan and is developed in the school system to address the child's present level of performance and how his or her disability impacts the child's function in the school environment and participation in the curriculum.

Case Seven: C. In the acute setting, children are frequently referred to occupational therapy services just prior to discharge. The OT and family identify strengths and weaknesses in the discharge environment and develop an intervention plan.

Worksheet 2: Developmental Positions

A. Supine	**(F)** Facilitates the development of head control, muscles of the trunk, back and hips, and balance.
B. Prone	**(A)** Encourages hands to reach and engage and encourages midline activities. Facilitates development of stomach muscles through body flexion in older infants. Facilitates extension in premature infants. Easy visual attention.
C. *Side-lying*	**(E)** Develops muscles of the trunk, back, and hips. Strengthens muscles of the arm. Allows the child to accept body weight to one side.
D. Prone on elbows	**(B)** Facilitates head control and helps develop muscles of the shoulders, arms, back, and hips. Facilitates hand-to-mouth activities. Facilitates development of flexor tone in premature infants.
E. Side sitting	**(C)** Facilitates hands together and makes it easier to touch or hold a toy. Facilitates hand and head at midline. Relaxes the child and requires less effort to move the body. Encourages extremity flexion and adduction. Develops the rib cage. Encourages rolling when reaching for toys.
F. Ring sitting	**(G)** Helps develop muscle control and strength in the shoulders, arms, hips, legs, and back. Helps to facilitate balance with weight shifting.
G. Four-point, quadruped	**(D)** Facilitates the development of muscles of the shoulders, arms, and back, head control, and the ability to weight shift when reaching.

Worksheet 3: Tone Questions

1. **D.**
2. **C.** This is the definition of strength. Tone and strength are not the same. Tone is the amount of resistance felt in the muscle during passive movement.
3. **B.** Tightness and shortening in the agonist muscle almost always produces weakness and overstretching of the antagonist muscle. Care must be given in treatment to address the tightness, weakness, and shortening of the agonist, as well as the lengthening and weakness of the antagonist muscle to provide appropriate biomechanical alignment of the joint and improve functioning.
4. **C.** Tapping and quick stroking are both facilitatory and would increase tone. Slow, firm massage strokes can help decrease tone but are more temporary in nature. The best answer is casting the arm. Casting the arm would provide a prolonged stretch and a longer lasting impact on UE tone. It will support the area in proper alignment during functional use of the UE and help to encourage more proper movement patterns.
5. **C.** Vibration is facilitatory and would increase tone. Handing the child's items in the left UE would not help to address the child's increased tone in his or her right UE and would encourage decreased use of the right UE. Weight-bearing through right side sitting while facilitating use of the left UE is the best way to inhibit tone in the right UE.
6. **C.** Using rotation of the trunk and bringing him into flexion will help to decrease his extensor tone and mimics the natural progress of coming from supine into sitting. Placing your hand behind the head of someone with extension patterns usually encourages them to push into extension. Pulling the child into sitting does not encourage active use of the abdominals through normal patterns. Option D does not facilitate the child to be active in any way, it would be very difficult with a 5-year-old, and it would become more difficult as the child grows.
7. **C.** You want to encourage increased trunk tone to provide increased stability for reaching against gravity. Slow swinging in circles in unsupported sitting on the swing would not help to address his decreased tone and trunk stability.

Having him reach overhead and off to the side is too much of a challenge at this time given his inability to reach above his center of gravity. Providing slow stroking and keeping him on a static surface would not help to increase his tone and stability.

Worksheet 4: Facilitating In-Hand Manipulation

1. B
2. A
3. D
4. D
5. A/S
6. C/S
7. B/S
8. A
9. A
10. A

Worksheet 5: Feeding Scenario

1. **Answer:** Consider changing to the Haberman nipple or thickening the formula to decrease the formula flow rate. If Jacob starts out sucking then stops, he is likely becoming disorganized by the formula entering the oral cavity. By slowing the formula down you can decrease the amount that is obtained per suck and can increase Jacob's ability to coordinate his suck/swallow/breathe pattern. Holding Jacob in a more upright position will also help to decrease the impact that gravity has on pulling the formula to the back of his mouth and increase time to coordinate his oral movements. You might also discuss increasing Jacob's oxygen slightly during the feeding process with the physician, which can help increase coordination as well.

2. **Answer:** Jennifer has low tone that is impacting her proximal stability and the strength of her mouth movements, resulting in poor nippling skills. Several things should be considered with Jennifer. Bundling could be tried to help improve her stability. Holding her in a semi-upright side-lying position will also provide her with more stability and decrease the impact of gravity pulling her mouth open. Using a soft nipple will help decrease the strength of suck required. Providing firm, steady jaw support will help to increase the stability of her oral

musculature. Chilling the nipple and/or formula will also help to increase alertness and the swallowing reflex.

3. **Answer:** Antoine needs to be positioned with more hip and knee flexion to help break up his extensor patterning. Although his parents might be able to hold him in their lap in more hip/knee flexion, it is unlikely that they will be able to feed him and manage his tone at the same time. It is also not age appropriate for Antoine to be held in his parent's lap for feeding. Antoine should be positioned in his wheelchair or a specialized feeding chair to facilitate hip and knee flexion and help break up his extensor patterning.

4. **Answer:** It is a good idea to recommend that the family provides Jessica with a pacifier each time she is receiving a tube feeding. This helps to keep her sucking pattern strong, albeit nonnutritive, and helps her associate the sucking process with becoming full. You might also recommend that they wipe Jessica's face before and after each tube feeding. Children with oral feedings receive a good amount of input to the facial area, with food getting on their face during the feeding process and having their faces wiped during and after the feeding process. Children with tube feedings do not have the challenge of food getting on their face during meals and therefore, often have decreased sensory input to the facial area.

5. **Answer:** Angelica demonstrates poor jaw control. It would be a good idea to use a three-point jaw support technique or support with your index or middle finger under her jaw and your thumb resting under her lower lip to provide improved lip closure. You should also be sure that Angelica is positioned well with good support being provided. You might try reclining her slightly so that there is not as much of a downward gravity pull on her jaw. Be sure to keep her head in alignment with her body and her chin tucked.

6. **Answer:** Have John's parents use a thickening agent to thicken the liquid they are presenting him in the cup. The slower movement of the liquid will give him more time to coordinate his arm movements and lip and tongue movements in presenting the liquid to the oral cavity. The thickened liquid will move more slowly, allowing John to prepare for the entrance of the liquid into his mouth. The thickened liquid is heavier and provides more input to the lips and tongue during movement. It is also more adhesive and

maintains more of a bolus formation, rather than the thin liquid that flows quickly and easily.

7. **Answer:** Try using Dycem or another nonslip product under Elijah's dish to keep it from moving during his attempts to get the food off the plate. Use a scoop bowl to provide a good edge to scoop the food against and to give Elijah a clue as to when to try to change the force used in the task. You might try placing some light cuff weights on Elijah's wrists to give him more input and help dampen his excess movement patterns, and/or try using a weighted utensil.

8. **Answer:** Try presenting Tiffany with a spoon that has a built-up handle. There are also many commercially available plastic molded children's spoons that are lighter and have adaptive handles where the child can slide his or her hand through, so a portion of the handle is in the palm and a portion goes around the dorsum of the hand. If needed, the bottom portion of this handle can also be built up to accommodate decreased grasping skills.

Worksheet 6: ADL

1. **C.** This activity works on the in-hand manipulation skills needed to manage the button through shifting and translating it in the hand and then on placing the button or penny into the buttonhole or slot of the penny bank.

2. **C.** Because of movement from the child's waist to overhead, you are working on taking the shirt off, but you could also address donning if, after completing the preceding task, you have the child put the hoops back over the head and around the waist after you take them off the post.

3. **B.** Zipping and buttoning require more pinch strength than gross grasp strength, which is truly what is addressed in tug of war. Brushing hair requires sustained grasp on the brush but not as much active grasp against resistance as is required in pulling up your pants.

4. **B.** This activity simulates putting an arm through a sleeve.

5. **A.** This activity addresses sustained pinch strength and mimics an arm moving during sustained pinch.

6. **C.** This works on a portion of buttoning, which is placing an object (e.g., button) into a slot (e.g., buttonhole).

7. **B.** Although the other statements might be true to a point and/or could be used appropriately during some point of treatment, the first place to start is evaluating the child and helping the parents address strategies based on issues the child is having with developing independence in toileting.

8. **A.** Although B is true, it would be better to help inhibit the ATNR pattern by bringing the baby's head into midline through rolling him or her into side-lying.

9. **C.** You are specifically addressing Luke pulling up his pants after they are on. The other activities help in getting his legs into the pants.

10. **B.** Although the other activities can be used to help with dressing, using sequencing cards is the best activity to help Jennifer put her clothes on in order.

Worksheet 7: Case Scenarios

1. **B.** This activity will provide proprioceptive input to the hands, arms, and trunk. It will help to increase stability and control. This activity will improve awareness of arm, hand, and finger movements. It provides vestibular input, which can help with postural–ocular control. Swinging will help with trunk strength and control and playing in rice and finger painting will increase tactile input; however, the obstacle course provides the most comprehensive input to address the student's issues.

2. **C.** This activity addresses both trunk and UE strength in a dynamic manner. It facilitates postural control and upright positioning to help free the hands for writing. Completing a puzzle in prone or side sitting is likely not enough of a challenge as this student can be in a more upright position. Sitting on a ball and doing a table top activity addresses proximal stability by using an unstable base, but does not provide as much input as the other activity.

References

Bazyk, S., & Case-Smith, J. (2010). School-based occupational therapy. In J. Case-Smith (Ed.), *Occupational therapy for children* (6th ed., pp. 713–743). St. Louis, MO: Mosby.

Bundy, A. C., Lane, S., Murray, E. A., & Fisher, A. G. (2002). *Sensory integration: Theory and practice* (2nd ed.). Philadelphia, PA: F. A. Davis Company.

Case-Smith, J. (2010). Development of childhood occupations. In J. Case-Smith (Ed.), *Occupational therapy for children* (6th ed., pp. 56–83). St. Louis, MO: Mosby.

Comprehensive Program in Sensory Integration. (2003). *Course manuals 1–4.* Torrance, CA: University of Southern California and Western Psychological Services (USC/WPS).

Dudgeon, B. J., & Crooks, L. (2010). Hospital and pediatric rehabilitation services. In J. Case-Smith (Ed.), *Occupational therapy for children* (6th ed., pp. 785–811). St. Louis, MO: Mosby.

Dunn, W. (1999). *Sensory profile user's manual.* San Antonio, TX: The Psychological Corporation.

Hunter, J. G. (2010). Neonatal intensive care unit. In J. Case-Smith (Ed.), *Occupational therapy for children* (6th ed., pp. 649–680). St. Louis, MO: Mosby.

Myers, C. T., Stephens, L., & Tauber, S. (2010). Early intervention. In J. Case-Smith (Ed.), *Occupational therapy for children* (6th ed., pp. 681–712). St. Louis, MO: Mosby.

O'Brien, J., & Williams, H. (2010). Application of motor control/motor learning to practice. In J. Case-Smith (Ed.), *Occupational therapy for children* (6th ed., pp. 245–274). St. Louis, MO: Mosby.

Parham, L. D., & Mailloux, Z. (2010). Sensory integration. In J. Case-Smith (Ed.), *Occupational therapy for children* (6th ed., pp. 325–372). St. Louis, MO: Mosby.

Schuberth, L. M., Amirault, L. M., & Case-Smith, J. (2010). Feeding interventions. In J. Case-Smith (Ed.), *Occupational therapy for children* (6th ed., pp. 446–473). St. Louis, MO: Mosby.

Wright-Ott, C. (2010). Mobility. In J. Case-Smith (Ed.), *Occupational therapy for children* (6th ed., pp. 620–648). St. Louis, MO: Mosby.

Special Practice Settings Days 22–24

Community Practice and Wellness

Susan Meyers

Learning Objectives

- Define community practice.
- Compare and contrast practice options as presented in this chapter.
- Describe considerations of safety that guide evaluation and intervention in community practice.
- Describe how the cultures of clients influence expectations of community practice.
- Describe the advantages of providing community therapy.
- Describe the three steps or processes that comprise intervention.

Key Terms

- *Community based*: Occupational therapy (OT) services that are focused on clients and families living independently within the home and community settings.
- *Health promotion*: Therapy aimed at improving control over behaviors that impact the health of individuals, both physically and mentally.
- *Prevention*: Therapy aimed at preventing or stopping illness or disability through promoting healthy lifestyle behavior modifications and practices.
- *Service delivery*: Standards and policies that guide consistent and quality healthcare services.
- *Wellness*: A healthy state, both physically and mentally.

Introduction

Community practice and wellness or health promotion includes people of all ages and abilities being offered occupational therapy services in locations where they live, work, and engage in community activities of value and interest. Practice can be with an individual in their natural environment or services designed to meet the needs of an entire community. Practice is client-centered, focused on occupational performance in context, and based on best evidence (Scaffa, 2014). Independent living in the least restrictive environment is a component of occupational therapy practice that addresses client participation in everyday occupations regardless of disability (American Occupational Therapy Association [AOTA], 2014).

Although there are different ways to define community practice, there is agreement that this practice occurs outside of an institutional setting and provides the field of occupational therapy with unique opportunities. Community practice is provided in a variety of locations: schools, homes, community centers, and work sites. Occupational therapist practitioners have an opportunity to learn about people in their natural environments rich with culture and interpersonal relationships. Engagement with an individual or agency may occur over a prolonged period enhancing understanding of challenges and their potential solutions (Shultz-Krohn & Pendleton, 2013). Therapeutic relationships usually extend to a client and a caregiver, teacher, and/or employer. An occupational therapy practitioner in community practice observes those who support or are in a position to facilitate positive outcomes, as well as those who may be barriers to the client's desired therapy outcomes. One of the most important aspects of community practice is providing a safe environment for clients. An occupational therapy practitioner brings knowledge and skills to modify environments and provide education and advocacy to enhance safety in occupational performance for clients, families, schools, and employers.

Practice Options

Working with Children

Early intervention provides services to children from infancy to age 3 years with the purpose of enhancing a child's development in a natural environment (Stephens & Tauber, 2005). Individual states are responsible for providing comprehensive services to children with an environmental or biological risk of developmental delay (Individuals with Disabilities Education Act of 2004 Amendments (P. L. 108-446), 2004). Occupational therapy services are usually provided in a child's home with the primary caregiver present. In an early intervention program, the occupational therapy practitioner may participate in an evaluation of a child, or may receive a referral for services from a developmental specialist if occupational therapy is needed to enhance the child's development. An occupational therapy practitioner arranges visits consistent with the needs of the child's caregiver in a home or preschool setting. Working closely with a mother or a teacher or both, and valuing their perspectives, an occupational therapy practitioner provides direct or consultative services (Lawler & Mattingley, 2014).

A preschool environment may be inclusive of children with differing abilities. An early intervention therapist may recommend a developmental preschool program to a parent whose child is "aging out" of early intervention. Preschool develops skills that help prepare a child for school with occupational therapy services aiding in the development of motor or social skills of a child with special developmental delays. Direct services may be provided in the preschool setting or via consultative services to a teacher who has the primary responsibility for fostering age-appropriate skills among his or her students.

Occupational therapists practice in schools that are inclusive of children with differing abilities. Both public and private schools employ occupational therapy practitioners work with children who have identified needs for occupational therapy services to enhance learning. An

occupational therapist or therapy assistant may work in a single school or travel to serve multiple schools. Occupational therapy in schools is designed to facilitate a child's ability to learn through inclusion in a general education curriculum (Individuals with Disabilities Education Act of 2004 Amendments (P. L. 108-446), 2004). Provision of therapies is determined by local school districts to be most efficacious for their constituents. Some schools hire their own occupational therapy practitioners while others contract with agencies to provide services. School occupational therapy practitioners work with teachers, parents, other therapists, and school personnel to provide services needed to facilitate learning. Individual, group, and consultative services may be provided. Time constraints and high numbers of clients may challenge occupational therapy practitioners working in school environments.

Working with Adults

There are many opportunities to work with adults in community settings including, but not limited to, the following: assisted living centers, community mental health programs, group homes, work environments, home health, and wellness programs (Meyers, 2010; Shultz-Krohn & Pendleton, 2013).

Assisted living settings help adults who need some help with either activities of daily living (ADL) or instrumental activities of daily living (IADL) skills or both while enabling them to maintain autonomy over much of their lives. The decision to relocate to an assisted living environment is often a choice made collaboratively between aging adults and their family members when independent living is no longer considered viable. The individual moves into an apartment or a single private room and remains "in charge" of many aspects of their daily living. Assistance is provided in areas such as home maintenance, transportation, and management of medicines. Meals and social activities are available on-site and community involvement is encouraged. Assisted living facility staff determines a person's eligibility for residence based on functional performance. An occupational therapy practitioner's focus with persons in independent living facilities is enhanced autonomy and safety. An occupational therapy practitioner most often is a consultant to an assisted living facility regarding safety factors that affect all residents or for assessment of an individual's functional performance. Persons living in assisted living may receive more traditional rehabilitation services from a home healthcare agency when challenges to their assistance level occur (Fisher, Atler, & Potts, 2007).

Community mental health services are provided to persons with chronic mental illness in their homes or day treatment centers (Shultz-Krohn & Pendleton, 2013). There are also a number of persons with chronic mental illness living in shelters and on the street. Assertive outreach is designed to take mental health services to the client in their homes or other living environments with the objective of reducing hospitalization and increasing client satisfaction (Peterson, Michael, & Armstrong, 2006). Through assertive outreach, an occupational therapy practitioner visits with a client in the client's preferred location, which may be the client's home. Within the natural living environment, an occupational therapy practitioner gains a better understanding of the challenges and barriers that influence a client's performance (Meyers, 2010). Community mental health centers provide day treatment including: meals, areas for performing ADLs such as hygiene activities, social and recreational activities, and assistance with the development of work skills.

The independent living movement has encouraged advocacy by parents of adult children unable to live without supervision in the community. As their children progressed through school programs that focused on skills that could be used for self-care and paid or volunteer work, living arrangements were sought to increase more independence. Group homes provide supervision as needed, while encouraging independence (Shultz-Krohn & Pendleton, 2013). Occupational therapists consult with the staff of group homes to develop individual programs to enhance residents' ADL and IADL skills.

Work Programs

Returning to work after an illness or injury or entering the workplace for the first time are important goals for many adults and provide motivation for rehabilitation (Johansson & Tham, 2006; Shultz-Krohn & Pendleton, 2013). Work is often associated with a person's identity, gives meaning and purpose to life, and provides structure for living. Sager and James (2005) studied injured workers and their rehabilitation process and found that injured workers wanted to return to meaningful, productive work roles. Although work hardening programs may reduce the effects of injury and build strength and endurance, it may not address a worker's motivation to return to work (Loisel et al., 2005). Occupational therapy

provided in a work site soon after injury that includes skilled intervention positively correlates with the worker's motivation to return to work. Rehabilitation in the workplace allows an occupational therapy practitioner to observe actual physical conditions and performance demands to facilitate a worker's transition from client to worker role (Shultz-Krohn & Pendleton, 2013). An occupational therapy practitioner's presence in a work site can help focus the attention of employers and insurers on the prevention of future injuries to clients and their coworkers (King & Olson, 2014; Lysaght, 2004).

Occupational therapists and occupational therapy assistants (OTAs) provide services in a client's home as a continuum of care following inpatient rehabilitation. There are many advantages to rehabilitation in the client's naturalistic environment including observations of physical and social supports or barriers to goal attainment. Services provided in clients' homes present opportunities for occupational therapy practitioners to collaborate with clients and their family or caregiver. Therapy occurs in clients' homes and the community using naturally occurring resources for ADL and IADL skills and recommending modifications to facilitate performance and enhance safety. Occupational therapy practitioners providing services in clients' homes must understand that control of the environment remains with clients and their client's families. Changes in the physical environment or costs associated with enhanced safety recommendations or both may be unwelcome. Scheduling conflicts with clients and performance of tasks inconsistent with cultural preferences may need to be negotiated (Shultz-Krohn & Pendleton, 2013).

Wellness Programs

Maintaining and improving health contain the costs of health care (Folland, Goodman, & Stano, 2007). Occupational therapy has opportunities to focus on wellness as individuals and communities take greater responsibility for their health (Baum, 2007). Wellness encompasses a person's perceived need and responsibility for engagement in occupations that provide satisfaction. Some examples of programs that enhance well-being and self-control include the following: obesity management, backpack awareness, aging in place, safe driving, and life coaching (Reitz, 2014). All of these focus on needs and interests of an individual or a group, which give them greater control of the activities and roles that give life meaning.

Obesity-related chronic health challenges, such as diabetes and cardiovascular disease, often result in premature death or a lifetime of disability. These health challenges may interfere with job performance, participation in family and community activities, and lead to chronic depression. Obesity is no longer a challenge that impacts adults alone, and has encroached into the lives of children and adolescents, interrupting normal development. Occupational therapists collaborate with others in their communities to develop and implement programs that increase physical activity and stress reduction for individuals or groups contending with these and other health-related challenges.

Most aging adults prefer to live independently in their own home (Siebert, 2003). Aging in place is a movement directed at older adults who wish to remain in their homes throughout their life span but need assistance to evaluate the safety of their home and education to modify their performance of ADLs and IADLs to meet their changing physical capacity (Bowen, 2001). Reducing hazards in a home through physical modifications may be most effective in preventing falls in homes of older adults (Bonder, 2014). Services for older adults are often provided by community agencies advocating for independent living.

Driving safely is a concern that primarily affects older adults but may also relate to an adult of any age who has had an illness or disability that affects performance of driving skills. Occupational therapy has moved to the forefront of this area by developing practice guidelines for driving and community mobility for older adults (AOTA, 2007; Stav, Arbesman, & Lieberman, 2008; U.S. Small Business Administration, 2015). The AOTA has collaborated with the American Association of Retired Persons and the Automobile Association of America in a program to recommend care modifications and driving services (Strzelecki, 2008).

Life coaching is offered by OTs in their communities with the goal of assisting clients to achieve wellness in challenging environments (Hawksley, 2007). An occupational therapy practitioner working as a life coach would assist a client to identify and plan steps to achieve goals, increase energy, and reduce stress (Yousey, 2001).

Community Considerations

There are two primary considerations that influence occupational therapy practitioners working in community practice, including an appreciation of culture as a factor in occupational performance and safety for the client and for the occupational therapy practitioners. Occupational therapy practice in the community occurs in contexts that reflect rich and diverse cultures. Culture is defined as a way of living that is reflective of values, attitudes, beliefs, ideas, and customs shared by a group of people (Black, 2014; Fitzgerald, Mullavey-O'Byrne, & Clemson, 1997). A client's culture influences occupational behavior standards and expectations (AOTA, 2014). Smaller communities may be composed of people aligned with a shared culture; however, as a community gets larger, cultural diversity expands. In larger urban centers, occupational therapy practitioners encounter people of different races, ethnicities, religions, socioeconomic statuses, and other social locations; therefore, practitioners must be prepared to engage respectfully with all clients. One of the greatest barriers to effective care in a multicultural environment is value conflicts between occupational therapy practitioners and clients (Fitzgerald et al., 1997). For example, in some cultures, aged adults are not encouraged in independent function since it is considered the responsibility of their children to provide such care.

An occupational therapy practitioner is a guest in a client's home and is advised to follow customs of the client and others living there (Black, 2014). Scheduling a visit in the community to gain maximum benefit to the client and OT team will involve collaborations with caregivers (Solet, 2014). Occupational therapists and assistants working in early intervention know that a visit during regular nap time is generally not productive, and an occupational therapy practitioner working in home health will know that having a caregiver present will facilitate understanding the support or limitations available to a client. During the first visit in a new environment, the OT identifies cultural artifacts that are important to the client. Fashion of dress is relevant to the client and OT. After observing cues from the environment, an occupational therapy practitioner may choose to modify his or her appearance to be viewed as acceptable to the client. Methods of meal preparation also can present a new challenge to an occupational therapy practitioner who is unfamiliar with dietary restrictions due to a particular custom or religious requirement. Understanding gender roles and age expectations within a culture also will influence therapy outcomes. It is ineffective to focus on IADLs that will never be performed by a client because of cultural taboos. Cultural and religious rituals are an important part of belonging and participating in society. Understanding the meaning and performance demands of rituals to enable participation by a client may be a major focus of occupational therapy (AOTA, 2014). Observing and listening without personal bias can be difficult; however, failing to understand another person's culture can be an obstacle to effective community practice (Royeen & Crabtree, 2006).

Awareness of socioeconomic status is another factor that is a component of a client's culture and social locations. Understanding challenges to performance takes into account that some individuals or communities lack resources to provide environmental modifications to accommodate differences in abilities. Individual clients may understand that home modifications or adaptive devices may facilitate performance of ADLs and IADLs, but lacking financial resources, they may refuse or ignore therapy recommendations. Understanding that financial limitations exist, and knowing if assistance would be acceptable to a client, marks the starting point for discussions about how best to meet a client's unique needs.

Safety

Living safely is an expectation for most people. Occupational therapy addresses safety of home and work environments through direct service and consultation and advocates for safe engagement through accessibility of public spaces, events, and transportation. Prevention of further harm through unsafe practices or environments is part of home health services. Working with older adults with a history of falls, OTs have been effective in assessing and reducing home hazards to prevent further injury (Rigby, Trentham, & Lotts, 2014). Occupational therapists assess safety hazards in homes by observing a client's caregiver performing ADLs and IADLs. Occupational therapy practitioners who usually travel to community sites by car may want to experience other modes of transportation to determine how easily their clients can move outside of their homes to the market, banks, medical and dental offices, and places of worship, for example. Discussion about valued roles will lead an occupational therapy practitioner to analyze performance demands and suggest modifications that may be made to enhance safety. A mother may value caring for a small child and need modifications to safely bathe her child. Shopping and money management are tasks where personal safety may be impaired by cognitive disabilities, and therapy can address these safety concerns (Tipton-Burton, McLaughlin, & Englander, 2013). Occupational

therapists address safety through community programs such as backpack safety programs, applying ergonomic principles in the workplace, and offering programs aimed at the prevention of violence.

There are personal safety concerns for any healthcare worker providing services in the community. Personal safety begins with vigilance and a keen awareness of the surroundings when going to and from a client's residence. There are safeguards for an occupational therapy practitioner that include visual identification as a home health provider with a name or a car tag or both, uniforms or scrubs, and employing a cell phone to contact a client or ask for assistance. Occupational therapists manage their personal safety through knowledge of their clients and their communities, as well as possessing confidence in their ability to get help when needed.

Screening and Assessments

The greatest advantage of providing community therapy is the opportunity to evaluate occupational performance in the client's natural environment where performance demands exist and physical and social barriers are evident. In schools, OTs observe classrooms for sensory distractions and how well children interact with their peers and teachers. In a work environment, an occupational therapy practitioner observes performance challenges such as the physical layout of a classroom and task performance and support that is available from coworkers and employers. An occupational therapy practitioner working in community practice is concerned with factors that will empower clients and facilitate occupational engagement (AOTA, 2014).

Evaluation of context of a client's occupational performance includes cultural factors such as gender and associated roles, age, faith tradition, race and ethnicity, and socioeconomic status (AOTA, 2014). Occupational therapists practicing in home health begin the evaluation by observing the client's surroundings. How a living space is decorated is an opening to a client's history, beliefs, and values. An occupational therapy practitioner can engage the client and his or her caregiver and family members in sharing the importance of certain objects and how they relate to rituals and occupational performance relevant to client-centered care. Therapy in the community includes sharing of stories and ideas, as well as problem-solving based on mutual respect. If an occupational therapy practitioner does not understand the values shared by a client and his or her family members, recommendations for therapy may be ignored.

Observation of the natural environment also takes into account physical structures such as internal space dimensions demarcated by walls and other physical barriers, objects (e.g., furniture and tools), and external space (e.g., entrances and walkways) (Shotwell, 2014). Discussing valued activities that include others and the client's access to these activities is an important component of evaluation in community practice. Most people get enjoyment and validation of themselves through social interactions. Evaluation of social interactions can be observed during usual social activities in a naturalistic context (Fisher & Griswald, 2010).

Occupational profiles give OTs information about clients' values, interests, and what they want and need to be able to do (AOTA, 2014). The Canadian Occupational Performance Measure along with observation of the performance of ADL and IADL tasks provides measures used for comparisons during intervention (Doig, Fleming, Kuipers, & Cornwell, 2010; Law et al., 2005; Shotwell, 2014). Integrating a client's functional performance, personal preferences, and community environment occurs through the process of activity analysis. The OT identifies assets and barriers that may advance or deter occupational performance. Sharing this information with a client and other persons of influence in the environment results in preliminary goals for intervention.

The exact manner of data collection is influenced by the needs of the client, the reason for therapy, and the frame of reference or model of practice or both that an occupational therapy practitioner employs. Formal and informal structured or unstructured assessment tools may also be used; however, standardized and criterion- or norm-referenced assessment tools provide objective data to support or justify continued need for occupational therapy services. Occupational therapists working with children utilize developmental assessments and observation of performance of age-appropriate tasks. Discussion with parents and teachers or surveys to be used at home may shed light on a child's performance deficits in different environments. Evaluation of adults using the Model of Human Occupation can identify current roles and those impaired or lost due to illness or injury and activities that support those roles (Solet, 2014; Tipton-Burton et al., 2013). These data paired with observation and performance in the client's natural environment help occupational therapy practitioners to identify barriers that need to be addressed (e.g., home modifications to enable role performance). Evaluation in the community is multidimensional, continuous, and responsive to a client's developing achievement of desired occupations.

Interventions

Collaboration focused on clients' self-management, education, and environmental modifications is key to successful community practice outcomes. Depending on the service delivery model, interventions often are directed at individual clients and their family members or other caregivers, employers and employees, or groups and populations within a particular community. Intervention involves a three-step process of planning, implementing, and reviewing outcomes that is dynamic and cyclical until therapy services are concluded (AOTA, 2014).

Planning interventions begin with a process of clinical reasoning in which evaluation results are integrated with practice models, frames of reference, and evidence-based practice (Scaffa, 2014). Occupational therapists and clients who collaborate in planning interventions increase clients' level of commitment to achieve their established goals (Doig et al., 2010). A client may need activities to occupy time, increase independence in living skills, and improve relationships with others. Interventions are discussed with a client around discrepancies between functional performance and goals. In the planning process, an occupational therapy practitioner may discover that a client is unable to recognize or accept that he or she may not return to former functional status or the client is resistant to an occupational therapy practitioner's recommendation (Wheeler, 2014).

In a continuum of care, a community-based occupational therapy practitioner addresses implementation of skills training along with assessment of naturally occurring barriers and available supports at the conclusion of an inpatient's therapy (Wheeler, 2014). The opportunity to modify the environment may be more effective to enhance client function than services directed at changing a client. Occupational therapists practicing in a community should be familiar with options to remove barriers that are acceptable and financially feasible. Universal design brings an array of products to retail stores for everyone to use to make their work safe and comfortable. Accessible design in new construction and added access to existing buildings and natural spaces eliminates barriers and enhances participation for persons of all abilities. Technology includes devices and products commercially available to make occupations easier for everyone. Using these devices opens opportunities for persons with disabilities to engage in activities at home, school, and work. Computers, smart pads, and phones have opened opportunities for clients and also to occupational therapy practitioners who use these devices as therapy tools (Rigby et al., 2014).

During home care visits or other community services provided by occupational therapy practitioners, home modifications are often recommended to enhance clients' safety (Bonder, 2014). Interventions may include durable medical equipment for performance of ADLs or reorganization of space for ease of performance of daily occupations. Challenges occur when a client or family member resists changes to their physical environment. A client can be tired, frustrated, and anxious about his or her future and be either actively resistant or passive about intervention strategies. These challenges can be managed within a therapeutic relationship. Occupational therapists must actively listen to client and family concerns, provide information, and negotiate a solution that satisfies a client's safety needs and family concerns (Taylor, 2014).

In community practice, intervention is reviewed as it continues and a client's functional abilities change. The dynamic process of intervention and disabling injury or illness requires an occupational therapy practitioner to continually observe performance and listen to a client or his or her caregiver and make modifications in intervention to satisfy goals or treatment.

Referrals and Discharge Considerations

Occupational therapists may provide community services through an organization that has multiple service providers, a structure for supervision, centralized billing, and routine methods of accountability. However, some OTs may opt for private practice as either a lone practitioner or with other service providers and will need to establish methods to monitor accountability. All practices must adhere to guidelines established by their funding sources such as Medicare or private insurance companies (Lohman, 2014). Independent practice requires understanding and compliance with all state and professional regulations for occupational therapy practitioners (Doherty, 2014). When a private practice under the auspices of an OT includes professionals such as physical or speech therapists, the manager of the practice

also assumes responsibility for compliance with regulations affecting these practitioners. For example, if a third party identifies fraudulent documentation or billing by an occupational therapy practitioner, it is the responsibility of the practice manager to report this to the respective licensing boards of the person who has committed this breach.

Management and Standards of Practice

In community practice, most OTs are responsible for scheduling visits and delivering and documenting services provided without direct supervision. Therefore, organization skills to effectively manage time to include direct service, travel to sites of delivery, and documentation are essential. For example, grouping client visits by common locations and establishing a daily routine for documentation and billing contribute to effective practice. Community OTs must plan for their own continuing education in their areas of practice to stay up to date with therapy techniques and documentation and to maintain professional and state credentials.

OTAs often are required by state regulations to have a specific amount and type of supervision by an OT. State regulations specify these requirements and it is the responsibility of both the OT and OTA to see that they are met and documented (Youngstrom, 2014). Community practice like all professional practices is guided by ethical considerations. In community practice where there may be little direct oversight, it is the occupational therapy practitioner's responsibility to adhere to a professional code of ethics.

Summary

Community practice and wellness include occupational therapy services delivered to persons with a variety of challenges at home, school, workplace, and community programs. The occupational therapy evaluation and intervention process can be most effective when delivered in a client's preferred environment where there are naturally occurring supports. Occupational therapy practitioners use their skills of observation and therapeutic use of self to establish a collaborative relationship with clients to create safe occupational performance in clients' preferred activities.

Chapter 31 Self-Study Activities (Answers Are Provided at the End of the Chapter)

Read the following case study and then answer the questions:

My first visit with Angie was a continuation of services from a community mental health program. Diagnosed with chronic severe depression, Angie was a regular participant in activities that provided socialization and volunteer work opportunities while living with her husband of 8 years in a one-bedroom apartment. Medication effectively controlled most of Angie's symptoms of depression and she was satisfied with her life until she developed symptoms of multiple sclerosis (MS). Her family physician began medication to mediate her MS symptoms but this resulted in less efficacy of the medication she took for her depression. She decided that she would prefer to stop taking the medication for MS and live with her symptoms, rather than fall into debilitating depression. My visit was to assess her function in her home and community since her gait had become unsteady and she feared falling.

Arriving at the entrance to her building, I observed that the exterior entrance had no steps or other barriers and her home was just past the main entrance. It was only upon entering her home that I observed her bathroom was located just inside the door but the rest of her living areas were two steps down from that level. Due to the placement of the bedroom door, there would be no possibility of a ramp to the bathroom; however, installing a railing and grab bars would make her home safer. During the first visit we discussed her valued roles as wife and homemaker. She had been independent in shopping and participating in community activities. I observed an open book and a full book case and we discussed our mutual love of reading. I asked her about her homemaking activities as we walked about her kitchen. Since Angie reported becoming fatigued as she cleaned her home and prepared meals, we discussed organizing her work space to conserve energy. Since Angie collaborated in problem-solving her challenges, she was eager to implement changes to make her home safer and simplify her work.

Angie experienced a rapid escalation of her MS symptoms, including weakness and urinary incontinence. The most distressing outcome for her was an inability to exit her home independently to engage in social activities and reading discontinuance due to blurred vision. This was the point where, despite use of a cane and a wheelchair to go out with her husband to visit family, Angie decided to try medication to alleviate her MS symptoms. Her primary physician and psychiatrist agreed to work together to try and give her relief from both the MS symptoms and subsequent depression. There was success with ameliorating the MS symptoms; for example, her urinary incontinence abated; her vision improved and she began reading again; and her depression was lessened. Her gait remained unsteady; however. Durable medical equipment was provided for use while she was alone in her home, including a standard walker, bedside commode (i.e., to decrease the need to use the steps up to her bathroom), and a wheelchair for use outside her home. Her husband was supportive and helped with her use of the bathroom when he was home. Her mother who lived nearby visits, often helping Angie with some personal and home care tasks. Angie continued to prepare meals and do laundry and enjoyed weekend and evening outings with her husband.

The focus of Angie's intervention was safety and maintenance of valued roles, leisure, and work activities. Collaboration with Angie, her husband, and her doctors would need to be continued as Angie's symptoms change. Note: Questions 1–2 are related to the aforementioned case.

1. The OT was responsible to deliver services, which kept Angie safe in her home. Where will he/she begin Angie's evaluation?
   A. With observation of the home environment
   B. With a conversation with Angie about her concerns
   C. With a conversation with Angie about her previous service providers regarding their concerns
2. The OT has determined that Angie will need adaptive equipment to be safe alone in her home. What should the OT consider in the recommendations?
   A. Acceptance of the suggested equipment by Angie and her husband
   B. The cost of the equipment
   C. Ease of use of the equipment
3. An OTA is working with a client learning to live alone in his own apartment for the first time. One therapy session focuses on meal

preparation and cleanup. At the conclusion of the meal, the client picks up the dirty pots and dishes and runs them under some cold water and sets them on the counter to dry. What is the next step the OTA might take to improve health and safety for the client related to kitchen cleanup?

A. Ask the client to describe any prior experience with kitchen cleanup either as a participant or as an observer.

B. Identify procedures to safely wash dishes and the importance of using soap and hot water.

C. Provide an opportunity to wash dishes with the client demonstrating safe dishwashing procedure.

D. Give the client a handout that describes procedures for safe dishwashing.

Chapter 31 Self-Study Answers

Question 1

Response "B" is the answer that stresses client-centered care. Angie's concerns relate to her needs to continue to perform the roles and activities that she considers important to her well-being. Response "A" is also important since addressing the home environment may help Angie achieve her goals; however, the occupational therapist should *begin* the evaluation through a conversation with the client.

Question 2

- Response "A" is the most appropriate answer; unless equipment is accepted (and wanted) by the client, it is unlikely to be used.
- In review of response "B," the cost of equipment may also be a consideration, but community-based OTs are likely to know of resources to pay for equipment that a client is unable to afford.
- Response "C" is also important because if equipment is difficult to use, it may be abandoned by clients. For example, mobility aids that do not fit into the client's primary mode of transportation may not ease participation in activities throughout the community.

Question 3

While responses "A," "B," and "C" will give useful information, answer "C" is the correct response.

That is, demonstration is the most effective method to improve safety in home management tasks. While working alongside the client to wash and dry dishes after a meal, the OTA can provide important information about the process and also food safety. It does not put the client "on the spot" to answer that he has not done this task previously or has not seen it done correctly. Working collaboratively on this task, the OTA has an opportunity to build rapport with the client and positively reinforce performance, which is likely to result in continued safe dishwashing practices.

Additional Considerations

- It would be helpful to have a discussion with the client about concerns that an occupational therapy practitioner might have with the client's kitchen cleanup process (e.g., hygiene in the kitchen and other areas of the home, and food-borne illness).
- What information about this particular client might help the OT construct an intervention process that would result in meal preparation? Consider cognitive ability, interest in task, and motivation.
- Consider other methods OT can use to improve this client's performance in food safety (e.g., local cooking groups the client may attend, use of technology to demonstrate and reinforce safe practice).

References

American Occupational Therapy Association. (2007). *Board and specialty certification.* Retrieved from https://www.aota.org/Education-Careers/Advance-Career/Board-Specialty-Certifications.aspx

American Occupational Therapy Association. (2014). *Occupational therapy practice framework: Domain & process* (3rd ed.). Bethesda, MD: AOTA Press/American Occupational Therapy Association.

Baum, C. (2007). Achieving our potential. *American Journal of Occupational Therapy, 61*(6), 615–623.

Black, R. M. (2014). Culture, race, ethnicity and the impact on occupation and occupational performance. In B. A. B. Schell, G. Gillen, & M. Scaffa (Eds.), *Willard & Spackman's occupational therapy* (12th ed., pp. 173–187). Philadelphia, PA: Wolters Kluwer Health/Lippincott Williams & Wilkins.

Bonder, B. (2014). Providing occupational therapy for older adults with changing needs. In B. A. B. Schell, G. Gillen, & M. Scaffa (Eds.), *Willard & Spackman's occupational therapy* (12th ed., pp. 541–552). Philadelphia, PA: Wolters Kluwer Health/Lippincott Williams & Wilkins.

Bowen, R. E. (2001). Independent living programs. In M. E. Scaffa (Ed.), *Occupational therapy in community-based practice settings* (pp. xxv, 414). Philadelphia, PA: F. A. Davis Company.

Doherty, R. F. (2014). Ethical practice. In B. A. B. Schell, G. Gillen, & M. Scaffa (Eds.), *Willard & Spackman's occupational therapy* (12th ed., pp. 413–424). Philadelphia, PA: Wolters Kluwer Health/Lippincott Williams & Wilkins.

Doig, E., Fleming, J., Kuipers, P., & Cornwell, P. L. (2010). Clinical utility of the combined use of the Canadian Occupational Performance Measure and Goal Attainment Scaling. *American Journal of Occupational Therapy*, 64(6), 904–914. Retrieved from http://www.ncbi.nlm.nih.gov/pubmed/21218681

Fisher, A. G., Atler, K., & Potts, A. (2007). Effectiveness of occupational therapy with frail community living older adults. *Scandinavian Journal of Occupational Therapy*, 14(4), 240–249. doi:10.1080/11038120601182958

Fisher, A. G., & Griswald, L. A. (2010). *The evaluation of social interaction*. Fort Collins, CO: Three Star Press.

Fitzgerald, H. M., Mullavey-O'Byrne, C., & Clemson, L. (1997). Cultural issues from practice. *Australian Journal of Occupational Therapy*, 44, 1–21.

Folland, S., Goodman, A. C., & Stano, M. (2007). *The economics of health and health care* (5th ed.). Upper Saddle River, NJ: Pearson Prentice Hall.

Hawksley, B. (2007). Work-related stress, work/life balance and personal life coaching. *British Journal of Community Nursing*, 12(1), 34–36. Retrieved from http://www.ncbi.nlm.nih.gov/pubmed/17353810

Individuals with Disabilities Education Act of 2004 Amendments (P. L. 108-446). (2004).

Johansson, U., & Tham, K. (2006). The meaning of work after acquired brain injury. *American Journal of Occupational Therapy*, 60(1), 60–69. Retrieved from http://www.ncbi.nlm.nih.gov/pubmed/16541985

King, P. M., & Olson, D. L. (2014). Work. In B. A. B. Schell, G. Gillen, & M. Scaffa (Eds.), *Willard & Spackman's occupational therapy* (12th ed., pp. 678–696). Philadelphia, PA: Wolters Kluwer Health/Lippincott Williams & Wilkins.

Law, M., Baptiste, S., Carswell, A., McColl, M., Polatajko, J., & Pollack, N. (2005). *Canadian occupational performance measure*. Ottawa, ON: Canadian Occupational Therapy Association.

Lawler, M. C., & Mattingley, C. (2014). Family perspectives on occupation, health and disability. In B. A. B. Schell, G. Gillen, & M. Scaffa (Eds.), *Willard & Spackman's occupational therapy* (12th ed., pp. 150–162). Philadelphia, PA: Wolters Kluwer Health/Lippincott Williams & Wilkins.

Lohman, H. (2014). Payment for services in the United States. In B. A. B. Schell, G. Gillen, & M. Scaffa (Eds.), *Willard & Spackman's occupational therapy* (12th ed., pp. 1051–1067). Philadelphia, PA: Wolters Kluwer Health/Lippincott Williams & Wilkins.

Loisel, P., Falardeau, M., Baril, R., Jose-Durand, M., Langley, A., Sauve, S., & Gervais, J. (2005). The values underlying team decision-making in work rehabilitation for musculoskeletal disorders. *Disability and Rehabilitation*, 27(10), 561–569. doi:10.1080/09638280400018502

Lysaght, R. M. (2004). Approaches to worker rehabilitation by occupational and physical therapists in the United States: Factors impacting practice. *Work*, 23(2), 139–146. Retrieved from http://www.ncbi.nlm.nih.gov/pubmed/15502294

Meyers, S. K. (2010). *Community practice in occupational therapy: A guide to serving the community*. Sudbury, MA: Jones and Bartlett Publishers.

Peterson, M., Michael, W., & Armstrong, M. (2006). Homeward bound: Moving treatment from the institution to the community. *Administration and Policy in Mental Health and Mental Health Services Research*, 33(4), 508–511. doi:10.1007/s10488-005-0013-3

Reitz, M. (2014). Health promotion theories. In B. A. B. Schell, G. Gillen, & M. Scaffa (Eds.), *Willard & Spackman's occupational therapy* (12th ed., pp. 574–587). Philadelphia, PA: Wolters Kluwer Health/Lippincott Williams & Wilkins.

Rigby, P., Trentham, B., & Lotts, L. (2014). Modifying performance contexts. In B. A. B. Schell, G. Gillen, & M. Scaffa (Eds.), *Willard & Spackman's occupational therapy* (12th ed., pp. 364–381). Philadelphia, PA: Wolters Kluwer Health/Lippincott Williams & Wilkins.

Royeen, A. M., & Crabtree, J. L. (2006). *Culture in rehabilitation: From competency to proficiency*. Upper Saddle River, NJ: Pearson Education.

Sager, L., & James, C. (2005). Injured workers perspectives of their rehabilitation process under the New South

Wales workers compensation system. *Australian Journal of Occupational Therapy, 52*, 127–135.

Scaffa, M. E. (2014). Occupational therapy interventions for organizations, communities and populations. In B. A. B. Schell, G. Gillen, & M. Scaffa (Eds.), *Willard & Spackman's occupational therapy* (12th ed., pp. 342–352). Philadelphia, PA: Wolters Kluwer Health/Lippincott Williams & Wilkins.

Shotwell, M. P. (2014). Evaluating clients. In B. A. B. Schell, G. Gillen, & M. Scaffa (Eds.), *Willard & Spackman's occupational therapy* (12th ed., pp. 281–301). Philadelphia, PA: Wolters Kluwer Health/Lippincott Williams & Wilkins.

Shultz-Krohn, W., & Pendleton, H. M. (2013). Application of the occupational therapy framework to physical dysfunction. In L. W. Pedretti, H. M. Pendleton, & W. Schultz-Krohn (Eds.), *Pedretti's occupational therapy: Practice skills for physical dysfunction* (7th ed., pp. 28–54). St. Louis, MO: Elsevier.

Siebert, C. (2003). Aging in place: Implications for occupational therapy. *OT Practice, 8*, 16–20.

Solet, J. M. (2014). Optimizing personal and social adaptation. In M. V. Radomski & C. A. T. Latham (Eds.), *Occupational therapy for physical dysfunction* (7th ed., pp. 925–954). Philadelphia, PA: Wolters Kluwer Health/Lippincott Williams & Wilkins.

Stav, W. B., Arbesman, M., & Lieberman, D. (2008). Background and methodology of the older driver evidence-based systematic literature review. *American Journal of Occupational Therapy, 62*(2), 130–135. Retrieved from http://www.ncbi.nlm.nih.gov/pubmed/18390007

Stephens, L. C., & Tauber, S. K. (2005). Early intervention. In J. Case-Smith (Ed.), *Occupational therapy for children* (4th ed., pp. 771–794). St. Louis, MO: Mosby.

Strzelecki, M. (2008). Driving the profession. *OT Practice, 13*(5), 9–11.

Taylor, R. (2014). Therapeutic relationships and client collaboration. In B. A. B. Schell, G. Gillen, & M. Scaffa (Eds.), *Willard & Spackman's occupational therapy* (12th ed., pp. 425–436). Philadelphia, PA: Wolters Kluwer Health/Lippincott Williams & Wilkins.

Tipton-Burton, M., McLaughlin, R., & Englander, J. (2013). Traumatic brain injury. In L. W. Pedretti, H. M. Pendleton, & W. Schultz-Krohn (Eds.), *Pedretti's occupational therapy: Practice skills for physical dysfunction* (7th ed., pp. 881–915). St. Louis, MO: Elsevier.

U.S. Small Business Administration. (2015). An official website of the United States Government. Retrieved from https://www.sba.gov

Wheeler, S. D. (2014). Providing occupational therapy for individuals with traumatic brain injury. In B. A. B. Schell, G. Gillen, & M. Scaffa (Eds.), *Willard & Spackman's occupational therapy* (12th ed., pp. 925–935). Philadelphia, PA: Wolters Kluwer Health/Lippincott Williams & Wilkins.

Youngstrom, M. J. (2014). Supervision. In B. A. B. Schell, G. Gillen, & M. Scaffa (Eds.), *Willard & Spackman's occupational therapy* (12th ed., pp. 1068–1087). Philadelphia, PA: Wolters Kluwer Health/Lippincott Williams & Wilkins.

Yousey, J. (2001). Life coaching: A one to one approach to changing lives. *OT Practice, 6*(1), 11–14.

Health Promotion and Wellness

Michael A. Pizzi

Learning Objectives

- Understand the link between health and occupation.
- Define health promotion and identify its relevance to occupational therapy practice.
- Identify three levels of prevention and apply them to occupational therapy practice.
- Apply health behavior theories to all areas of practice.

Key Terms

- *Health promotion*: Social and environmental interventions that are used to help others increase control and thereby improve their health status.
- *Prevention*: The process of stopping a health risk or injury from occurring.
- *Well-being*: The state of being healthy.
- *Wellness*: The state of being in good physical and psychosocial health.

Health and Occupation

"Health is the essential foundation that supports and nurtures growth, learning, personal well-being, social fulfillment, enrichment of others, economic production, and constructive citizenship" (Jenkins & Pan American Health Organization, 2003, p. 3). Occupational therapists (OTs) have always been concerned about the health, well-being, and quality of life of individuals, communities, and populations, particularly, as it relates to and impacts participation in one's self-chosen and favored occupations.

Occupational balance is important to promoting health. The founders of the occupational therapy profession emphasized a unique human need to balance work, rest, play, and sleep and to utilize occupation as a preventive or protective factor from illness (Dunton, 1915; Meyer, 1922). Others believed that habit development and healthy habits strengthen a person's ability to engage in daily life (Slagle, 1934).

What Is Health Promotion?

According to the World Health Organization (WHO, 1986), health promotion is defined as follows:

> The process of enabling people to increase control over and to improve health. To reach a state of complete physical, mental and social well-being, an individual or group must be able to identify and realize aspirations, to satisfy needs, and to change and cope with the environment. Health is therefore seen as a resource for everyday living, not the object of living. Health is a positive concept emphasizing social and personal resources, as well as physical capabilities. Therefore health promotion is not just the responsibility of the health sector, but goes beyond healthy lifestyles to well-being. (p. 5)

Leading a healthy life is not just about extending life, but rather enabling a person to actively engage in that life. Participation in what is important and meaningful to an individual, and in the context of where people work, play, laugh, and love, is crucial to sustaining daily living (WHO, 1986). OTs and occupational therapy assistants (OTAs) have a vital role to play in promoting health and well-being for individuals, communities, organizations, and society.

According to the American Occupational Therapy Association (AOTA) position paper, *Occupational Therapy in the Promotion of Health and Well-being*, the following are three areas that OTs and OTAs can facilitate these critical aims:

1. To promote healthy lifestyles;
2. To emphasize occupation as an essential element of health promotion strategies; and
3. To provide interventions, not only with individuals, but also with populations (AOTA, 2013, p. S50).

Examples of these critical aims include (1) developing healthy eating and activity routines for schoolchildren to promote a healthy lifestyle; (2) engaging the well elderly in cognitive, physical, and social occupations within their living environments; and (3) creating a community-based arts program for self-expression and emotional/mental well-being for women impacted by breast cancer and their families (AOTA, 2013).

Healthy People 2020 (United States Department of Health and Human Services, 2014) supports the promotion of health and well-being of all of society by addressing the gaps and needs of the health of all individuals. Some of the leading health indicators included are mental, physical, and environmental health, as well as social determinants of health. Social determinants include factors such as education, neighborhood safety, prevention services, employment, and access to healthy foods. Research is needed to assess if these social determinants of health can be positively impacted through universal preventive OT programming.

OT and Prevention

There are three levels of prevention (AOTA, 2013) in which OTs and OTAs can intervene. These can be found in **Table 32-1**.

Under a public health model, there are three levels or tiers of intervention one may take to promote health and well-being: universal, targeted/at-risk, and intensive (Arbesman, Bazyk, & Nochajski, 2013). At the universal level (Tier 1), promotion of physical and emotional health for the whole population is considered. Promotion efforts focus on optimizing health, building competencies and strengths, and designing environments to help individuals, communities, and populations thrive and to be healthy. Targeted services (Tier 2) focus more specifically on the prevention of illness, disease, and disability. At this level, it is important for OTs to be aware of the conditions that place people at risk for illness and embed

Table 32-1 Levels of Prevention

Prevention Stage	Description	Example
Primary	"Education or health promotion efforts designed to prevent the onset and reduce the incidence of unhealthy conditions, diseases, or injuries" (AOTA, 2013, p. S48).	Education to wear helmets while riding bicycles or motorcycles and the creation of safe hazard-free playgrounds.
Secondary	Aims are to prevent or alter disease or disability possibilities.	Smoking cessation and healthy weight management.
Tertiary	Preventing further progression of an illness or disability.	Rehabilitation.

Data from American Occupational Therapy Association, 2013; United States Depart-ment of Health and Human Services, 2014.

strategies to prevent health challenges. At the intensive state (Tier 3), therapy services focus on people who are already ill or disabled or both. At this level, given the holistic nature of OT, it is important for OT intervention to focus on both the physical and the emotional causes and consequences of illness or disability. These tiers reflect the three levels of prevention and are another way to explore how to recognize and implement health promotion strategies.

These levels or tiers are crucial for occupational therapy practitioners to understand in this era of healthcare delivery. The profession is well versed in the tertiary or intensive level of care. However, there are opportunities to expand our professional role in health care by including OT services in primary care, which includes either primary and secondary prevention or universal and targeted levels.

Theories of Health Promotion and Health Behavior Change

Occupational therapy theories, models of practice, and frames of reference primarily focus on a person's ability to regain function and how people can adapt to changing life circumstances. While not specifically or directly related to health and well-being, they "explain human behavior in relation to health and occupational performance" (Reitz, Scaffa, & Pizzi, 2010, p. 22). From a health promotion and wellness perspective, understanding health and health behavior is necessary to enable maximal participation in daily occupations. All behaviors in which people are engaged are impacted by health, just as health status is affected by occupational participation. Thus, it is crucial to understand theories that can be used to create more evidence in health promotion and wellness-focused OT services. Two models are discussed here that are commonly used in health behavior change: the Health Belief Model (HBM) and the Transtheoretical Model (i.e., Stages of Change).

Health Belief Model

The HBM was developed by social psychologists (Rosenstock, 1974). It is based on how one's perceptions of self and the environment impact their health behaviors. Mediating health behaviors is based on certain beliefs; **Table 32-2** presents the model's list of beliefs with their definitions along with the cues to action.

A person would take action and is more likely to change his or her health behaviors when there is sufficient motivation to change and a person believes that (1) one is susceptible to an illness; (2) the health event impacts one's life in a negative way; (3) taking actions are beneficial; (4) benefits of action outweigh barriers; and (5) there are cues for action that are in evidence and noted by the person (Rosenstock, 1974). Regarding cues to action, when the readiness to make a health behavior change is high, the cue can be simple and low level

Table 32-2 HBM Beliefs and Definitions

Belief	Description
Perceived susceptibility	The risk perception of contracting a disease.
Perceived severity	How serious one perceives a health problem would be.
Perceived benefits	An action stage, where the person weighs the resources and availability of such to reduce the threat of illness.
Perceived barriers	The costs or negative aspects if one engages in a health behavior.
Cues to action	These are the internal and external cues that empower one to initiate a health behavior.

Data from Rosenstock, 1974.

Table 32-3 HBM in Action

Concept	Condom Use Education Example
1. Perceived Susceptibility	Youth believe they can get STDs or HIV or become pregnant.
2. Perceived Severity	Youth believe that the consequences of getting STD or HIV or becoming pregnant are significant enough to try to avoid.
3. Perceived Benefits	Youth believe that the recommended action of using condoms would protect them from getting STD or HIV or becoming pregnant.
4. Perceived Barriers	Youth identify their personal barriers to using condoms (i.e., condoms limit the feeling or they are too embarrassed to talk to their partner about it) and explore ways to eliminate or reduce these barriers (i.e., have them practice condom communication skills to decrease their embarrassment level).
5. Cues to Action	Youth receive reminder cues for action in the form of incentives (e.g., pencils with a printed message) or reminder messages (e.g., messages in the school newsletter).
6. Self-Efficacy	Youth are confident in using a condom correctly in all circumstances.

HIV, human immunodeficiency virus; STD, sexually transmitted disease.
Data adapted from Resource Center for Adolescent Pregnancy Prevention, 2015.

(e.g., a coaching phone call or a billboard). Self-efficacy, or one's belief in one's self and actions, is realized when barriers are overcome and the person feels confident they can carry out the health behavior. Finally, there are modifying variables, or client factors, that can determine adopting a certain behavior (e.g., religious preferences and values). **Table 32-3** provides an example of the HBM in action.

Transtheoretical Model

The Transtheoretical Model, better known as the Stages of Change Model, is based on the fact that change does not often occur at a specific rate or in a linear fashion, but is individual. It was developed by Prochaska and DiClemente (1982). There are five stages to this model, as can be seen in **Table 32-4**.

Should relapse occur, as when a person dealing with alcohol abuse begins to drink again, then the cycle resumes (see **Figure 32-1**).

Table 32-4 Transtheoretical Model Stages of Change

Stage	Definition
Precontemplation	Not yet acknowledging there is a problem or issue.
Contemplation	Acknowledgment of a problem but not sure if the person wishes to make changes.
Preparation	Getting ready to change.
Action	Changing the behavior.
Maintenance	Maintaining the behavior.

Data from Prochaska and DiClemente, 1982.

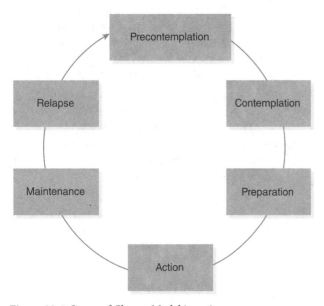

Figure 32-1 Stages of Change Model in action.

The following is an example of the Stages of Change Model in action:

> Mary does not realize that her smoking behaviors may have contributed to her stroke (i.e., precontemplation). The OT or OTA, seeing her through home care for example, introduces the consequences of smoking and educates her about smoking and its effects on one's bodily systems, its potential for causing a second stroke, as well as the impact of secondary smoke on others. Mary begins to think about changing her behaviors but admits difficulty (i.e., contemplation). The OT or OTA says there are alternatives, such as reducing the number of cigarettes or changing the environments where she smokes. Mary begins to prepare to redesign her life to eliminate smoking (i.e., preparation). Mary begins to cut her smoking by one cigarette per week, and only smokes on her deck (i.e., action). After 6 months, Mary has quit smoking and plays solitaire instead, as her OT suggested, whenever she has the urge to smoke (i.e., maintenance).

Screening and Assessments

Many health promotion or health and wellness assessments are available, and most of them are disease specific. "It is important from a health promotion perspective to differentiate between the constructs of health and functional status. Many assessments of health status include items that measure function. As a result, these tools are negatively biased against persons with disabilities" (AOTA, 2013, p. S48). There are only two occupational therapy assessments that directly address health and occupation. Those are the Pizzi Health and Wellness Assessment (PHWA) and the Pizzi Healthy Weight Management Assessment (PHWMA). Both are semistandardized, criterion-referenced interviews.

Pizzi Health and Wellness Assessment

The only published health-specific, occupation- and client-centered assessment is the PHWA (Pizzi, 2001). This assessment has been modified since its original publication and consists of six health areas (i.e., occupational, social, family, physical, mental/emotional, and spiritual) that are rated on a Likert scale to gain the client's perspective of his or her health status. Under each topic, the client answers three occupation-based questions in each category on the questionnaire (or via an interview). The occupational therapy practitioner asks clients which area(s) they wish to improve, if they are satisfied with their level of health in each area, and if they are ready to make changes. Together, the client and the OT develop a treatment plan based on each area of health. There is also a significant other version, where the significant other rates and discusses the occupation and health of their loved one. This assessment can be administered by both an OT and an OTA, with the OTA reviewing the assessment data with the OT and collaborating with the client on achievable and measurable goals.

Pizzi Healthy Weight Management Assessment

Developed in 2013, this assessment has theoretical foundations in the Stages of Change Model using occupational therapy constructs from the Occupational Therapy Practice Framework and the obesity literature. The assessment has a child/youth version and a parent/caregiver version. In 2014, Pizzi developed an adult version and a caregiver/significant other version. Self-ratings on a Likert scale tell OTs if a person wants to and is ready to make a change in a certain occupational area, and how stressful making that change would be for the person. The person is involved in their own goal planning by asking them to provide the top areas in which they would like to make change and if they perceive that they require assistance in making that change. This client-centered approach helps people realize there is a level of self-responsibility for goal achievement, with the OT or OTA facilitating and supporting that positive change. The child/youth version can be administered for ages 10–21 years. The parent/caregiver version can be administered to any caregiver concerned about weight issues with their child. Caregivers can be anyone involved with the active care of a child, including, for example, parents, grandparents, foster parents, and nannies. The adult version (i.e., 21 years old and above) is for any person wishing to create a healthy weight management lifestyle. The significant other version provides OTs with data that may signify occupational environmental challenges for weight management.

Both the PHWA and the PHWMA have demonstrated clinical utility. The PHWA and PHWMA are undergoing psychometric testing and both have demonstrated face and content validity.

SF-36

The SF-36 (2014) is a commonly used health assessment that measures a person's health and well-being in both the physical and mental health areas. It is a generic measure that can be used with adults. It is a valid and reliable norm-referenced tool; however, it is not occupation or client centered. Rather, it does provide OTs with a health profile of a client that can be helpful information to use in conjunction with an occupational profile. OTs often use the tool to analyze health data in conjunction with OT data.

Interventions

The following interventions reflect areas of primary, secondary, and tertiary prevention or the universal, targeted, and intensive levels. All interventions would be occupation based and client centered. The client can be defined as an individual, community, population, or organization. While some interventions are preventive

in nature, others may be less obvious; for example, helping a community cope with a natural disaster through occupation-focused interventions can help to ameliorate further mental health challenges.

Primary and universal interventions (i.e., individual):

- Educational programming for home health aides on strategies to prevent falls for their elderly clients;
- Bullying seminars to grade schoolers and their teachers and ways to implement them in the classroom, at the bus stop, and in other places throughout the school-district;
- Stretching programs for injury prevention.

Primary and universal interventions (i.e., populations):

- Cultural sensitivity training for local parent–teacher organizations;
- Physical activity community programming for elders with sedentary lifestyles;
- Consulting with an organization on implementing ergonomically correct work stations;
- Community programming on healthy eating and habit development for parents of children who are overweight.

Secondary prevention and targeted interventions (i.e., individuals):

- Healthy cooking classes for children addressing weight issues;
- Prevention of pressure ulcers for clients who are wheelchair users;
- Smoking cessation programs for people who have experienced a stroke;
- New parent training for teen parents.

Secondary prevention and targeted interventions (i.e., populations):

- Resilience training for communities impacted by natural disasters; and
- School-wide interventions for those experiencing grief after the loss of a classmate.

Tertiary prevention and intensive interventions (i.e., individuals):

- Cognitive retraining with individuals with traumatic brain injury;
- Interventions that facilitate social skills for a child diagnosed with autism; and
- Caregiver support groups for those dealing with cancer.

Referrals and Discharge Considerations

In the area of wellness and health promotion, the OTs may refer clients to appropriate healthcare professionals based on screening and assessment results. Once the client or client group have achieved their stated goals, discharge from services gradually occurs.

Management and Standards of Practice

Ethical dilemmas can arise when practicing under a health and wellness umbrella. Often, health promotion assessment and interventions may occur in nontraditional settings where there may be little to no supervision. It is often up to the occupational therapy practitioner to determine the ethically and morally right thing to do, armed with knowledge of the AOTA Code of Ethics (AOTA, 2015) and the practice act in one's state. The OT and OTA must be aware that health and leading a healthy lifestyle is not valued by some clients, which is the right of every individual. Value conflicts between what the OT deems is good and right related to a client's health and health behaviors is not always aligned with the client's values. The OTA has special considerations of requiring OT supervision, even if indirectly, and is required to follow through with obtaining the state-designated level of supervision.

Summary

OTs and OTAs have important roles to play in the promotion of health and well-being of individuals, communities, populations, and society. Primary, secondary, and tertiary prevention are areas in which occupation- and client-centered interventions can be implemented so that all people can participate in daily life to the fullest. Having knowledge in theories that underlie those interventions is essential to help ensure efficacious OT services.

Chapter 32 Self-Study Activities (Answers Are Provided at the End of the Chapter)

1. Maria is a 32-year-old corporate executive with two children aged 4 and 6 years. She was recently divorced and lives in an upscale suburban neighborhood with her children. She employs a nanny who cares for her children 60–70 hours per week. Although she works many hours, she is experiencing financial difficulties. Due to her recent divorce and having full custody of her children who she does not see as often as she would like, Maria is exhibiting signs of depression. Despite this, she is still able to function at work and home. What stage of prevention should the OT address?

2. You are working in the community with adults who are overweight and obese and who wish to change their weight status. Fill out the Health Belief Model table:

Belief	Description Related to an Adult Who Is Overweight or Obese
Perceived susceptibility	
Perceived severity	
Perceived benefits	
Perceived barriers	
Cues to action	

3. What are some potential self-efficacy issues such a person may experience that could lead to not changing health behaviors?

Chapter 32 Self-Study Answers

1. Maria, at the individual level, is at the secondary prevention/at-risk targeted stage. Maria is already experiencing depression but can still function. The goal is for Maria to maintain her functional abilities at home and work and not spiral into further depression. Further depression will alter her ability to participate in meaningful life occupations and roles. Should this happen, she will be in the tertiary prevention or intensive stage.

2. You are working in the community with adults who are overweight and obese who wish to change their weight status. Fill out the Health Belief Model table:

Belief	Description Related to a Child Who Is Overweight or Obese
Perceived susceptibility	Understanding that continuing to overeat could lead to greater weight gain.

Perceived severity	Overeating can cause multiple physical challenges in the future and acknowledges the child's current weight is not healthy.
Perceived benefits	Changing eating habits and food intake, eating healthier, developing an exercise routine, and becoming mentally stronger.
Perceived barriers	Tough to lose weight but taking action, one day at a time, one meal at a time, one walk around the block daily, could be more beneficial to future health than not engaging in these behaviors; acknowledging the difficulty of losing weight but learning cognitive behavioral techniques.
Cues to action	Daily meditations, positive self-talk, written goals and food diaries, and having a weight coach.

3. Poor experiences with weight loss may include:
- Being bullied as a child leading to social isolation and poor self-worth
- Poor body image
- Seeing media images that do not reflect an individual's life experiences

References

American Occupational Therapy Association. (2013). Occupational therapy in the promotion of health and well-being. *American Journal of Occupational Therapy, 67*(Suppl. 6), S47–S59. doi:10.5014/ajot.2013.67S47

American Occupational Therapy Association. (2015). Occupational therapy code of ethics. *American Journal of Occupational Therapy, 69*(Suppl. 3), 6913410030. doi:10.5014/ajot.2015.696S03

Arbesman, M., Bazyk, S., & Nochajski, S. M. (2013). Systematic review of occupational therapy and mental health promotion, prevention, and intervention for children and youth. *American Journal of Occupational Therapy, 67*(6), e120–e130. doi:10.5014/ajot.2013.008359

Dunton, W. R. (1915). *Occupation therapy: A manual for nurses.* Philadelphia, PA: WB Saunders.

Jenkins, C. D., & Pan American Health Organization. (2003). *Building better health: A handbook of behavioral change.* Washington, DC: Pan American Health Organization, Pan American Sanitary Bureau, Regional Office of the World Health Organization.

Meyer, A. (1922). The philosophy of occupation therapy (Vol. 1): Archives of occupational therapy. *American Journal of Occupational Therapy, 31*(10), 639–642.

Pizzi, M. (2001). The Pizzi holistic wellness assessment. *Occupational Therapy in Health Care, 13*(3–4), 51–66. doi:10.1080/J003v13n03_06

Prochaska, J. O., & DiClemente, C. C. (1982). Transtheoretical therapy: Toward a more integrative model of change. *Psychotherapy: Theory, Research & Practice, 19*(3), 276–288.

Reitz, S. M., Scaffa, M. E., & Pizzi, M. A. (2010). Occupational therapy conceptual models for health promotion practice. In M. E. Scaffa, S. M. Reitz, & M. Pizzi (Eds.), *Occupational therapy in the promotion of health and wellness* (pp. 22–45). Philadelphia, PA: F. A. Davis.

Resource Center for Adolescent Pregnancy Prevention. (2015). *Theories & approaches.* Retrieved from http://recapp.etr.org/recapp/index.cfm?fuseaction=pages.theoriesdetail&PageID=13

Rosenstock, I. M. (1974). Historical origins of the health belief model. *Health Education Monographs, 2*(4), 328–335.

SF-36. (2014). *SF-36 Health survey scoring demonstration.* Retrieved from http://www.sf-36.org/demos/SF-36.html

Slagle, E. C. (1934). The occupational therapy programme in the state of New York. *Journal of Mental Science, 80,* 639–649.

United States Department of Health and Human Services. (2014). *Healthy People 2020.* Retrieved from https://www.healthypeople.gov

World Health Organization. (1986). *The Ottawa charter for health promotion.* Retrieved from http://www.who.int/healthpromotion/conferences/previous/ottawa/en/

Occupational Rehabilitation and Ergonomics, and Low Back Pain

Regina Parnell and Jane Pomper DeHart

Learning Objectives

- Define functional capacity evaluation (FCE), ergonomic assessment, job site evaluation, work hardening, work conditioning, job coaching, light duty programming, and work tolerance screening.
- Choose the most appropriate discipline for the client based on previous rehabilitation outcomes.
- Describe the purpose for FCE, ergonomic assessment, job site evaluation, work hardening, job coaching, work tolerance screening, and light duty programming.
- Describe the components of a FCE, ergonomic assessment, job site evaluation, work hardening, work conditioning, job coaching, work tolerance screening, and light duty programming.
- Describe what attributes make up a challenging client.
- Describe the components of proper documentation.
- Describe the rationale and indications for the use of lumbar supports.
- Recognize the levels of education needed to promote proper health and awareness of the occupational therapist's (OT's) role in decreasing days away from work to the client, work employer, supervisor, and employer's upper management.

Key Terms

- *Ergonomic assessment*: Assessment tools designed to evaluate the ergonomic risk factors associated with a job. It considers job tasks, the work environment, body regions used in a task, and functional task requirements (AIHA Ergonomic Committee, 2011).

- *Functional capacity evaluation (FCE)*: A systematic process for assessing a client's physical and functional work-related abilities. More than 55 FCEs are available and vary in their measures of physical and psychological factors. Many require training to achieve competency in administration and interpretation (Rice, 2014).
- *Job analysis*: A systematic evaluation of the physical, cognitive, and psychosocial aspect of a job, which involves visiting the jobsite and observing the workers performing their job tasks. This includes measuring equipment, placement of equipment and supplies, and interviewing workers and supervisors. Job analysis provides information that is critical for workers with disabilities to be successful in their return to work (Rice, 2014).
- *Job site evaluation*: The evaluation of a worker's ability to complete specific critical job tasks associated with their occupation (Rice, 2014).
- *National Institute for Occupational Safety and Health (NIOSH)*: A division of the Centers for Disease Control and Prevention which provides national and world leadership to prevent workplace illnesses and injuries. It conducts training and provides resources based on research and interventions focused on maintaining worker safety and ergonomics (Centers for Disease Control and Prevention [CDC], 2015).
- *Occupational information network (O*Net)*: Free online database of jobs, which provides standardized descriptions of hundreds of occupations (Ha, Page, & Wietlisbach, 2013).
- *Work conditioning*: Rehabilitative treatment focuses on the remediation of physical and cognitive skills the worker needs to function at their job or employment setting. It follows acute care and precedes work hardening (Rice, 2014).

- *Work hardening*: A multidisciplinary approach to interventions designed to maximize the worker's ability to return to their job or employment setting. It encompasses the full spectrum of employee functions including communication, psychosocial skills, physical skills, and vocational needs (Rice, 2014).
- *Workman's compensation*: A system of paid benefits provided to workers who have job-related injuries or illnesses (Kaskutas, Snodgrass, & American Occupational Therapy Association [AOTA], 2009).
- *Work-related musculoskeletal disorders*: Any injury or condition resulting from exposure to a work environment, work tasks, or work conditions (CDC, 2013).

Introduction

This chapter provides the background information required to return clients back to work in a work setting, and how to properly document outcomes for work, clinical, insurance, and legal systems. This chapter will also provide guidance on how to communicate with work supervisors, upper management of employers, and the union when placing the worker back into a work setting.

History of Occupational Therapy and Rehabilitation

Work has always been a core tenet of occupational therapy as the founding practitioners focused on the moral and ethical treatment of those with mental illness (Christiansen & Haertl, 2014). The need for physical rehabilitative therapy developed largely secondary to the return of wounded soldiers following World War I (Christiansen & Haertl, 2014). Legislations such as the Vocational Education Act of 1917, the Civilian Rehabilitation Act of 1920, the Social Security Act of 1935, and the Vocational Rehabilitation Act of 1943 emerged to support the presence of occupational therapy practitioners in work-related rehabilitation (Ha et al., 2013). By the 1980s, occupational therapy practitioners were employed in industrial rehabilitation and work hardening clinics, holistically treating injured workers with the goal of returning them to productive employment (Ha et al., 2013). Additional laws such as the American

with Disabilities Act, the Occupational Safety and Health Administration government regulations, and payment sources for workers' compensation continue to shape the practice of occupational therapists (OTs) and occupational therapy assistants (OTAs) in employment settings (AOTA, 2016; Ha et al., 2013). Today, OTs utilize a variety of assessments and treatment modalities to address the needs of the employee with acute or chronic work-related disorders (Ha et al., 2013). Also, OTs are often consulted about ergonomic issues at various types of work sites (Ha et al., 2013). The following three sections present information about work-related disorders, assessments, and intervention approaches.

Common Work Disorders

Workplace injuries and illnesses may be permanent or transient. These health conditions range from physical conditions affecting the muscles, nerves, and tissues to psychosocial conditions, which can impair the person's ability to engage in work (Rice, 2014). Three broad categories of work-related disorders are discussed below.

- *Musculoskeletal disorders*: One of the most common work-related complaints is low back pain. Additional sites of injury include upper extremity joints including incidences of tendinopathies (Kaskutas et al., 2009). Neuromuscular work disorders have multiple causes including mechanical demands of job tasks, workplace climate, poor body mechanics, and personal factors such as age, gender, and physical conditioning (Duff, 2004a). The signs and symptoms of these disorders are varied and range from dull aches to sharp pains. The onset can be acute or chronic with episodic bouts of symptoms. Recovery can be slow even with treatment (Duff, 2004b).
- *Visual disorders*: Clients may develop eyestrain or perceptual and coordination challenges due to engagement in work tasks. Changes in the structure of the eye may also emerge (Sanders, 2004). Visual and perceptual difficulties may be related to environmental exposure on the job, as well as conditions such as light intensity. Age and anatomy and physiology may also present risk factors (Sanders, 2004). Signs and symptoms vary but typically include pain, burning, spasm, blurred vision, and changes in eye shape or color (Sanders, 2004).

- *Psychosocial*: Clients may also develop anxiety, depression, or adjustment disorders in response to job demands (Erez, 2008). Clients who have experienced trauma on the job may experience fear that interferes with their return to work. Psychological stress at work may be attributed to the physical or social environment, role demands, or the course of treatment for disabilities (Edwards, 2004). Symptoms may include those associated with anxiety, depression, and somatization. Clients may avoid certain work-related tasks and experience difficulty completing tasks or compromise safety protocols (Erez, 2008).

Work Rehabilitation

Occupational therapists employed in work rehabilitation settings focus on various interventions designed to facilitate the client's independent function at work. Goals include a timely return to work, satisfaction in their worker role, remediation and prevention of future illness, or negative psychosocial consequences due to unemployment (AOTA, 2016).

Screening and Assessments of Acute Work Injuries

- *Occupational profile*: An occupational profile must be completed and should include a history of the disorder, as well as results from assessments such as pain evaluations, sensibility tests, and a functional evaluation (Chisholm & Schell, 2014). A variety of assessments can be used to assess work performance with the majority falling into the category of functional capacity evaluation (FCE) (Rice, 2014).
- *Functional capacity evaluations*: According to Rice (2014), the purpose of an FCE is to determine the appropriateness of a job assignment. FCEs allow goals to be developed for return to work while establishing a functional baseline and identifying various limiting factors and restrictions for returning to work including prognosis, frequency and duration, and the necessity for additional services (e.g., vocational rehabilitation, specialized physical therapy (PT)/OT/OTA, and job site evaluation). An FCE examines the client's current physical abilities and their essential workplace tasks (Rice, 2014). A general evaluation of physical

and cognitive abilities is where the OT assesses range of motion, strength, and subjective pain complaints, followed by a functional portion where the OT runs through several tests to assess sitting, standing, walking, squatting, and lifting (i.e., floor to waist, waist to waist, waist to shoulder, and waist to overhead). Additional tests include pushing and pulling, carrying bilaterally and carrying unilaterally, kneeling, crawling, and fine motor tasks (e.g., gripping and pinching). Safety practices during work evaluations are also assessed (Rice, 2014).

Goal setting and recommendations are a part of the documentation process that include noting inconsistencies in performance, symptom magnification, nontest behavior, goals, and recommendations (Rice, 2014).

Interventions for Acute Work Injuries

Modalities commonly used during the acute injury phase include cryotherapy, transcutaneous electrical nerve stimulation, paraffin, and fluidotherapy. Treatment approaches incorporate isometrics, controlled loading, and progressive stress (Duff, 2004b). Work hardening and conditioning approaches are implemented in response to conclusions drawn from functional vocational evaluations (Rice, 2014); both are described below.

Work Conditioning Versus Work Hardening

Work conditioning is discipline specific, focuses on the remediation of physical and/or cognitive challenges, and generally follows acute care (Rice, 2014). As an intervention, its narrow focus is on the functional skills needed for a specific employment setting (Rice, 2014). Work conditioning occurs at least three days a week, if not daily, and four hours per day (i.e., on average) in the clinic (AOTA, 2016). Circuit training is often used to restore musculoskeletal and cardiovascular conditioning, as well as correct body mechanics while performing work tasks (AOTA, 2016).

Work hardening incorporates a multidisciplinary approach to prepare the employee for return to work and is designed to follow the rehabilitative processes initiated in work conditioning (Rice, 2014). Treatment is typically five days a week, two to four hours each day and includes multiple services such as psychosocial counseling, ergonomics, job coaching, and other transitional work programs (AOTA, 2016). Sandoval and DeWeese

(2014) recommend the following factors for occupational therapy practitioners to consider when evaluating the appropriateness of potential clients for work conditioning or work hardening programs:

- Does the injured worker have medium to heavy job demands instead of sedentary job tasks?
- Is the worker ready to begin job-specific endurance and conditioning exercises?
- Is the worker ready to adhere to requirements of body mechanics?
- Can the worker follow work safety protocols?
- Is there only a minimal need for manual treatment modalities?
- Has the worker demonstrated progress throughout the acute phase of their injury?
- Is the worker motivated to return to work?

Related Programming

Additional strategies can assist with the evaluation and treatment of workers with injuries that impact their ability to return to work. They are as follows:

- *Work simulation*: Be creative. Break the job or jobs down into specific parts and work those in order to achieve total job duty. A combination of multiple performance requirements such as strength, agility, and balance is typically included (Rice, 2014).
- *Work tolerance screening*: Intensive screening occurs over a one- to two-day evaluation where the physical demands of work are simulated in a controlled setting (Eisenhower Medical Center, 2016). This assists in determining an individual's ability to return to his/her previous job and/or whether the worker can perform critical demands of a new job prior to the development of a formal vocational plan.
- *Light/modified duty programming*: Involves the development of a program to help prevent lost workdays and reduce workers' compensation claims and payouts. This is accomplished through education, recognition, and commitment of all employees, supervisors, upper management, and medical staff, as well as the safety department (Hall, 2000).
- *Job coaching*: On-site job coaching occurs with an employee and/or employer upon the employee returning to work in order to provide

documentation of compliance or noncompliance with recommendations to return to work safely with or without restrictions (Job Accommodation Network, 2013). The occupational therapy practitioner will also assist with implementation of proper body and lifting mechanics with an emphasis on correct utilization of work techniques (AOTA, 2016).

Job coaching, work tolerance screening, and light/modified duty programming are additional areas in occupational rehabilitation that require continuing education and training.

Therapeutic Use of Self

Clients in work rehabilitation programs can exhibit a wide range of physical and interpersonal responses to treatment (Rice, 2014). While many clients will be motivated and actively engaged in their goal setting, some clients will struggle to create or achieve reasonable treatment goals for return to employment (Rice, 2014). The Intentional Relationship Model may be useful in effectively navigating a client's interpersonal and occupational engagement challenges (Taylor, 2014). The OT can enlist any or all of the six therapeutic modes (i.e., advocating, collaborating, empathizing, encouraging, instructing, and problem-solving) of relating to clients (Taylor, 2014). The OT practitioner uses interpersonal reasoning throughout the therapy process to determine which mode(s) to enlist to best support the client's needs and efforts (Taylor, 2014).

Documentation

To justify the need for work hardening/work conditioning, the documentation differentiates from general occupational therapy. For example, goals should focus on maximizing the level of function required to return to work safely and in a timely manner. Further, objectives for remediation and prevention of future injury should be addressed, as well as issues related to unemployment (AOTA, 2016). There needs to be careful tracking of outcomes with specific and focused work goals based on very specific and focused evaluations (AOTA, 2016). It is also important to ensure that all third-party payer forms are completed accurately (Smith, 2013). The AOTA

(2016) provides general guidelines for strong documentation which includes the following:

- Write legible notes.
- Be timely with documentation.
- Only include necessary details related to treatment and progress.
- Document all important conversations with related parties.
- Be direct and to the point (examples below):
  - Activity was discontinued by the client due to complaints of pain. However, no changes in technique or signs of increased effort such as . . . were noted.
  - The client reports he/she cannot perform because of pain. However, there is no objective basis to limit the client from performing the activity. Returning to work involving performance of that activity would be unsuccessful because of a client's subjective limitations. Return to work involving . . . would be more successful.
  - Due to the inconsistencies noted, it is impossible to determine objective capabilities. However, there are some reasonable suggestions for rehabilitation management.

Low Back Pain

Client Education: Chronic Pain

Individuals with chronic pain face quality of life challenges due to persistent physical and psychological discomfort. Client education is recommended as one component of pain management, which may aid in their return to function and independence despite the presence of chronic pain. **Table 33-1** provides basic information on low back pain and examples of health content appropriate for client education.

Ergonomics

Ergonomics is the study of work and is a discipline which draws from a number of fields of study in order to create a system for prevention, evaluation, and management of safety and comfort throughout all areas of occupation (Jacobs et al., 2002). **Table 33-2** outlines common ergonomic principles used to assess or prevent typical work hazards.

Table 33-1 Back Pain Concepts and Details

Concepts	Details
Basic information	Basic spinal anatomy.
	Basic body lifting mechanics instruction.
	Home exercise program.
	Posture reeducation.
	Pain management techniques.
Advanced information	Neutral spine concept.
	Emphasize critical need for spinal stabilization.
Home exercise program	Spinal stabilization and total body reconditioning.
Lumbar back braces and belts	NIOSH recommendations (i.e., recommended not mandatory).
Lifting, carrying, and twisting	Keep the load close.
	Keep the load off the floor.
	Keep the torso as vertical as possible with proper lumbar curvature.
	Do not jerk or move fast with loads.
	Avoid side lifting and twisting, especially with heavy loads.
	Ergonomic programs to reduce risks related to lifting tasks.

Data from Centers for Disease Control and Prevention, 2015; Grangaard, 2013.

Workstation Design

The appropriate placement of workstation components can support work efficiency and limit the risks of work-related injuries. **Table 33-3** presents a list of ergonomic guidelines for creating a workstation that promotes good posture and minimizes muscle and eyestrain.

Youth Ergonomics

Although this chapter pertains to adults, occupational therapy practitioners play a significant role in wellness and health promotion in regard to ergonomics for children. While it is possible to modify basic ergonomic principles to accommodate growing children and small children, adolescents have unique ergonomic needs based on their developmental status and childhood occupations. **Table 33-4** outlines important ergonomic factors and solutions to consider when assessing work environments commonly associated with children.

Table 33-2 General Ergonomic Principles

	Principles	Worker Risks	Work Solutions
1	Work in neutral positions	Awkward positions place stress on joints, muscles, bones, and nerves.	Make handles longer, change the position of the work surface, and use left- or right-handed tools.
2	Reduce excessive force	Muscle fatigue and risk of injury.	Use mechanical assistance to move heavy items or power tools (i.e., especially for torque).
3	Keep everything within easy reach	Discomfort, muscle strain, fatigue, and risk of injury.	For routine and repeated activities, maintain supplies in front of the client. Items used for occasional tasks can be placed outside of the neutral zone.
4	Work at proper heights	Shoulder fatigue, neck, and back strain.	Adjust the surface to work at elbow height for precise work or lower the surface 4–5 inches for heavy work.
5	Reduce excessive motions	Onset of fatigue early in the work day; injury or errors in task processes.	Use power tools and align surfaces to minimize movement. Implement/utilize conveyer assist or gravity assist.
6	Minimize fatigue and static load	Standing, reaching, and holding items for extended periods of time leads to muscle fatigue, cramping, strain, and pain.	Change the angle of the work surface, use extenders for tools, and use footrests and fixtures to hold parts.
7	Minimize pressure points (e.g., contact stress)	Soft tissues are at risk of injury.	Assure proper fit/grip for tools, pad or contour edges, eliminate physical barriers to completing tasks, and use mechanical assist.
8	Provide clearance	Bumping the head, knees, and toes.	Have head clearance clearly marked, allow space for knee clearance when sitting, and foot clearance when on ladders. Have a clear view of the work space/path and utilize clutter-free and slip-resistant floors.
9	Move, exercise, and stretch	Muscle shortening, fatigue, poor conditioning, and poor circulation.	Take rest breaks from strenuous tasks, movement breaks for sedentary tasks, and alternate sitting and standing if possible.
10	Maintain comfortable environment	Temperature extremes affect work performance, the body works harder to maintain temperature, and affected sensation may increase the risk for errors.	Maintain a comfortable temperature and wear protective clothing (e.g., gloves) when needed.
11	Maintain appropriate lighting and noise levels	Eye irritation, work errors, or falls. High decibels cause ear pain, fatigue, and increased distractibility.	Avoid glare. Use task lights, use protection for higher decibel noise levels, and use visual cues to communicate as needed.
12	Make display and controls understandable	Eyestrain and mistakes with reading dials or controlling a task.	Use high contrast colors and shapes, large displays, and compatibility with direction indicators (e.g., up = higher and down = lower).
13	Work organization	Abnormal circadian rhythm, fatigue, and risk of physical injury due to the frequency of job tasks.	Adhere to work–rest cycles, body mechanics protocols, ergonomic principles, and job safety practices.

Data from MacLeod, 2008; UAW-Ford National Joint Committee on Health Safety & University of Michigan Center for Ergonomics, 1988.

Referrals and Discharge Considerations

Clients are referred from a number of sources including medical providers, insurance companies, attorneys, and state agencies (AOTA, 2016). Planning and discharge begins with the initial assessment. Occupational therapy practitioners evaluate the fit between the job demands and the client's work capacities. Recommendations are made regarding return to work needs for accommodations or modifications of the job site or job tasks (see the Occupational Information Network for standardized job descriptions). Clients who are making progress in therapy may continue in treatment even if they return to work.

Table 33-3 Ergonomic Desk Analysis

Work Component	Ergonomic Design
Computer desk	The desk surface has adequate room for computer, keyboard, and mouse placement. It is adjustable and has adequate leg clearance. It minimizes awkward positions and exertion.
Computer chair	Supports the lower back, legs, buttocks, and arms. Reduces exertion, contact stress, and awkward body positioning. It is adjustable and positioned so the feet rest comfortably on the floor.
Document holder	Place the document holder close to the user and the computer monitor to reduce the risk of awkward head and neck postures, as well as eyestrain.
Keyboards	The keyboard should be centered and at an elbow height. The keyboard tray should be adjustable. The keyboard should also be of an appropriate size to accommodate the user. Ergonomic keyboards promote neutral wrist postures.
Monitors	The top of the monitor should be positioned just above eye level and 20–40 inches from the eye to the computer screen. The monitor should be adjustable and have an antiglare screen.
Telephones	Phones should be positioned close to avoid repeated reaching or shoulder, arm and neck pain, and to allow for hands-free use (e.g., speaker or headset).
Mouse	The computer mouse should have a comfortable design, which may be used by either hand.
Wrist/palm support	A support may be used to increase comfort and reduce muscle fatigue while facilitating neutral wrist angles.

Data from Occupational Safety and Health Administration, 2016.

Table 33-4 Ergonomic Guidelines for Children

	Design	Supervision	Child's Practice
1	*Backpacks*: Wide adjustable straps, compartments, and child size.	Attend to the child's complaints. Weight should not exceed 10% of the child's weight.	Position straps below shoulders, resting on hips, and hold heavy items closest to the body.
2	*School workspace*: Use a range of child-sized furniture.	Inquire about the child's comfort and advocate for furniture modifications.	Use proper body mechanics, take breaks, and keep frequently used supplies within reach.
3	*Handwriting*: Use a workstation with neutral positioning for the back, hip, knee, and ankle (i.e., approximately 90°–90°–90°).	Allow 2-min breaks after 20–30 min of writing.	Take frequent writing breaks.
4	*School computer stations*: Use adjustable monitor stands and antiglare screens.	Allow and encourage children to take breaks.	Take frequent breaks and stretch.
5	*Home computer stations*: Adjust to the youth's size, support the back and seat with pillows, and use a smaller keyboard and mouse.	Monitor computer time and provide reminders to take frequent breaks.	Take frequent breaks and stretch.
6	*Laptop computers*: Provide an external keyboard and mouse, as well as a lightweight laptop.	Place the laptop on a stable surface at eye level (i.e., 12–18 inches from the body), and limit computer time.	Advocate for an external keyboard and mouse, take frequent breaks, and avoid positions that cause strain.
7	*Homework space*: Use sturdy work surfaces, task lighting, and appropriate sized furniture.	Monitor for good work practices.	Choose sturdy work surfaces, adjustable chairs, and good lighting.
8	*Video games and television*: Provide a youth-sized chair, turn off vibration options if present, adjust the screen to the proper height, and use proper lighting.	Provide parameters for these activities.	Stretch periodically, use good posture, and hold controls lightly.
9	*Fitness*: Design play areas inside and outside of the home, and buy toys that promote fitness.	Provide age-appropriate chores, plan family activities, and advocate for physical education in schools.	Incorporate physical activity into daily routines, limit computer and TV time, and find physical options to relieve boredom.
10	*Sports and performing arts*: Manufacture aesthetically pleasing equipment, wheeled equipment, instrument bags, and youth-sized equipment and environments.	Monitor youth complaints, ensure proper fit of equipment, provide down time, and alternate among activities.	Perform warm-ups, stretches, cool-downs, and notify parents if pain is present.

Data from Jacobs et al., 2008.

Clients who have plateaued in therapy are discharged and referred to the next phase of occupational rehabilitation or other health services (Kaskutas et al., 2009).

Management and Standards of Practice

The OT works closely with the OTA in various practice settings to provide rehabilitative treatment to clients with work-related disorders. Supervision and mentoring from the OT should match the current competency and support the advancing proficiency of the OTA (AOTA, 2016). Both the OT and OTA should adhere to ethical practice standards, as well as any legal requirements outlined in state practice acts, regulatory bodies, and payment entities (AOTA, 2016).

Chapter 33 Self-Study Activities (Answers Are Provided at the End of the Chapter)

Case Scenario One

A 42-year-old male with a rotator cuff tear and repair is a tool and dye maker on a machine in which he loads parts from a pallet on the floor, and places them into the machine (i.e., the client reaches into the machine). The reach into the machine is approximately 16 inches, and the weights vary from 2 to 20 pounds. The client also has to close the sliding door (i.e., that sticks from time to time), and must push a mechanical lever up and to the right to start the machine. What "exercises" and/or education will help the client with his job?

Case Scenario Two

Which of the following most appropriately reflects proper documentation?

A. The client cannot lift 20 pounds.
B. The client complains of pain constantly and is, therefore, magnifying.
C. The client exhibits trunk stiffening and cannot control appropriate faulty body and postural mechanics. The client has been instructed on proper maintenance of body mechanics over a 50-minute period and remains unable to demonstrate proper control.
D. The client drops the box and could not explain his inability to hold it; he is therefore malingering.

Case Scenario Three

The physician asks you to dispense a lumbar support to his client. The client is returning to work in one week. His job is in the heavy category as defined by the U.S. Department of Labor. This is defined as lifting on an occasional basis with weight up to and exceeding 100 pounds independently. The physician says it will help protect his back. What should be the OT's response to the physician?

Case Scenario Four

You are asked to educate an employer on minimizing work injury claims and possible lost workdays. Please list some suggestions that you would discuss with management and supervisors versus employees themselves.

Chapter 33 Self-Study Answers

Case Scenario One

1. Perform body mechanics instruction.
2. Teach the client appropriate abdominal bracing, hip hinging, joint protection, and trunk posture.
3. Perform lifting tasks from the floor with weight ranging from 2 to 20 pounds with good body mechanics.
4. Perform outward reaching over distances of 6 to 16 inches with weight ranging from 2 to 20 pounds while focusing on proper body and lifting mechanics.
5. Use Thera-Band® to simulate the motions needed to push the lever to start the machine and/or use Baltimore Therapeutic Equipment (BTE) (i.e., work simulator equipment/isokinetic machine) to help simulate the work task.

Case Scenario Two

C is the correct answer. It describes the most objective findings that explain why things are occurring. Choices a, b, and d have no significant objective measures to back up the documentation.

Case Scenario Three

The OT practitioner would state that the client requires education on the use of the brace. This education will include a discussion on the brace being a psychological aid and that it is to be used as an adjunct with proper body and lifting mechanics. The client must realize that it will not prevent low back injury. The OT practitioner would also discuss proper problem-solving skills with regard to testing weight and the importance of requesting assistance when needed.

Case Scenario Four

With management and supervisors, the OT must discuss the need to allow individuals to report claims in order to identify potential risks. Begin with education on proper body and lifting mechanics, pain management techniques, and additional ergonomic interventions. The OT should also discuss workplace politics and attitudes as they relate to how the employees/supervisors may react to injuries. With regard to the employees, it is important to discuss fatigue avoidance, stretching, and exercises rather than disease processes.

References

AIHA Ergonomic Committee. (2011). *Ergonomic assessment toolkit*. Retrieved from https://www.aiha.org/get-involved/VolunteerGroups/Documents/ERGOVG-Toolkit_rev2011.pdf

American Occupational Therapy Association. (2016). *Work rehabilitation*. Retrieved from http://www.aota.org/About-Occupational-Therapy/Professionals/WI/Work-Rehab.aspx

Centers for Disease Control and Prevention. (2013). *Work-related musculoskeletal disorders (WMSD) prevention*. Atlanta, GA: USA.gov. Retrieved from http://www.cdc.gov/workplacehealthpromotion/implementation/topics/disorders.html

Centers for Disease Control and Prevention. (2015). *Ergonomics and musculoskeletal disorders*. Retrieved from https://www.cdc.gov/niosh/topics/ergonomics/

Chisholm, D., & Schell, B. A. B. (2014). Overview of the occupational therapy process. In B. A. B. Schell, G. Gillen, M. Scaffa, & E. Cohn (Eds.), *Willard & Spackman's occupational therapy* (12th ed., pp. 266–280). Philadelphia, PA: Wolters Kluwer Health/Lippincott Williams & Wilkins.

Christiansen, C., & Haertl, K. (2014). A contextual history of occupational therapy. In B. A. B. Schell, G. Gillen, M. Scaffa, & E. Cohn (Eds.), *Willard & Spackman's occupational therapy* (12th ed., pp. 9–34). Philadelphia, PA: Wolters Kluwer Health/Lippincott Williams & Wilkins.

Duff, S. (2004a). Pathomechanics of MSDs. In M. J. Sandors (Ed.), *Ergonomics and the management of musculoskeletal disorders* (2nd ed., pp. 63–87). St. Louis, MO: Butterworth Heinemann.

Duff, S. (2004b). Treatment of MSD and related conditions. In M. J. Sandors (Ed.), *Ergonomics and the management of musculoskeletal disorders* (2nd ed., pp. 89–131). St. Louis, MO: Butterworth Heinemann.

Edwards, D. (2004). Pscyhosocial factors. In M. J. Sandors (Ed.), *Ergonomics and the management of musculoskeletal disorders* (2nd ed., pp. 265–279). St. Louis, MO: Butterworth Heinemann.

Eisenhower Medical Center. (2016). *Industrial rehabilitation*. Rancho Mirage, CA: Author. Retrieved from https://www.emc.org/health-services/occupational-health/industrial-rehabilitation/

Erez, A. B. H. (2008). Psychosocial factors in work-related musculoskeletal disorders. In K. Jacobs (Ed.), *Ergonomics for therapists* (3rd ed., pp. 123–136). St. Louis, MO: Mosby Elsevier.

Grangaard, L. (2013). Low back pain. In H. M. Pendleton & W. Schultz-Krohn (Eds.), *Pedretti's occupational therapy: Practice skills for physical dysfunction* (7th ed., pp. 1091–1109). St. Louis, MO: Elsevier.

Ha, D., Page, J., & Wietlisbach, C. (2013). Work evaluations and work programs. In H. M. Pendleton & W. Schultz-Krohn (Eds.), *Pedretti's occupational therapy: Practice skills for physical dysfunction* (7th ed., pp. 337–380). St. Louis, MO: Elsevier.

Hall, R. (2000). *Light duty, limited duty or modified duty assignments*. Retrieved from http://www.workforce.com/articles/light-duty-limited-duty-or-modified-duty-assignments

Jacobs, K., Bhasin, G., Bustamante, L., Buxton, J. C., Chiang, H. Y., Greene, D., . . . Wieck, A. (May 27, 2002). *Everything you should know about ergonomics and youths but were afraid to ask. Occupational Therapy Practice*, 11-14, 16-19.

Job Accommodation Network. (2013). *Accommodation and compliance series: Job coaching in the workplace.*

Retrieved from https://askjan.org/media/downloads /JobCoachingA&CSeries.pdf

Kaskutas, V., Snodgrass, J., & American Occupational Therapy Association. (2009). *Occupational therapy practice guidelines for individuals with work-related injuries and illnesses*. Bethesda, MD: American Occupational Therapy Association.

MacLeod, D. (2008). *10 Principles of ergonomics*. Retrieved from http://www.danmacleod.com/ErgoForYou/10 _principles_of_ergonomics.htm

Occupational Safety and Health Administration. (2016). *Computer workstations eTool*. Retrieved from https:// www.osha.gov/SLTC/etools/computerworkstations /checklist.html

Rice, V. J. B. (2014). Restoring competence for the worker role. In M. V. Radomski & C. A. T. Latham (Eds.), *Occupational therapy for physical dysfunction* (7th ed., pp. 870–908). Philadelphia, PA: Wolters Kluwer Health/Lippincott Williams & Wilkins.

Sanders, M. (2004). Job design. In M. J. Sandors (Ed.), *Ergonomics and the management of musculoskeletal disorders* (2nd ed., pp. 230–264). St. Louis, MO: Butterworth Heinemann.

Sandoval, G., & DeWeese, C. (2014). *Expediting the return to work process using work conditioning/hardening*. Retrieved from http://www.rehabpub.com/2014/07 /expediting-return-work-process-using-work -conditioninghardening/

Smith, J. (2013). Documentation of occupational therapy services. In H. M. Pendleton & W. Schultz-Krohn (Eds.), *Pedretti's occupational therapy: Practice skills for physical dysfunction* (7th ed., pp. 117–139). St. Louis, MO: Elsevier.

Taylor, R. (2014). Therapeutic relationship and client collaboration. In B. A. B. Schell, G. Gillen, M. Scaffa, & E. Cohn (Eds.), *Willard & Spackman's occupational therapy* (12th ed., pp. 425–436). Philadelphia, PA: Wolters Kluwer Health/Lippincott Williams & Wilkins.

UAW-Ford National Joint Committee on Health Safety & University of Michigan Center for Ergonomics. (1988). *Fitting jobs to people: The UAW-Ford ergonomics process job improvement guide*. Detroit, MI: UAW-Ford National Joint Committee on Health and Safety.

Wheelchair Seating and Mobility

Diane Thomson and Patricia Tully

Learning Objectives

- Describe the core concepts of the Human Activity Assistive Technology (HAAT) model.
- Identify necessary assessment areas of wheelchair seating and mobility evaluation.
- Identify the necessary standard measurements associated with wheelchair seating and mobility evaluation.
- Describe the four types of postural deformities.
- Describe how to determine an appropriate mobility device for clients according to their functional activity level.
- Apply knowledge of wheelchair seating and mobility evaluation and assessment to chapter self-study activities.

Key Terms

- *Durable Medical Equipment (DME)*: A category of Medicare benefits.
- *Fixed deformity*: "A permanent change taking place in the bones, muscles, capsular ligaments, or tendons that restricts the normal range of motion of the particular joint and affects the skeletal alignment of the other joints" (Cook & Polgar, 2014, p. 462).
- *Flexible deformity*: "Appearance of a deformity as a result of increased tone and muscle tightness causing the person to assume certain postures, externally applied resistance in the opposite direction allows movement of the joint and reduction in the "'deformity'" (Cook & Polgar, 2014, p. 462).
- *Hemi-height wheelchair*: A wheelchair that has the same features of a standard wheelchair and provides a seat to floor height of 17 to 18 inches and is typically used by someone who needs a lower seat to floor height due to short stature or to allow the client to place their feet on the ground to self-propel.
- *Medicaid*: A state health care funding source.
- *Medicare*: A federal health care funding source.
- *Pelvic obliquity*: "One side of the pelvis is higher than the other when viewed in the frontal plane" (Cook & Polgar, 2014, p. 466).
- *Pelvic rotation*: "One side of the pelvis is forward of the other side with rotation in a lateral plane" (Cook & Polgar, 2014, p. 466).
- *Power mobility device (PMD)*: A PMD is defined as a class of wheelchairs that includes a power wheelchair or a power-operated vehicle, such as a motorized scooter.
- *Power-operated vehicle (POV)*: A PMD that is operated by a tiller style input device (e.g., a motorized scooter).
- *Power wheelchair*: A wheelchair propelled by an electric motor; a component of Medicare DME benefits.
- *Pressure injury*: Previously labeled pressure ulcer, is an injury to the skin and/or underlying tissue usually over a bony prominence as a result of pressure, or pressure in combination with shear (National Pressure Ulcer Advisory Panel [NPUAP], 2016).
- *Pressure injury stages*: Provide definitions of pressure injuries and concise staging descriptions based on the amount of anatomic tissue loss in a pressure injury (NPUAP, 2016).
- *Pressure redistribution*: Goal or outcome of seating technology that results in a change in the distribution of pressure to relieve areas of high pressure (Cook & Polgar, 2014, p. 466).

- *Pressure relief*: Removing or reducing pressure under bony prominences to decrease a client's risk of developing a pressure injury.
- *Recline wheelchair*: A standard wheelchair that allows changing the seat-to-back angle, as well as the lower extremity joint angles using the leg rests.
- *Scoliosis*: "Lateral or rotational curvature of the spine" (Cook & Polgar, 2014, p. 468).
- *Shearing*: "The process of deep structures moving in the direction of applied force while superficial structures remain immobile" (Cook & Polgar, 2014, p. 468).
- *Standard height manual wheelchair*: Weighs more than 36 pounds, has a seat to floor height greater than 19 inches, and does not have features to accept specialized seating or client positioning.
- *Tilt-in-space wheelchair*: Tilt-in-space refers to changing the orientation of a client sitting in a wheelchair, while maintaining the hip, knee, and ankle angles.
- *Ultra-lightweight wheelchair*: Categorized by Medicare as a K5 manual wheelchair and considered custom due to multiple adjustment options (e.g., seat options and adjustable center of gravity) and weight under 30 pounds.
- *Weight shifts*: A method of performing pressure relief (e.g., the client shifts weight laterally or anteriorly or performs a push-up using the side panel arm rests).
- *Windswept deformity*: One hip is adducted and the other hip is abducted (Cook & Polgar, 2014, p. 470).

Introduction

This chapter will describe the process for assessing a client for an appropriate wheelchair by evaluating relevant physical, environmental, social, cognitive, and psychological factors. Case studies have been provided to allow for a better understanding of the concepts presented. These will provide an opportunity to reinforce the learning of the preceding concepts, as well as applying the knowledge acquired.

Human Activity Assistive Technology Model

"The HAAT model shares many features of other models that integrate activity (occupation), the person, and the environment" (Cook & Polgar, 2014, p. 7). These models include the WHO's ICF (World Health Organization [WHO], 2015) and Person-Environment-Occupational Performance (Baum & Christiansen, 2005). "The model describes someone (human) doing something (activity) in a context using AT" (Cook & Polgar, 2014, p. 7). The basic principles of this model start with studying human performance versus behavior within a context while completing an activity. This gives useful conclusions to address how technology is working for the subject. This also provides the context for how assistive technology can be useful in the facilitation of performance during specific activities. The model places the human first by assuring the technology meets the needs of the client, rather than trying to adapt the client to the technology. "The HAAT model is depicted as an integration of the human, activity, and AT, nested in context" (Cook & Polgar, 2014, p. 41).

When looking at the model, an occupational therapist (OT) can look at each aspect in isolation; however, identifying the connections makes the end result of the activity complete. "The activity or need is identified first, followed by the aspects of the human that affect the ability to perform and engage in the activity. The contextual influences that affect human performance of that activity are then considered. The AT design and recommendations come last, signifying technology's place to enable activity participation and engagement" (Cook & Polgar, 2014, p. 41). Following this path, the activity or the task the client needs to complete is identified first. Once identified, the client's actions and the human potential needed to perform the task(s) are taken into consideration. Lastly, the OT must consider the client who is completing the activity and what areas of human performance will affect the client's ability to carry out the activity (i.e., context). These items should be determined within a thorough assessment of the client, including visual, auditory, sensory, and neuromusculoskeletal function. The context looks at the setting in which the activity will be performed, as well as social, cultural, temporal, and physical context. Following the completion of the above steps, the OT will have the information that is necessary to implement assistive technology required to complete identified tasks.

Evaluation

The International Classification of Functioning, Disability, and Health (ICF) model is a framework developed by the WHO for measuring health and disability at both individual and population levels (WHO, 2015). It is referenced in this chapter because it provides a framework (e.g., terminology and concepts) for incorporating the individual, the activity, the technology, and the environment into the service provision process.

There are many components to consider during a wheelchair assessment that vary based on the sequence in which they are addressed in relation to client-specific needs (Arledge et al., 2011). Three main categories should be addressed based on the ICF, which include body structures and functions, activities and participation, and environment and current technology (Arledge et al., 2011). Additionally, assessments may range from simple screening to a comprehensive evaluation of all ICF categories (Arledge et al., 2011). The following section will describe the assessment of proper seating and positioning, as well as assistive technology required for client mobility.

History and Physical Examination

Client history and physical examination entails gathering complete and accurate information about a client's past and present health history (e.g., symptoms, primary and secondary diagnoses, date of onset and history of progression, mechanism of injury if applicable, medical history and environmental considerations). Diagnoses and functional status should describe limitations, especially if they will affect seating, positioning and/or function, or provide justification for a client's wheelchair or equipment needs. It is also important to consider body systems (e.g., cardiovascular, respiratory, and digestive systems), as systemic involvement may affect a client's ability to safely ambulate or propel the wheelchair. Any recent or upcoming surgeries that may affect seating should also be documented (e.g., intrathecal baclofen pump placement or tendon release surgery). For example, flap surgeries are of significant importance due to the importance of skin integrity. If a surgery, which may change posture, positioning, or range of motion (ROM), is upcoming, the wheelchair assessment may need to be postponed until after the surgery (i.e., keeping issue healing time in mind when applicable). If conditional factors and context are not considered, the prescribed wheelchair may not be the appropriate equipment upon delivery.

Cognitive and Visual Status

Cognitive and visual deficits can have a direct effect on the effective and safe use of any wheelchair, especially a power wheelchair. Memory and problem-solving deficits (e.g., following commands and topographical orientation) and visual deficits (e.g., as neglect and field cuts) may impact effective and safe function with the device in specific or multiple environments. However, cognitive and visual deficits, including partial or complete blindness, should not rule out independent use of a wheelchair. More pronounced deficits will require a more detailed assessment for determination of safe equipment use, as well as identifying training needs once a device is prescribed.

Sensation and Skin Integrity

Sensation is of major importance for clients using a wheelchair secondary to the consequences of skin breakdown (e.g., infection, morbidity, and mortality). A somatosensory assessment must be completed to determine whether a client has intact, impaired, or absent sensation and the implications for the seating system. Moreover, a history and/or presence of pressure injuries, including the location and stage of the injury, are a necessary aspect of a seating and positioning assessment. The NPUAP (2016) defines a pressure injury as damage to a specific area of skin or soft tissue that is the result of prolonged pressure and/or shearing, which can present as either intact or open skin. Pressure injuries are staged as described in **Table 34-1**; documenting the stage and description of a pressure ulcer (i.e., when applicable) will be necessary to properly address a client's seating needs and to justify necessary equipment (e.g., accommodative cushion and seating system).

Principles of Seating for Postural Control

It is important to recognize that proximal stabilization near the center of a client's body—specifically the pelvis as a key point of control—will facilitate posture and control of the extremities (Cook & Polgar, 2014). Therefore, alignment and stabilization of the pelvis are normally the first areas addressed when positioning a client. The trunk can be addressed after proper positioning of the pelvis,

Table 34-1 Stages and Descriptions of Pressure Injuries

Stage	Description
Stage I	Defined as intact skin with nonblanchable redness of a localized area; usually over a bony prominence.
Stage II	Defined as partial thickness loss of the dermis presenting as shallow and open with a red pink wound bed; without slough.
Stage III	Defined as full-thickness tissue loss. Subcutaneous fat may be visible but bone, tendon, and muscles are not exposed.
Stage IV	Defined as full tissue loss with exposed bone, tendon, or muscle, and in the presence of unstageable wounds. These are defined as full-thickness skin or tissue loss in which the actual depth of the injury may be obscured by slough and/or eschar in the wound bed.

Note: Deep tissue injury is a purple or maroon localized area of discolored intact skin or blood-filled blisters due to damage of underlying soft tissue from pressure and/or shear.

Data from: NPUAP (2016).

followed by head and neck positioning (Cook & Polgar, 2014). Proper positioning, movement, and support of the upper extremities is also a critical factor for any seating system (Cook & Polgar, 2014). By and large, positioning can greatly increase or decrease the function of a client's body systems, functional mobility and reach (i.e., proper positioning is essential).

Posture Control Evaluation

A common understanding regarding postural alignment is to have the client sit as close to 90° of flexion at the hips, knees, and ankles as possible (i.e., 90, 90, 90). This is a point of reference to work from; however, 90, 90, and 90 is not necessarily obtainable by all clients. That is, "a client who is forced by the design of a wheelchair or seating system to sit continuously in one position will be uncomfortable and unable to reposition for tasks" (Bunning, 2009, p. 854). Accordingly, a physical motor assessment should be completed to determine the ability to transfer, bilateral symmetry, and ROM throughout the spine and pelvis, as well as signs of pressure or shear, and other factors that may affect sitting (Bunning, 2009).

A comprehensive mat evaluation should be completed on every client. This assessment is multifaceted and is

essential in prescribing appropriate seating and positioning. When using the HAAT model, the functional use of the body can be assessed with the knowledge of the activity the client would like or needs to perform. The determination of function will lead to the seating and positioning necessary to complete the activity, and therefore will determine the assistive technology required. Although a mat is the preferred location for this assessment, it may also be completed on a similar firm and flat surface. The following items should be tested in supine and sitting.

Head and Neck Position

When looking at the head and neck position, the OT should determine if the client can maintain adequate head control to interact with the environment. If a client is unable to maintain adequate head control, the OT will document postural deformities (e.g., flexed, extended, rotated, laterally flexed, and hyperextension), if and how a given deformity affects other body regions (e.g., the trunk or pelvis) and recommendations for accommodative positioning. Although an upright and forward facing position of the head is preferable, tolerance of this position must be assessed. It should also be determined if the head position changes the visual field, induces spasms, or increases agitation. Headrest and overall positioning options can be recommended from these findings.

Upper Extremity Function

When looking at the upper extremities, active range of motion (AROM) and passive range of motion (PROM) for all planes of motion will be evaluated with limitations noted. Manual muscle testing should be performed if it is not contraindicated. Gross motor coordination, as well as dexterity/fine motor coordination, should also be determined. During this assessment, the functional use of the upper extremities will be established for propulsion of the mobility device being prescribed. The presence of abnormal muscle tone or primitive reflexes, and how these findings impact a client's function is also documented. Manual versus power wheelchair, use of a scooter, safe use of a joystick versus the need for specialty controls, and a specific joystick handle are some of the options that will be decided by upper extremity function. The style of armrest (e.g., arm pad versus arm trough, and height adjustable) will also be determined by these findings.

Trunk Position

The trunk should be assessed while the client is seated on a firm and flat surface, and postural deformities should be documented (e.g., kyphosis, lordosis, scoliosis, and trunk rotation). It should also be noted if postural asymmetries are fixed or flexible. Static and dynamic movements and associated findings (e.g., muscle spasms and abnormal muscle tone), as well as the impact on client positioning and function, are also assessed in the seated position. The overall findings (e.g., postural deformities, spasms, abnormal muscle tone, and functional movement) will assist the OT with backrest and cushion selection, as well as other wheelchair components as discussed below.

Pelvis Position

Pelvic positioning is extremely important because the position of the pelvis will affect all other seated postures. Postures to note include anterior or posterior pelvic tilt, pelvic obliquity (i.e., as described by the low side), and pelvic rotation, as well as fixed or flexible deformities. Flexible postural deformities can be determined while assessing the deformity through positioning changes, posture, and balance. Pelvic position findings will be used to select the backrest and seat cushion, as well as other components of the wheelchair as discussed below.

Hip and Foot Position and Lower Extremity Function

Positioning of the hip will affect positioning of the pelvis, which is determined and documented during the assessment of lower extremity and pelvic ROM. It should also be noted that an abducted or adducted hip joint and/or a windswept deformity (i.e., specifically for children with cerebral palsy) may be indicative of a hip dislocation. ROM should be assessed with the client supine on a mat with the hips placed in flexion and the knees flexed to determine the functional seating position. PROM and AROM should be assessed for all planes of lower extremity motion and manual muscle testing should be completed if not contraindicated. Hamstring flexibility deficits should be documented to address proper positioning of the lower extremities (e.g., pressure redistribution and positioning). Foot position (e.g., neutral,

dorsi-flexed, plantar-flexed, inverted, and everted) and ROM are also measured and documented in this position. Lower extremity ROM, strength, and endurance will be critical determinants for bilateral lower extremity self-propulsion, the use of a hemiparetic technique (e.g., one arm and one leg on the same side of the body), or justification for a power wheelchair.

Spasticity and Muscle Tone

Although spasticity and abnormal muscle tone are evaluated throughout the mat assessment, the location, effect on function, and effect on seating should be determined and clearly documented to prescribe and justify the mobility device being recommended.

Measuring the Client

After completing functional positioning and ROM assessments, measurements of the client need to be taken for the proper size of the equipment being recommended. These measurements should be taken on a firm, flat surface such as a mat (Buck, 2011; Cook & Polgar, 2014). The following is a list of necessary measurements:

- Hip width
- Hip to popliteal fossa
- Shoulder width
- Chest width
- Chest depth
- Knee to heel
- Inferior angle of scapula to mat
- Axilla to mat
- Top of shoulder to mat
- Top of head to mat
- Elbow to mat
- Elbow to wrist and finger tip
- Foot length and width

When learning how to measure, a common approach is to add 2 inches to the measured hip width and take away 2 inches from the measured seat depth. Clinically, there are many practical and functional implications that must be interpreted by the OT when performing wheelchair seating and mobility assessments. For example, the risk of postural deformities or pressure injuries due to incorrect positioning, or increased shoulder pain or overuse injuries secondary to inappropriate seat width and depth.

Activities and Participation

Basic and Instrumental Activities of Daily Living Status and the Use of a Mobility Device

Basic activities of daily living (BADLs) are defined as "activities oriented toward taking care of one's own body" (American Occupational Therapy Association [AOTA], 2014, p. S19). These activities include bathing, toileting, dressing, swallowing/eating, feeding, and functional mobility. Instrumental activities of daily living (IADLs) are "activities to support daily life within the home and community that often require more complex interactions than those used in BADLs" (AOTA, 2014, p. S19). These activities include care of others, care of pets, child-rearing, driving and community mobility, financial management, and home management. BADLs and IADLs in regard to mobility-related activities of daily living (MRADLs) are an essential part of any wheelchair justification. The Department of Health and Human Services (2011) describes MRADLs as toileting, feeding, dressing, grooming, and bathing in the customary locations of the home. While this is important in the overall assessment of the individual, it is irrelevant if they cannot get to the customary location of the home independently, safely, and in a timely manner. The movement from point A to point B to perform or participate in the activity is a critical piece of evidence that must be evaluated to demonstrate a mobility limitation (Piriano, 2010). When addressing activities of daily living (ADLs), it should be noted how each activity is completed, where they are completed, and how much assistance is required to complete them. It should also be noted how each activity would be assisted by a recommended mobility device.

Environment and Current Technology

Current Wheelchair Seating and Mobility

If a client does not have equipment for wheeled seating, it should be noted, as well as any ambulatory device the client may be using. If a wheelchair is being used for mobility, the make, model, size, and age of the wheelchair, along with the propulsion method should be identified. The cushion, backrest, and necessary accessory items should also be noted in the same manner. The device should then be evaluated for safety and any repairs that may be required. Necessary repairs should be documented to determine whether the wheelchair should be repaired or replaced. If replacement is identified as most appropriate (e.g., cost-effective), the OT and the client should discuss likes versus dislikes of the current system to assist with the determination of a new wheelchair that will allow for increased function in the client's environment.

Home Environment

It is necessary to determine function, as well as accessibility essential for the completion of MRADLs within the client's home environment. The type of dwelling should be noted (e.g., house, apartment, senior living center, assisted-living, and long-term care). For example, if the client lives in a senior living center, accessibility information such as the location of the dining and laundry rooms and the client's mailbox should be identified (i.e., as applicable). Equally, if a client lives in a house, apartment, or condominium, similar information will need to be identified, including wheelchair accessibility within and to the home (e.g., ramp, stairs, and mechanical lift). If stairs are present, the number of stairs should be noted, as well as how the client is currently managing the stairs (e.g., gluteal bumping, ambulating, and family assistance). To best determine accessibility within the home environment, the durable medical equipment supplier or OT may be required to complete a home visit. This is often the best opportunity to complete a trial of the prescribed wheelchair. The OT should evaluate the client's functional abilities within the home with a focus on how the physical environment enables or constrains function (Rigby, Stark, Letts, & Ringaert, 2009).

Transportation and Community Involvement

Significant issues in determining the appropriate wheelchair are transportation and community access. In regard to transportation, it is important to know if the client is a passenger or an independent driver, as well as the type of vehicle in which they are being transported. If they are an independent driver, the OT should also note how they are driving and if they drive from a wheelchair or a car seat. Important considerations for those who drive from the wheelchair include visual field and functional reach. The OT should also document if a client was formally driving or is planning to return to or become an independent driver, as this will likely affect wheelchair and equipment recommendations. When applicable, necessary adaptations to the vehicle should be documented (e.g., ramps, lifts, tie downs, lock-down systems, and hand controls). Transfer needs within the vehicle are also important to document, which includes how and/or who is placing the wheelchair into the vehicle. Community access should look at school, work, IADLs, and leisure activities, including the environments where these actions take place.

Clinical Criteria

After the above factors are assessed and documented, specific clinical criteria will assist with the determination of the appropriate equipment, as well as assist with the justification required for the equipment. Clinical criteria include:

- Mobility limitations causing an inability to participate in MRADLs.
- An inability to ambulate safely or functionally, and/or cognitive or sensory deficits that can be accommodated to allow for the safe use of a mobility device necessary to participate in MRADLs.
- The ability or potential ability to safely use the mobility device.
- Environmental support for the use of the mobility device.
- Sufficient function or ability to use the recommended equipment (e.g., the least restrictive device).

Equipment Recommendations

Psychosocial Issues—Rejection of Equipment

Rejection of equipment or technology abandonment is identified as "when the consumer stops using a device even though the need for which the device was obtained still exists" (Cook & Polgar, 2014, p. 113). Phillips and

Zhao (1993) identified four factors that significantly relate to the abandonment of technology: (1) failure of providers to take consumers' opinions into account, (2) easy device procurement, (3) poor device performance, and (4) changes in consumers' needs or priorities. Accordingly, the OT must consider psychosocial issues when determining the correct equipment for a client. Taking the HAAT model into consideration, each part of human, activity, and assistive technology intertwines with context. The context in which the individual uses the equipment (e.g., environment and activity) will determine continued and long-term utilization of the equipment. This context additionally includes the social context of peers and strangers, as well as a client's self-image. A negative self-image and the loss of independence can lead to other psychosocial issues. With such factors considered, equipment that was determined in concert with the client and the client's wants and needs can decrease psychosocial risks. Lastly, clients must agree they will use the recommended equipment for it to be a proper recommendation.

Mobility Skills and Balance

Mobility skills include, but are not limited to, ambulation, wheelchair propulsion, transfer technique, and function. During a wheelchair assessment, the type of transfer performed, as well as the safety and amount of assistance required, should be considered as the OT chooses the most appropriate equipment. This information will assist in identifying the appropriate wheelchair components on, and frame style of, the prescribed wheelchair.

Ambulation is the first step. If the client can safely and functionally ambulate without a device on a routine and regular basis, no wheeled mobility should be provided. For an evaluation of functional ambulation, consider all ADLs the person will perform while walking. For example, this may include tasks of divided attention and carrying necessary objects. To function without the assistance of another person or device, a client must be able to walk and carry objects within the home environment, which includes the ability to attend to distractions (e.g., ambient noises and a visual field with a variety of items or obstacles in it).

If the client is unstable without a device, determination of a cane or walker for safety is the next step in the mobility assessment. "Functional ambulation integrates ambulation into ADLs and IADLs. By using an occupation-based approach, the OT assesses the client's abilities within the performance context and with an understating of the client, habits, routines, and roles" (Bolding, Adler, Tipton-Burton, & Verran, 2013, p. 239). Within the determination of functional ambulation, ambulation of household distances and history of falls should also be noted. If the client has a history of falls, frequency and cause are important factors. Subsequent injuries should be stated. Medical contraindications associated with a diagnosis, such as fatigue associated with multiple sclerosis or amyotrophic lateral sclerosis, may also be justification for wheeled mobility, despite completing functional ambulation at the time of the assessment. Functional ambulation should be independent with no assistance from a caregiver, including caregiver supervision for safety. If the client is unable to functionally ambulate on their own, with or without an assistive device, then wheeled mobility should be the option chosen.

Once ambulation has been assessed and ruled out as the main form of independent self-mobility, the manual wheelchair assessment would be the next step. Within this step, each type of manual wheelchair should be considered. The client should use a manual wheelchair on a trial basis to assess their ability to functionally propel on multiple surfaces, including tile, carpet, and over thresholds. The trials should take into consideration the time of day when the person is most fatigued and would need the greatest mobility assistance. If a manual wheelchair is the most appropriate option, delineation between frame styles is necessary. Basic considerations include frame style (i.e., folding frame versus rigid frame), frame seat to floor height (i.e., standard height wheelchair frame versus hemi-height wheelchair frame), and frame weight (i.e., standard, lightweight, and ultra-lightweight frames). If it is not possible, nor reasonable to self-propel a manual wheelchair, a scooter or power-operated vehicle (POV) is the next consideration.

In order to safely use a scooter/POV, the use of bilateral upper extremities with fine motor coordination is a necessity. The client should also be able to safely transfer onto the captain style seat safely, and maneuver around the tiller style control device. Supportive positioning is not possible within this device, so postural issues that required support would rule out a POV. If these qualifications cannot be met, then a power mobility device may be the next consideration.

When considering power mobility, the lower level devices must be ruled out as nonfunctional for the client. For power mobility, a client must be able to demonstrate safe and functional use as determined by the therapy team, caregivers, and client themselves. Considerations will include frame style, seating system needs (e.g., positioning and power seating functions), and a driver input device.

It is important to understand the difference between a group 2 power wheelchair and a group 3 power wheelchair. These are groupings used by Medicare and are dependent on the features of the wheelchair. A group 2 power wheelchair can accommodate one power option at a time and not all models can address this need. It can accommodate off the shelf backrests and cushions for positioning needs. These wheelchairs typically have smaller drive wheels and are less stable with decreased shock absorption, which additionally increases vibration throughout the wheelchair. This could increase spasms and muscle tone for some individuals. The group 3 power wheelchairs have the ability to upgrade an electronics system allowing for increased programming of the wheelchair, as well as the ability to continue to utilize the wheelchair for a person with a progressive diagnosis. Medicare requires the individual to have a mobility limitation due to a neurologic condition, myopathy, or congenital skeletal deformity. This type of wheelchair has increased the ability to address positioning needs. It has larger drive wheels with increased shock absorption, which reduces vibration throughout the wheelchair, as well as vibratory effects perceived by the client.

Significant to all these choices, manual wheelchair, scooter, and power wheelchair considerations, the ability to perform independent, adequate, and functional weight shifts or pressure redistribution is a necessity. Examples of these weight shifts include safe standing, lateral/anterior lean, and push-up techniques. With the manual wheelchair and scooter, the person must be able to perform their own weight shifts with an appropriate frequency and time frame throughout regular and routine use of the equipment. The manual wheelchair and the POV have no ability to assist with weight shifts. Within a power wheelchair, power tilt, power recline, and power-elevating leg rests are all positioning options that may be used for pressure redistribution. Some group 2 power wheelchairs have the ability to add a power seating system. Stability and client needs should be considered as this system is limited to one power seating option.

Group 3 power wheelchairs or rehabilitation seating provides the ability for increased stability, decreased vibration, single and multiple power functions, and the ability to utilize specialty controls.

Determining Items for the Seating System

A seating system does not just consist of a wheelchair. Each component placed within a system addresses a postural or functional need. A seating system consists of the wheelchair, backrest, cushion, trunk supports, pelvic supports, leg rests, armrests, headrests, and other parts. Not all of these parts may be needed for every wheelchair and the assessment is used to determine the appropriate components for each client. The following will describe the types of components available; however, this is not a comprehensive list.

Manual Wheelchairs

Manual wheelchairs are classified into different groups by the Paralyzed Veterans Administration Recommendations for Preservation of Upper Limb Function. The standard wheelchair is designed for short-term hospital or institutional use, weighs greater than 35 pounds, and is not adjustable. The lightweight wheelchair weighs 30–35 pounds and has minimal adjustability. The ultra-lightweight or custom manual wheelchair weighs less than 30 pounds, and has several options of adjustability for client positioning and functional mobility.

The standard and lightweight wheelchairs are folding frame wheelchairs. However, ultra-lightweight wheelchairs can have either a folding or a rigid frame. Other categories of manual wheelchairs include a tilt-in-space and/or a reclining wheelchair. These chairs are commonly used for individuals who are unable to propel a manual wheelchair, cannot use a power wheelchair, have poor postural control, and/or are unable to reposition themselves for weight shifts. This style of wheelchair can also include a combination of tilt and recline.

When determining the use of a manual wheelchair versus a power wheelchair for a client, it is important to address questions such as, "Does the user have sufficient strength and endurance to propel the chair at home and in the community over varied terrain, and what will be the long-term effects of the propulsion choice" (Bolding et al., 2013, p. 244).

Power Wheelchairs

POVs/scooters might be used for a client who has difficulty walking or a decreased ability to propel a manual wheelchair. If this individual displays full AROM of both upper extremities and has no positioning needs, the scooter might be the right mobility device. They should also be able to transfer safely onto the device and display the cognitive skills to use it safely. Home access is also a deciding factor as a scooter has a longer wheelbase than a power wheelchair. This wheelbase increases the turning radius of the device.

Decreased upper extremity function, trunk stability, skin integrity, or safety with transfers may be a determining factor in moving into a power wheelchair option. The first power wheelchair option is a consumer power wheelchair, which has limited client positing capabilities (e.g., can only accommodate one power positioning actuator) and is less stable as compared to higher end options. A consumer power wheelchair also possesses less capable shock absorption, which may increase tone or spasticity in some individuals. For individuals with issues such as increased positioning needs, the need for multiple power seat functions, and limited upper extremity function that would require specialty controls, a power wheelchair with rehabilitation seating would be most appropriate.

Power wheelchairs are designed in three different configurations: rear-wheel drive, mid-wheel drive, and front-wheel drive. Within a rear-wheel-drive configuration, the wheelchair is more stable at top speeds and therefore can reach a higher speed than mid- or front-wheel chairs. The disadvantage is the larger turning radius. The mid-wheel-drive wheelchair has the smallest turning radius. It is ideal for maneuvering in small places and is more stable than front-wheel drive at top speeds. The disadvantage of this wheelchair is the front and rear casters. These can get caught up on curbs or rough terrains. The front-wheel-drive wheelchair is ideal for rough terrains and climbing curbs. The disadvantages of this wheelchair are the slow top speed and it often has a higher learning curve for use.

Each model can accommodate a stationary seat or power tilt, power recline, and/or power-elevating leg rests or foot platforms. These will be used for postural control, positioning, pressure redistribution, and functional tasks.

Seat Cushions

When determining the appropriate seat cushion, diagnosis, skin integrity, postural deformities, positioning needs, sensation, and the weight of the client should be considered. Cushions should distribute pressure evenly, provide a stable support surface for the pelvis and thighs, function effectively in different climates, dissipate heat and moisture, and manufactured using lightweight and durable materials. Medicare divides seat cushions into several basic groups. The most common include general use cushions, skin protection cushions, positioning cushions, and some combination of skin and positioning cushion features together. The skin protection and positioning cushions come in multiple materials such as foam, gel, fluid, and air. Each of these has different characteristics that may interact with each individual differently, impacting their body structures, positioning, and function, along with their engagement within the environment.

Backrests

The purpose of a backrest is to promote pelvic posture, increase spinal extension, decrease lateral trunk leaning, enhance cardiopulmonary function, provide support to decrease reliance on the upper extremities to maintain upright positioning, increase functional reach, provide a base for neck and head control, increase efficiency of wheelchair propulsion, substitute for weak or absent muscles, and decrease the risk of postural deformities. The backrest can also provide a point of relaxation, as well as provide the support and stabilization needed for dynamic movement to increase function. When determining the backrest for a client, diagnosis, postural deformities/positioning needs, back height, lateral support, and back angle should be considered. Each of these may be different for each client depending on the needs of each individual.

Documentation and Funding Issues

Documentation should be client-specific and refer to the client's identified challenges and goals, while providing a clear account of the client's physical, functional, and environmental needs. Documentation should also include limitations of any equipment currently used by the client, the intended goals of the new wheelchair and seating technology, the recommendations made based on the assessment, and the rationale for those

recommendations (Arledge et al., 2011). This information is gathered within the wheelchair seating and mobility assessment and used to pursue funding for equipment.

Medicare Considerations

Medicare is administered by the federal government, and the rules are the same for every state in the nation. [It] is a health insurance program for four groups: (1) individuals age 65 years or older; (2) people of all ages who meet the standards of disability under the Social Security Act; (3) the disabled children of persons who had been working and who became disabled themselves, died, or retired at age 65 years; and (4) people with end-stage renal disease. (Cook & Polgar, 2014, p. 61)

Medicare reimbursement for assistive technology is based on eligibility, coverage, and medical necessity, and excludes items and features deemed as being unnecessary (i.e., for personal comfort, convenience, or custodial care).

Medicaid Considerations

The primary goal of Medicaid is to provide medical assistance to persons in need and to furnish them with rehabilitation and other services to help them gain or maintain independence. Medicaid is not a federally mandated program. Instead, states must elect to participate and express their desire to do so by submitting a state plan for medical assistance to CMS. (Cook & Polgar, 2014, p. 60)

Other Reimbursement Sources

Other sources of funding may be private insurance that is obtained through employment or private purchase. Vocational rehabilitation services, service clubs, private foundations, or other volunteer organizations may also be funding sources for assistive technology.

Referrals and Discharge Considerations

OTs work closely with qualified and trained wheelchair vendors for wheeled seating and mobility services, and refer to appropriate healthcare professionals for any additional recommendations as needed. Whether wheeled seating and mobility services are specialized or a part of the client's initial treatment plan, discharge most often occurs once the client is functional and independent with their wheeled seating and mobility equipment. If the client was receiving occupational therapy for additional areas of occupation, treatment may continue even after function and independence in wheeled seating and mobility has been achieved.

Management and Standards of Practice

Wheelchair seating and mobility evaluation and recommendations are part of an OT's treatment plan, which includes training necessary to ensure the client is functional and capable of performing their necessary MRADLs, client-equipment safety precautions and final fitting, and delivery of the equipment.

Occupational therapy practitioners should teach their clients about routine and regular cleaning and follow-up maintenance for their equipment, who to schedule follow-up appointments with, and to routinely have their equipment reassessed by their physicians and clinicians for its fitness and functioning.

Outcome measures are necessary in order to compare seating and mobility technology (e.g., existing vs. recommended) at the individual level, its impact on quality of life, and to evaluate the effectiveness of the overall service delivery structure and process (Cook & Polgar, 2014).

When addressing standards of practice, it is important for an OT to follow the Occupational Therapy Code of Ethics (Code). The first principle in the Code states that occupational therapy personnel must address the well-being and safety of all clients (AOTA, 2015). One of the related standards of conduct focuses on the importance of education and training to ensure competence and services within the occupational therapy's scope of practice (AOTA, 2015). Although introductory wheelchair seating and positioning education is provided within the curriculum of OT education, it should be noted that not all clients will be able to sit within a basic system. It is important to receive further education for intermediate and advanced seating systems to decrease the risk of potential medical issues for individuals being served.

Other ethical situations that may arise include providing documentation that would lead a funding source to pay for an unnecessary device or allowing documentation to be completed by someone other than the therapist with the therapist signing off in agreement. All documentation should be truthful and written by the evaluating clinician. Documentation cannot be accurately completed without a full evaluation of the client by the OT.

Due to the evaluative nature of wheelchair seating and positioning, the occupational therapy assistant (OTA) must be aware of licensure and regulatory guidelines surrounding the area of seating and mobility. For instance, the Rehab Engineering and Assistive Technology Society of North America (RESNA) has Assistive Technology Practitioner and Seating and Mobility Specialist certification for both the OT and the OTA. However, state licensure, payer requirements, and scope of practice will dictate the practitioner requirements for seating and mobility care. As with any evaluation process, an OT and OTA should follow the standard rules and regulations according to their professional licensure. Together, they collaborate on specific goals written into the client's treatment plan. The OTA should give input, and document accordingly, on the equipment's impact on the client's function, ability to perform ADLs, and the capability to use trialed equipment as observed during client treatment sessions. An OTA must consult with the OT regarding any modifications made to the equipment.

After the evaluation process is complete, further training for use of the device can be completed by the OTA, and they can also provide information during this time in regard to fitness and functioning for the OT to further address upon reevaluation.

Summary

There are many goals to consider when evaluating and prescribing wheeled seating and mobility. These goals include special attention to posture, comfort, respiration, skin integrity, prevention of further injury and deformity, while addressing existing conditions (Dudgeon, Deitz, & Dimpfel, 2014). In addition, it is critical to facilitate vision readiness, limb use, functional access, and performance throughout various environments, while paying special attention to cosmetics (Dudgeon et al., 2014).

Understanding the implications of proper versus improper seating will allow the therapist to minimize risk factors for medical issues for each client. Completing a comprehensive physical and functional evaluation will provide the needed information to address the needs of each individual.

Chapter 34 Self-Study Activities (Answers Are Provided at the End of the Chapter)

1. A 20-year-old client presents to a clinic with a diagnosis of T4 paraplegia and a history of ischial pressure injuries that are currently closed.
   A. Would you recommend a manual or power wheelchair and why?
   B. What are the advantages and disadvantages of a folding frame wheelchair versus a rigid frame wheelchair?
   C. List three cushion types that may be appropriate for this client?

2. A 65-year-old with C6 tetraplegia, who has used a manual wheelchair for 15 years, presents to the clinic with complaints of bilateral shoulder pain, as well as increased fatigue due to a recent diagnosis of congestive heart failure.
   A. What type of wheelchair would you recommend and why?
   B. What are the pros and cons of a power-operated wheelchair compared to a manual wheelchair for this individual?
   C. What environmental considerations should you take into consideration?

3. A 41-year-old woman with multiple sclerosis is able to ambulate with a walker; however, she reports multiple falls, and shortness of breath during and immediately following walking short distances. She lives alone in a house with two steps to enter. She has had two exacerbations in the last six months with significant progression of her disease and weakness in her bilateral upper and lower extremities.
   A. What factors are important to address within her environment before providing a wheelchair?
   B. What cognitive considerations should be made before providing a wheelchair?

   C. What are the psychological considerations (e.g., willing to accept transition of walker vs. manual wheelchair vs. scooter or power wheelchair)?
   D. Using principles of the HAAT, what are the major issues surrounding the client that affect her use of a wheelchair?

4. An 8-year-old boy with cerebral palsy presents to the clinic with his parents for a wheelchair evaluation. He is unable to ambulate and has only used a stroller with his parents pushing him prior to this evaluation.
   A. What environments should be considered?
   B. What developmental issues should be considered?
   C. What type of wheelchair will increase his function and activity during his life roles?
   D. From whom is the information for the evaluation gathered?

5. A 70-year-old male with expressive aphasia and left-sided hemiparesis post stroke comes to the clinic with his 80-year-old wife. It is noted he is using a cane and his wife's physical assistance to help him come into the clinic, and has many bruises on his hemiparetic arm which is hanging at his side. His wife communicates for him as his challenges with aphasia and apraxia make it difficult for him to communicate in the new clinic environment. She reports he remains in his lazy boy recliner all day, and requires her help to move about the home to perform tasks such as going to the bathroom.
   A. What is the best method of evaluation for this client?
   B. What type of mobility device will increase his function and safety for MRADLs?
   C. What postural concerns would you look at for this man?
   D. What environmental access questions would be important for this couple?

6. Label the following parts of a standard wheelchair using the provided figure (**Figure 34-1**).

Seat back	Mag wheel	Arm rest pad	Caster
Rear tire	Caster fork	Side panel	Footplate
Hand rim	Heel loop	Seat upholstery	Crossbar
Wheel lock	Push handles	Leg/foot rest	

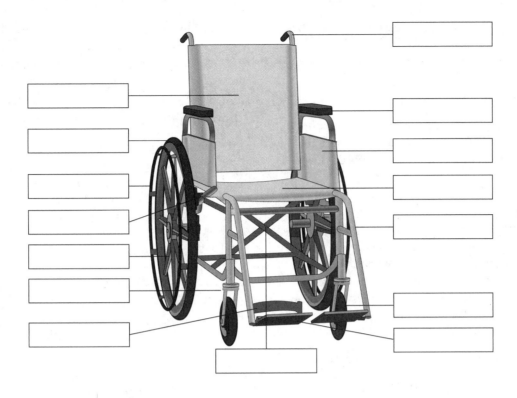

Figure 34-1

Chapter 34 Self-Study Answers

Question 1

A. Recommend a manual wheelchair secondary to a young male with no upper extremity issues. The manual wheelchair will allow for increased accessibility. At this level, he should be able to adequately perform pressure relief and position changes, as well as higher level wheelchair skills, such as wheelies, fall recovery, and stair bumping.

B. An advantage of the folding frame wheelchair is that it will fold for easy transport. A disadvantage is that it is heavier than a rigid frame and it has more movable parts, which cause increased maintenance issues. An advantage of the rigid frame wheelchair is that it is lighter in weight than a folding frame wheelchair, requires less maintenance, is easier to transport, and has fewer movable parts, which decrease the shock to the shoulder joint and spine. A disadvantage is that it does not have removable parts, such as

footrests, which may make it more difficult for some clients to perform transfers because it limits the ability to place the feet on the ground.

C. Three cushion types that may be appropriate for the client are air filled, dense foam with fluid overlay, and viscoelastic foam.

Question 2

A. A power wheelchair is recommended secondary to the cardiac and respiratory issues he is facing with the congestive heart failure, as well as shoulder overuse injuries.

B. A power wheelchair will decrease the stress on his shoulders and heart, will conserve energy, and provide increased function and independence. It could pose accessibility issues within the home and community, as well as transportation issues. A manual wheelchair will increase the current shoulder overuse injury, as well as his risk for heart attack and stroke due to the new diagnosis. His current environment is set up for a manual wheelchair to decrease accessibility issues.

C. Environments to address would be home, transportation, work (i.e., if not retired), community, and family environments he frequents.

Question 3

A. Accessibility into and throughout the home (e.g., ramp and doorways), life roles (e.g., work, family, leisure interests, BADLs, IADLs, MRADLs), and transportation needs.
B. Problem-solving, memory, safety/judgment, and topographical orientation.
C. Mood/coping skills and accepting the progressive nature of the disease. The therapist will need to address issues of mobility with the client's present and future needs, as well as a discussion with the client to develop an understanding and acceptance of the recommended device.
D. Human: lives alone, cognitive status?
E. Activity: life roles?
F. AT: What device will be used (e.g., manual wheelchair, scooter, or power wheelchair)?
G. Context: Where will the device be utilized (e.g., home, work, or community)?

Question 4

A. Home, school, and playground/community.
B. Piaget's stages of human development (i.e., concrete operations). Children begin logical thinking surrounding concrete objects and activities. Can complete complex tasks with several steps forward and backward (e.g., using a dial in one direction to turn speed up and opposite direction to turn speed down). Can classify and sort objects by characteristics. Realizes multiple solutions for problem-solving.
C. A power-operated wheelchair with a power seat elevator will allow for increased interactions with peers and increased mobility throughout all environments. Limitations may include transportation of a power wheelchair by the parents, ability to

install ramps at home for access, and the child's ability to safely maneuver the wheelchair.
D. Child, parents, caregiver, teacher, school-based clinicians, and wheelchair supplier.

Question 5

A. What is the best method of evaluation for this client? Considering the client's aphasia and apraxia, a functional movement evaluation will be the most direct form of evaluation. Trialing the recommended equipment with the client will give you the clearest information.
B. What type of mobility device will increase his function and safety with MRADLs? The client requires the use of an assistive device and assistance from his wife. The bruising on his hemiparetic arm may indicate he is on blood thinners and/or may have poor sensation on that side. He may also have left neglect. A manual wheelchair would be the first consideration. Evaluation of a hemi-height wheelchair would be important to see if he can propel himself within the home.
C. What postural concerns would you look at for this man? Support of his hemiparetic side is important. This may require a cushion and backrest that facilitate improved posture, along with an arm trough or lap tray to support his impaired arm. Sensation will also need to be assessed on his hemiparetic side, and consideration of a pressure redistributing cushion. He may also display postural deformities such as a pelvic obliquity and scoliosis.
D. What environmental access questions would be important for this couple? It will be important for this client to be able to transfer in and out of the wheelchair to his lazy boy recliner, push himself around the home, and move in and out of the bathroom. It is also important to consider transportation and the wife's ability to get the wheelchair in and out of the car effectively.

Question 6

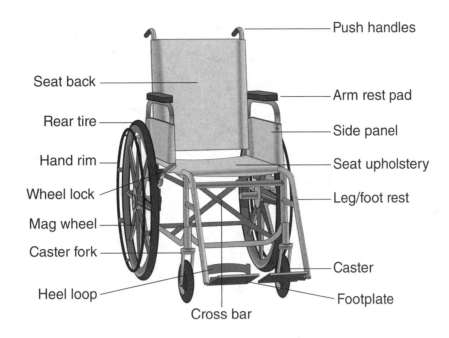

Push handles

Seat back

Arm rest pad

Rear tire

Side panel

Hand rim

Seat upholstery

Wheel lock

Leg/foot rest

Mag wheel

Caster fork

Caster

Heel loop

Footplate

Cross bar

Figure 34-2

References

American Occupational Therapy Association. (2014). Occupational therapy practice framework: Domain and process (3rd ed.). *American Journal of Occupational Therapy, 68*(Suppl. 1), S1–S48. doi:10.5014/ajot.2014.682006

American Occupational Therapy Association. (2015). Occupational therapy code of ethics. *American Journal of Occupational Therapy, 69*(Suppl. 3). doi:10.5014/ajot.2015.696S03

Arledge, S., Armstrong, W., Babinec, M., Dicianno, B. E., Digiovine, C., Dyson-Hudson, T., & Stogner, J. (2011). *RESNA wheelchair service provision guide*. Retrieved from http://www.resna.org/sites/default/files/legacy/resources/position-papers/RESNAWheelchairService ProvisionGuide.pdf

Baum, C. M., & Christiansen, C. (2005). Person-environment-occupation-performance: An occupation-based framework for practice. In C. Christiansen, C. M. Baum, & J. Bass-Haugen (Eds.), *Occupational therapy: Performance, participation, and well-being* (3rd ed., pp. 243–259). Thorofare, NJ: SLACK.

Bolding, D., Adler, C., Tipton-Burton, M., & Verran, A. (2013). Mobility. In H. M. Pendleton & W. Schultz-Krohn (Eds.),*Pedretti's occupational therapy: Practice skills for physical dysfunction* (7th ed., pp. 233–294). St. Louis, MO: Elsevier.

Buck, S. (2011). *More than 4 wheels: Applying clinical practice to seating, mobility, and assistive technology.* Milton, ON: Therapy NOW!

Bunning, M. E. (2009). Assistive technology and wheeled mobility. In E. B. Crepeau, E. S. Cohn, & B. A. B. Schell (Eds.), *Willard & Spackman's occupational therapy* (11th ed., pp. 850–867). Philadelphia, PA: Wolters Kluwer Health/Lippincott Williams & Wilkins.

Cook, A. M., & Polgar, J. M. (2014). *Assistive technologies: Principles and practice* (4th ed.). St. Louis, MI: Elsevier/Mosby.

Department of Health and Human Services. (2011). *Fact sheet: Power mobility (PMDs): Complying with documentation and coverage requirements*. Retrieved from https://www.cms.gov/Research-Statistics-Data-and-Systems/Monitoring-Programs/CERT/Downloads/PMD_DocCvg_FactSheet_ICN905063_Sept2011.pdf

Dudgeon, B. J., Deitz, J. C., & Dimpfel, M. (2014). Wheelchair selection. In M. V. Radomski & C. A. T. Latham (Eds.), *Occupational therapy for physical dysfunction* (7th ed., pp. 495–519). Philadelphia, PA: Wolters Kluwer Health/Lippincott Williams & Wilkins.

National Pressure Ulcer Advisory Panel. (2016). *Pressure injury stages*. Retrieved from: http://www.npuap.org /resources/educational-and-clinical-resources /npuap-pressure-injury-stages/

Phillips, B., & Zhao, H. (1993). Predictors of assistive technology abandonment. *Assistive Technology, 5*(1), 36–45. doi:10.1080/10400435.1993.10132205

Piriano, J. (2010). *Clinical and documentation demands for mobility-related activities of daily living*. Retrieved from http://www.hme-business.com/Articles/2010 /09/01/Minding-MRADLs.aspx

Rigby, P., Stark, S., Letts, L., & Ringaert, L. (2009). Physical environments. In E. B. Crepeau, E. S. Cohn, & B. A. B. Schell (Eds.), *Willard & Spackman's occupational therapy* (11th ed., pp. 820–849). Philadelphia, PA: Wolters Kluwer Health/Lippincott Williams & Wilkins.

World Health Organization. (2015). *International classification of functioning, disability and health (ICF)*. Retrieved from http://www.who.int/classifications/icf /icf_more/en/

Assistive Technology, Driver Rehabilitation, Home, and Community Mobility

CHAPTER
35

Donna Case

Learning Objectives

- Define assistive technology (AT).
- Define universal design.
- Recognize the role of AT on facilitating participation in meaningful occupations.
- Determine the importance of appropriate AT selection and provision.
- Recognize basic AT solutions for optimal safety and independence in activities of daily living and instrumental activities of daily living.
- Describe the different conceptual framework models that driver rehabilitation specialists use.
- Describe the importance of the International Classification of Functioning, Disability, and Health on the field of AT and driver rehabilitation.
- Describe the role that driver strategies and driving tactics may play in optimizing driver, passenger, and pedestrian safety.

Key Terms

- *Certified driver rehabilitation specialist (CDRS)*: Assists clients of all ages and abilities to explore transportation solutions for drivers with disabilities.
- *Infrared (IR)*: Invisible radiant energy that can be used to remotely control electronics.
- *QWERTY layout*: The keyboard layout based on the original keyboard where the top left row of the keyboard from left to right reads Q-W-E-R-T-Y.
- *Universal design*: Accessibility of all environments for people with and without disabilities.
- *Word prediction*: A feature that predicts a word or word phrase based on input of limited characters.

Introduction

This chapter includes: (1) An overview of assistive technology (AT) and how it promotes occupation, and (2) driver rehabilitation, home, and community mobility. Determining a definition of AT can be difficult as every federal law defines AT differently. However, most laws contain portions of the following definition of AT: "any item, piece of equipment, or product system, whether acquired commercially off the shelf, modified, or customized, that is used to increase, maintain, or improve functional capabilities" (Individuals with Disabilities Education Improvement Act of 2004, p. 2652). AT can be used for habilitation or rehabilitation and may be used in combination. AT changes rapidly and can therefore make it difficult to stay current in practice. In addition, AT overlaps with technology utilized by people without known disabilities and thus can become more accessible to clients with disabilities. Occupational therapy practitioners should focus on characteristics of technology and matching it with the strengths and needs of the client.

Universal Design

Universal design is the design of products, environments, or teaching so that the majority of people can use it without the need for specialized design or adaptation. It grew out of the accessible design movement that focused on designing environments for persons with disabilities. While the accessible design movement focused solely on principles to facilitate access for clients with disabilities, universal design benefits all people. AT can utilize both accessible and universal design principles (Cook & Polgar, 2015).

Determining Appropriate Assistive Technology

Core to occupational therapy is the focus on the client as he or she functions within the environment. When an occupational therapist (OT) assesses the need for AT, the client is central to the process. The OT must address the environments in which the client customarily finds him or herself, what specific task(s) is important to a given situation, and what is needed by the client to be able to accomplish the desired tasks (Zabala, 2010). A key indicator for the identification of need for AT appears when there is a disconnect between what the client wants or needs to be able to do and the natural or environmental supports that exist. Clients with disabilities should be presented with an array of options that include low, medium, and high-tech options (Cook & Polgar, 2015).

Assistive Technology and Screening and Driver Rehab/Community Mobility Team Members

Various professionals are included in a client's treatment team with varying specialties based on the client's needs. These professionals may include the following:

- OT practitioners who may work as an AT practitioner (ATP) or certified driver rehabilitation specialist (CDRS).
- Speech and language pathologist.
- MSW (i.e., a social worker).
- Audiologist.
- Nurse.
- Physician.
- Seating and mobility specialist (may be an OT, occupational therapy assistant [OTA], physical therapist, or physical therapy assistant).
- Teacher or vocational counselor.
- Rehabilitation engineer.
- Suppliers (Cook & Polgar, 2015).

AT Screening and Assessments

Conceptual frameworks that are used by rehabilitation professionals play a key role in underpinning their evaluation procedures and guiding their observations, decisions, and intervention processes. The models that are most relevant for AT, home evaluation, and driver rehabilitation, include the following:

- Model of Human Occupation (Kielhofner & Janice, 1980).
- Student, Environments, Tasks, and Tools (SETT) Framework (Zabala, 2016).
- Person, Environment, Occupation Model (Law et al., 1996).
- Canadian Model of Occupational Performance (Law et al., 1990).

AT Interventions

AT assessment and intervention practice in occupational therapy is driven by the goals of the client, the strengths and needs of the client, and the environmental supports or barriers that need to be addressed in order to accomplish the overall goal(s). Structured interviews and questionnaires serve as important assessment tools in the identification of occupational performance within daily roles (Cook & Polgar, 2015). Successful AT provision addresses, but is not limited to, sensation, range of motion, strength, endurance, coordination, cognition, and culture to determine the most efficient and available AT devices for each specific client. Positioning, trunk, and pelvic control impact a client's interaction with AT and must be considered. When connecting the client with AT, the characteristics that are required by the client to complete the desired task should be matched to the properties of a specific AT device (Cook & Polgar, 2015).

Computer Access

AT has changed most rapidly in the area of computer access. Previously, most accommodations or AT solutions were added on to existing information exchange technology. In recent years, more accessibility solutions are included in new devices at the time of purchase. When determining computer access for clients with disabilities, it is important to begin with the basic modifications (Cook & Polgar, 2015). All computers, tablets, and most smartphones have accessible features built within their operating systems and occupational therapy practitioners should look into what is available before determining additional modifications or if AT is required. Computer access may be divided into categories as described in detail below.

Input Accommodations

Input addresses how the client accesses and controls what information is delivered to the device. Input can be achieved through several means including direct or indirect selection.

Direct Selection

Keyboards: There are a variety of mechanical keyboards commercially available (e.g., ergonomic, one handed, wireless, and alternative keyboard such as IntelliKeys); the most commonly used is the QWERTY layout keyboard (Anson, 2013; Bunning, 2014; Cook & Polgar, 2015). In contrast, the availability of touch screens facilitates on-screen keyboards (Anson, 2013; Bunning, 2014; Cook & Polgar, 2015).

Mouse: The most commonly used mouse has two buttons (i.e., left and right) and a movement sensor that allows the user to move a cursor on the computer screen. Movements are right, left, forward, and backward. A variety of adaptations include trackballs, foot mouse, and touchless. Mainstream technologies such as touch screens provide on-screen arrow keys and allow for swiping and tapping (Anson, 2013; Bunning, 2014; Cook & Polgar, 2015).

Indirect Selection

This manner of input is generally slower than direct selection and for this reason, direct selection is usually chosen if possible.

Scanning: The scanning selection set is presented on a display and each item is highlighted in a systematic manner. When the desired choice is highlighted, the client activates the selection through a variety of switch options (Cook & Polgar, 2015).

Speech recognition: Developed for clients with limited ability to access information technology, speech recognition technology has become a mainstream solution for individuals without known disabilities. This category is generally referred to as speech to text. Both platforms include a version of speech to text within its accessibility features. Some clients with disabilities are able to successfully interact with the information technology using input selection, while others may require additional software such as Dragon® NaturallySpeaking (Anson, 2013; Bunning, 2014; Cook & Polgar, 2015).

Rate enhancement: Allowing clients to generate a greater number of characters than the number of selections that are made, the most common rate enhancement is word prediction or word completion. Every operating system offers this enhancement, but for some clients a separate software program with greater opportunity for customization is required (Anson, 2013; Bunning, 2014; Cook & Polgar, 2015).

Output Accommodations

Output accommodations generally addresses the outcome of what is input on an information system. Output accommodations are built into most operating systems for clients with a variety of impairments and should be assessed first. Some clients require additional hardware and software to accommodate their desire for output information. Cook and Polgar (2015) describe these accommodations as follows:

- *Screen or text enlargement*: Utilized by clients without known disabilities and are essential for clients with visual impairments. When enlarging the screen or text the client's viewing section focus narrows.
- *Text to speech*: Developed for clients with visual impairments but has proved useful for clients with learning disabilities and those for whom English is a second language.
- *Braille displays and embossing tools*: Accommodations that are added to information technology after purchase.
- *Adaptive cursors or signals*: Included in the accommodation section of most operating systems.
- *Auditory signals*: Can be added to visual signals for clients with visual impairments.

Augmentative and Alternative Communication Devices

Augmentative and alternative communication (AAC) devices allow clients who have difficulty with expressive language to communicate with others. Options range from very low-tech devices such as paper and pencil, alphabet boards, American Sign Language, and gestures to high-tech devices that generate speech. The following must be considered when determining the appropriate AAC device.

Speech: Synthesized speech is generated electronically by the AAC device. The voice may require familiarity with it to understand what is actually being said. Digitized speech is recorded human speech that is recalled when the user desires to communicate a specific word, thought, or sound.

Display: A static display consistently displays the same menu for the user regardless of the situation or environment. A dynamic display is one in which the selection set that is presented to the user changes as new choices are made, and has potential for unlimited conversation.

Dedicated or nondedicated devices: Dedicated devices are designed only for communication purposes. Nondedicated devices have an AAC component but also provide other features (e.g., iPads, smartphones, and tablets; Cook & Polgar, 2015).

Environmental Access

Electronic aids to daily living (EADLs) promote client independence in a variety of areas (Anson, 2013) that are powered by electricity or infrared waves. This technology was initially developed to allow clients with physical impairments to have access to, and control of, their environment. Mainstream technology has advanced through the use of smart house technology controlled within the actual environment or from a remote access such as a smartphone or tablet. EADLs allow clients to answer the telephone, operate the television and radio, turn the lights on and off, lock and unlock doors, and adjust the temperature. Retrofitting a home for a client requiring EADLs is generally accomplished with a system such as the X-10 where appliances and items are plugged into a receiver while the control unit is linked to each item by a specified receiver address. Newer homes are being built with technologies that allow users to connect with all smart devices without the need for external hardware (Cook & Polgar, 2015).

Closed captioning: Closed captioning was developed for clients with auditory impairments and can also be utilized by consumers in loud areas, or clients for whom English is a second language. The Television Decoder Circuitry Act of 1990 requires that all televisions sold have inbuilt circuitry that allow for closed captioning without the need for an additional accommodation (National Association of the Deaf, n.d.). The Telecommunications Act of 1996 requires all television broadcasters to provide closed captioning (Federal Communications Commission, n.d.).

Closed-circuit television (CCTV): CCTV is most appropriate for clients with visual impairments and acts as a magnifier that uses a mounted camera to project magnification of a piece of paper onto a television screen.

Braille note takers: New technologies have made it possible for clients with low vision to take notes and either download them or print them from a Braille printer through the use of Braille note takers.

Wheelchair seating and mobility: Refer to Chapter 34 for information on mobility and locomotion.

Specialized training: ATP certification occurs through the Rehabilitation Engineering and Assistive Technology Society of North America (RESNA). This certification is voluntary and provides a level of expertise and commitment to the AT area of practice. The Association for Driver Rehabilitation Specialists (ADED) offers credentialing for CDRSs. Continuing education is critical for all OTs and OTAs practicing in the area of AT and driver rehabilitation (Cook & Polgar, 2015).

Funding

Funding for AT is derived from a variety of sources. Federal legislation such as the Individuals with Disability Education Act of 2004 requires school systems to provide AT if a client needs it in order to participate in their educational program. Federally mandated vocational rehabilitation is provided for clients who require AT in order to gain or maintain employment. Medicaid and Medicare provide funding for specific AT within designated environments. While each funder has different requirements, the OT works with the team to determine eligibility for specific AT needs (Cook & Polgar, 2015). Additional legislation that impacts the provision of AT includes the Rehabilitation Act of 1973, which mandates rehabilitation technology as a primary benefit in a client's plan of care. The expansion of AT services and devices is provided through the Assistive Technology Act of 1998. The Americans with Disabilities Act of 1990 applies AT to the five basic areas of reasonable and necessary accommodations. Finally, the Developmental Disabilities Assistance and Bill of Rights Act offers grants to advocacy programs for clients with AT needs (Cook & Polgar, 2015).

Reimbursement

Medical insurance coverage is highly variable; however, documentation must demonstrate medical or reasonable necessity. A letter of medical or reasonable necessity provides a rational and justification for the recommended AT. The following information should be included in a letter of medical necessity:

- Client's roles and occupational performance.
- Results from the client/family interview.
- Trial results of the recommended device.
- Cost analysis of alternative devices with a list of pros and cons.
- How this device will enhance the client's occupational performance (Cook & Polgar, 2015).

Driver Rehabilitation, Home, and Community Mobility

Driving is an important symbol of adult autonomy and independence. The independent community mobility afforded by driving has a major influence on a client's quality of life. Most drivers with functional impairments have similar needs to drive and to maintain their community mobility, as do clients in the general population. The professional services of driver rehabilitation specialist (DRSs) can be invaluable in helping people with physical and/or cognitive limitations to maintain their community mobility while protecting the safety of the client driver and the public at large.

Driver Rehabilitation Screening and Assessments

Programs offering clinical evaluations provide key information that can be used by the driver rehabilitation team members. They also help to identify clients who are at risk, and provide concrete data to support decisions to discontinue the evaluation process before the client has received an on-road evaluation. Mental abilities such as reaction time, visual acuity, decision-making, judgment, and planning are included in either the office or clinic examination to establish the safety and capabilities of the driver (American Occupational Therapy Association, 2016). Programs offering clinical evaluations and simulator assessments offer many advantages including the following:

- The capability to assess client responses to challenging stimuli, including animate and inanimate obstacles.

- How the client copes during variable inclement and clement weather conditions.
- Topographical orientation in familiar and unfamiliar environments.
- Night driving performance.

Simulators may also bridge the gap between clinical and on-road evaluations by providing a tangible way for clients to practice driving skills after narrowly failing a clinical or on-road evaluation. Programs offer comprehensive driver rehabilitation evaluations and more help to ensure that the client is provided with a comprehensive driver evaluation. After the comprehensive evaluation has been completed, additional services should include driver training and/or addressing alternative community mobility as a critical instrumental activities of daily living (IADLs; Dickerson & Schold, 2016). Alternative community mobility may include assisting clients and their caregivers with identifying viable and safe alternatives to driving, or riding as a passenger in motor vehicles.

Balancing Injury Risk and a Client's Desire to Drive

Evaluating drivers with functional impairments should include reliable screening (i.e., filtering out) of those whose driving performance would present an unacceptable risk to the drivers themselves, prospective passengers, pedestrians, and public and private property (Dickerson & Schold, 2016).

International Classification of Functioning, Disability, and Health (ICF)

The ICF provides a standard lexicon (i.e., universal vocabulary) for describing interrelationships between health, disability, functioning, and other related issues such as driving (World Health Organization, 2001). The full version of the ICF has two parts: Part 1: Functioning and Disability and Part 2: Contextual Factors. Part 1 is subdivided into "Body Functions and Structures" and "Activities and Participation." Part 2 is subdivided into "Environmental Factors" and "Personal Factors." This classification system may help DRSs to describe more consistently the nature and extent of client challenges and related factors (World Health Organization, 2001). Risk management frameworks assert that driving is a hazardous activity, that is, driving a vehicle in ordinary traffic is an inherently hazardous activity for drivers, passengers, and pedestrians alike. Crash risk varies according to the age and/or medical condition of the driver. Crash risk increases with increasing age beyond approximately 75–80 years of age (AAA, 2011).

Primary Team Members

Driver Rehabilitation Specialist

The DRS plays a central role in providing efficacious driver rehabilitation in addition to community mobility services to clients and their caregivers. DRSs work with ancillary team members to ensure that clients achieve their driver rehabilitation goals and/or community mobility goals.

Clients and Caregivers

The client is at the center of the driver rehabilitation team. It is mutually beneficial for the client, DRS, and other team members when a client's full participation in the decision-making process is encouraged and expected. The caregiver often "fills in the blanks" and provides valuable insight that the client may be lacking or unwilling to provide.

Vehicle Modifier

The vehicle modifier is also known as the mobility equipment dealer or vendor. The vehicle modifier plays a primary role in the provision of driver rehabilitation and community mobility services. Vehicle modifiers do much more than their name implies. For example, they often help the client and DRS identify the optimal vehicle type and vehicle modifications that maximize the client's safety as a driver or passenger after efficiently accessing or exiting a vehicle. Reputable mobility equipment dealers are members of the National Mobility Equipment Dealer's Association (National Highway Traffic Safety Administration, 2007).

Driving Retirement or Cessation

When it is determined that a client is no longer able to drive safely with or without restrictions, the DRS should be compelled to assist his or her client with identifying and using community mobility resources for dependable alternative transportation (Opp, 2016). Access to dependable alternative transportation is an essential IADL and is

necessary to fully empower clients who no longer drive (Dickerson & Schold, 2016). Alternative transportation options are often unfamiliar to clients and caregivers who have relied on driving a motor vehicle as their primary, and more often their sole, method of transportation.

Home and Accessibility

The Americans with Disabilities Act of 1990 was enacted as a civil rights legislation that addresses a variety of domains that impact clients with disabilities including employment, participation in state and local government services, and programs, and public accommodations (Kornblau, 2013). One of the most successful portions includes increasing the accessibility of public environments for persons with mobility impairments (Sabata, 2014). As people age or develop an injury or trauma, they may fear that they will be unable to remain in their home. There are a number of tools that can assist OTs with evaluating home environments and making appropriate recommendations for optimal safety and independence.

- Creating accessible homes provides a quick checklist on accessible home features (Kansas State University Agricultural Experiment Station and Cooperative Extension Service, 1996).
- The Home Fit Guide provides a checklist on accessible home features as well (AARP, 2008).
- Tox Town is an interactive website that enables users to identify potential toxic hazards within their homes and communities (NIH U.S. National Library of Medicine, n.d.).

Home evaluations and recommendations for modifications and equipment (e.g., durable medical equipment and assistive devices) complement AT consultation and recommendations. For example, OTs can recommend an environmental control unit through AT consultation while AT services can help identify the need for home evaluations. The following list provides an outline of commonly assessed areas included in an OT home evaluation:

Entrances:

- Doorway openings
- Locks and door handle types
- Ramp specifications (e.g., rise and run ratios, turning platforms, handrails, surface type, and portable versus permanent)
- Thresholds

Kitchens:

- Cabinets (e.g., height, depth, width, locations, shapes, and handle types)
- Cook tops (e.g., gas or electric, control knob location, and adaptive devices)
- Counter space (e.g., height, depth, width, location, shape, and types)
- Fire extinguishers (e.g., types and locations)
- Ovens/microwaves (e.g., types and locations)
- Refrigerator (e.g., types, storage variations, and locations)
- Sinks (e.g., height, depth, width, location, shape, types, disposal location, insulated pipes, and faucet handle types)

Bathrooms:

- Water heater temperature
- Center floor drain
- Faucet types
- Floor spaces (e.g., turning radii)
- Grab bars
- Heating lamps
- Nonslip flooring
- Shower head types
- Shower types (e.g., roll-in or step-in shower)
- Toilets and bidets (e.g., height and types)
- Tub types (e.g., old-fashioned-style tubs, standard tubs, and specialty walk-in tubs)

Bedrooms:

- Beds (e.g., sizes, types, locations, and transfer aids)
- Bedroom locations
- Closets (e.g., types, sizes, locations, and rod types)
- Furniture placement
- Light switches (e.g., locations and types)

Hallways:

- Hallway width
- Lighting

Laundry room:

- Washers and dryers (e.g., styles and types)
- Sorting and folding tables (e.g., types, sizes, locations, permanent, or portable)

Indoor and outdoor stairways:

- Handrails
- Safety strips
- Color contrast

- Light switches (e.g., locations and types)
- Step specifications

Alarm systems:

- Call for help systems
- Door knobs
- Doors (e.g., types and sizes)
- Electrical outlets (e.g., types and locations)
- Evacuation plans
- Extension cords
- Fire extinguishers (e.g., types and locations)
- Flooring (e.g., surface types and color contrast)
- Light switches (e.g., locations and types)
- Indoor and outdoor maintenance plans
- Phones (e.g., type and location)
- Smoke and carbon monoxide detectors (e.g., types and locations)
- Thermostats (e.g., types, height, and locations)
- Water temperature
- Windows (e.g., sizes, types, and locations)

Referrals and Discharge Considerations

Individuals requiring occupational therapy services for AT, driving, and home evaluations may require a prescription from a doctor indicating the need for the specified services. Individual insurances dictate how many therapy sessions will be paid. AT, driving, and home evaluations can occur in as little as one session, but may require training for specific tasks. Discharge from driver rehabilitation may occur when a client is found unsafe to drive, when the client is able to resume driving, or when the vehicle has been modified and deemed safe and functional.

Management and Standards of Practice

Occupational therapy practitioners working in these areas of practice should work within the constraints of a team. As stated previously, team members may vary but always include the client and their support system. OTAs who are skilled within these practice areas are valuable team members and may provide training in the use of AT or specific accommodations suggested for the client.

Chapter 35 Self-Study Activities (Answers Are Provided at the End of the Chapter)

Match the following legislation with its impact on the provision of AT equipment and services (Cook & Polgar, 2015):

1. _____ Rehabilitation Act of 1973, as amended 2. _____ Assistive Technology Act of 1998 3. _____ Americans with Disabilities Act of 1990 4. _____ The Developmental Disabilities Assistance and Bill of Rights Act 5. _____ Individuals with Disabilities Education Act Amendments of 2004	**A.** Provides grants to states for developmental disability councils, university-affiliated programs, and protection and advocacy activities for people with developmental disabilities. **B.** Every child, under this law, has a right to free and appropriate education. Includes children with disabilities to be educated with their peers. Allows AT devices and services for students 3–21 years old. **C.** Section 508 mandates equal access to electronic office equipment for all federal employees; mandates rehabilitation technology as a primary benefit to be included in an individual's written rehabilitation plan. **D.** Prohibits discrimination on the basis of disability in employment, state and local government, public accommodations, commercial facilities, transportation, and telecommunications, all of which affect the application of AT. **E.** Addressed for the first time in legislation, the expansion of AT devices and services, and mandates consumer-driven AT services.

Match the following accessibility features with its appropriate term (Cook & Polgar, 2015):

6. _____ Display and Readability 7. _____ Sounds and Speech 8. _____ Keyboard Options 9. _____ Mouse Options 10. _____ Accessibility Utility	**A.** QWERTY **B.** SnapTo **C.** Text-to-Speech **D.** Screen Resolution **E.** Narrator

Match each device with the appropriate consumer requirements (Cook & Polgar, 2015):

11. _____ Standard Keyboards 12. _____ Standard Computer Displays 13. _____ Standard Mouse Control	**A.** The consumer must be able to read text, decipher graphics or icons, locate and follow a small mouse cursor, have good figure-ground perception, and distinguish color. **B.** The consumer must be able to demonstrate range of motion, strength, coordination, and timing. **C.** The consumer must be able to hold or make controlled contact, move, and stop the mouse cursor at a desired location, and activate a button at the appropriate time.

Place in order the correct steps in the service delivery process, beginning with the first (1) and ending with the last (6) (Cook & Polgar, 2015):

14. _____ Initial Evaluation 15. _____ Recommendations and Report 16. _____ Follow-along 17. _____ Implementation 18. _____ Referral and Intake 19. _____ Follow-up

Chapter 35 Self-Study Answers

1. C
2. E
3. D
4. A
5. B

6. D
7. C
8. A
9. B
10. E
11. B
12. A
13. C
14. 2
15. 3
16. 6
17. 4
18. 1
19. 5

References

AAA. (2011). *Senior driving: Facts and research*. Retrieved from http://seniordriving.aaa.com/resources -family-friends/conversations-about-driving /facts-research

AARP. (2008). *The AARP home fit guide*. Retrieved from http://assets.aarp.org/www.aarp.org_/articles /families/HousingOptions/200590_HomeFit_rev 011108.pdf

American Occupational Therapy Association. (2016). *Driving evaluations by an occupational therapist*. Retrieved from https://www.aota.org/practice/productive-aging /driving/clients/evaluate/eval-by-ot.aspx

Anson, D. (2013). Assistive technology. In H. S. K. McHugh Pendleton & S.-K. Winifred (Eds.), *Pedretti's occupational therapy: Practice skills for physical dysfunction* (pp. 427–449). St. Louis, MO: Elsevier/ Mosby.

Bunning, M. E. (2014). Technology for remediation and compensation of disability. In M. V. Radomski & C. A. T. Latham (Eds.), *Occupational therapy for physical dysfunction* (7th ed.). Baltimore, MD: Wolters Kluwer Health/Lippincott Williams & Wilkins.

Cook, A. M., & Polgar, J. M. (2015). *Assistive technologies: Principles and practice* (4th ed.). St. Louis, MO: Elsevier/Mosby.

Dickerson, A., & Schold, E. (2016). *Driving and transportation alternatives for older adults*. Bethesda, MD: American Occupational Therapy Association. Retrieved from http://www.aota.org/about-occupational -therapy/professionals/pa/facts/driving-transportation -alternatives.aspx

Federal Communications Commission. (n.d.). *Telecommunications Act of 1966*. Retrieved from https://transition .fcc.gov/telecom.html

Individuals with Disabilities Education Improvement Act of 2004 (IDEA 2004), Pub. L. No. 108-446, 20 U.S.C. 1400 et seq. (2004). Retrieved from http://idea.ed.gov /download/statute.html

Kansas State University Agricultural Experiment Station and Cooperative Extension Service. (1996). *Creating accessible homes*. Retrieved from http://www .maraisdescygnes.k-state.edu/home-family-money management/energy-and-housing/energy-housing -information/creatingaccessiblehomes.pdf

Kielhofner, G. B., & Janice, P. (1980). A model of human occupation, part 1: Conceptual framework and content. *American Journal of Occupational Therapy, 34*(9), 572–581.

Kornblau, B. L. (2013). Americans with Disabilities Act and related laws that promote participation in work, leisure, and activities of daily living. In H. S. K. McHugh Pendleton & S.-K. Winifred (Eds.), *Pedretti's occupational therapy: Practice skills for physical dysfunction* (7th ed., pp. 381–411). St. Louis, MO: Elsevier/Mosby.

Law, M., Baptiste, S., McColl, M., Opzoomer, A., Polatajko, H., & Pollock, N. (1990). The Canadian occupational performance measure: An outcome measure for occupational therapy. *Canadian Journal of Occupational Therapy, 57*(2), 82–87.

Law, M., Cooper, B., Strong, S., Stewart, D., Rigby, P., & Letts, L. (1996). The person–environment–occupation model: A transactive approach to occupational performance. *Canadian Journal of Occupational Therapy, 63*(1), 9–23.

National Association of the Deaf. (n.d.). *Television decoder circuitry act*. Retrieved from https://nad.org/issues /civil-rights/television-decoder-circuitry-act

National Highway Traffic Safety Administration. (2007). *Adapting motor vehicles for older drivers*. Retrieved from https://www.nhtsa.gov/sites/nhtsa.dot.gov/files /documents/hs810732.pdf

NIH U.S. National Library of Medicine. (n.d.). *Tox town: Environmental health concerns and toxic chemicals where you live, work, and play*. Retrieved from http:// toxtown.nlm.nih.gov/index.php

Opp, A. (2016). *Behind the wheel: Occupational therapy and older drivers*. Retrieved from https://www.aota .org/about-occupational-therapy/professionals/rdp /articles/older-drivers.aspx

Sabata, D. (2014). Optimizing access to home, community, and work environments. In M. Vining Rodomski & T. L. Catherine (Eds.), *Occupational therapy for physical dysfunction* (7th ed.). Baltimore, MD: Lippincott Williams & Wilkins.

World Health Organization. (2001). *ICF: International classification of functioning, disability and health*. Geneva, Switzerland: Author.

Zabala, J. (2010). *The SETT framework: Straight from the horse's mouth*. Paper presented at the Special Education Council of Alberta Teacher's Association, Alberta, Canada.

Zabala, J. (2016). *Sharing the SETT framework*. Retrieved from http://www.joyzabala.com/

Documentation, Management, Reimbursement, and Working with a COTA Days 25–27

Documentation of Occupational Therapy Practice

Deborah Loftus

Learning Objectives

- Explain the purpose and methods for correct occupational therapy documentation.
- Describe Occupational Therapy Practice Framework III terminology as it relates to documentation.
- Write appropriate and measurable client-centered goals.
- Apply information of applicable regulations, guidelines, and reimbursement systems as they relate to the documentation of occupational therapy practice.
- Demonstrate basic knowledge in the following types of documentation: screening, initial evaluation, intervention plan, progress reports, daily progress notes (e.g., SOAP), narrative notes, and discharge reports. Documentation should be relevant and understandable; in addition, goals should be measurable and achievable.
- Apply the guidelines for the documentation of the occupational therapy practice.

Key Terms

- *Assessments*: A tool used to evaluate a client that contributes to the entire evaluation.
- *Client-centered goal*: A goal that is based on a client's needs and wants.
- *Clinical reasoning*: The ability to problem-solve and make decisions through the various areas of a client's plan of care.
- *Evaluation*: A comprehensive review that leads the occupational therapist (OT) toward a client-centered treatment plan.
- *Evidence-based practice*: The ability to use literature to support practice.
- *Intervention plan*: The plan of care that guides the occupational therapy process.
- *Protected health information (PHI)*: PHI contains information about health, health care, and payment that is linked to an individual.
- *Skilled intervention*: Services that only a qualified OT or occupational therapy assistant can provide.

Introduction

This chapter will describe the fundamental elements of the occupational therapy documentation process. Occupational therapy documentation self-study worksheets and corresponding answer keys are provided at the end of the chapter to help reinforce learning and retention of key information.

Occupational Therapy Practice Framework

The Occupational Therapy Practice Framework: Domain and Process III (OTPF III) is a summary of interconnected principles that describe occupational therapy practice. It is essential for the occupational therapist (OT) and occupational therapy assistant (OTA) students to review and understand the OTPF III document in preparation for the National Board for Certification in Occupational Therapy® exam. According to the OTPF III, occupational therapy is defined as "the therapeutic use of everyday life activities (occupational) with individuals or groups for the purpose of enhancing or enabling participation in roles, habits, and routines in home, school, workplace, community, and other settings" (American Occupational Therapy Association [AOTA], 2014, p. S1).

In the OTPF III, the importance of occupation-based intervention plans is emphasized. Within the OTPF III the roles of OTs and OTAs are delineated. The initial vision of the framework was based on the premise of therapeutic occupations as a way to heal illness and furthermore, maintain health. The framework is meant to act as a guide for occupational therapy practice along with evidence-based practice and relevant knowledge within the identified areas of practice.

The OTPF III is divided into two main areas: (1) the domain of occupational therapy and (2) the process of occupational therapy (Sames, 2015).

Domain of Occupational Therapy

Within the domain section in the OTPF III are five main areas of occupational therapy practice with subcategories within each area (AOTA, 2014):

1. Occupations are defined as the "daily life activities in which people engage" (AOTA, 2014, p. S9). Within the area of occupations are eight subcategories that are essential to understand:
   i. Activities of daily living (ADLs)
   ii. Instrumental activities of daily living (IADLs)
   iii. Rest and sleep
   iv. Education
   v. Work
   vi. Play
   vii. Leisure
   viii. Social participation
2. Client factors
   i. Body structures
   ii. Body functions
   iii. Values, beliefs, and spirituality
3. Performance skills
   i. Motor skills
   ii. Process skills
   iii. Social interaction skills
4. Performance patterns
   i. Habits
   ii. Routines
   iii. Roles
   iv. Rituals
5. Contexts and environments, which include six subcategories:
   i. Cultural contexts
   ii. Physical environments
   iii. Social environments

   iv. Personal contexts
   v. Temporal contexts
   vi. Virtual contexts (AOTA, 2014)

The client's occupational identity, well-being, health, and participation in life are based on the domain. It is important to know that all aspects of the domain are of equal value and they all interact to affect client outcomes (AOTA, 2014). These areas are described in more detail in Chapter 5.

The Occupational Therapy Documentation Process

The basic components of the occupational therapy documentation process include four main areas as listed in AOTA's 2013 Documentation Guidelines (AOTA, 2013):

1. *Screening*: This includes documenting the referral source and demonstrating the rationale of why an occupational therapy evaluation and treatment is needed.
2. *Evaluation*: The in-depth report that includes data gathered throughout the evaluation process depends on the guidelines of the payer, facility, and state or federal laws. Specific types of standardized and/or nonstandardized assessments that will be focused on for interventions will be included in the evaluation. It is important to document if the client needs skilled instruction in this area.
3. *Intervention*: The intervention plan documents specific goals and the various intervention approaches that will be used to achieve the client's targeted outcomes. A daily note is also required that documents the treatment between the client and the occupational therapy provider. In a daily note, or sometimes called a progress note, the client's response to treatment is recorded. It is important to document the client's progress toward their goals and if modifications of the treatment plan are needed. Occupational therapy practitioners are encouraged to be as specific as possible when writing these notes (e.g., level of assistance needed, the amount of cueing needed, and how the client tolerated each task). OTs must use the correct wording and terminology to justify continuing skilled services and the level of complexity of the services provided by OT practitioners (Morreale &

Borcherding, 2013). Medicare and many other payers do not reimburse for occupational therapy services that are nonskilled in nature, or not necessary for the client's current condition. According to the Centers for Medicare and Medicaid Services (2012), *skilled* services have very explicit criteria and are performed by qualified professionals, including occupational therapy students and OTAs under the OT's supervision. They require professional education, decision making, and highly complicated skills with a knowledge base that are reflective of a high level of competence. *Nonskilled* services are defined as those that are typically routine or maintenance types of therapy, which could be carried out by nonprofessional personnel, caregivers, or family members. Specifically, the Centers for Medicare and Medicaid Services (2012) reports that services must be reasonable and necessary. The level of complexity or the condition of the client shall be such that the services required can be safely and effectively performed only by a qualified therapist, and a client's clinical condition requires the skills of a therapist. More information related to Medicare and Medicaid documentation, including definitions and rules and regulations, can be found at the CMS website (www.cms.gov).

4. *Outcomes*: The discharge report is a summary of the occupational therapy services provided and the outcomes achieved between the initial evaluation and discharge. It is important to include the client's goal status on this report.

The OTPF III gives a detailed description of the building blocks of occupational therapy practice. Understanding the importance of this framework is essential to fully understand and appreciate how important the use of occupation is within the context of occupational therapy service provision.

Guidelines for Documentation

The Guidelines for Documentation of Occupational Therapy (AOTA, 2013) is another essential publication that is important to review when studying for the board exam. It describes the importance of the documentation of occupational therapy services and the need to have thorough and accurate documentation whenever professional services are provided to a client, including 15 fundamentals on what should be included in each type of documentation (AOTA, 2013):

1. *Client identification*: Make sure the client's full name, and case number if applicable, is on every page of all necessary documentation (e.g., initial evaluation, reevaluations, daily notes, and discharge reports). Abbreviations of client names are not appropriate when recording occupational services and are not accepted by many insurance companies.

2. *Date*: Obvious information such as the complete date (i.e., month, day, and year) and time is essential information that must be present on all documentation. This information serves to show the chronological order in which events occur during treatment. The time of day may be required for inpatient acute and rehabilitation documentation.

3. *Type of document*: The type of encounter an OT practitioner has with a client (i.e., initial evaluation or a daily progress note) and the facility, company, or agency through which the occupational services are being rendered should appear on each piece of documentation provided, as well as the type of note that is being written.

4. *Signature*: The treating practitioner's full name followed by the professional designation (e.g., Jane Doe, OTR/L) should appear on each documented note to identify the person who saw the client for the corresponding treatment date.

5. *Placement of signature*: All notes must have the signature line at the end of the note to prevent tampering of documentation.

6. *Countersignature*: OTs may be required to countersign the signatures of OTAs and OT students. This may be necessary secondary to state and facility regulations when OTAs and students are assisting with treatment. The countersignature also provides documentation of the supervision that is required by some jurisdictions.

7. *Compliance*: It is essential that all occupational therapy practitioners are in direct compliance with all laws, regulations, as well as employer and payer requirements.

8. *Terminology*: Facilities vary on acceptable and recognized terminology. Prior to completing an organization's documentation process, confirm what is considered to be acceptable terminology.

9. *Abbreviations*: OTs and OTAs may use abbreviations that are approved by their facility. Note that abbreviations that are used in one facility may not be used in another.

10. *Corrections*: Errors should typically be corrected by drawing a single line with a black pen through the word(s) in error and writing the OT practitioner's initials above or next to the line. Erasing or scribbling is not accepted on occupational therapy notes, may not be accepted by insurance carriers, and would not be valid in a court of law. However, it is always prudent to confirm the documentation policies used within a given healthcare system, clinic, or setting.

11. *Technology*: Individual facilities vary when it comes to dictating the policies and procedures applicable to the use of technology in occupational therapy documentation. It is the OT practitioner's responsibility to maintain compliance with documentation policies.

12. *Record disposal*: Federal and state laws, in combination with facility regulations, determine the appropriate method for disposing occupational therapy documentation when it is no longer needed.

13. *Confidentiality*: OTs and OTAs must possess knowledge of all federal, state, and individual facility rules in regard to confidentiality, including the 2015 AOTA Code of Ethics. According to the Health Insurance Portability and Accountability Act (HIPPA, 1996), the practitioner has a responsibility to protect confidential information from unauthorized access. Accordingly, OT documentation must remain objective and nonjudgmental.

14. *Record storage*: Variability exists from facility to facility regarding record storage and retention. OTs practitioners must obey all federal, state, and facility regulations when storing occupational therapy documentation. In most instances, charts must be kept in a locked or secure storage cabinet and/or room per regulations of various accrediting bodies, such as the Commission on the Accreditation of Rehabilitation Facilities (CARF) or the Joint Commission on the Accreditation of Healthcare Organizations (JCAHO).

15. *Clinical reasoning and expertise*: All documentation must ensure the safe and effective delivery of care by an occupational therapy practitioner, and is achieved by utilizing clinical reasoning and expertise.

Principles of Good Documentation

Documentation acts as a permanent, legal document that is the primary method of communication used to report exactly what occurred during the therapy session. It is essential that the clinician providing the occupational therapy services complete all documentation, and if this does not occur, it is considered fraudulent. It should also be noted that all occupational therapy documentation (i.e., computerized or written) may undergo a legal review. Reimbursement for occupational therapy services is dependent on correct, well-written documentation that justifies the need for skilled intervention. Documentation is the vehicle with which OTs and OTAs demonstrate the value of their intervention. Many times the thoroughness of the therapist's documentation dictates if therapy is reimbursable by the insurance companies. It is important to know that the client's diagnosis or prognosis should not be used as the only rationale for why occupational therapy services are indicated. Confidentiality must be maintained throughout the documentation processes. Documentation of medical necessity may be needed to determine client access to continued occupational therapy services (Smith, 2013).

Three Main Purposes of Documentation

The three main objectives of documentation are as follows:

1. Communicates the rationale for why occupational therapy services are appropriate by utilizing the occupational therapy clinician's clinical reasoning and professional judgment that indicate the need for skilled intervention.

2. Provides information about the client from the unique perspective of the occupational therapy provider.

3. Documents a sequential record of the client's health condition, the occupational therapy services provided, the client's response to treatment, and therapeutic outcomes (AOTA, 2013).

Best practices in documentation should be followed when documenting any type of occupational therapy service, including:

- Relevant information
- Clear, concise, and in-depth information

- Standard language
- Correct spelling
- Approved abbreviations
- Signature with credentials at the end of the document
- Reflection of the Occupational Therapy Practice Framework

Main Components of Documentation

The main components of occupational therapy documentation include the following:

1. Initial evaluation
   a. Client information
   b. Referral information; reason for referral or physician's order
   c. Occupational profile
      i. Occupational history and experiences
      ii. Activities, routines, and roles
      iii. Interests, values, and needs
   d. Assessments that are performed with a client should be selected by the OT based on a review of the client's chart, previous documentation, and/or findings from the initial evaluation.
      i. Standardized tests (e.g., grip strength)
      ii. Nonstandardized tests (e.g., narrative reports)
   e. Summary and analysis
   f. Therapy recommendations
2. The collaborative establishment of goals between clients and therapists
   a. Short- and long-term goals
      i. *Measurable*: When writing goals, the OT must select measurable variables (e.g., range of motion measured using a goniometer and grip strength measured using a dynamometer) in order to document a client's progress, or lack of progress.
      ii. *Occupation based*: The fundamental values of the occupational therapy profession are based on the idea that participation in occupation is essential for a person to acquire health, wellness, and life satisfaction. Goals need to be based on the client's relevant occupations as their primary means to create meaningful goals.
      iii. *Functional*: As OTs it is necessary that we show that our services result in functional changes in our clients. It is typical that

reimbursement sources require the demonstration of improvement in function to receive payment for rendered occupational therapy services (Sames, 2015).
      iv. *Client centered*: All occupational therapy goals should be based on the client's needs. Developing client-centered goals should be a collaborative effort between the treating therapist and the client.
      v. *Time based*: Long- and short-term goals need to have an end point. This is necessary to enable the therapist to know when to reevaluate goals and assess if the goal is met or needs to be modified or discontinued.
   b. Another tool for remembering the essential parts of goal writing is using the SMART system. Each letter of the word SMART stands for an important aspect of goal writing described below (Sames, 2015).
      i. *Significant*: Ensure that goal writing is a collaborative effort between the therapist and the client, thereby making it significant and meaningful to the client.
      ii. *Measurable*: When writing any goal it is important for the OT to write it in measurable terms in order to keep track of the client's progress or lack of progress. The therapist also needs to document with specific descriptive words such as "the client will be able to put on and button their coat independently" to ensure the goal is obtainable. If the therapist wrote, "the client will improve with dressing," then the goal is vague and may never be met.
      iii. *Achievable*: The therapist must use their clinical judgment to find the "just right" challenge when creating goals. The goal may be difficult; however, not impossible for the client to achieve.
      iv. *Related*: It is essential that the goal has a connection to the client's occupational needs and that short-term goals relate to each other.
      v. *Time limited*: Long- and short-term goals need to have an end point. This is necessary to enable the therapist to know when to reevaluate goals and assess if the goal is met or needs to be modified or discontinued.

   c. RHUMBA is another tool that can be useful in organizing the therapist's information to ensure effective documentation. Each letter of the word RHUMBA identifies something that the therapist should remember when writing goals.

      R: Relevant: To ensure a goal is relevant, make sure it is meaningful and functional for the client.

      H: How long: A timeline is an essential piece of information that should be included in all goals. For example, how long does the OT expect it to take to reach the goal?

      U: Understandable: A good way to make a goal is understandable is to make sure that anyone filling out for an OT as a practitioner should be able to easily understand the plan and goals that you had intended for the client to complete.

      M: Measurable: A measurement of function including progress, maintenance, or decline must be included in a goal statement. An example of a measurement would be the level of independence, accuracy, or duration.

      B: Behavioral: The task must have measurable occurrences or outcomes that must be observed (i.e., something the OT can see the client do or hear the client say), not inferred.

      A: Achievable: Similar to the SMART system, having the goal achievable means the therapist must use their clinical judgment to find the "just right" challenge when writing goals. The goal may be difficult; however, not impossible for the client to achieve within their individual circumstances.

3. Intervention plan

   i. Performance skills (e.g., motor, process, or communication/interaction skills)

   ii. Performance patterns (e.g., habits, routines, or roles)

   iii. Context (e.g., cultural, physical, or social)

   iv. Activity demands (e.g., space demands and social demands)

   v. Client factors/participation (e.g., body functions and structures)

4. Progress reports showing skilled interventions are needed to document each occupational therapy session with the client. Many types of note styles are available to create a progress report, including checklist notes, narrative notes, and descriptive notes.

   a. The SOAP note is a type of note that is commonly used as it summarizes the treatment session utilizing the following criteria:

      i. *Subjective*: This section of the note reports the client's perspective on their condition. For example, if the client tells the OTA "my shoulder really hurt last night and it prevented me from sleeping," it would be important to document this information in the subjective portion of the SOAP note. This allows the OTA to convey important information by recording the client's own description. It is acceptable to quote or summarize what the client actually said in this section.

      ii. *Objective*: All objective and measurable data that are obtained during an OT session should be recorded in this section of the SOAP note. An example would be "the client engaged in 30 minutes of therapy focusing on bilateral upper extremity active range of motion and functional mobility. The client needed moderate verbal cues to position herself appropriately for reaching objects in the upper cabinets and freezer. The client was able to transfer 5 small cans from one upper cabinet to another upper cabinet with fatigue rated 7/10 on a 0–10 scale. No reports of pain were noted."

      iii. *Assessment*: This portion of the SOAP note includes the therapist's skilled interpretation of the client's progress, limitations, and expected outcomes from occupational therapy services.

      iv. *Plan*: In this section of the SOAP note, the therapist documents the specific treatment that they intend on pursuing to achieve the client's goals. Any recommendations that the OTA may have for the client (e.g., installing grab bars) should be included in the plan.

   b. *Checklist notes*: This type of note allows for a lot of information to be communicated with less time spent documenting, as the therapist will typically check boxes with the appropriate information already completed.

c. *Narrative notes*: This type of note reads similar to a first person story written by a clinician that describes a specific clinical event or situation, in paragraph format. An example would be writing about a treatment with a client that illustrates how an OT intervention made a difference in client outcomes or describes the client's progress toward a particular goal (Sames, 2015, p. 188).

d. *Discharge report*: A necessary piece of documentation that must include the client's progress or lack of progress from the beginning to the end of occupational therapy services. The discharge report, sometimes referred to as the discontinuation summary, serves as the final phase of occupational therapy services. In certain settings, such as acute care, discharge planning may begin immediately.

Management and Standards of Practice

Many legal and ethical considerations need to be made when documenting occupational therapy services. It is important to realize that all health records are considered legal documents and can be used as evidence in any type of legal proceeding or litigation process. Government payers can review clinical documentation and billing records at any point, even years after a client is discharged (Sames, 2015, p. 468). Occupational therapy practitioners must be thorough and accurate with their documentation (e.g., an undocumented event or situation reported by an OT or OTA is not admissible as evidence in the court of law). This is especially true when safety issues arise such as client falling or hurting themselves. According to Sames (2015, p. 67), it is important to "document only what you see, hear, touch, or smell" and avoid documenting interpretations. A good example would be if someone reported to an OTA that a client fell; however, the OT did not see it. In such instances, the OTA should include the details of the specific person who told them that the client fell, along with all pertinent details, as opposed to reporting only that "the client fell."

One of the laws that OT practitioners are required to comply with is the Health Insurance Portability and Accountability Act (HIPPA, 1996). This law protects the confidentiality of all client information in many different ways. The law covers many aspects of confidentiality from preventing OTs and OTAs from talking to a coworker in a public place about a client's functional status, to protected health information that may be stored on a computer that needs to be password protected.

Medicare fraud is another important area to understand when documenting occupational therapy services. "Fraud is the deliberate concealment of the facts from another person for unlawful or unfair gain" (Fremgen, 2006, p. 125). Medicare fraud or abuse is typically an action that causes additional costs to Medicare. Some examples would be submitting documentation that is false for payment, or billing for occupational therapy services that are not provided by a licensed therapist, such as a student. The best policy when it comes to documentation is to be truthful and precise and as detailed as possible (Sames, 2015, p. 83).

Occupational therapy practitioners typically refer to both OTs and OTAs, as they both have expertise in the practice of occupational therapy. However, it is ultimately the role of the OT to ensure that all documentation is completed in compliance with state, facility, and reimbursement regulations and standards. Unless it is required by state law, employer, or is a reimbursement requirement, AOTA (2013) does not require that an OT cosign documentation written by the OTA. Some states do require a cosignature by the OT, as well as a log of the visits that were supervised. When working with occupational therapy and OTA students, all documentation needs to be cosigned by a supervisor to ensure the note was written correctly and includes all necessary information (Sames, 2015, pp. 94–95). OTs are responsible for developing the treatment plan and are fundamentally responsible for service delivery. However, once the evaluation is completed and the treatment plan devised, the OT makes the decision about who will execute the treatment plan (i.e., OT or OTA) (Egan & Dubouloz, 2014, p. 40). Occupational therapy managers typically are expected to manage the overall documentation process of the department they are overseeing, and complete intermittent reviews of documentation of services for quality control and reimbursement purposes.

Summary

It is important to know that different organizations may have their own documentation formats. Irrespective of the system or format used to document occupational therapy services, the OT must be certain they conform to federal and state laws, as well as reimbursement source requirements. Ultimately, it is the responsibility of the OT to be aware of and abide by all documentation requirements, including professional, ethical, and practice standards (Sames, 2014, p. 474).

Chapter 36 Self-Study Activities (Answers Are Provided at the End of the Chapter)

1. Review commonly used abbreviations and fill out the blanks with the correct abbreviation (right column).

Upper extremity _____

Lower extremity _____

Both upper extremities _____

Left upper extremity _____

Right upper extremity _____

Both lower extremities _____

Left lower extremity _____

Right lower extremity _____

Distal interphalangeal joint _____

Metacarpophalangeal joint _____

Proximal interphalangeal joint _____

Fracture _____

Active assistive range of motion _____

Active range of motion _____

Functional range of motion _____

Passive range of motion _____

Range of motion _____

Wheelchair _____

Within functional limits _____

Within normal limits _____

Motor vehicle accident _____

Open reduction, internal fixation _____

Rheumatoid arthritis _____

Spinal cord injury _____

Traumatic brain injury _____

Total hip replacement _____

Transient ischemic attack _____

Diagnosis _____

History of _____

Durable medical equipment _____

Short-term goal _____

Long-term goal _____

As needed _____

Activities of daily living _____

Twice a day _____

Above knee amputation _____

Standby assistance _____

Contact guard assistance _____

Home exercise program _____

Non–weight-bearing _____

2. Match the information related to the documentation process with the correct term for its use.

1. Checklist note _____

2. Narrative note _____

3. Discharge report _____

4. Performance skills _____

5. Performance patterns _____

6. Context _____

7. Activity demands _____

8. Client factors _____

A. Motor, process, communication, and interaction skills.

B. Body functions and structures.

C. Type of note that allows for a lot of information to be communicated with less time documenting, as typically the therapist or assistant will check boxes with the appropriate information already completed.

D. Cultural, personal, physical, social, temporal, and virtual.

E. Habits, routines, ritual, and roles.

F. Type of note that reads similar to a first person story written by a clinician that describes a specific clinical event or situation, in paragraph format.

G. Space and social demands.

H. A necessary piece of documentation that must include the client's progress or lack of progress from the beginning to the end of occupational therapy services.

Chapter 36 Self-Study Answers

Question 1

Upper extremity	UE
Lower extremity	LE
Both upper extremities	BUE
Left upper extremity	LUE
Right upper extremity	RUE
Both lower extremities	BLE
Left lower extremity	LLE
Right lower extremity	RLE
Distal interphalangeal joint	DIP
Metacarpal phalangeal joint	MP
Proximal interphalangeal joint	PIP
Fracture	Fx
Active assisted range of motion	AAROM
Active range of motion	AROM
Functional range of motion	FROM
Passive range of motion	PROM
Range of motion	ROM
Wheelchair	WC
Within functional limits	WFL
Within normal limits	WNL
Motor vehicle accident	MVA
Open reduction, internal fixation	ORIF
Rheumatoid arthritis	RA
Spinal cord injury	SCI
Traumatic brain injury	TBI
Total hip replacement	THR
Transient ischemic attack	TIA
Diagnosis	Dx
History of	Hx
Durable medical equipment	DME
Short-term goal	STG
Long-term goal	LTG
As needed	PRN
Activities of daily living	ADL
Twice a day	b.i.d.
Above knee amputation	AKA
Standby assistance	SBA
Contact guard assistance	CGA
Home exercise program	HEP
Non–weight-bearing	NWB

Question 2

1. C
2. F
3. H
4. A
5. E
6. D
7. G
8. B

References

American Occupational Therapy Association. (2013). Guidelines for documentation of occupational therapy. *American Journal of Occupational Therapy, 67*(Suppl. 1), S1–S48.

American Occupational Therapy Association. (2014). Occupational therapy practice framework: Domain and process (3rd ed.). *American Journal of Occupational Therapy, 68*(Suppl. 1), S1–S48.

Centers for Medicare and Medicaid Services. (2012). Medicare and Medicaid statistical supplement. Baltimore, MD. Retrieved from https://www.cms.gov/Research-Statistics-Data-and-Systems/Statistics-Trends-and-Reports/MedicareMedicaidStatSupp/2012.html

Egan, M., & Dubouloz, C. (2014). Practical foundations for practice: Planning, guiding, documenting and reflecting. In M. V. Radomski & C. A. T. Latham (Eds.), *Occupational therapy for physical dysfunction* (7th ed., pp. 25–43). Philadelphia, PA: Wolters Kluwer Health/Lippincott Williams & Wilkins.

Fremgen, B. F. (2006). *Medical law and ethics* (2nd ed.). Upper Saddle River, NJ: Pearson/Prentice Hall.

Health Insurance Portability and Accountability Act of 1996 (HIPPA). P. L. No. 104-191. Stat. 1938. (1996).

Morreale, M. J., & Borcherding, S. (2013). *The OTA's guide to documentation: Writing SOAP notes* (3rd ed.). Thorofare, NJ: SLACK.

Sames, K. M. (2014). Documentation in practice. In B. A. B. Schell, G. Gillen, & M. Scaffa (Eds.), *Willard & Spackman's occupational therapy* (12th ed., pp. 466–475). Philadelphia, PA: Wolters Kluwer Health/Lippincott Williams & Wilkins.

Sames, K. M. (2015). *Documenting occupational therapy practice* (3rd ed.). Boston, MA: Pearson.

Smith, J. (2013). Documentation of occupational therapy services. In L. W. Pedretti, H. M. Pendleton, & W. Schultz-Krohn (Eds.), *Pedretti's occupational therapy: practice skills for physical dysfunction* (7th ed., p. xviii). St. Louis, MO: Elsevier.

Management and Business Fundamentals in Occupational Therapy

Denise Hoffman

Learning Objectives

- Identify management roles in occupational therapy practice.
- Differentiate between leadership, supervision, management, and administration.
- Describe the process of management and the impact on occupational therapist's (OTs) productivity and work day management.
- Describe common quality improvement measures.
- Describe how outcome measures are necessary to managing occupational therapy delivery of care.
- Distinguish competency and professional development.

Key Terms

- *Leadership*: Taking responsibility for directing and motivating individuals toward a common goal.
- *Mission*: The focus and purpose of a specific organization.
- *Plan–do–check–act cycle*: A quality management approach used to solve problems including identifying and analyzing the issue, developing, testing, and checking how effective the solution was, and implementing the solution into practice.
- *Quality of care*: Services that are provided in a safe and effective manner consistent with the rules and regulations of professional boards.
- *Role delineation*: Identifying and distinguishing tasks based on the skill set of specific professionals.
- *SWOT analysis*: The identification and analysis of the strengths, weaknesses, opportunities, and threats of an organization.
- *Vision*: The eventual outcome or accomplishment of a specific organization.

Introduction

This chapter is divided into two categories: competency and direct management. The Centennial Vision describes the future direction of occupational therapists (OTs) as individuals who are "strengthening our capacity to influence and lead" (American Occupational Therapy Association [AOTA], 2007, p. 614). Competency and direct management leadership skills are necessary to build the path of promoting quality evidenced-based practice.

Occupational therapy management encompasses the role of the practitioner in a position of leadership responsible for planning, organizing, staffing, directing, and controlling the environment to foster a safe and effective delivery of care for the consumer and practitioner (Braveman, 2009, 2014). Manager's responsibilities are a well-orchestrated balance of multitasking, delegating, quality control, and mentoring which can be difficult without a foundational knowledge of fiscal awareness, conflict resolution skills, and an awareness of state and federal regulatory practice guidelines (Braveman, 2009).

Occupational therapy leaders partake in responsibility demands within supervisory, managerial, and administrative roles. To thoroughly identify the manager's role in occupational therapy, one must examine and distinguish between a supervisor, manager, and administrator. Supervisors have the least responsibilities within the organization required to facilitate staff feedback and interpersonal skills, mentor staff, and support administrative policies (Braveman, 2009). Managers are in the middle tier of the leadership team, advocating for occupational therapy departmental resources, fostering continuing education, and professional growth opportunities, while administering performance evaluations for staff (Braveman, 2009). An administrator engages in the role of the highest tier of the leadership team that strategically plans the organization, creates policies and procedures, and creates organizational and departmental budgeting while establishing quality control and assurance metrics (Braveman, 2009).

The occupational therapy manager is in the middle of the leadership triad with communication and responsiveness to both the administration and supervisors in the organization. The manager has to balance clinical competency and ethical practice without influential external factors such as reimbursement, productivity, or organizational demands that may impact the professional outcomes and cohesiveness of staffing (Glennon & VanOss, 2010).

Competency

Competency is a means to ensure that the OT practitioner is capable and trained to perform their job responsibilities. Basic competency includes completing course work through an accredited occupational therapy program, passing the National Board for Certification in Occupational Therapy (NBCOT®) exam, obtaining state licensure, and meeting employment requirements (Braveman, 2009).

Managers maintain organizational accreditations, outline job descriptions, create retention incentives, and measure practitioner skill sets through annual performance evaluations and competencies for employees. Continuing to construct opportunities for professional growth through continuing education and program development allows managers to increase professional and organizational competency among staff (Braveman, 2009).

Professional Development

Professional development fosters safe and effective delivery of care. Professional development can be obtained from taking weekend courses, online classes, reading professional journals, case studies, or mentoring with expert OTs. Management is responsible for providing the vehicle to access and guide one toward a learning environment that is equally beneficial for the consumer, practitioner, and facility. Practitioners must develop and demonstrate clinical, ethical, and legal competency to demonstrate professional growth and sustainability. The AOTA identifies knowledge, clinical reasoning,

interpersonal skills, performance skills, and ethical reasoning as the top five competency focus areas for new practitioners (AOTA, 2003). For additional readings on these competencies, go to http://www.aota.org/pdt/index.asp.

Job Responsibility

Occupational therapy manager's responsibilities include budgeting, staffing, competency, and policy responsibilities. Due to reimbursement, federal and state, and societal shifts, occupational therapy managers need to be change agents to sustain viable quality in practice. Creating the environment that lends itself to flexibility and staff engagement is ideal for best practice and positive client outcomes (Thomas, 2011).

Evidenced-Based Practice

Occupational therapy managers incorporate evidenced-based practice in an organization's delivery of care to increase and sustain competency in the workplace. Five strategies have been created to drive evidenced-based practice: formulate questions, search and sort the evidence, critically appraise the evidence, apply the practice, and self-evaluate. There are different types of rigor in research that will aid managers in choosing the best type of research to validate the treatment and competency ranging from level 1 (e.g., unbiased control group/strong research-based evidence) to level 5 (e.g., expert opinion) (Abreu & Chang, 2011; Braveman, 2006).

Self-Assessment

Identification of tools and resources for self-awareness and self-assessment is necessary for competency measures demonstrating best practice within professional and organizational settings (Foss, 2011). Through self-assessment, the occupational therapy manager must be competent to deliver constructive feedback and the practitioner needs to be prepared on how to process and apply the information.

Direct Management

Occupational therapy management is the process of planning, organizing, directing, and controlling employees in an organization to achieve and promote quality of practice and positive client outcomes (Braveman, 2014). A common management method of quality assurance and quality management is the plan–do–check–act (PDCA) technique to encompass a progress monitoring system managing clients, employees, and the organization (Braveman, 2006).

Legislation and Legal Management

Legislative policies create a platform for health care, education, and social systems to allow consumer accessibility, development of reimbursement fees, and assurance of quality and safety of care (Lamb, Meir, & Metzler, 2011). Federal and state regulations manage the scope of practice for practitioners (AOTA, 2014). The Department of Health and Human Services regulates health policies in the United States that impact occupational therapy, as does as the Centers for Medicare and Medicaid Services (Lamb et al., 2011).

Advocacy

Writing letters to representatives, attending state and/or federal Capitol Hill Day, presenting at staff meetings, and volunteering and maintaining membership on state and federal occupational therapy organizations are ways to support and advocate for the occupational therapy profession and populations serviced by occupational therapy (Lamb et al., 2011).

Accreditation Guidelines

Facilities, schools, hospitals, and private practices voluntarily adhere to accreditation guidelines that may require the practitioner to maintain yearly competencies for continued practice in those settings. The following accreditation programs help to increase consumer protection and demonstrate higher learning skills among practitioners (Kramer & Harvison, 2011; Lamb et al., 2011).

- *JCAHO*: Joint Commission on Accreditation of Healthcare Organizations: The largest, volunteer, nonprofit, private program for accredited health care (Lamb et al., 2011).
- *CARF International*: Commission on Accreditation of Rehabilitation Facilities: Private, nonprofit organization that accredits outpatient human services and medical rehabilitative programs all over the world (Lamb et al., 2011).

- *CHEA*: Council for Higher Education Accreditation: Private organization to promote and protect students in academia and recognize higher education (Kramer & Harvison, 2011).

Policies and Guidelines

Each state establishes their policies and scope of practice. Managers who oversee multiple states are responsible for policies in each state. Awareness of occupational therapy assistant (OTA) supervision, evaluation and interventions, paperwork, and delivery of care are guidelines identified in professional state policies (Lamb et al., 2011).

Reimbursement

Refer to Chapter 38.

Licensure

State licensure is a process that regulates the competency of an OT practitioner who demonstrates completion of accredited academic coursework, fieldwork rotations, and the NBCOT® exam. Fees and specialty requirements will vary from state to state; hence, adherence to individual state requirements is the practitioner's responsibility. Review your individual state guidelines for clarification on your process by searching for "State OT Statutes and Regulations" and "Model Practice Act Final" at http://www.aota.org.

Risk Management

Risk management in occupational therapy is a process that an organization utilizes to identify and assess risks involved in management, delivery, and outcomes of consumer care with current or new programs (Braveman, 2014). Identification of factors that impact budgets, technology, and staffing plays an integral part of organizational success, but the initial investment to validate cost, effectiveness, and outcome measures is risk management (Braveman, 2014). Providing mechanisms in place to assess risk factors is needed to increase viability and sustainability of a business with initial strategic planning organizations that will identify, assess, and implement the resources and tools to promote best practice (Braveman, 2014).

Quality Improvement

Quality improvement fosters a sense of change and problem-solving strategies to increase productivity, staff engagement, fiscal responsibility, and positive population outcomes (Braveman, 2006). However, being an agent of change can foster resistance without the gradual execution, resources, and evidence to support change. With dynamic changes in health care and education, new policies and procedures are demanding quality improvement plans to increase efficiency, reimbursement, and the delivery of care (Braveman, 2006).

Electronic medical records (EMRs), new technology, and updated equipment, as well as annual performance reviews formulate a plan toward quality improvement in an organization. Continually reassessing the plan and adapting to necessary changes in quality improvement is necessary through program development and staffing management strategies (Braveman, 2006, p. 254).

Program Development

Developing new programs and emerging practice is often created out of a quality improvement assessment, increasing productivity, changing delivery or type of services, and sustaining current policy and procedures (Braveman, 2006). The Occupational Therapy Practice Framework: Domain and Process guides the manager and practitioner on internal and external factors that promote quality health care (AOTA, 2014). A synthesis of program development strategies, emerging practice missions, visions, and theory-based knowledge promotes an effective and successful approach to new areas of practice and organizational projects (AOTA, 2014; Braveman, 2006).

Occupational therapy entrepreneurs face financial dilemmas with startup funds, equipment, and technology demands and are required to develop risk management protocols to justify the new business (Braveman, 2006). Formulating a vision to a viable business requires analysis of business systems, competition, financial means, and clinical knowledge. The Small Business Administration and Service Corps of Retired Executives are two resources that can aid entrepreneurs in developing a business plan and managing risks with a new business or new program (Score Association, 2016; U.S. Small Business Administration, 2016).

Outcome Measures

Outcome measures are used in practice to identify client success and satisfaction with their delivery and quality of care (Foss, 2011). Occupational therapy managers implement standardized assessments to objectively gather this data. Data collection tool such as the Functional Independence Measure (FIM) is a common tool used to evaluate rehabilitation outcomes (Foss, 2011). Performance reviews are common assessments to measure employee outcomes (Glennon & VanOss, 2010).

Scope of Practice

The Occupational Therapy Framework III guides occupational therapy practice and includes the domain and process categories for practitioner management of delivery of care (AOTA, 2014). This document identifies differences between the OT and OTA, evaluation and intervention processes, and practice requirements (AOTA, 2014). This combination educates the consumer, payer, and referral specialist on the scope of practice for occupational therapy. Each state has an individualized scope of practice that illustrates their specific societal, healthcare, and educational needs for occupational therapy. For your state's scope of practice, go to: www.aota.org and search "MSRSOTA.pdf."

Accountability Process

Management is required to identify strengths and weaknesses in order to develop a global business plan that accounts for organizational growth. A SWOT analysis is commonly used to identify internal and external strategies for organization management (Score Association, 2016; U.S. Small Business Administration, 2016). Review Table 37-3 in the end of the chapter self-study activities to understand and apply the process of organizational analysis.

Technology Monitoring

With the growing demand and dynamic changes in technology, resources are readily available for creating new policies on confidentiality and technology usage (Braveman, 2014). Managers have to be abreast of confidentiality policies and procedures regarding electronic mediums for communication, as well as for documentation. EMRs, electronic billing, and budgeting data will require the manager to initially purchase the equipment, and the software to sustain current practice documentation (Braveman, 2014). With the evolution of technology, managers have to decipher staffing needs for training and implementation of new technology within the organization (Braveman, 2009).

Documentation Guidelines

Universal documentation standards include assessments, a plan of care development, reassessment, and daily note documentation to meet the needs of the facility and reimbursement guidelines. Documentation has traditionally been in written paper format but has migrated to more EMR formats comprising of dropdown boxes and narrative reporting (Braveman, 2014). EMRs allow for a digital version of a client's medical chart.

Management and Standards of Practice

It is every practitioner's ethical responsibility to maintain current knowledge of federal, state, institutional, and international regulations that guide the highest level of service delivery and practice of occupational therapy (AOTA, 2015b). With changes in health care and regulatory demands, OTAs are in a higher demand for direct care, which places OTs in supervisory roles and creating greater opportunities to engage in evaluations (AOTA, 2015b). Therefore, there is an ethical concern about supervision that has and will continue to rise between OT and OTA collaboration. The OT and OTA role delineation requires clear discernment prior to servicing any clients because every state defines supervision differently (AOTA, 2009). OTs and OTAs should develop a "supervision and partnership" relationship including documentation with the amount, frequency, and level of supervision, which fosters professional growth, as well as ensures the highest level of care and protection for the consumer (AOTA, 2009, p. 797). Lack of awareness regarding professional knowledge and competencies in health care, regulatory reforms or organizational changes is unethical and may impact the safety of the consumer and the practitioner (AOTA, 2015b).

Types of Leadership

With the diversity in practice settings, health care, and educational changes, utilization of different leadership theories throughout management is needed to increase effective results, outcomes, and success in the workplace. The following three leadership styles are commonly displayed in occupational therapy; however, these are not reflective of all the behaviors utilized; hence attention to one's individual practice setting and personal skills may reflect additional styles. *Situational leadership* encompasses a triad of directing, coaching, and delegating responsibilities to change behaviors and achieve task completion (Winston, 2015). *Transformational leadership* is a process to motivate individuals and create opportunities to achieve changes (Bowyer, 2015). *Servant leadership* guides the organization toward serving and altruistic behaviors rather than authoritative behaviors (Dunbar, 2015). Professional responsibilities by occupational therapy practitioners to obtain basic leadership competencies and understand various theories and types of leadership styles are needed to effectively manage day-to-day operations and maintain competencies that will impact the management of day-to-day business.

Summary

This chapter outlines the key components in management for best practice in occupational therapy. This is a guide to foster your understanding of the basic requirements and scope of direct management and competencies for a new practitioner. Utilize the matching activities and case studies to complete your preparation for the NBCOT® exam.

Chapter 37 Self-Study Activities (Answers Are Provided at the End of the Chapter)

Match the term (right column) with the correct definition (left column). See **Table 37-1**.

Advocacy and legislation have impacted the profession of occupational therapy linking consumer awareness, accessibility, and safety to improving more meaningful, functional lives at all ages. Match the

Table 37-1 Terms and Definitions

Definition		Term
1. Highest leadership position in an organization responsible for policy and procedural development, organizational strategic planning, budgeting, and quality control and assurance measures.		**A.** Management process
2. Formulates questions, searches and sorts the evidence, critically appraises the evidence, applies to practice, and self-evaluates.		**B.** Supervisor
3. A nonprofit credentialing agency that works along with state regulatory bodies and provides information on credentials, professional conduct, and certification renewal.		**C.** Manager
4. A quality improvement strategy identifies the process that needs improvement, data collection, assessment of the new process, and implementation of the data and results. All four components increase a fluid and concise plan to address client success and quality of care (Braveman, 2006).		**D.** Administrator **E.** Competency **F.** CHEA **G.** Evidenced-based practice
5. Planning, organizing, directing, and controlling.		**H.** Self-assessment
6. Person responsible for facilitating staff feedback and interpersonal skills, mentoring staff, and supporting administrative policies.		**I.** Practice framework domains **J.** JCAHO
7. Advocates for occupational therapy departmental resources, fosters continuing education and professional growth opportunities, while assessing performance measures of staff.		**K.** CARF **L.** ACOTE
8. Completing course work through an accredited occupational therapy program, passing the NBCOT® exam, obtaining state licensure, and meeting employment requirements.		**M.** SWOT **N.** Documentation
9. Accreditation Council for Occupational Therapy Education®: Sets standards for education of all OT and OTA students (Kramer & Harvison, 2011).		**O.** Quality improvement **P.** Medicare Part B
10. Justifies the need for treatment, demonstrates progress toward goals, and justifies the service was skilled therapy (AOTA, 2009).		**Q.** NBCOT® **R.** PDCA
11. Strategic planning for a business or new department identifying the strengths, weaknesses, opportunities, and threats to the new programming (Score Association, 2015; U.S. Small Business Administration, 2015).		
12. Plan-do-check-act management process to monitor quality and quality improvement (Braveman, 2006).		
13. Occupations, client factors, performance skills, performance patterns, contexts, and environments (AOTA, 2014).		
14. Joint Commission on Accreditation of Healthcare Organizations: The largest, volunteer, nonprofit, private program to accredit health care (Lamb et al., 2011).		
15. Insurance that covers outpatient occupational therapy but with a cap of $1,940 per calendar year for occupational therapy services; limiting the beneficiary to receive all the necessary therapy within these financial parameters (AOTA, 2015a).		
16. Commission on Accreditation of Rehabilitation Facilities: Private, nonprofit organization that accredits outpatient human services and medical rehabilitative programs all over the world (Lamb et al., 2011).		
17. Council for Higher Education Accreditation: Private organization to promote and protect students in academia and recognize higher education (Kramer & Harvison, 2011).		
18. Reflection journaling, client and peer feedback, client outcomes, performance observations, and audit of documentation (Foss, 2011).		

description or definition (right column) with the laws that have influenced the profession (left column); see **Table 37-2** (Lamb et al., 2011).

Case Studies

Case Study 1

Read the case study and answer the provided questions.

Chris, an OT, has been practicing for only 1 year at a skilled nursing facility when his manager resigned and the facility asked Chris to take over the management position immediately. He would be responsible for budgeting, organizational competency execution, and maintaining quality management, as well as staffing management and client care 20% of the time. He is the only licensed OT because the remaining two department staff are OTAs with over 15 years of experience and a new graduate who has passed the NBCOT® certification exam, but does not have a state license. In the last staff meeting Chris learned his facility was out of compliance with organizational competencies such as employee performance reviews and chart audits.

- Is Chris qualified for this position?
- What is Chris's first responsibility if he takes this position?
- How much delegation can he provide to the OTA and the new graduate?

- What is Chris's obligation to maintain clinical and organizational competency?

Case Study 2

Read the case study and answer the provided questions.

Pat is a new graduate from an OTA program who has already received her license and she has accepted a full-time employment opportunity at an outpatient rehabilitation facility with an experienced OT, Chris. He is already supervising three other OTAs with over 1 year experience. In a meeting between Pat and Chris, supervision was discussed, including documentation of time, frequency, and ways to communicate. Pat is competent in her skills and feels the level of supervision is unfair in comparison to the other OTA she is working with and has requested less direct, one-on-one supervision. Pat has seen the other OTAs perform evaluations when Chris is getting too busy and she has inquired with Chris about the rules at the facility for OTAs to perform evaluations.

- Is Pat objective in her comparison and is this a reasonable request for the safety of the client and Pat to have less supervision?
- When one OT is on staff, and they are overwhelmed with evaluation referrals, can experienced OTAs perform the evaluations under the direction of the OT?

Table 37-2 Descriptions and Laws

Law		Description or Definition
1. Education for All Handicapped Children of 1975 and Individuals with Disabilities Education Act		A. A pivotal law for occupational therapy providing accessibility in public facilities, accommodations from employers, and independent living supports for individuals.
2. Medicare part B		B. A law protecting an individual's health insurance if they lose or change jobs and provides security measures for private health records.
3. Americans with Disabilities Act of 1990		C. A plan to provide free public education to children with physical and mental disabilities.
4. Health Insurance Portability and Accountability Act of 1996		D. A type of insurance that provides occupational therapy benefits in freestanding outpatient facilities.
5. Balanced Budget Act of 1997		E. A healthcare reform, including habilitative and rehabilitative therapy, that allows preexisting conditions to receive coverage for care and services from occupational therapy.
6. Patient Protection and Affordable Care Act of 2010		F. A prospective fee schedule for occupational therapy services was set, skilled nursing facilities began evaluating and offering occupational therapy services, and a cap was placed on outpatient Medicaid occupational therapy.

Lamb et al., 2011

Chapter 37 Self-Study Answers

Table 1

1. D
2. G
3. Q
4. O
5. A
6. B
7. C
8. E
9. L
10. N
11. M
12. R
13. I
14. J
15. P
16. K
17. F
18. H

Table 2

1. C
2. D
3. A
4. B

5. F
6. E

Answers to Case Study 1

When accepting a job promotion, increased responsibilities, or your first job position, one must complete a thorough assessment of the job performance requirements and your professional skill set. Chris would have to be a graduate of an accredited occupational therapy program, pass this NBCOT® certification exam, possess a current state license, and be current with state continuing education requirements (AOTA, 2003). Furthermore, Chris should complete a SWOT analysis to identify his clinical competencies, risk factors, and outcome of the promotion (Score Association, 2016; U.S. Small Business Administration, 2016). See **Table 37-3** for Chris's SWOT analysis; items on the right column are individual reflections and may not be a reflection of every new manager.

First Job Responsibility

Chris would need to address insufficiencies in both staff and organization deficiencies simultaneously. Facilities are required to maintain CARF certification and/or JACHO, including documentation, internal audits, consumer protection measures, outcome management, and employee competencies (Lamb et al., 2011). Using a formal procedural model can help a manager organize a strategic plan of action that will

Table 37-3 SWOT Analysis	
Strengths	• Chris has a B.S. in business management
	• Chris has a goal of entering management
	• Chris has always received excellent performance reviews
	• Chris is a member of his state occupational therapist association and AOTA
	• The facility has a management leadership program Chris would be enrolled in with a mentor because the facility has several facilities throughout the state
Weaknesses	• Chris has only 1-year clinical experience
	• Chris would be addressing organizational and employee competency issues immediately; therefore, he may not have the immediate skills to address these incompetencies
Opportunities	• Management position opening, fulfill his desire to be in a management position
	• Opportunities to connect and utilize state and national organizations and their resources
	• An opportunity to use knowledge from his B.S. degree in business management
Threats	• Time: Can he obtain the organizational and clinical competencies to successfully manage an occupational therapy department
	• Competency deficiencies with staff and organization that have to be addressed immediately
	• Learning curve of a new position. . . is there time to accommodate
	• Frustration and burnout early in his career

guide a manager through the different phases of solving a problem (Braveman, 2006). Establishing target outcomes and dates to accomplish these deficiencies is necessary to avoid fiscal penalties, as well as protecting the consumer delivery of care (Braveman, 2006). Chris would then need to direct his OT to their state government website licensure board to complete necessary documentation and paperwork for licensure to work. (Review your individual state guidelines for clarification on your process by searching for "State OT Statutes and Regulations" and "Model Practice Act Final" at http://www.aota.org.) Depending on state laws the new graduate may not be able to work without a state license or would require additional supervision.

Delegation Responsibilities

Chris is fortunate to have an OTA with experience who can provide feedback on previous successful management strategies. The OTA cannot perform evaluations but can assist with increased responsibility of program development and execution, such as directing group therapy sessions, in services to other staff, and increased responsibility of equipment and supply management (Glennon & VanOss, 2010). The OTA can also perform assessments after demonstrating service competency. Chris is short staffed as his position is vacant and his OT is not licensed. He will need to continue all evaluation assessments until his OT is licensed, unless his state practice defines otherwise. After his OT is licensed, Chris can delegate all evaluations to that therapist and open his time up for management.

Obligation to Maintain Clinical and Organizational Competencies

It is every OT's responsibility to maintain clinical, professional, and ethical competencies (AOTA, 2003). Employers may not provide practitioners with all the clinical or management information; therefore, supporting professional advocacy, maintaining professional state and national memberships, as well as seeking employee resources are ways to ensure competencies (Glennon & VanOss, 2010). Chris must ensure competencies of the facility to protect consumer safety, increase positive outcomes, and adhere to insurance guidelines. A skilled nursing facility must maintain competencies guided by federal and state regulations that manage the scope of practice for practitioners (AOTA, 2014). The Department of Health and Human Services regulates health policies

in the United States that impact occupational therapy, as well as the Centers for Medicare and Medicaid Services (Lamb et al., 2011). Policies and procedures establish order and viability of a profession, and should not be viewed as a hurdle, but rather as a means to facilitate best practice.

Answer to Case Study 2

According to the Code of Ethics from the AOTA (2015b), it is the OT's professional and ethical responsibility to maintain competency and knowledge on all regulatory, state, and federal guidelines regarding the occupational therapy supervision of OTAs. Chris is responsible for all the delivery of care he provides and the delivery of care performed by the OTAs under his direction and his plan of care (AOTA, 2009). Chris must exercise daily clinical judgment and the ability to execute procedural justice for the overall safety of the consumer and practitioner by providing more supervision for a new graduate (AOTA, 2015b). With new graduates, AOTA (2010) recommends a minimum of three to five hours of direct contact of close supervision and co-signatures alone are not sufficient for supervision requirements. Ultimately, it is the OT's professional responsibility to sign off on daily documentation and the delivery of care; hence if there are any deficiencies in the service of care from the OTA, Chris would be responsible (AOTA, 2009). Every state has different practice guidelines that outline the supervision collaboration between the OT and the OTA; however, Chris must follow the most stringent guideline set forth from the state, organization, federal or international regulations to protect himself, the OTA, and the consumer (AOTA, 2015b).

Second, it is unethical for Chris to allow OTAs to perform evaluations despite the shortage of his time. The OTA may assist with portions of the evaluation following state guidelines, but Chris is ultimately responsible for the evaluation. Pat has a valid and ethical concern that needs to be addressed and corrected to follow all regulations (e.g., state, federal, and organizational). Health care is continuously changing; therefore, having access to the changes and knowledge of how to address demands will prevent unethical practice to occur and protect the highest quality of service delivery for the practitioner and consumer. Chris could discuss his need for an on-call OT with his manager to balance demands of the influx of client referrals while managing the departmental budget and adhering to ethical practice.

References

Abreu, B. C., & Chang, P. J. (2011). Evidence-based practice. In K. Jacobs & G. L. McCormack (Eds.), *The occupational therapy manager* (5th ed., pp. 331–347). Bethesda, MD: AOTA Press.

American Occupational Therapy Association. (2003). *Professional development tool.* Retrieved from http://www.aota.org/education-careers/advance-career/pdt.aspx

American Occupational Therapy Association. (2007). American Occupational Therapy Association's Centennial Vision and Executive Summary. *American Journal of Occupational Therapy, 61*(6), 613–614.

American Occupational Therapy Association. (2009). Guidelines for supervision, roles, and responsibilities during the delivery of occupational therapy services. *American Journal of Occupational Therapy, 63,* 797–803.

American Occupational Therapy Association. (2010). *OT/OTA partnerships: Achieving high ethical standards in a challenging health care environment. Advisory opinion for the Ethics Commission.* Retrieved from https://www.aota.org/-/media/Corporate/Files/Practice/Ethics/Advisory/OT-OTA-Partnership.pdf

American Occupational Therapy Association. (2014). Occupational therapy practice framework: Domain and process (3rd ed.). *American Journal of Occupational Therapy, 68*(Suppl. 1), S1–S48.

American Occupational Therapy Association. (2015a). *Advocacy reports.* Retrieved from www.aota.org/Advocacy

American Occupational Therapy Association. (2015b). Occupational therapy code of ethics. *American Journal of Occupational Therapy, 69*(Suppl. 3). doi:10.5014/ajot.2015.696S03

Braveman, B. (2006). *Leading & managing occupational therapy services an evidence-based approach.* Philadelphia, PA: F. A. Davis Company.

Braveman, B. (2009). Management of occupational therapy services. In H. S. Willard, E. B. Crepeau, E. S. Cohn, & B. A. B. Schell (Eds.), *Willard & Spackman's occupational therapy* (11th ed., pp. 914–927). Philadelphia, PA: Wolters Kluwer Health/Lippincott Williams & Wilkins.

Braveman, B. (2014). Management of occupational therapy services. In B. A. B. Schell, G. Gillen, & M. E. Scaffa (Eds.), *Willard & Spackman's occupational therapy* (12th ed., pp. 1016–1030). Philadelphia, PA: Wolters Kluwer Health/Lippincott Williams & Wilkins.

Bowyer, P. (2015). Tansformational leadership theory and the model of human occupation. In S. B. Dunbar & K. Winston (Eds.), *An occupational perspective on leadership: Theoretical and practical dimensions* (2nd ed., pp. 25–34). Thorofare, NJ: SLACK Incorporated.

Dunbar, S. B. (2015). Servant leadership and the person-environment-occupation model. In S. B. Dunbar & K. Winston (Eds.), *An occupational perspective on leadership: Theoretical and practical dimensions* (2nd ed., pp. 49–57). Thorofare, NJ: SLACK Incorporated.

Foss, J. J. (2011). Mentoring and professional development. In K. Jacobs & G. L. McCormack (Eds.), *The occupational therapy manager* (5th ed., pp. 237–251). Bethesda, MD: AOTA Press.

Glennon, T., & VanOss, T. (2010). Identifying and promoting professional behavior. *OT Practice*, 13–16.

Kramer, P., & Harvison, N. (2011). Accreditation related to education. In K. Jacobs & G. L. McCormack (Eds.), *The occupational therapy manager* (5th ed., pp. 577–588). Bethesda, MD: AOTA Press.

Lamb, A., Meir, M., & Metzler, C. (2011). Federal legislative advocacy. In K. Jacobs & G. L. McCormack (Eds.), *The occupational therapy manager* (5th ed., pp. 441–454). Bethesda, MD: AOTA Press.

Score Association. (2016). *Score for the life of your business.* Retrieved from https://www.score.org

Thomas, J.V. (2011). Reimbursement. In K. Jacobs & G. L. McCormack (Eds.), *The occupational therapy manager* (5th ed., pp. 385-406). Bethesda, MD: AOTA Press.

U.S. Small Business Administration. (2016). *An official website of the United States Government.* Retrieved from https://www.sba.gov

Winston, K. (2015). Situational leadership and occupational therapy. In S. B. Dunbar & K. Winston (Eds.), *An occupational perspective on leadership: Theoretical and practical dimensions* (2nd ed., pp. 15–24). Thorofare, NJ: SLACK Incorporated.

Reimbursement

Denise Hoffman

Learning Objectives

- Distinguish the differences between federal, state, third-party payers, and private payers.
- Compare and contrast between Medicare and Medicaid reimbursement.
- Describe documentation required for occupational therapy practice.
- Describe the importance of diagnosis and procedural coding.
- Identify the appeals process for claim denials.
- Summarize documentation requirements for reimbursement.

Key Terms

- *Centers for Medicare and Medicaid Services (CMS)*: The federal agency that oversees and administers reimbursement for Medicare and Medicaid services.
- *Durable medical equipment (DME)*: Assistive or adaptive medical equipment ordered by healthcare professionals.
- *Fee schedule*: Fees listed by health insurance plans used for payment to providers.
- *Fraud*: When a healthcare professional purposefully falsifies services provided.
- *Network*: A group of healthcare organizations (e.g., professionals and hospitals) that provide services under a contractual agreement.
- *Out of network provider*: A healthcare organization (e.g., professional and hospital) that is not under contractual agreement to provide services, which may or may not be reimbursable.

Introduction

This chapter will review knowledge on insurance and reimbursement in occupational therapy practice in the United States. The content in this chapter highlights reimbursement knowledge identified in the Accreditation Counsel Standards for Occupational Therapy Education and the Standards of Practice in Occupational Therapy (American Occupational Therapy Association [AOTA], 2016).

The history of reimbursement for healthcare services dates back to the 1700s with the federal Marine Hospital, which evolved into the first insurance provider in 1929 with Blue Cross Blue Shield; however, insurance did not grow substantially until the twentieth century with the expansion of the healthcare and insurance industry (Lohman, 2014). Legislative changes have impacted reimbursement and occupational therapy services in the United States. In 1965, Medicare expanded to include occupational therapy services. In 1978, the Individuals with Disabilities Act (IDEA) was enacted to provide free education to children with disabilities, and in 2010 the Patient Protection and Affordable Care Act was activated increasing coverage for the uninsured (Braveman, 2009). The IDEA is legislation that outlines the free education to all children regardless of disability with the inclusion of infants and toddlers (Braveman, 2009).

Third-party payers are governmental and private insurance companies that pay the medical provider for services rendered (Braveman, 2009). Individuals may seek insurance coverage through employment, self-funding, or private insurance plans. Employees may pay for their insurance with pretaxed wages but would be responsible for additional deductibles, copayments, coinsurance, or out of pocket expenses. Deductibles are set out of pocket expenses the individual is responsible to cover for medical care prior to coverage of medical benefits activation.

Coinsurance is a fixed percentage an individual or secondary insurance pays to cover medical expenses, whereas copayments are a fixed amount the individual or secondary insurance pays to cover medical expenses (Braveman, 2009; Lohman, 2014; Thomas, 2011).

Medicare

The largest federally funded payer for occupational therapy services in the United States is Medicare (Department of Health and Human Services Center for Medicare and Medicaid Services, 2015). The Centers for Medicare and Medicaid Services of the Department of Health and Human Service manages this massive organization. Individuals over 65 years of age and individuals under 65 years of age with specific disabilities are eligible to apply for Medicare. Hospitals, facilities, and private practices are required to be in a network-contracted provider (e.g., rather than out of network provider) in order to receive reimbursement.

Dual enrollment occurs when an individual has coverage from both Medicare and Medicaid for medical expenses (Braveman, 2009; Lohman, 2014; Thomas, 2011).

Medicaid

Medicaid is a mutually federal and state-funded program that considers eligibility for individuals with disabilities or low income. Eligibility and benefits coverage vary from state to state, but there is mandatory and optional coverage depending on the state adoptions. Reviewing your state adoption plan is necessary as each state may have various straight, Health Managed Organization, or Prospective Payment Plan options.

The Children's Health Insurance Program (CHIP)

The CHIP is one type of Medicaid program that offers insurance to children who are not already covered with a family income that is 200% below the poverty level. This allows children with disabilities to receive medical care such as outpatient occupational therapy services. Not all Medicaid plans will have the same coverage of benefits, and different plans may require prior authorizations; therefore, identifying these parameters will be state specific. Refer to each state's website or go to www.insure kidsnow.gov for more information.

Workers' Compensation

This unique program offers reimbursement for expenses accrued due to work-related injuries through employment, state, or federally funded programs depending on the place of employment. Most workers' compensation programs have specific providers, referral processes, and documentation that is required for occupational therapy reimbursement eligibility; therefore, adhering to the employer's policy is necessary for coverage (Braveman, 2009). Workers' compensation covers wage compensation, medical treatment including occupational therapy services, and vocational training (Thomas, 2011).

Private Payers

Legislation and consumer-driven demands have accelerated a change in private insurance plan options in the United States. The demand has influenced awareness on emerging practice areas such as autism and an overall increase in occupational therapy referrals. Employers are offering a wider variance in cost and benefit options to employees. Occupational therapists (OTs) must consider many factors when providing services to consumers with private insurance to secure payment for services rendered.

Other Insurance Plans

Additional healthcare plans have evolved out of societal demands and changing needs. In 1975, the IDEA, a federal and state-funded program, was enacted covering services for children with disabilities to receive free and appropriate education including school-based occupational therapy services (Lohman, 2014).

Throughout history, occupational therapy has played a vital role in the recovery and healthcare delivery system for our active service individuals, as well as our veterans. The Veterans Program offers medical, mental health, and rehabilitative services to all veterans, and Tricare offers the same benefits for active duty service members and their families (Braveman, 2009).

Documentation Requirements

Occupational therapy documentation defines interventions provided, records progress, and outlines future plans of service (AOTA, 2014, 2015b). All regulatory providers require basic paperwork consisting of an initial evaluation report with a plan of care, daily documentation, and progress notes or recertification. Some insurance providers may require an initial prior authorization letter to justify the need and frequency of occupational therapy services. Medicaid plans vary among states, and commercial or private insurance plans may have different requirements for authorization to cover occupational therapy services; hence verifying individual's benefits prior to the start of care is recommended for every insurance provider (Braveman, 2009).

Prior Authorization

Depending on the payer, a prior authorization is needed that would include the dates of service, diagnosis code, procedural codes, and plan of care. Additional paperwork including a prescription may be requested depending on the payer. Understanding common procedural coding (CPT) will help to request prior authorization for the type of treatment that is being delivered (Braveman, 2009; Thomas, 2011). General awareness of the International Statistical Classifications of Disease (ICD) codes, which is the universal diagnosis coding system, is needed to aid in providing the correct diagnosis to the payer source for prior authorization (Department of Health and Human Services Center for Medicare and Medicaid Services, 2015; Lohman, 2014, p. 1060).

Prescription Referral

Our national association articulates in our scope of practice that although it is not a requirement of the AOTA, a prescription is required by most third-party payers for reimbursement. Occupational therapy services are regulated by laws and payer policies that must be followed for reimbursement (AOTA, 2015a).

Diagnosis and Procedural Coding

Identifying a universal diagnosis code to use for occupational therapy claims and documentation is necessary for classification of the client's condition, deficits, or disability. These diagnoses are derived from the ICD codes, or more commonly referred to as ICD coding (AOTA, 2015a). Additionally, current procedural terminology (CPT) coding is necessary to classify the type of treatment for billers to receive correct reimbursement. CPT codes delineate the type of service delivery from evaluations to specific intervention procedures and are determined after the ICD coding of a diagnosis occurs. CPT codes range from 97,000 to 97,999 and are frequently timed codes based on an eight-minute rule (Lohman, 2014; Thomas, 2011). Billable time using CPT codes may vary within settings such as school-based intervention in comparison to outpatient services; therefore, consult with your organization or agency to find out the specific billing procedures necessary to ensure that accurate policy and procedures are followed.

Claim Submission

Electronic claim submission for occupational therapy services is the primary mode of transmission; however, in specific circumstances, approval for paper submission is allowed. A CMS 1500 is a claim submission for documentation in outpatient freestanding occupational therapy facilities (Department of Health and Human Services Center for Medicare and Medicaid Services, 2015). A CMS 1450 (UB-04) is a claim submission for documentation of occupational therapy performed in hospitals and skilled nursing facilities (Department of Health and Human Services Center for Medicare and Medicaid Services, 2015).

Appeals Process

Every regulatory agency has a policy and procedure for filing, documenting, and completing an appeal to a denied claim. Claims are denied for various reasons including, but are not limited to, insufficient documentation, lack of medical necessity, or exhausted benefits. Regulatory payers have an appeal process outlined in their policy and procedure manuals. Filing an appeal is not a guarantee of coverage and is time-consuming for the organization and OT practitioner. Clients are often on hold for long durations while the appeal process is completed.

Management and Standards of Practice

The collaboration between OTs and occupational therapy assistants (OTA) is to ensure the highest quality of service for each client while fostering professional competency among the employees (AOTA, 2015a). OTs are responsible for educating OTAs on interventions, as well as the documentation and billable CPT codes for reimbursement (AOTA, 2015a). Knowledge of current regulatory providers that prohibit OTAs to provide treatment must be followed and practiced consistently by all OTs (Lohman, 2014). It is also important to note that occupational therapy aides are not licensed providers and cannot perform the same responsibilities as an OTA; hence their time is not billable (AOTA, 2015a).

Summary

Reimbursement is fundamental to the survival of any medical organization. Proper documentation and understanding of ICD and CPT coding is critical to increasing fluidity of prior authorization and delivery of care. Gaining a global understanding of insurance benefits will increase continuity of care, awareness of covered benefits, and decrease high out of pocket expenditures for the client.

Additional Reimbursement Resources

- American Occupational Therapy Association: http://www.aota.org
- Blue Cross Blue Shield Association: http://www.bluecares.com
- Centers for Medicare and Medicaid Services: http://cms.hhs.gov
- Insure Kids Now: http://www.insurekidsnow.gov

Chapter 38 Self-Study Activities (Answers Are Provided at the End of the Chapter)

Self-Study Activity I

Match the best answer (right column) with the corresponding definition (left column). See **Table 38-1** for description and matching answers for reimbursement.

Table 38-1 Reimbursement Descriptions

1. _____ Who is paying for occupational therapy services?	A. A fixed amount the individual or secondary insurance pays to cover medical expenses
2. _____ Who is the target population that can receive insurance?	B. Set out of pocket expenses paid by the individual prior to coverage of insurance for medical expenses
3. _____ Covered and excluded services in an insurance plan are called?	C. Set fee schedule by insurance companies to pay providers
4. _____ What is a deductible?	D. Eligible consumer
5. _____ What is a coinsurance?	E. A contractual agreement with an insurance payer to accept fee schedule, as well as to adhere to policy, documentation, and reimbursement guidelines
6. _____ What is a copayment?	F. Federal, state, workman's compensation, private, and/or self-payers
7. _____ What is dual enrollment?	G. Insurance benefits
8. _____ Fee for service is?	H. Enrollment in Medicare and Medicaid plans to cover medical expenses
9. _____ In network status is?	I. A fixed percentage an individual or secondary insurance pays to cover medical expenses

Data from Braveman 2009, Lohman 2014, Thomas 2010.

Table 38-2 Scope of Practice and Department of Health and Human Services

1. _____ Medicare Part A impacts occupational therapy because?	**A.** Predetermined fee for service for individuals receiving outpatient occupational therapy services
2. _____ Medicare Part B impacts occupational therapy because?	**B.** Total allowed amount for reimbursement for outpatient occupational therapy services per person per year
3. _____ $1,940.00 Cap applies to what?	**C.** Reimbursement for occupational therapy services received while hospitalized, at a skilled nursing facility, or receiving hospice care
4. _____ International Statistical Classification of Disease codes—Tenth Revision—Clinical Modification/Procedure Coding System (ICD-10-CM/PCS)	**D.** A law that protects the privacy and security of an electronic exchange of client information
5. _____ Diagnostic and Statistical Manual of Mental Disorders Fifth edition	**E.** Established coding system for orthotics and prosthetics and durable medical equipment for Medicare providers that is used in occupational therapy services
6. _____ Healthcare Professionals Advisory Committee	**F.** The newest uniform coding system for the OT to use in billing to define the diagnosis they are treating
7. _____ Health Insurance Portability and Accessibility Act (HIPPA)	**G.** The newest mental health manual defining mental health conditions incorporated in the ICD-10-CM/PCS

Data from American Occupational Therapy Association, 2015a; Department of Health and Human Services Center for Medicare and Medicaid Services, 2015; Thomas, 2010.

Self-Study Activity 2

Locate the AOTA Scope of Practice, Thomas (2011), and the Department of Health and Human Services "Next generation of coding" resources, then match the best answer (right column) with the best definition (left column); see **Table 38-2**.

Case Study 1

With an increase in private insurance utilization, understanding preauthorizations, out of network fees, visit and procedural coding, billing, and documentation is necessary for reimbursement and is the responsibility of each OT practitioner; not just the facility or organization. Why?

Case Study 2

Trey is an experienced OTA in a hand therapy clinic and started working with a new employee, Bailey, a licensed OT with minimal splinting experience. They are working in an outpatient facility connected to a local hospital. A reimbursement issue arises when a new order for a wrist cock up splint is ordered. The clinic has no supplies nor does Bailey, and she does not feel competent in making the splint. She informs

Trey that, "we do not get reimbursed for the splint material, and I do not have time or feel comfortable making this splint, so why don't you try and make it?" She informs Trey to go next door to the hospital and borrow material for the splint and then informs him not to bill for his time. Trey has concerns borrowing materials and not billing for his time. Are Trey's concerns valid?

Chapter 38 Self-Study Answers

Self-Study Activity 1 Answers

1. F
2. D
3. G
4. B
5. I
6. A
7. H
8. C
9. E

1. C
2. A
3. B
4. F
5. G
6. E
7. D

Case Study 1 Answers

Insurance companies offer a variety of plan options; therefore, basic knowledge of Blue Cross Blue Shield will not guarantee that you as the OT, with every employer that offers Blue Cross Blue Shield, will have the same visit limitations, coding acceptance, copayment, or deductibles. There are several plans within the Affordable Care Act that offer a bronze, silver, and gold plan with varying deductibles and covered benefits. Prior knowledge and authorization may be necessary to inform you as the provider how much reimbursement will be. Oftentimes, without prior authorization coverage, reimbursement will not be provided. Managers often monitor these plans and authorizations to prevent time-consuming appeals or lack of payment, which impacts budgeting and staffing costs. Furthermore, specific plans may only cover services within the dates on a progress note or plan of care and specific procedural coding. Keeping current documentation and utilization of correct procedural coding for treatment is necessary to ensure payment and sustainability of your job with an organization (Braveman, 2009; Thomas, 2011).

Case Study 2 Answers

Yes! It is the ethical responsibility that the supervising OT is competent in all procedures, modalities, and splinting techniques they are supervising over the OTA (AOTA, 2015a). Therefore, the OTA should not have made the splint because of ethical supervision concerns. Second, devaluing the role of an OTA (i.e., stating their time is not billable) does not demonstrate professionalism toward the OT or OTA collaboration (AOTA, 2015a). Any skilled therapy time spent with a client delivered by the OT or OTA is billable time, therefore underbilling, not charging for services is insurance fraud. There are CPT codes that are not covered by insurance such as splinting materials;

hence borrowing from another cost center is not ethical. When splinting or services are not covered, organizational rules should be established and well understood by all parties including all therapists and the consumer prior to the start of care.

References

American Occupational Therapy Association. (2014). Occupational therapy practice framework: Domain and process (3rd ed.). *American Journal of Occupational Therapy, 68*(Suppl. 1), S1–S48. doi:10.5014/ajot.2014.682006

American Occupational Therapy Association. (2015a). *Scope of practice Q & As*. Retrieved from http://www.aota.org/Practice/Manage/Scope-of-Practice-QA.aspx

American Occupational Therapy Association. (2015b). Standards of practice for occupational therapy. *American Journal of Occupational Therapy, 69* (Suppl. 3), 6913410057. doi:10.5014/ajot.2015.696S06

American Occupational Therapy Association. (2016). *Accreditation council for occupational therapy education (ACOTE®) standards and interpretive guide*. Retrieved from http://www.aota.org/-/media/corporate/files/educationcareers/accredit/standards/2011-standards-and-interpretive-guide.pdf

Braveman, B. (2009). Management of occupational therapy services. In E. B. Crepeau, E. S. Cohn, & B. A. B. Schell (Eds.), *Willard & Spackman's occupational therapy* (11th ed., pp. 914–927). Philadelphia, PA: Wolters Kluwer Health/Lippincott Williams & Wilkins.

Department of Health and Human Services Center for Medicare and Medicaid Services. (2015). *ICD-10-CM/PCS the next generation of coding*. Retrieved from https://www.cms.gov/Medicare/Coding/ICD10/downloads/ICD-10Overview.pdf

Lohman, H. (2014). Payment for services in the United States. In M. E. Scaffa, B. A. B. Schell, G. Gillen, & E. S. Cohn (Eds.), *Willard and Spackman's occupational therapy* (12th ed., pp. 1051–1067). Philadelphia, PA: Lippincott Williams & Wilkins.

Thomas, J. V. (2011). Reimbursement. In K. Jacobs & G. L. McCormack (Eds.), *The occupational therapy manager* (5th ed., pp. 385–405). Bethesda, MD: AOTA Press.

Research

Rosanne DiZazzo-Miller and Moh H. Malek

Learning Objectives

- Compare and contrast between the three major categories of research (i.e., quantitative, qualitative, and mixed methods).
- Define mixed methodology.
- Define threats to validity typically present in research.

Key Terms

- *Bias*: "Anything that produces systematic error in a research finding" (Vogt & Johnson, 2011, p. 28).
- *Reliability*: The extent to which a measure produces consistent results.
- *Statistical significance*: The probability that an observed effect is not occurring by chance, usually expressed with a *p*-value (i.e., alpha level) of less than 0.05 (i.e., $p < 0.05$).
- *Validity*: "The degree to which an instrument or test accurately measures what it is supposed to measure" (Vogt & Johnson, 2011, p. 415).

hallmark of research is that studies need to be empirical, which means that the conclusions drawn are verifiable and often refers to the results of the statistical analyses. For example, in quantitative research, if there is a statistically significant ($p < 0.05$) difference between two groups (e.g., Group A and Group B), then the investigator must accept the alternative hypothesis (e.g., observations resulted in a real effect). Conversely, if there is no statistically significant ($p > 0.05$) difference between Group A and Group B, then the investigator must accept the null hypothesis (e.g., observations did not result in a real effect). However, prior to beginning any research venture, an appropriate research question must be formulated, followed by choosing a feasible research design that appropriately controls for bias, so that it is plausible to conclude that the results of the study are due to the effects of the independent variable (Blessing & Forister, 2013). Using the PICO format as suggested by Gutman (2010), a thorough research question should include the clinical population (P), intervention (I), description of comparison or control group (C), and outcome measure (O).

Introduction

As a whole, information derived from research studies has the potential to influence the treatment of clinical populations. Although a single study does not result in treatment or policy changes, it may lead to research that contributes to determining the efficacy or harm of interventions in the long term. All empirical research should possess qualities that are systematic and objective. The term systematic refers to a deliberate approach for answering the research question, whereas objective refers to anything that produces preventable error in the research findings (Trochim, Donnelly, & Arora, 2016). Another

Quantitative Methodology

The measurement of outcomes using objectively acquired numerical data distinguishes quantitative research methods from others. Quantitative methods can be used to describe populations, show trends, predict relationships, and are often used to examine cause-and-effect relationships among variables (Portney & Watkins, 2009; Trochim et al., 2016). Quantitative designs include single-subject, cross-sectional or longitudinal, survey, secondary analysis, meta-analysis, quasiexperimental, and randomized controlled studies (Portney & Watkins, 2009; Trochim et al., 2016). While quantitative methods need to be systematic and objective, it is equally important to control for extraneous variables, which may influence the outcome variable.

The distinction between experimental and quasiexperimental research resides in whether or not random assignment was used by the investigator, when placing participants in either the control or experimental group. It is important to note that with certain research questions it is not practical or ethical to have random assignment. For example, if an investigator is examining the effect of stroke on balance and mobility, would it be possible and/or ethical to randomize healthy individuals into either an experimental group (e.g., induce stroke) or a control group (e.g., no stroke induced)? Of course, the response is a profound "no"; however, the research question can still be answered. Using a quasiexperimental design, the investigator could recruit clients poststroke (i.e., the experimental group) and healthy individuals (i.e., the control group) matched for age and gender. Thereafter, functional assessments can be performed on both groups and then statistically compared to determine whether or not balance and mobility is affected after a stroke.

Regardless of whether your research design is true experimental or a quasiexperimental, the investigator must control for internal and external validity. Internal validity refers to whether the independent variable (e.g., the treatment or program) caused the change in the dependent variable (e.g., the effect or outcome). The threats to internal validity, therefore, compromise the investigator's ability to conclude that the independent variable resulted in changes in the dependent variable. Not having groups equivalent at baseline (i.e., selection) may be a potential threat to internal validity. For example, if there is a statistically significant mean difference between the experimental and control groups on the preintervention assessment, then this influences the results of the postintervention results. Another example of a threat to internal validity is experimental mortality, which is more often likely in studies with clinical populations rather than with healthy populations. Thus, if you start with 50 participants per group and at the end of the study have 1 group with only 10 participants remaining, this may influence the results of your study.

External validity refers to whether or not the results of a study can be generalized to the larger population. The questions that a researcher needs to consider are, "How representative is my sample of the population of interest?" and "How widely do the findings apply?" For example, if your study consists of 20- to 30-year-old men, then the results cannot be extended to 50- to 60-year-old men or even 20- to 30-year-old women. The point here is

Table 39-1 Quantitative Statistical Analyses

Method	Purpose
Descriptive statistics	Provides information on the study sample's central tendency, variability, skewness, and kurtosis through a summary of statistics such as mean, median, standard deviation, and sample distribution.
Chi-square	No assumption of distribution. Compares actual numbers with expected numbers among groups by examining the relatedness or independence of two categorical variables (independent variables [IV] and categorical dependent variables [DV]).
t-tests	Various types of t-tests measure the distance and significance within a group or between-group means. Commonly used to compare mean score of two groups on a continuous variable.
Analysis of variance (ANOVA)	An extension of the t-test that measures differences in group means. Controls for Type I error in place of analyzing data through multiple t-tests.
Multivariate analysis of variance	Similar to ANOVA except there are several DVs, such as comparing groups to different but related DVs.
Analysis of covariance	Measures differences in group means similar to ANOVA; however, the third variable is labeled a covariate, and has an effect on the DV. This is used to control for possible effects of an additional variable that may impact the effect of the IV. The effect or covariate is, in essence, removed.
Repeated measures	ANOVA with the additional capability of measurement across time or condition.
Correlation	Tests relationships in exploratory studies to explore the strength of a relationship between two continuous variables.
Regression	An extension of correlation used to predict a set of IVs on one continuous dependent measure.

Data from Portney and Watkins, 2009; Tabachnick and Fidell, 2007; Trochim and Donnelly, 2008.

that the conclusions of your study can only be applied to the population that is represented in your sample.

Table 39-1 provides a brief overview of various types of statistical analyses along with their corresponding purpose.

Qualitative Methodology

A deeper understanding of various phenomena is the goal of qualitative methods, where it is predominantly used to understand insight, feelings, and perspectives of specific populations, and is thereby more descriptive and exploratory in nature (Carr, 1994; Portney & Watkins, 2009; Trochim et al., 2016). Qualitative investigations center on various methods of inquiry including ethnography, grounded theory, phenomenology, discourse analysis, and case study design (Munhall & Chenail, 2008; Richards & Morse, 2013). See **Table 39-2**. In qualitative inquiry, behavior and emotion are observed and analyzed for emerging themes (Richards & Morse, 2013). This process is time intensive and usually involves individuals or small groups of people. While qualitative findings are typically viewed as less generalizable, results can inform and enhance understanding of client experiences (Myers, 2000).

Phenomenology and ethnography are common qualitative methods of inquiry, where purposeful, snowball, convenience, or theoretical sampling seeks to ensure valid representation rather than randomization (Hasselkus & Murray, 2007; Holthe, Thorsen, & Josephsson, 2007; Richards & Morse, 2013). Ethnography is useful to study the various subgroups of people, with a focus on lives that are impacted by a disability (Law et al., 1998). The goal of

ethnographers is to tell the story of daily life within a specific subgroup that is derived from participants' personal meaning and the manner in which they relate to their daily life (Willis & Trondman, 2000). Although participant observation is the most traditional method of ethnographic data collection, various other methods such as focus groups, unstructured interviews, and the study of documents and photographs help us gather rich data from the field (Richards & Morse, 2013). However, the duration of focus groups has been controversial among ethnographers and phenomenologists. Ethnographers argue that focus groups of 1–1.5 hours are too short to gather meaningful data, while phenomenologists are more concerned about the absence of the one-on-one interaction between the researcher and the participant (Agar & MacDonald, 1995; Bradbury-Jones, Sambrook, & Irvine, 2009).

Ethnographers are also concerned that focus groups occur outside of the natural setting where daily life takes place (Holthe et al., 2007). Conversely, an advantage of focus groups over participant observation is the intense focus on a topic in a limited time period, and the data

Table 39-2 Qualitative Methods of Inquiry, Purpose, Strategies, and Data Analysis

Qualitative Method	Purpose	Strategies	Data Analysis
Ethnography	Immersion and engagement with culture/group under study. Focus on detailed description versus explanation—Observational type questions	Unstructured recorded interviews, observation, field notes, videos, photos, and genograms	Thematic categorizations, search for inconsistencies/contradictions, and generate conclusions about what and why
Grounded theory	Inductive approach—New data direct research with constant comparison of observations. Goal is emerging theory—Process type questions	Recorded interviews, observations, field notes, and diaries	Constant comparative analysis, detailed knowledge, and time trajectory
Phenomenology	Seeks to understand life experiences through a thorough examination of each case—Meaning of phenomena	Recorded interviews, focus groups, literature, poetry, and films	Intensive individual examination, systematic, reflective study of lived experiences through reading, reflection, and writing
Discourse analysis	Draws from sociolinguistics and cognitive psychology to understand communications—Social construction	Detailed examination of text/language used in everyday life, recorded interviews, documents, diaries, and documentaries	Coding, conversation analysis, and notations with a focus on sequence and underlying meanings. Includes an examination of social and cultural contexts of text/language
Case study	Examination of one or more cases in order to provide an in-depth description of a social phenomenon—Illustration of experience	Observation, field notes, recorded interviews, and/or focus groups of a single or small group of similar cases	Focus is on roles and relationships, and physical and social contexts. Connections rather than categories of data are sought

Data from Kielhofner, 2006; Munhall and Chenail, 2008; Richards and Morse, 2013.

gathered from the interactions between focus group participants that would not occur in individual interviews (Bradbury-Jones et al., 2009; Morgan, 1997). Data analysis for both methods is inductive—where the researcher allows for the emergence of ideas and themes rather than a previous theory (Clarke, 2009). In phenomenology, participants' stories are examined verbatim, through the emic (i.e., the insider) experience and etic (i.e., the outsider) interpretation, with triangulation of data (i.e., using different sources of information to increase validity) (Clarke, 2009). A primary threat to qualitative methods of inquiry centers on the researcher misinterpreting the meaning expressed by study participants, or if the researcher substitutes it with their own (Kielhofner, 2006). In fact, both methods require researcher reflexivity—the practice of acknowledging the influence of the researcher's own knowledge on the study itself—a threat throughout all qualitative studies (Blair & Robertson, 2005). Analysis with ethnography includes a rich description through reading notes and coding or diagramming patterns, whereas phenomenological analysis is centered on exploring themes and meaning through reflective writing (Richards & Morse, 2013). The final product of both typically includes a written account where ethnography's focus is on participant insight and attitudes, and phenomenology's focus is on describing and interpreting the lived experiences (Bradbury-Jones et al., 2009; Holthe et al., 2007). Both methodologies provide insight and understanding into the experience, which can inform the development of quantitative measures (Byers & Wilcox, 1991).

Case studies—either multiple or singular—are commonly used in practice to describe a social phenomenon or in some cases, as a means to generate theory (Creswell, 2014; Munhall & Chenail, 2008). Case studies provide an avenue for clinicians to gather outcomes on how interventions can make a difference in real-world scenarios. Grounded theory utilizes a process of constant comparative analysis where the main goal is to generate theory (Munhall & Chenail, 2008).

Mixed Methodology

Ponterotto (2005) discusses a paradigm shift toward a more inclusive reliance on both quantitative and qualitative methods—a noted change from the dominating world of quantitative science. Rather than treating these two methods as separate, when intertwined they can inform each other on various aspects of research and practice (Johnson & Onwuegbuzie, 2004), resulting in triangulation

or the combination of research methods (Jick, 1979). An example of sequential triangulation (Creswell, 2014) can be seen in the development and administration of a quality of life survey for a specific subgroup. Qualitative inquiry and analysis are required to develop the appropriate questioning. Further, quantitative inquiry can target a large sample where data analysis can provide numerical data to test the survey framework and provide generalizability to various subgroups (Trochim et al., 2016). Therefore, it is important that we understand the implications of both methods of inquiry and the critical role they play in illuminating each other together, rather than apart. Regardless of the methodological approach, the research question informs the research method, which informs the type of data collected, pursuant analyses, and ultimate contribution toward evidence-based practice (Hammell, 2002).

Management and Standards of Practice

Evidence drives occupational therapy practice. According to the most recent Accreditation Council for Occupational Therapy Education 2011 Standards, "the rapidly changing and dynamic nature of contemporary health and human services delivery systems requires the occupational therapist (OT) to possess basic skills as a direct care provider, consultant, educator, manager, researcher, and advocate for the profession and the consumer" (AOTA, 2012, p. S6). Therefore, it is important for OT practitioners to understand basic research principles even if they do not identify as a researcher. Practitioners, regardless of their research background or interests, must base practice on evidence or knowledge as opposed to trial and error for the benefit of current and future clients (Depoy & Gitlin, 2011). Furthermore, this basic knowledge provides OT practitioners with the ability to appraise or critically evaluate published research in order to decide if it is contextually relevant. Occupational therapy assistants can assist with data collection on a research team and provide their unique perspectives under the supervision of an OT.

Chapter 39 Self-Study Activities (Answers Are Provided at the End of the Chapter)

1. Review the following terms and match them with their corresponding definition.

Term	Definition
A. Bias **B.** Clinical trial **C.** Correlation **D.** Ethnography **E.** Experimental study **F.** Generalizability **G.** Hawthorne effect **H.** Inclusion/exclusion criteria **I.** Institutional review board **J.** Likert scale **K.** Member checking **L.** Nonparametric statistics **M.** Parametric statistics **N.** Phenomenology **O.** Qualitative research **P.** Quantitative research **Q.** Quasiexperimental **R.** Random sample **S.** Random assignment **T.** Reliability **U.** Triangulation **V.** Validity	**1.** _____ The investigation of a culture through study of its members and systematic data collection and analysis.
	2. _____ Also called the "observer effect" where participants change their behavior because they are being observed.
	3. _____ When data, interpretations, or conclusions are tested with a member of the group from which they were obtained.
	4. _____ A qualitative method of inquiry based on perceptions of lived experiences.
	5. _____ A general method of inquiry used to investigate phenomenon.
	6. _____ A statistical method where the data are ordinal (i.e., ranking order), and are not required to be normally distributed, and therefore does not make any assumptions about parameters.
	7. _____ The extent to which a measure tests what it is supposed to test.
	8. _____ A controlled study using human participants designed to evaluate the effectiveness of an intervention.
	9. _____ Research that is similar to experimental research without the random assignment to treatment or control group.
	10. _____ A relationship between two variables.
	11. _____ A qualitative strategy used to facilitate validation of data through cross verification from two or more sources.
	12. _____ The process where scientists performing the research influence the results.
	13. _____ The extent to which a measure produces consistent results.
	14. _____ A statistical method where data result from a probability distribution and make inferences about the parameters.
	15. _____ The method of selecting a study sample from a population in such a way that every possible sample that could be chosen has a predetermined probability of being selected.
	16. _____ The extension of research findings and conclusions on a study population to a larger population.
	17. _____ The creation of study groups where each participant is assigned to a research group based on chance in hopes to eliminate confounding variables.
	18. _____ Criteria that either qualify or disqualify potential participants from participating in a research study.
	19. _____ A formal, systematic process for obtaining quantifiable data in numerical form for analyses to test for relationships.
	20. _____ A group of peers that examine research proposals to ensure it is ethical and safe for participants.
	21. _____ A scale that typically includes a neutral point and five or seven points of agreement/disagreement toward a statement.
	22. _____ A study where participants are assigned to an intervention or control group to evaluate the effects of an intervention.

Data from: Depoy and Gitlin (2011); Munhall and Chenail (2008); Trochim and Donnelly (2008).

Chapter 39 Self-Study Answers

Question 1

1. D
2. G
3. K
4. N
5. O
6. L
7. V
8. B
9. Q
10. C
11. U
12. A
13. T
14. M
15. R
16. F
17. S
18. H
19. P
20. I
21. J
22. E

References

Agar, M., & MacDonald, J. (1995). Focus groups and ethnography. *Human Organization, 54*(1), 78–86.

American Occupational Therapy Association. (2012). 2011 Accreditation Council for Occupational Therapy Education standards. *American Journal of Occupational Therapy, 66,* S6–S74. doi:10.5014/ajot.2012.66S6

Blair, S. E. E., & Robertson, L. J. (2005). Hard complexities—Soft complexities: An exploration of philosophical positions related to evidence in occupational therapy. *British Journal of Occupational Therapy, 68*(6), 269–276.

Blessing, J. D., & Forister, J. G. (2013). *Introduction to research and medical literature for health professionals* (3rd ed.). Burlington, MA: Jones & Bartlett Learning.

Bradbury-Jones, C., Sambrook, S., & Irvine, F. (2009). The phenomenological focus group: An oxymoron? *Journal of Advanced Nursing, 65*(3), 663–671. doi:10.1111/j.1365-2648.2008.04922.x

Byers, P. Y., & Wilcox, J. R. (1991). Focus groups: A qualitative opportunity for researchers. *The Journal of Business Communication, 28*(1), 63–79.

Carr, L. T. (1994). The strengths and weaknesses of quantitative and qualitative research: What method for nursing? *Journal of Advanced Nursing, 20*(4), 716–721. Retrieved from http://www.ncbi.nlm.nih.gov/pubmed/7822608

Clarke, C. (2009). An introduction to interpretative phenomenological analysis: A useful approach for occupational therapy research. *British Journal of Occupational Therapy, 72*(1), 37–39.

Creswell, J. W. (2014). *Research design: Qualitative, quantitative and mixed methods approaches* (4th ed.). Thousand Oaks, CA: SAGE Publications.

Depoy, E., & Gitlin, L. N. (2011). *Introduction to research: Understanding and applying multiple strategies* (4th ed.). St. Louis, MO: Elsevier.

Gutman, S. A. (2010). Reporting standards for intervention effectiveness studies. *American Journal of Occupational Therapy, 64*(4), 523–527. Retrieved from http://www.ncbi.nlm.nih.gov/pubmed/20825122

Hammell, K. W. (2002). Informing client-centered practice through qualitative inquiry: Evaluating the quality of qualitative research. *British Journal of Occupational Therapy, 65*(4), 175–184.

Hasselkus, B. R., & Murray, B. J. (2007). Everyday occupation, well-being, and identity: The experience of caregivers in families with dementia. *American Journal of Occupational Therapy, 61*(1), 9–20. Retrieved from http://www.ncbi.nlm.nih.gov/pubmed/17302101

Holthe, T., Thorsen, K., & Josephsson, S. (2007). Occupational patterns of people with dementia in residential care: An ethnographic study. *Scandinavian Journal of Occupational Therapy, 14,* 96–107.

Jick, T. D. (1979). Mixing qualitative and quantitative methods: Triangulation in action. *Administrative Science Quarterly, 24*(4), 602–611.

Johnson, R. B., & Onwuegbuzie, A. J. (2004). Mixed method research: A research paradigm whose time has come. *Educational Researcher, 33*(7), 14–26.

Kielhofner, G. (2006). *Research in occupational therapy: Methods of inquiry for enhancing practice.* Philadelphia, PA: F. A. Davis Company.

Law, M., Stewart, D., Letts, L., Pollock, N., Bosch, J., & Westmoreland, M. (1998). *Guidelines for critical review of qualitative studies.* Retrieved from http://www.musallamusf.com/resources/Qualitative-Lit-Analysis-pdf.pdf

Morgan, D. L. (1997). *Focus groups as qualitative research* (2nd ed.). Newbury Park, CA: SAGE Publications.

Munhall, P. L., & Chenail, R. (2008). *Qualitative research proposals and reports: A guide* (3rd ed.). Sudbury, MA: Jones and Bartlett Publishers.

Myers, M. (2000). Qualitative research and the generalizability question: Standing firm with proteus. *The Qualitative Report, 4*(3/4). Retrieved from http://nsuworks.nova.edu/tqr/vol4/iss3/9/

Ponterotto, J. G. (2005). Qualitative research in counseling psychology: A primer on research paradigms and philosophy of science. *Journal of Counseling Psychology, 52*(2), 126–136. Retrieved from http://xa.yimg.com/kq/groups/17264267/175124790/name/QualitativeResearchParadigmsandPhilosophyofScience.Ponterotto%282005%29article.pdf

Portney, L. G., & Watkins, M. P. (2009). *Foundations of clinical research: Applications to practice* (3rd ed.). Upper Saddle River, NJ: Prentice Hall.

Richards, L., & Morse, J. M. (2013). *Readme first for a user's guide to qualitative methods* (3rd ed.). Thousand Oaks, NJ: SAGE Publications.

Tabachnick, B. J., & Fidell, L. S. (2007). *Using multivariate statistics* (5th ed.). Boston, MA: Pearson.

Trochim, W., Donnelly, J. P., & Arora, K. (2016). *Research methods: The essential knowledge base*. Mason, OH: Cengage Learning.

Vogt, W. P., & Johnson, B. (2011). *Dictionary of statistics and methodology: A nontechnical guide for the social sciences* (4th ed.). Thousand Oaks, CA: SAGE Publications.

Willis, P., & Trondman, M. (2000). Manifesto for ethnography. *Ethnography, 1*(5–16).

The OT and OTA: Working Together for Optimal Client Outcomes

Susan Robosan-Burt

Learning Objectives

- Compare and contrast the roles of the occupational therapist (OT) and the occupational therapy assistant (OTA) in the occupational therapy process.
- Identify the responsibilities of the OT in the occupational therapy process.
- Identify the responsibilities of the OTA in the occupational therapy process.
- Identify the professional behaviors that impact the OT and OTA partnership.
- Describe the levels and methods of supervision in general practice settings.
- Identify the elements that foster an effective OT and OTA partnership.
- Identify the distinct value of the OT and OTA partnership.
- Identify the ethical principles that apply to the OT and the OTA partnership.

Key Terms

- *Code of Ethics*: A public document that addresses the most prevalent ethical concerns of the occupational therapy profession.
- *Guidelines*: A document that outlines general principles for the delivery and documentation of occupational therapy services.
- *Roles and responsibilities*: A guideline that defines and outlines specific roles and responsibilities for OTs and OTAs during the delivery of occupational therapy services.
- *Standards*: A document that defines standards for practice and continued competency.

- *Supervision*: A process and partnership within the practice of occupational therapy that is developed to ensure the safe and effective delivery of occupational therapy services and client-centered care.

Description

When working in a setting where there are occupational therapists (OTs) and occupational therapy assistants (OTAs), efficacious and evidence-based practice requires a collaborative relationship. The relationship is based on respect and trust similar to the therapeutic relationship we establish with our clients. Similarly, a professional rapport is established between occupational therapy practitioners when previous experience, skills, strengths, and weaknesses are identified to establish a client-centered partnership. Development of this professional partnership can additionally foster a mutually satisfying and collaborative relationship. The American Occupational Therapy Association (AOTA) defines the relationship between the OT and the OTA as a partnership. The term occupational therapy practitioner is utilized in this chapter and refers to both OTs and OTAs (AOTA, 2014b).

A partnership develops over time and is enhanced by a mutual and shared desire and commitment to the clients and groups served. True signs of a good leader include making a concerted effort to foster the strengths of others by recognizing their knowledge, skillsets, and values, as well as providing support and encouragement. Supervision is a leadership quality that requires additional responsibilities and takes time to develop in order to obtain the needed knowledge and skills. Equally, continued time and effort are essential to maintain an effective occupational therapy practitioner partnership.

Role Delineation

The AOTA states that an OT is autonomous and able to deliver occupational therapy services independently—without supervision. The AOTA also states that an OTA delivers occupational therapy services with supervision by, and in partnership with, an OT (AOTA, 2014a). As we continue advancing as a profession toward the AOTA's Centennial Vision of being science-driven and globally connected, we must continue to focus on providing evidence-based care and add to that knowledge base by participating in ongoing and new research projects. The role of the OTA in research is to review and apply professional literature, participate in the data collection process, and contribute to the research process (AOTA, 2014a; Solomon, 2003). This is another example of an opportunity for collaboration and partnership between the OT and OTA, which enhances the occupational therapy process and client outcomes.

Provision of Client-Centered Care

The OT is accountable for all aspects of care and ensures that the occupational therapy process is safe and effective (AOTA, 2014b, 2015b). The OTA plays an essential role in carrying out this process. Throughout the occupational therapy process, practitioners are engaged in clinical reasoning, which requires effective written and verbal communication. Collaboration is essential when an OT is working with an OTA. The OT must understand her or his role and responsibilities, as well as those of the OTA. Additionally, an OT must be knowledgeable about OTA education and training. The Accreditation Council for Occupational Therapy Education Standards may be utilized as a reference for OTA entry-level education and competencies. The OT determines when to delegate responsibilities to the OTA based on competency. The OTA must assure that they are competent to carry out the responsibilities delegated to them by the OT (AOTA, 2015a).

Practitioner Responsibilities

The following responsibilities are outlined in the AOTA's Standards of Practice for Occupational Therapy

(AOTA, 2015b). These reflect the minimally accepted standards of practice and levels of contribution and participation by the OTA. The OTA can contribute to all aspects of the occupational therapy process. See the guidelines for supervision, roles, and responsibilities during the delivery of OT services and the AOTA Code of Ethics for further information (AOTA, 2014a, 2015b). The following chapter sections outline the responsibilities assumed by the OT and the OTA during the occupational therapy process.

Screenings and Assessments

The OT is responsible for directing the screening, evaluation, and reevaluation process, as well as all related documentation. The OTA contributes to the screening, evaluation, and reevaluation process in partnership with the OT. The OT is responsible for the interpretation of the assessment results; however, both practitioners contribute to timely and accurate documentation of client screening, evaluation, and reevaluation.

Intervention Planning, Implementation, and Review

The OT is responsible for directing the development, documentation, and implementation of the intervention plan. The OT and the OTA collaborate to develop the intervention plan, as well as articulating the plan's rationale when establishing effective intervention strategies. Additionally, both practitioners contribute to the timely and accurate documentation of OT services.

Intervention implementation: The OT and the OTA are responsible for providing direct client care and to ameliorate challenges identified and documented during the evaluation and development of the intervention plan, respectively. Practitioners are also responsible for accurately documenting the services they have provided in a timely and effective manner. Practitioners must understand the expectations for documentation and billing of occupational therapy services used by individual facilities or healthcare systems where they are employed, contracted or provide OT services.

Intervention review: The OT is responsible for determining if occupational therapy services should be continued without changes, continued but modified, or discontinued. The OTA contributes to the process of intervention review.

Outcomes: The OT is responsible for selecting, assessing, and interpreting the outcomes, as well as directing the outcome process. The OTA contributes to the assessment of the safety and effectiveness of the occupational therapy services provided and the outcomes achieved. Both practitioners contribute to the documentation.

Transition or discontinuation plan: The OT is responsible for the transition or discontinuation plan and corresponding documentation. The OTA contributes to the plan by documenting or articulating the client's needs, goal status, performance, and resources. Both practitioners contribute to the documentation and transition or discharge plan (AOTA, 2014a).

Professional Behaviors

Professional behavior is expected in health care. In fact, professional behavior could be considered a prerequisite and facilitator of clinical reasoning. Examples of professional behaviors necessary for the delivery of effective client-centered care include a positive attitude, flexibility in thoughts and actions, effective communication skills (i.e., written and verbal), and a respectful demeanor (Glennon & Van Oss, 2010).

Supervision

Entry-level OTs can supervise an OTA. They must have knowledge of the supervisory process and the responsibilities associated with providing effective supervision that is consistent with AOTA's Code of Ethics (AOTA, 2015c; Youngstrom, 2014). Supervision is a collaborative process in which the OT and the OTA facilitate an ongoing relationship that is established on trust, mutual respect, and effective written and verbal communication. OTs and OTAs develop a plan for supervision and mutually share in the responsibility of establishing a plan that reflects a collaborative partnership, as well as helping to ensure that effective supervision is provided when necessary. The OT is responsible to ensure that the level of supervision is appropriate. The OTA is also responsible for determining if the supervision level and frequency established is appropriate, as well as for requesting and obtaining supervision based on competency (AOTA, 2014a, 2015a). The plan must be developed specifically to meet the needs of the clients and practitioners while adhering to facility policies, state licensure laws, regulatory bodies, and third-party payer guidelines.

When establishing a supervisory plan, it is important to communicate successful learning styles and methods of supervision. Trust is mutually developed and established throughout the process. The OT and OTA must be respectful and knowledgeable of their respective roles, and cognizant of the amount of experience and skills each practitioner contributes based on areas of practice. Clinical reasoning and discussion can enhance professional knowledge, partnership, and the ability to directly apply the provision of occupational therapy services. The benefit of this partnership in the delivery of client-centered care is enhanced by effective supervision. Both practitioners must agree on the supervisory plan, as well as how the plan will be structured. Documentation and maintenance of records related to supervision and outcomes may be mandated by the facility or state licensure law. Both practitioners must be knowledgeable of the supervision guidelines as outlined in the state licensure law. Supervision must meet facility, reimbursement, legal, and ethical requirements. The most stringent guideline is the guideline to follow. Therapists must have knowledge and access to facility policies, state licensure laws, public health codes, reimbursement guidelines, and the AOTA Code of Ethics. A lack of knowledge is not an excuse for making an error in judgment as it pertains to the law. The AOTA Code of Ethics is a public statement that helps promote and maintain professional conduct within the membership (AOTA, 2015c).

An OT with more than 1 year of experience can supervise fieldwork students at both the OT and OTA levels. The OT working with an OTA and supervising students is responsible for modeling the partnership of the OT and OTA (AOTA, 2015a; Youngstrom, 2014).

Levels of Supervision

Direct or line of sight: For this level of supervision, the OT will be in the area when the OTA is providing occupational therapy services. This level of supervision would be appropriate for an OTA who is a new graduate, acquiring a new skill, recently entered a new area of practice, or when establishing service competency.

General supervision: For this level of supervision, the OT may not be on site; however, they may be available by telephone or other means of electronic transmission. This level of supervision would be appropriate for an OTA who has established service competency in the area of practice.

Methods of Supervision

- *Delegation versus authoritative*: Delegation is when a mutual trust is established and the task is assigned to the OTA. Authoritative is providing a task to an OTA in a direct manner and expecting the OTA to complete the task.
- *Collaborative*: A respect of others' skills, knowledge, passion, and areas of expertise.
- *Clinical reasoning*: The process of documenting competence on service delivery including performance and judgment throughout assessments and interventions.
- *Observation*: Providing time in the OTA's schedule to observe the OT's interventions.
- *Written*: The provision of inheritance notes for the caseload.
- *Modeling*: Showing the proper implementation of an intervention with client or a new assessment.
- *Demonstration*: Utilizing a new piece of equipment or demonstrating desired behaviors.
- *Teaching*: Instruction on a new assessment, providing verbal and visual instructions to meet the individual learning style (AOTA, 2014a).

Supervision requires effective communication between the OT and the OTA and between the OT practitioners and a client's family and interdisciplinary care team members, in order to provide effective evidence-based client-centered care. The following are five areas that contribute to effective supervision:

- *Comprehensive collaboration*: This includes clinical reasoning and a discussion of best practice.
- *Communication*: Both written and verbal forms of communication contribute to effective supervision.
- *Coordination*: Scheduling, not just clients, but time for discussion and the clinical reasoning process is important with supervisory relationships.
- *Commitment*: Serving the public, the provision of best practice and evidenced-based care, as well as serving your profession are important attributes of an effective supervisor.

- *Contribution*: Effective supervisors also participate in sharing knowledge and participating in continued professional development (AOTA, 2014a).

It is important for OTs to advocate for the time required to provide the level of supervision and collaboration required for safe and effective client-centered care.

Competency

Continuing competence is part of lifelong learning. Practitioners assess current competence and plan for professional growth. Both OTs and OTAs must be prepared to be lifelong learners, incorporating evidence-based practice and best practice into the provision of occupational therapy services (AOTA, 2015a). "The occupational therapist and the occupational therapy assistant demonstrate and document service competency for clinical reasoning and judgment during the service delivery process, as well as for the performance of specific techniques, assessments, and intervention methods used" (AOTA, 2014a, p. S19). The OT must establish current competence and be knowledgeable of the OTA's level of competency and skill.

Additionally, the OT must be knowledgeable of the possibility that a partnership may not always be that of similar years or areas of practice. It is the responsibility of the OTA as well to have this knowledge of the OT providing supervision. The OT must ensure that the OTA has competency in the areas that will be required specific to the facility and client population. An OT cannot establish service competency in an area for which they are not competent. Competency is established when the OT determines the OTA can perform a given or requested task and acceptable and predictable outcomes are achieved (AOTA, 2015a; Youngstrom, 2014).

The AOTA has established five standards for continuing competence as they are used to assess, maintain, and document continued competency. Each standard has elements that relate directly to the partnership of the OT and OTA, and describe how there are shared values and knowledge that guide roles and responsibilities (AOTA, 2015a). Standards for Continuing Competence are described in **Table 40-1**.

OTs are also encouraged to participate in continued professional development and seek out mentors and peer

Table 40-1 Standards for Continuing Competence

Knowledge	Demonstrate expertise in your responsibilities and integration of AOTA documents, legislative, legal, and regulatory issues into all areas of practice.
Critical reasoning	Demonstrate the proper use of inductive and deductive reasoning during clinical reasoning and decision-making specific to roles, context, and responsibilities.
Interpersonal skills	Utilize effective communication methods, implement feedback to modify one's own professional behavior, demonstrate collaboration, and the ability to develop and sustain positive and productive interprofessional and team relationships.
Performance skills	Demonstrate current evidence-based practice, therapeutic use of self, and quality improvement processes that optimize client outcomes.
Ethical practice	Understand and adhere to the Code of Ethics.

Data from American Occupational Therapy Association, 2015c.

supervision for professional growth (AOTA, 2014a). Continuing education requirements vary among state licensure boards; however, it is required for national certification.

Documentation

Documentation must be timely, complete, and accurate. Practitioners working as a collaborative team may not have the time to discuss a previous treatment session and it is imperative that documentation is available to the practitioner who will be providing occupational therapy services. The signature and credentials of those practitioners contributing to the delivery of occupational therapy services must be on the documentation for the services provided. Cosignature on documentation by the supervising OT is required only if mandated by the facility, state law, regulatory body, or third-party payer. The OT and the OTA are responsible for the

knowledge of facility policies, state licensure law, regulatory mandates, and reimbursement guidelines as it relates to the documentation of occupational therapy services.

Advocacy

Advocacy is a part of our everyday practice; we advocate for our clients. Additionally, we must advocate for ethical practice, which includes effective supervision such as scheduling, productivity, and assisting or providing information regarding staffing. Practitioners must identify and articulate the distinct value of the provision of occupational therapy services, as well as the distinct value of the partnership between the OT and the OTA and the impact on client care and productivity.

Legal Responsibilities

It is the responsibility of all licensed practitioners to assure that they are adhering to their applicable state practice act and licensure law in order to protect the public.

Management and Standards of Practice

The OT is responsible for all aspects of the occupational therapy process. If there is a partnership with an OTA, supervision is required. It is the responsibility of both practitioners to have knowledge of roles and responsibilities, as well as facility policies, state licensure laws, regulatory body, and reimbursement guidelines. Additionally, practitioners can follow the AOTA Occupational Therapy Code of Ethics as a guide for ethical conduct (AOTA, 2015c).

Chapter 40 Self-Study Activities (Answers Are Provided at the End of the Chapter)

1. Match the following terms to the correct definition.

Terms	Definitions
A. Partnership	**1.** _____ include evidence incorporated into practice and quality improvement measures to prevent practice errors and optimize client outcomes.
B. Collaborative supervision	**2.** _____ provided in line of sight; appropriate for a new graduate.
C. Knowledge	**3.** _____ for occupational therapy practice requires that the practitioners identify and articulate the distinct value of the provision of occupational therapy services, as well as the distinct value of the partnership between the OT and the OTA and the impact on client care and productivity.
D. Written	**4.** _____ supervision requires the OT to be in the area when the OTA is providing occupational therapy services.
E. Supervision	**5.** _____ is the relationship between the OT and the OTA.
F. Supervisory plans	**6.** _____ is demonstrating the expertise in your responsibilities and integration of AOTA documents, legislative, legal, and regulatory issues into all areas of practice.
G. Modeling	**7.** _____ is respecting others' skills, knowledge, passion, and areas of expertise.
H. Competency	**8.** _____ must be timely, complete, and accurate.
I. Interpersonal skills	**9.** _____ occurs when you provide time in the OTA's schedule to observe the OT's interventions.
J. General	**10.** _____ is obtained when an OTA and an OT perform the task and same outcomes are achieved.
K. Advocacy	**11.** _____ utilizes effective communication methods, use feedback to modify one's own professional behavior, demonstrate collaboration, and the ability to develop and sustain positive and productive team relationships.
L. Line of site	**12.** _____ inheritance notes for the caseload is an effective method of supervision.
M. Documentation	**13.** _____ are mutually established between the OT and the OTA.
N. Critical reasoning	**14.** _____ supervision appropriate for an OTA who has established service competency in the area of practice.
O. Performance skills	**15.** _____ understands and observes the Code of Ethics and Ethical Standards.
P. Observation	**16.** _____ is showing the proper implementation of an intervention with a client or a new assessment.
Q. Ethical practice	**17.** _____ demonstrates inductive and deductive reasoning for decision-making and problem-solving skills specific to roles and responsibilities.

2. Answer the multiple-choice questions based on the following:

Sara is an OTA and has been working in the school system for six months; previously she was working in a pediatric outpatient clinic for 3 years. Maria, an OT, is Sara's supervisor and has been since she started at the school system. Maria and Sara meet once a month; this month Maria cancelled their meeting. Maria asked Sara to write up a review of her caseload and instead of meeting in person Maria would just sign the document.

1. Meeting to review clients on Sara's caseload is an example of:
   - **A.** Collaboration
   - **B.** Clinical reasoning
   - **C.** Direct supervision
   - **D.** General supervision

2. What should Sara do?
   A. Write the review of her caseload and have Maria sign it
   B. Do nothing
   C. Document the conversation
   D. Attempt to reschedule meeting
   E. Both C and D
3. Instead of meeting in person what other option was there for Sara and Maria to collaborate regarding students on her caseload?
   A. Telephone
   B. Text
   C. Email
   D. Facebook

Chapter 40 Self-Study Answers

1. Terms and Definition Answers
   1. O
   2. E
   3. K
   4. L
   5. A
   6. C
   7. B
   8. M
   9. P
   10. H
   11. I
   12. D
   13. F
   14. J
   15. Q
   16. G
   17. N
2. Multiple-choice question answers
   1. D. General supervision (i.e., the OT may not be on site; however, they may be available by telephone or other means of electronic transmission). This level of supervision would be appropriate for an OTA who has established service competency in the area of practice. The review of the caseload includes clinical reasoning and collaboration on treatment interventions and goals.

2. D. Both the OT and the OTA are responsible for the supervisory process.
3. A. Text, email, and Facebook would be a violation of confidentiality.

References

American Occupational Therapy Association. (2014a). Guidelines for supervision, roles, and responsibilities during the delivery of occupational therapy services. *American Journal of Occupational Therapy, 68,* S1–S48.

American Occupational Therapy Association. (2014b). Occupational therapy practice framework: Domain and process (3rd ed.). *American Journal of Occupational Therapy, 68*(Suppl. 1), S1–S48. doi:10.5014/ajot.2014.682006

American Occupational Therapy Association. (2015a). Standards for continuing competence. *American Journal of Occupational Therapy, 69*(Suppl. 3), 6913410055p1–6913410055p3. doi:10.5014/ajot.2015.696S16

American Occupational Therapy Association. (2015b). Standards of practice for occupational therapy. *American Journal of Occupational Therapy, 69*(Suppl. 3), 6913410057p1–6913410057p6. doi:10.5014/ajot.2015.696S06

American Occupational Therapy Association. (2015c). Occupational therapy code of ethics. *American Journal of Occupational Therapy, 69*(Suppl. 3), 6913410030p1–6913410030p8. doi:10.5014/ajot.2015.696S03

Glennon, T., & Van Oss, T. (2010). Identifying and promoting professional behavior. *OT Practice, 15*(17), 13–16.

Solomon, A. (2003). Utilizing and contributing to research. In A. Solomon & K. Jacobs (Eds.), *Management skills for the occupational therapy assistant* (pp. 135–154). Thorofare, NJ: SLACK Incorporated.

Youngstrom, M. J. (2014). Supervision. In M. E. Scaffa, B. A. B. Schell, G. Gillen, & E. S. Cohn (Eds.), *Willard and Spackman's occupational therapy* (12th ed., pp. 1068–1087). Philadelphia, PA: Lippincott Williams & Wilkins.

Wrapping up the Review Day 28

CHAPTER 41

Fifteen Days and Counting

Rosanne DiZazzo-Miller

Learning Objectives

- Identify an appropriate date and time to schedule your examination.
- Construct a time frame schedule using Table 41-1 as an example.
- Analyze correct and incorrect answer choices following the completion of practice examination questions.

It is now time for you to use the online content and begin taking practice examinations. You will begin the practice test section of exam preparation, calculate domain areas, and identify and review challenging areas of study. **Table 41-1** presents an example of a suggested time frame for completing the remaining portion of your exam preparation.

We hope you enjoyed your 45-day journey through this book. It is our hope that we have provided you with the guidance and materials needed to successfully pass the NBCOT® examination and become a COTA®. Remember—confidence is everything. If you are prepared, then you are ready. Know that! Take a deep breath, stand up tall, and walk into that room knowing you've done all you could possibly do, and perform confidently.

Table 41-1 Suggested Time Frame	
Day 31	• Try to get at least eight hours of uninterrupted sleep every night if you can! Remember, there are 200 multiple-choice questions. Some of these will have three answer options and others will four answer options. Either way, there is only one correct answer. In addition to these questions, there are also six option multiple answer questions with three correct and three incorrect answer options. You have four hours to take the examination. This averages out to approximately a little over one minute for each question.
	• Make sure to frequently refer back to the question that is presented and focus on exactly what the question is asking. Is it asking what is best for the caregiver, the occupational therapy assistant (OTA), or the client? Is it asking about best practices related to intervention or assessment, what the OTA should do first, or is it asking what remedial or compensatory strategy is most appropriate? Students report that this is the most common mistake they make when taking the National Board for Certification in Occupational Therapy (NBCOT®) examination (i.e., students become distracted by the amount of information presented instead of focusing on the key words of the specific question). The latter, and running out of time, is why practice exams are so important.
	• Locate the testing center where you will be taking the test. Once you know the day and time, make sure to plan a visit on that same day and time of the week. This will allow you to better understand traffic and drive time during the time of day you will be leaving to take your test. Also, walk in and sit in the lobby for a moment. Take a look around so that the day of your test will not be your first visit to the testing center. This will help decrease anxiety levels on test day.
	• Take your first practice test. Locate a quiet room with computer access to simulate as closely as possible the testing environment. Sit through an entire four-hour block of time and complete Exam 1.
	• Review any content that was difficult during your practice test and take notes to revisit.
Day 32	• Calculate the domain areas and review the area(s) that are the most challenging to you. Remember to make sure to focus on answering exactly what the question asks, and do not get sidetracked by options that sound good or additional information presented in the questions.
	• Review correct and incorrect answers.

(continues)

Table 41-1 Suggested Time Frame (*continued*)

Day 33	• Continue review work from Exam 1 including correct and incorrect answers, as well as the six option multiple answer questions.
Day 34	• Locate a quiet room with computer access to simulate the testing environment and take Exam 2.
	• If confident after this second practice test, schedule your test, but give yourself enough time to complete your exam preparation.
Day 35	• Calculate the domain areas and review the area(s) that are the most challenging to you. Remember to make sure to focus on answering exactly what the question asks, and do not get sidetracked by options that sound good or additional information presented in the questions, yet have nothing to do with what the question asks.
	• Review correct and incorrect answers.
	• Complete the stress scale and reflection.
Day 36	• Continue review work from Exam 2 including correct and incorrect answers, as well as the six option multiple answer questions.
Day 37	• Again, locate a quiet room with computer access to simulate the testing environment and take Exam 3.
	• Schedule the test if you feel ready and if you have not done so already.
Day 38	• Calculate the domain areas and review the area(s) that are the most challenging to you. Remember to make sure to focus on answering exactly what the question asks, and do not get sidetracked by options that sound good or additional information presented in the questions.
	• Review correct and incorrect answers.
	• Did you visit the test site yet? If not, make sure to do so this week!
Day 39	• Continue review work from Exam 3 including correct and incorrect answers, as well as the six option multiple answer questions.
Day 40	• Locate a quiet room with computer access to simulate the testing environment and take Exam 4.
	• Schedule the test if you feel ready and have not done so already.
	• Complete the stress scale and reflection.
Day 41	• Calculate the domain areas and review the area(s) that are the most challenging to you. Remember to make sure to focus on answering exactly what the question asks, and do not get sidetracked by options that sound good or additional information presented in the questions.
	• Review correct and incorrect answers.
Day 42	• Continue review work from Exam 4 including correct and incorrect answers, as well as the six option multiple answer questions.
Day 43	• Final review should focus on any remaining areas of difficulty.
Day 44	• Congratulations, you have completed a rigorous 45 days of test preparation! Rest assured in your knowledge and ability. Continue reviewing until you are confident with the results, and then REST!
	• We recommend the following steps be taken to optimize your success:
	◦ Get a good night's sleep and wake up rested and confident that you are ready to take the exam! Studies have shown that it is not enough to simply get one good night's sleep the night before an exam. Remember to get several nights of restorative sleep heading up to the exam (i.e., at least eight hours of uninterrupted sleep).
	◦ Maintain a positive attitude, especially in the days leading up to the exam. In other words, think positive, and stay calm, cool, and collected.
	◦ Maintain good nutritional habits throughout your exam preparation, especially on the days leading up to, and the day of, the exam. Proper nutrition and good hydration can make a big difference in recall and test performance.
	◦ Stop studying one to two days prior to taking the exam. Cramming will not help you, and spending a day or two decompressing and relaxing will go a long way to help you get mentally prepared for the big day. Identify activities that you enjoy and that help you to relax, and do them without feeling guilty!
	◦ Lastly, we recommend taking the exam shortly after you have completed your test preparation, keeping in mind the importance of feeling confident in your knowledge and ability prior to taking the exam. In other words, if you need more time to review questions and answers or specific domains or chapter content, it is important that you take that time. However, remember that total exam preparation time should range somewhere between four and six weeks. Waiting longer than six weeks makes it more difficult to hold on to all the material you've covered.
Day 45	• Down time! Think of one or two relaxing activities and do them.

Advice from Our Item-Writing Specialist

Sara Maher

Learning Objectives

- Identify the key components of multiple-choice questions.
- Develop a systematic approach to reading and answering multiple-choice questions.
- Recognize strategies that are less useful during the licensing examination.
- Learn how to be best prepared on the day of the examination.

Key Terms

- *Answer*: Correct response to a multiple-choice exam question.
- *Distractor*: Incorrect options in a multiple-choice exam question.
- *Item writer*: The person who creates a multiple-choice question.
- *Stem*: The question (or problem) posed at the beginning of each multiple-choice question.

Introduction

Multiple-choice question examinations are one of the most common ways to test knowledge, especially for licensure examinations of healthcare professionals. Most of us have taken a variety of multiple-choice questions in a variety of different venues. The tips on the following pages are designed to help you look at multiple-choice questions with better clarity and perhaps help you to improve your scores on the board examination. Remember, no book chapter can guarantee you a successful score on the examination. Successfully passing any examination comes from knowledge, experience, and time well spent studying. However, the tips that follow may help you to approach each question systematically, thereby improving your chances of successfully navigating a correct answer.

Anatomy of a Multiple-Choice Question

To better prepare to answer a multiple-choice question, it is sometimes helpful to understand how questions are constructed. Every multiple-choice question is composed of several sections: the question or problem (i.e., the stem), the correct response (i.e., the answer), and a list of possible, but incorrect options (i.e., distractors). For the board examination, the stem will usually appear as a complete question followed by a list of one correct or BEST answer and two or three incorrect or inferior alternatives (i.e., distractors) (Burton, Sudweeks, Merill, & Wood, 1991).

An item writer (i.e., the person who creates a multiple-choice question) approaches each question with a distinct plan. The stem is the foundation of the item, and as such, should be written so that the test taker could come up with an answer without reading any of the responses (Burton et al., 1991). A well-constructed stem is critical for each question. The purpose of each distractor is to be realistic enough to grab the attention of test takers who do not understand the material well enough to rule out all options. Distractors appear as plausible responses for these individuals. However, each distractor must also be "wrong" enough to make them appear implausible for test takers who understand the material well. Only the correct answer should appear plausible to these test takers (Burton et al., 1991).

In this book, all item writers submitted multiple-choice questions as shown in **Figure 42-1**. Review

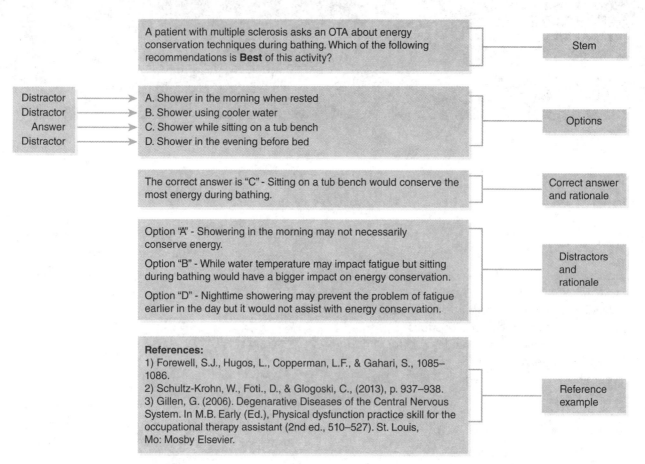

A patient with multiple sclerosis asks an OTA about energy conservation techniques during bathing. Which of the following recommendations is **Best** of this activity?

Stem

Distractor
Distractor
Answer
Distractor

A. Shower in the morning when rested
B. Shower using cooler water
C. Shower while sitting on a tub bench
D. Shower in the evening before bed

Options

The correct answer is "C" - Sitting on a tub bench would conserve the most energy during bathing.

Correct answer and rationale

Option "A" - Showering in the morning may not necessarily conserve energy.

Option "B" - While water temperature may impact fatigue but sitting during bathing would have a bigger impact on energy conservation.

Option "D" - Nighttime showering may prevent the problem of fatigue earlier in the day but it would not assist with energy conservation.

Distractors and rationale

References:
1) Forewell, S.J., Hugos, L., Copperman, L.F., & Gahari, S., 1085–1086.
2) Schultz-Krohn, W., Foti., D., & Glogoski, C., (2013), p. 937–938.
3) Gillen, G. (2006). Degenarative Diseases of the Central Nervous System. In M.B. Early (Ed.), Physical dysfunction practice skill for the occupational therapy assistant (2nd ed., 510–527). St. Louis, Mo: Mosby Elsevier.

Reference example

Figure 42-1 Anatomy of a multiple-choice question.

Figure 42-1 as we will use this figure to break down a question into its parts.

As you look at Figure 42-1, you will see a stem followed by four options or distractors. On the board examination, multiple-choice questions will have either three (i.e., A, B, and C) or four (i.e., A, B, C, and D) distractors. An important component of each question appears at the bottom of the diagram where one or more textbooks support each question. For the exam taker, this has several implications. First, while questions may be developed in the minds of an item writer, each question and distractor must be validated by textbook references. Second, textbooks are a great reference to study for the board examination. Textbooks, and not other items such as an instructor's notes or journal articles, must support the answer and distractors. Finally, a team who looks to ensure that references are correct reviews each question on the examination. This helps to ensure that multiple eyes review each question. With this basic understanding of the anatomy of a question, let's look at specific strategies to assist test takers in answering questions.

Test-Taking Strategies

The first strategy for any question is to read the stem thoroughly (Black, 1999; Ludwig, 2004; Towns & Robinson, 1993). It is often helpful to read the stem carefully, looking for key words such as FIRST, MOST, and BEST and so on as these are critical to answering the question correctly. Read the stem several times while covering the options and see if you can come up with the correct answer on your own (Burton et al., 1991; Ludwig, 2004). In Figure 42-1, three key phrases in the stem should stand out: (1) Stage 3 Parkinson's disease, (2) MOST APPROPRIATE, and (3) initial intervention. A reader of the question should think about the signs/symptoms that are typical for someone in Stage 3 Parkinson's disease, as well as the MOST APPROPRIATE, initial treatment.

Next, look at all of the options. Many exam takers get an answer wrong simply by not reading all options and overlooking a BETTER answer (Black, 1999; Ludwig, 2004). If we look at Figure 42-1 again, we see options that range from being in a wheelchair to driving. If we understand that Stage 3 Parkinson's disease involves postural instability and mild to moderate functional disability, we could rule out option (a) as involving a greater extent of disability, and option (d) which seems to indicate a person with relatively high functioning. Between the two choices left, option (c) involves stability, a key component identified in someone with Stage 3 Parkinson's disease. However, without the knowledge of what Stage 3 Parkinson's disease involves, a test taker must then rely on taking an educated guess for the answer.

If you come across a question that you do not think you know the answer to, slow down, and reread the question and options (Towns & Robinson, 1993). Sometimes a reader misses a key word at first glance when first reviewing a question; a second look may make all of the difference. Do not spend too much time on any one question as this may make you feel anxious for questions that follow (Ludwig, 2004). Instead, take an educated guess by eliminating incorrect or absurd responses (Black, 1999; Ludwig, 2004; Towns & Robinson, 1993). From Figure 42-1, for example, a reader might assume that Stage 3 Parkinson's disease is not the beginning stage, and could thereby rule out option (d) which indicates a person with relatively high functioning; leaving only three remaining options to choose from. Mark questions that you are not sure about and come back to them after you have finished those questions that you have better knowledge of (Ludwig, 2004; Towns & Robinson, 1993).

Finally, you can engage in test-wise strategies that will help improve your overall examination scores. First, pay attention to the time. By optimal time management you avoid spending too much time on one particular question (Towns & Robinson, 1993). It is better to get one question wrong than to lose points on other questions that you know the answer to simply because you ran out of time. Second, check each section of the test after you have completely finished it (Ludwig, 2004; Towns & Robinson, 1993). This can help the test taker to catch mistakes that were made originally such as marking the incorrect option when first answering a question, or skipping a question completely. A common question from test takers is "Should answers be changed during the question review?" Always remember that changing a multiple-choice question answer and guessing on the multiple-choice question are not the same. Advice you may have heard telling you to never change the first response on a multiple-choice examination is one of the most noted testing myths or urban legends in higher education. Specifically, the majority of time an answer is changed based on substantive reasoning, it is changed from the incorrect to the correct answer, and most test takers who change their answers improve their test scores (Bauer, Kopp, & Fischer, 2007; Fischer, Hermann, & Kopp, 2005; Geiger, 1997; Higham & Gerrard, 2005; Ludwig, 2004; Ludy, Benjamin, Cavell, & Shallenberger, 1984).

Some authors also advocate for implementing strategies that take advantage of idiosyncrasies in the construction of a multiple-choice question. Such strategies include looking for only options that are grammatically aligned with the stem, are longer than other options, or are located in the middle of a range of options (e.g., selecting the middle range if a group of ages are presented) (Towns & Robinson, 1993). However, with the board examination every attempt is made to minimize inconsistencies between the correct answer and all of the distractors. The item writer and editors look for these idiosyncrasies and attempt to eliminate them so each test taker is tested on his or her knowledge base and not on the ability to recognize idiosyncrasies in a particular question's construct. Try not to waste time on picking out subtle errors in the construction of a multiple-choice question as this can take precious time away from actually answering questions that you know or making an educated guess on the questions that you do not know the answer to.

Examination Day

The time has come to actually sit for the exam. On the night before the exam, take a little time to gather all of the material that you will need for the exam such as written confirmation from the testing site, directions to the testing site, appropriate clothing (e.g., the room temperature may be cool), photo identification, and tissues and so on. Plan to arrive at least 30 minutes earlier than the exam is scheduled as this will give you time to utilize the restroom and take care of any last-minute details, as well as giving yourself a minute to release any panic and tension. Some people like to walk briskly for a few minutes before entering the examination room, while others like to sit and practice a few deep-breathing techniques. Practice whatever activity best helps you feel mentally alert and less anxious. Before you get into the examination room, ask the testing proctor any questions that you might have about the facility. This can include information such as where the restroom is and where a water fountain is located and so on.

Once you are in the examination room, read the directions carefully for the examination and follow them diligently. As you begin to answer questions, answer the easiest questions first while marking the more difficult questions for later. Mark difficult questions that begin to take up too much of your time and return to them at a later time. However, it is suggested that you select an answer that you believe is the best answer in case you run out of time and cannot return to unanswered questions at a later time. Use your time wisely. Keep an eye on the timer so you can keep yourself at a good pace. Do not forget to take the time to read each question thoroughly, including each option. You will have all of the time allocated to you to finish the examination, so take advantage of the time allocated. Before you turn in the test, fight the urge to leave as quickly as possible. Instead, review the test questions that you can and give your answers one final thorough glance.

Conclusion

By understanding how multiple-choice exam questions are constructed, as well as helpful test-taking strategies to utilize for your upcoming board examination, you may increase your chances of successfully navigating correct answers. Strategies that may help during your upcoming examination include thoroughly reading each question and options, making educated guesses when an answer is not known, paying close attention to time management, and not being afraid to change your original answer. Be thoroughly prepared on examination day and take steps to reduce your anxiety such as arriving early and releasing tension prior to sitting in the examination room. Once your examination is over, take time to celebrate the victory of having completed the examination. The score will come at a later time, but for now enjoy the fact that you actually sat for and completed the board examination.

References

Bauer, D., Kopp, V., & Fischer, M. R. (2007). Answer changing in multiple choice assessment change that answer when in doubt—And spread the word! *BMC Medical Education, 7*, 28. doi:10.1186/1472-6920-7-28

Black, J. (1999). Hints for taking multiple choice examinations. *Plastic Surgical Nursing, 19*(3), 166, 170. Retrieved from http://www.ncbi.nlm.nih.gov/pubmed/10765304

Burton, S. J., Sudweeks, R. R., Merill, P. F., & Wood, W. (1991). *How to prepare better multiple-choice items: Guidelines for university faculty (M. S. Thesis).* Department of Instructional Science, Brigham Young University, Provo, UT.

Fischer, M. R., Hermann, S., & Kopp, V. (2005). Answering multiple-choice questions in high stakes. *Medical Education, 39*, 890–894.

Geiger, M. A. (1997). An examination of the relationship between answer changing, testwiseness, and examination performance. *The Journal of Experimental Education, 66*(1), 49–60.

Higham, P. A., & Gerrard, C. (2005). Not all errors are created equal: Metacognition and changing answers on multiple-choice tests. *Canadian Journal of Experimental Psychology, 59*(1), 28.

Ludwig, C. (2004). Preparing for certification: Test-taking strategies. *MEDSURG Nursing, 13*(2), 127–128. Retrieved from http://www.ncbi.nlm.nih.gov/pubmed/15119427

Ludy, T., Benjamin, J., Cavell, T. A., & Shallenberger, W. R. (1984). Staying with initial answers on objective tests: Is it a myth? *Teaching Psychology, 11*(3), 133–141.

Towns, M. H., & Robinson, W. R. (1993). Student use of test-wiseness strategies in solving multiple-choice chemistry examinations. *Journal of Research in Science Teaching, 30*(7), 709–722.

Life After the Exam

Rosanne DiZazzo-Miller

Learning Objectives

- Differentiate between state licensure and the National Board for Certification in Occupational Therapy (NBCOT®).
- Identify the appropriate steps to take to complete state licensure.
- Classify the steps for NBCOT certification renewal.
- List the steps that need to be taken in order to obtain state licensure.

Introduction

After you take the board examination there are some important steps that you need to take.

State Licensure

First you need to apply to your state regulatory board immediately after passing the examination to apply for state licensure. This is crucial! Send your application and payment as soon as possible.

NBCOT® Certification

National Board for Certification in Occupational Therapy (NBCOT®) certification requires professional development units (PDUs) for all practicing occupational therapy assistants (OTAs) who are registered with the NBCOT®. Search "professional development units" on the NBCOT home page (National Board for Certification in Occupational Therapy, 2015) and you will be provided with forms, guidelines, calculators, and additional tools to help you identify and keep track of your own PDUs,

which will facilitate the renewal process that occurs approximately every 3 years.

Renewal

You will also be responsible for maintaining both your state licensure and NBCOT certification. Remember that both are separate from each other and may have different requirements to maintain membership. On both your state license and NBCOT® registration cards, there will be an expiration date. Approximately two months prior to expiration, each agency will send you a notification to renew your license and registration. Make sure to follow up with them if you do not receive anything; also make certain your contact information is always current with both agencies, including address, phone, and name changes. Make a habit of keeping verification of payment and application receipts.

What If?

What if you do not pass? This question is on everyone's mind and no one wants to say it, but it is a possibility. First, although expensive, it would not be the end of the world. Back in the day, you could only have three strikes and you were out—that is not the case today. If at first you do not succeed—learn from your mistakes and keep trying. Here's how:

1. First, keep your chin up, be strong, and learn as much from this experience as you can. It is okay to feel sad, but do not be discouraged. There are many great OTAs who have had to repeat this examination. The most common reason for performing poorly on the examination is test-taking

strategies that result in confusion while attempting to answer the questions being asked. Don't lose sight of the end goal by being consumed with disappointment. Each day you work toward retaking your examination puts you one day closer to becoming an OTA.

2. Next, review your letter (i.e., if you have not burned it already) and take note of the domain areas that presented the most challenge to you.

3. Make sure that your new study plan focuses specifically on those areas. If you need more explanations on what those areas cover, make sure to review the "NBCOT® Practice Analysis" (National Board for Certification in Occupational Therapy, 2012).

4. Follow the steps for reapplying on the "NBCOT® website" (National Board for Certification in Occupational Therapy, 2015).

5. There is a waiting period prior to retaking the examination. Map out a new study plan with a calendar and give yourself enough time to practice and feel confident in your review before scheduling your retake. Remember that at this point if you are confident with your knowledge, your focus should be on reading and answering questions. Make certain you are confident with test-taking strategies (see Chapters 2, 3, and 43) before retaking the examination.

The final chapter of this book, Chapter 44, provides you with a supportive story in case you need one, and lessons learned from a student who had to retake her examination. Do what you need to do to keep going. Work out your aggressions in a kickboxing class, watch *The Blind Side, Rocky, Rudy, Marshall, The Pursuit of Happyness*, or any other film or speech that might help inspire you, but whatever you do—do not give up. Keep at it. You did not get to this point to throw it away over one test. As Mary Anne Radmacher (2009) once said,

> "Courage doesn't always roar. Sometimes courage is the quiet voice at the end of the day saying 'I will try again tomorrow.'"

References

National Board for Certification in Occupational Therapy. (2012). *2012 Practice analysis of the certified occupational therapy assistant: Executive summary.* Retrieved from http://www.nbcot.org/assets /candidate-pdfs/2012-practice-analysis-executive-cota

National Board for Certification in Occupational Therapy. (2015). *Connected. Current. Certified.* Retrieved from http://www.nbcot.org/

Radmacher, M. A. (2009). *Courage doesn't always roar.* San Francisco, CA: Conari Press.

Online Practice Examination Preparation Days 29–45

Back on the Horse

Jenna Tolmie and Rosanne DiZazzo-Miller

Introduction

There is an old Japanese proverb that says, "Fall seven times and stand up eight." Now, whether it is one, two, or eight—this is in essence, what some people may need to do in order to get through the task of passing their board examination.

Throughout the years, I (Rosanne) have had students approach me who did not pass the board examination on their first attempt. My response to them has been consistent. I would always say, "It's okay to be sad today. Eat what you want. Do what you want. Say what you want. But come tomorrow, shake it off, pull yourself up by your boot straps, and get back to work!"

When Jenna was a student, that is exactly what she did and yes, lived to tell about it. If you need a little more encouragement or to simply know you are not alone, read Jenna's story to keep you going.

Jenna's Story

One of the biggest obstacles upon graduating from an occupational therapy program was the fear and anxiety of taking a licensing examination, at least that was the case for me. During your Master's program you go day by day, studying the course material, passing the course examinations, completing numerous hours of fieldwork placement, but that one thing that always lingered in the back of my mind was where do I even begin to study for a licensing examination? Do I only study the board examination book? Do I go back to my school notes? Should I take an online course? These are all questions I asked myself while beginning to prepare for the examination. When preparing, I am sure you will find yourself asking friends, students, and coworkers about the test itself. One person may tell you it is as easy as can be. Another person may tell you it is nearly impossible, as it

covers such a wide range of material including items you may not have focused on during your Master's program. For me, I tried to move beyond the fear and anxiety that was instilled in me by asking friends simple questions about the examination, which only left me drowning in fear and feeling that the test was a mysterious puzzle that only lucky people and expert test takers can pass successfully. Having experienced this anxiety first hand, and being one of those "unlucky" people the first time around, I wanted to share my experiences with you. Instead of instilling fear into those taking the test, I aim to encourage, give each of you faith in yourself, and the understanding that hard work, dedication, managing your anxiety, and taking the time to successfully study and prepare for this examination will lead you to success.

The three things you need to succeed and pass this examination are:

1. Preparation
2. Organization
3. Practice

In order to prepare for this examination, you started on the right track by purchasing this examination preparatory book. Study each area of the book and continue to study the areas you are least familiar with.

The biggest factor that kept me from believing in myself was the continuous anxiety and fear that came along with preparing for a licensing examination. Study and learn ways for you to manage your anxiety. Reducing test anxiety is not something you can take care of the night before the test by simply having a movie night with friends, enjoying a nice dinner out, or a healthy breakfast on the morning of the examination. Although all of these may help you feel more at ease, reducing your anxiety takes much more preparation. It is something you need to incorporate into your study plan, so that all the techniques you used to reduce test anxiety will become second nature during the day of the examination. A lot of people who feel test anxiety will try to avoid it, which is exactly what I did the first time around. You hope and think it will just go away, but unfortunately it does not, especially the day of the examination. In preparing for the examination, take time in the morning to complete activities you enjoy that relax you; go to the gym, yoga, shopping, massage, whatever it may be that helps reduce your anxiety before jumping into a day's worth of studying. Know all the basic facts about the examination prior to scheduling the examination (e.g., how many questions are on the test, style of the test, how much time you have to take the test, how the test is scored, topics covered on the test, what the questions look like, and location of the testing facility). When you feel anxious and overwhelmed with the amount of material, take a break. Do not overdo it. When my mind became overwhelmed, I frequently found myself no longer retaining the information. Going for a walk, meeting a friend for lunch, or a simple five-minute break to listen to music with good deep breathing techniques can rest your mind.

The first time I prepared for this examination, I found myself studying for 10 to 12 hours a day. I found myself so consumed with studying, poor eating habits, and not taking the appropriate amount of breaks all the while thinking that this was the best thing for me; however, I was very wrong! Both your mind and body need a break. Come up with a study plan each day of chapters to conquer, with time to review in between. The study calendar provided in this book is a great way to start. Modify the calendar if necessary to meet your goals. Most people tell you to take this examination like a full-time job. I do agree with this statement; study hard during the week, but remember to combine it with the appropriate breaks. Follow your study plan and include days off to give your mind a rest. This is where the stress busters and journal reflections come in handy from Chapter 1.

Staying organized is also very helpful when preparing for this examination. Create a clear, targeted study plan with a time frame and chapters to be met each week leading up to the examination. I found sticking to that study plan to be very helpful. This keeps you on track in the days leading up to the examination. Make sure you leave time to review all your notes at least a week prior to the examination. You will need time to study and review after making notes and reading each chapter of this book.

My first time taking the examination I did not leave myself enough time to PRACTICE! Make sure you utilize and take advantage of the practice examinations. However, keep in mind not to get discouraged if you do not pass or score low on the online examinations. Practice the test for time management, ways to reduce

examination anxiety (e.g., breathing techniques and resting your mind during the test), and familiarize yourself with the type of questions the examination presents.

Time management is KEY. If you are able to successfully manage your time while taking this examination, it will also help you reduce the anxious feelings that may rise during the examination. For me, I found myself rapidly clicking through a number of the last few questions left as I knew I was about to run out of time. Taking multiple practice examinations will help reduce the chances of this.

Another strategy that also helped me overcome this examination was once I learned and studied all the material, I found myself thinking, What if I was this patient, what would I need help with? What would this person look like to me? What troubles/difficulties would I have and need help with? Envision yourself as the patient and put forth all your knowledge about the diagnoses or the case being presented to you.

An additional piece of advice to include in your studying is the examination environment. Distractions will arise the day of the examination as there are other students taking a variety of other examinations in the same room. Practice using earplugs to reduce outside noise. I found myself very distracted by the headphones each learning facility had, which were often too big and did not fit properly or comfortably, and only minimally reduced the noise of others typing or clicking next to me. Practice with comfortable earplugs if you are easily distracted by noise. Also, try taking a couple of practice examinations in a public setting such as a library to help you prepare.

Lastly, multiple-choice examinations are not for everyone, some people are good at multiple-choice examinations; others are better at practical examinations. Either way, you have come this far, so please do not give up if you are unsuccessful the first time around. Remember, you have worked so hard to get where you are today and there is a light at the end of the tunnel. If it was not for my dad instilling this motto continuously in my head growing up, "Winners never quit and quitters never win" I may have been one of those quitters and not be where I am today. Failing at first does not mean you will be a poor therapist, but rather, once you succeed and pass, it shows perseverance and dedication to this profession. It demonstrates hard work and commitment to get back up on your feet and learn from your mistakes the first time around, which has only helped me become a better therapist.

Today I am employed in my "dream job" specializing in the pediatric population. If I had given up rather than overcome my fear, anxiety, and hopelessness after initially being unsuccessful, I would not be the therapist that I am today.

INDEX

Note: Page numbers followed by 'f' and 't' represent figures and tables respectively.